HYPOXIC RESPIRATORY FAILURE IN THE NEWBORN

HYPOXIC RESPIRATORY FAILURE IN THE NEWBORN

From Origins to Clinical Management

Edited by

Shyamala Dakshinamurti

Section Editors

Steven H. Abman
Po-Yin Cheung
Satyan Lakshminrusimha
Patrick J. McNamara
William K. Milsom

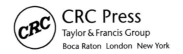

CRC Press
Taylor & Francis Group
Boca Raton London New York

CRC Press is an imprint of the
Taylor & Francis Group, an **informa** business

CRC Press
Boca Raton and London
First edition published 2022

by CRC Press
6000 Broken Sound Parkway NW, Suite 300, Boca Raton, FL 33487-2742
and by CRC Press

2 Park Square, Milton Park, Abingdon, Oxon, OX14 4RN

© 2022 Taylor & Francis Group, LLC

CRC Press is an imprint of Taylor & Francis Group, LLC

ISBN: 9780367493998 (hbk)
ISBN: 9781032078182 (pbk)
ISBN: 9780367494018 (ebk)

DOI: 10.1201/9780367494018

Typeset in Warnock Pro
by KnowledgeWorks Global Ltd.

CONTENTS

PART 1: THE ORIGINS OF HYPOXIA TOLERANCE
Edited by William K. Milsom

PART 2: FETAL HYPOXIA AND NEONATAL TRANSITION
Edited by Satyan Lakshminrusimha

PART 3: BIOLOGY OF HYPOXIC RESPIRATORY FAILURE IN THE NEONATE
Edited by Steven H. Abman

PREFACE

Babies with hypoxic respiratory failure were always the sickest in the newborn ICU. As a neonatology trainee, I would sit at their bedsides on call nights, watching their seesawing oxygen saturations, all our whirring, thumping machines a poor substitute for the safety and sanity of the uterus; willing their fist-sized hearts to pump a little longer, while we figured out a better way to push oxygen into them.

Yet, at these same oxygen levels, a fetus would have thrived. What failed these infants was the elemental transition process from fetus to newborn; the key to be born and to live in this world.

The genesis of this book can be traced back to those rollercoaster call nights. Also to the writings of evo-devo stalwarts Stephen Jay Gould and Sean Carroll; to serendipitous lectures by the inimitable John West on how the elephant lost its pleural space, and Paul Ponganis on the origins of the diving reflex, which felt like bathing one's brain in pure logic; and a chance meeting with Bill Milsom on a mountain in Mongolia. Clear connections can be made from human evolution to the process of our emergence as creatures capable of independent life. The poet Mary Oliver urged, *Pay attention / Be astonished / Tell about it.* This applies to scientists and clinicians too. There is a compelling poetry to physiology that lurks beneath the myriad details.

Gathered here is a collection of reviews by masters in their fields, highlighting the pathways of hypoxia and pulmonary hypertension from the population to the organism and the cell and drawing together international expertise in diagnosis and treatment. I am grateful to my august co-editors for their tremendous insights and enthusiasm in bringing this collection of knowledge together. And as always, delighted and illuminated by Satyan Lakshminrusimha's illustrations.

It must be acknowledged that this book was conceived before, but written during the COVID-19 pandemic. There has been no scientific connection established between COVID and neonatal pulmonary hypertension. But there is an affective connection, in writing about hypoxic respiratory failure at a crystalline moment when the world is struggling with the toll of hypoxic respiratory failure. I thank all the contributing authors for their commitment to this project despite this pressure.

Every book requires a village; in particular, the organizational skills of project managers Nathalie Buissé and Sophia Mbabaali from the George & Fay Yee Centre for Healthcare Innovation, and the Medical Sciences editorial desk at Taylor & Francis/CRC Press.

I thank my family for their support during the compilation of this volume, including eagle-eyed proofreading, and for their gifts of science, mountains and words.

Half a century ago, my cousin Sanjay died of hypoxic respiratory failure soon after birth. How much we have learned since then. To him and every blue baby since, this effort is in memory.

Shyamala Dakshinamurti

EDITOR

Dr Shyamala Dakshinamurti is a neonatologist and biomedical researcher, Professor of Pediatrics and Physiology at the University of Manitoba, Canada, and member of the Biology of Breathing theme, Children's Hospital Research Institute of Manitoba. She is research director for the University of Manitoba's Neonatology fellowship program, and a scientific organizer of the annual Canadian National Perinatal Research Meeting. Dr Dakshinamurti's research is on the hemodynamics of the neonatal pulmonary circuit and the physiology of hypoxia during circulatory transition. She is also a writer interested in science communication.

SECTION EDITORS

Dr Steven H. Abman is Professor of Pediatrics and Director of the Pediatric Heart Lung Center at the University of Colorado Anschutz School of Medicine and the Children's Hospital Colorado, USA. Having trained in Pediatric Pulmonary and Critical Care Medicine, Dr. Abman has had a long-standing interest in the developing lung circulation and pulmonary hypertension in diverse settings, as reflected by his clinical and laboratory-oriented research. He is currently Director of the Pediatric Pulmonary Hypertension Network (PPHNet), Executive Vice-Chairman for the BPD Collaborative and President of the American Pediatric Society.

Dr Po-Yin Cheung is a neonatologist of the Northern Alberta Neonatal Program of Alberta Health Services and a full Professor in the Departments of Pediatrics, Pharmacology and Surgery at the University of Alberta, Canada. He is also an Honorary Clinical Professor of the Department of Paediatrics and Adolescent Medicine at the University of Hong Kong and Honorary Consultant at the NICU of the HKU-Shenzhen Hospital. Dr. Cheung is a clinician-scientist and conducts both clinical and basic science research in neonatal hypoxia-reoxygenation injury and neonatal transition.

Dr Satyan Lakshminrusimha is a neonatologist and the Dennis and Nancy Marks Chair and Professor of Pediatrics at the University of California at Davis, Sacramento, USA. His areas of research interest include optimal oxygenation in neonatal lung injury, neonatal resuscitation, and pulmonary hypertension. Dr Lakshminrusimha enjoys drawing medical illustrations, for which he has developed an international reputation, and has developed mobile apps of neonatal illustrations and infographics.

Dr Patrick J. McNamara is a staff neonatologist and Director of the Division of Neonatology at the University of Iowa Stead Family Children's Hospital and Professor of Pediatrics and Internal Medicine, University of Iowa, USA. He is the current chair of the PanAmerican Hemodynamic Collaborative, Pediatric Academic Society Neonatal Hemodynamics Advisory and Neonatal Hemodynamics (TnECHO) Special Interest Group at the American Society of Echocardiography. His clinical and research interests include myocardial performance in the settings of a hemodynamically significant ductus arteriosus, pulmonary hypertension, and targeted neonatal echocardiography.

Dr William K. Milsom is a comparative physiologist and Emeritus Professor of Zoology at the University of British Columbia, Canada, best known as an authority on the evolution of respiratory processes in vertebrates. He has received the highest awards presented by the Canadian Society of Zoologists (the Fry Medal), the Comparative and Evolutionary Physiology Section of the American Physiological Society (the August Krogh Distinguished Lecture), and the Society for Experimental Biology (UK) (the Bidder Lecture), the three major societies in his discipline. He has also served as the President of the Canadian Society of Zoologists and as President of the International Congress of Comparative Physiology and Biochemistry. In 2012, Dr Milsom received the Distinguished Service Award from the Canadian Society of Zoologists in recognition of contributions to the well-being of zoology in Canada beyond the call of duty.

CONTRIBUTORS

Steven H. Abman
Division of Pulmonary Medicine
Department of Pediatrics
University of Colorado and Children's Hospital Colorado
Aurora, CO

Kurt H. Albertine
Division of Neonatology and Pulmonary
Department of Internal Medicine
University of Utah
Salt Lake City, UT

Karel Allegaert
Department of Development and Regeneration, Department of
    Pharmaceutical and Pharmacological Sciences
KU Leuven
Leuven, Belgium
and
Department of Clinical Pharmacy, Erasmus MC
Rotterdam, The Netherlands

Gabriel Altit
Division of Neonatology
Department of Pediatrics
McGill University and Montreal Children's Hospital
Montreal, QC, Canada

Pieter Annaert
Department of Pharmaceutical and Pharmacological Sciences
KU Leuven
Leuven, Belgium
and
Department of Clinical Pharmacy
Erasmus MC
Rotterdam, The Netherlands

Judy L. Aschner
Department of Pediatrics
Hackensack Meridian School of Medicine
Nutley, NJ
and
Department of Pediatrics
Albert Einstein College of Medicine
Bronx, NY
and
Joseph M. Sanzari Children's Hospital
Hackensack University Medical Center
Hackensack, NJ

Michelle Baczynski
Department of Respiratory Therapy
Mount Sinai Hospital
Toronto, ON, Canada

Anjali Y. Bhagirath
Children's Hospital Research Institute of Manitoba
Winnipeg, MB, Canada

Adrianne Rahde Bischoff
Department of Pediatrics
University of Iowa Stead Family Children's Hospital
Iowa City, IA

Jason Boehme
Department of Pediatrics
University of California, San Francisco
San Francisco, CA

R. Dale Brown
Departments of Pediatrics and Medicine
Cardiovascular Pulmonary Research Laboratories
University of Colorado
Anschutz Medical Campus
Aurora, CO

Emily Callan
Department of Pediatrics
Children's Hospital of Wisconsin
Milwaukee, WI

Nicholas R. Carr
Division of Neonatology
University of Utah School of Medicine
Salt Lake City, UT

Aravanan Anbu Chakkarapani
Neonatology and Clinical Pediatrics
Sidra Medicine and Weill Cornell Medicine
Doha, Qatar

Po-Yin Cheung
Division of Neonatal-Perinatal Care
Department of Pediatrics
University of Alberta
Edmonton, AB, Canada

Shyamala Dakshinamurti
Section of Neonatology, Department of Pediatrics
Department of Physiology
University of Manitoba
Children's Hospital Research Institute of Manitoba
Winnipeg, MB, Canada

Cassidy Delaney
Department of Pediatrics
School of Medicine
University of Colorado
Anschutz Medical Campus
Aurora, CO

Nolan DeLeon
Children's Hospital Research Institute of Manitoba
Winnipeg, MB, Canada

Contributors

Yvonne A. Dzal
Department of Biology and Centre for Forest Interdisciplinary
    Research
University of Winnipeg
Winnipeg, MB, Canada

Germán Ebensperger
Programa de Fisiopatología
Instituto de Ciencias Biomédicas (ICBM)
Facultad de Medicina
International Center for Andean Studies (INCAS)
Universidad de Chile
Putre, Chile

Yasser Elsayed
Section of Neonatology
Department of Pediatrics
University of Manitoba
Winnipeg, MB, Canada

Candice D. Fike
Department of Pediatrics
University of Utah Health
Salt Lake City, UT

Mark K. Friedberg
Cardiology
The Hospital for Sick Children
Toronto, ON, Canada

Csaba Galambos
Pathology
Anschutz Medical Campus
Aurora and Children's Hospital Colorado
Aurora, CO

Harry Gee
Obstetrics and Gynaecology
Birmingham Women's Hospital
Birmingham, United Kingdom

Jason Gien
Neonatal/Perinatal Medicine
University of Colorado
Anschutz Medical Campus
Aurora, CO

Regan E. Giesinger
Department of Pediatrics
University of Iowa
Iowa City, IA

Andrew W. Gill
Department of Paediatrics
University of Western Australia
Perth, Australia

M. Ruth Graham
Department of Anesthesiology, Perioperative and Pain Medicine
University of Manitoba
Winnipeg, MB, Canada

Emilio A. Herrera
Programa de Fisiopatología
Instituto de Ciencias Biomédicas (ICBM)
Facultad de Medicina
International Center for Andean Studies (INCAS)
Universidad de Chile
Putre, Chile

Allyson Hindle
Integrative Physiology
University of Nevada
Las Vegas, NV
and
Anesthesia Center for Critical Care Research
Massachusetts General Hospital
Boston, MA

Stuart B. Hooper
Obstetrics and Gynaecology Monash Health
Monash University
Melbourne, Australia

Amish Jain
Department of Pediatrics
University of Toronto
Toronto, ON, Canada
Mount Sinai Hospital
Toronto, ON, Canada

Robert P. Jankov
Departments of Pediatrics and Cellular and Molecular Medicine
University of Ottawa and Children's Hospital of Eastern Ontario
    Research Institute
Ottawa, ON, Canada

Richard Keijzer
Division of Pediatric Surgery
Department of Surgery
University of Manitoba and Children's Hospital Research
    Institute of Manitoba
Winnipeg, MB, Canada

Roberta L. Keller
Department of Pediatrics
University of California
San Francisco, CA

Stephen T. Kempley
Royal London Hospital and Barts and the London School of
    Medicine
London, United Kingdom

Martin Keszler
Department of Pediatrics
Women and Infants Hospital of Rhode Island
Providence, RI

Afif El Khuffash
Department of Neonatology
The Rotunda Hospital and School of Medicine
Royal College of Surgeons in Ireland
Dublin, Ireland

John P. Kinsella
Division Pediatrics–Neonatology
Children's Hospital Colorado
Colorado Fetal Care Center
USC Health–Neonatal Intensive Care Unit
Anschutz and Children's Hospital
Aurora, CO

Martin Kluckow
Neonatology, Department of Pediatrics
University of Sydney and Royal North Shore Hospital
Sydney, Australia

Girija Ganesh Konduri
Division of Neonatology
Department of Pediatrics
Medical College of Wisconsin and
Children's Research Institute
Milwaukee, WI

Satyan Lakshminrusimha
Department of Pediatrics
UC Davis Children's Hospital
Sacramento, CA

W.L. Amelia Lee
Barts and the London School of Medicine
London, United Kingdom

Philip T. Levy
Division of Newborn Medicine
Boston Children's Hospital
and
Department of Pediatrics
Harvard Medical School
Boston, MA

Aníbal J. Llanos
Programa de Fisiopatología
Instituto de Ciencias Biomédicas (ICBM)
Facultad de Medicina
International Center for Andean Studies (INCAS)
Universidad de Chile
Putre, Chile

Peter M. MacFarlane
Department of Pediatrics
Case Western Reserve University
Cleveland, OH

Emin Maltepe
Department of Pediatrics
University of California, San Francisco
San Francisco, CA

Patrick J. McNamara
Department of Pediatrics and Internal Medicine
University of Iowa Stead Family Children's Hospital
Iowa City, IA

William K. Milsom
Department of Zoology
The University of British Columbia
Vancouver, BC, Canada

Souvik Mitra
Department of Pediatrics
Dalhousie University and IWK Health Center
Halifax, NS, Canada

Catherine Morgan
Division of Pediatric Nephrology
Department of Pediatrics
University of Alberta
Edmonton, AB, Canada

Josef Neu
Division of Neonatology
Department of Pediatrics
University of Florida
Gainesville, FL

Eric B. Ortigoza
Division of Neonatal-Perinatal Medicine
Department of Pediatrics
UT Southwestern Medical Center
Dallas, TX

Allison S. Osborne
Department of Pediatrics
Rainbow Babies & Children's Hospital and Case Western
    Reserve University
Cleveland, OH

Christina M. Pabelick
Departments of Anesthesiology and Perioperative Medicine and
    Physiology and Biomedical Engineering
Mayo Clinic, Rochester
Rochester, MN

Graeme R. Polglase
Perinatal Transition Group
The Ritchie Centre
Department of Obstetrics and Gynaecology
Monash University and Hudson Institute of Medical Research
Victoria, Australia

Fabiana Postolow
Section of Neonatology
Department of Pediatrics
University of Manitoba
Winnipeg, MB, Canada

Y.S. Prakash
Departments of Anesthesiology and Perioperative Medicine and
    Physiology and Biomedical Engineering
Mayo Clinic
Rochester, MN

Roberto V. Reyes
Programa de Fisiopatología
Instituto de Ciencias Biomédicas (ICBM)
Facultad de Medicina
International Center for Andean Studies (INCAS)
Universidad de Chile
Putre, Chile

Danielle R. Rios
Clinical Associate Professor
University of Iowa
Iowa City, IA

Nicola J. Robertson
Perinatal Neuroscience and Neonatology
EGA Institute for Women's Health
University College London
London, England

Ola D. Saugstad
Department of Pediatrics
University of Oslo
Oslo, Norway
and
Ann and Robert H. Lurie Children's Hospital of Chicago and
    Northwestern University Feinberg School of Medicine
Chicago, IL

Arvind Sehgal
Monash Newborn
Monash Children's Hospital
Melbourne, Australia
and
Department of Pediatrics
Monash University

María Serón-Ferré
Programa de Fisiopatología
Instituto de Ciencias Biomédicas (ICBM)
Facultad de Medicina
International Center for Andean Studies (INCAS)
Universidad de Chile
Putre, Chile

Divyen K. Shah
Royal London Hospital
Barts and the London School of Medicine
London, United Kingdom

Prakesh S. Shah
Division of Neonatology, Department of Pediatrics
Mount Sinai Hospital
Toronto, ON, Canada

Tatum Simonson
Division of Pulmonary, Critical Care, & Sleep Medicine
Department of Medicine
University of California San Diego School of Medicine
San Diego, CA

Dominique Singer
Division of Neonatology and Pediatric Critical Care Medicine
University Medical Center Eppendorf
Hamburg, Germany

Anne Smits
Department of Development and Regeneration
KU Leuven
Leuven, Belgium
Neonatal Intensive Care Unit
University Hospital Leuven
Leuven, Belgium

Robin H. Steinhorn
Rady Children's Hospital
UC San Diego
San Diego, CA

Kurt R. Stenmark
Departments of Pediatrics and Medicine
Cardiovascular Pulmonary Research Laboratories
University of Colorado
Anschutz Medical Campus
Aurora, CO

Edwin W. Taylor
School of Biosciences
University of Birmingham
Birmingham, United Kingdom

Payam Vali
Department of Pediatrics
UC Davis Children's Hospital
Sacramento, CA

Maximo Vento
Department of Pediatrics
Health Research Institute La Fe
Valencia, Spain

Stephen Wedgwood
Department of Pediatrics
UC Davis School of Medicine
Sacramento, CA

Dany E. Weisz
Department of Pediatrics
University of Toronto
Sunnybrook Health Sciences Centre
Toronto, ON, Canada

David F. Wertheim
Department of Networks and Digital Media
Kingston University
London, United Kingdom

Jason Williams
Department of Biochemistry and Molecular Genetics
University of Colorado Anschutz Medical Campus, Aurora
Aurora, CO

Michelle J. Yang
Division of Neonatology
University of Utah School of Medicine
Salt Lake City, UT

Bradley A. Yoder
Division of Neonatology – Department
    of Pediatrics
University of Utah
Salt Lake City, UT

Hui Zhang
Departments of Pediatrics and Medicine
Cardiovascular Pulmonary Research Laboratories
University of Colorado Anschutz Medical Campus
Aurora, CO

Faith Zhu
Department of Pediatrics
University of Toronto
Toronto, ON, Canada

INTRODUCTION

Shyamala Dakshinamurti, William K. Milsom, Satyan Lakshminrusimha, Steven H. Abman, Po-Yin Cheung and Patrick J. McNamara

Contents

We have all been hypoxic.

We have craved oxygen since the day one of our eukaryotic ancestors first swallowed an aerobic mitochondrial bacterium and then, seduced by the prospect of multicellularity, began feeding its hungry cytochromes oxygen.

Nearly a century ago, Sir Joseph Barcroft postulated "the Everest *in utero*," a fetal environment in the womb comparable to the most hostile environmental conditions faced by adventurous mankind. Subsequently, expeditions reaching the summit of Everest mapped out the limits of human tolerance for hypoxemia. Fetal tolerance for intrauterine hypoxia arises from evolutionarily conserved physiological mechanisms, the antecedents of which can be learned from diving mammals or species at high altitudes. In whimsy we say, the fetus remembers when it was a turtle or a diving seal; then it is born and forgets. It's not merely whimsy; several chapters in this book recast Just So Stories in the form of stringently tested comparative physiology. The response to hypoxia in animals living in extreme environments illuminates how the human fetus handles its hypoxemic state, and why the human newborn suddenly cannot. The physiological changes seen during the transition from intrauterine to extrauterine life can be read as retracing the evolution and development of hypoxia tolerance, critical to biological study and clinical practice alike; while postnatal hypoxia creates a multisystem cliffhanger.

The conventional terminology "persistent pulmonary hypertension of the newborn," as with the term it once replaced, "persistent fetal circulation," is currently under siege. It is not necessarily persistent; it is not only in the newly born; it has bounced from one WHO classification category to another while remaining among the most rapidly progressive vasculopathies. The term "acute pulmonary hypertension" is more accurate, but it fails to capture the arrest of pulmonary circuit adaptation as a uniquely neonatal circumstance, triggered by hypoxia, inflammation, or pressure phenomena at a profoundly vulnerable moment of development. We, therefore, group these closely related pathophysiologies under the umbrella definition "hypoxic respiratory failure of the newborn," examine common pathways of disease, distinguish distinct natural histories and then differentiate PPHN (if that's what we should still call it) from other pulmonary hypertensions presenting during infancy.

This book covers the broad ground: The origins of hypoxia adaptation, the impact of oxygen on the circulatory transition at birth, the biochemistry of hypoxia in the pulmonary circulation, and the diagnosis and clinical management of hypoxic respiratory failure. In other words: What we once were; why we have been protected; what happens when that protection is lifted; how to diagnose when we have entered the maelstrom; what to do next, and what we still don't know. The impact of hypoxia is not limited to the lung; the "collateral damage" of hypoxia on other systems is reviewed, in addition to cardiovascular effects. Common threads run the length of the volume; you may want to read with multiple bookmarks in hand. The diving reflex appears in various forms in every section, as do cardiorespiratory coupling and reactive oxygen species. The introductions to each section of the book are gathered below, to highlight their internal connectivity.

The past decades have brought substantial advances in the care of pulmonary hypertension in the newborn. For the sake of our patients and their families, we must learn more, to do better.

Part 1: The origins of hypoxia tolerance

William K. Milsom

The inverse relationship between mass-specific metabolic rate and body size is well established across all animal taxa. Thus, mammals are born with a high demand for oxygen that increases progressively with the development of thermoregulatory capacity. In the human infant, this is accompanied by a loss (or resetting) of tolerance to hypoxia. The primary responsibility of the newborn to hypoxia is a reduction in metabolic rate, and this ability also decreases progressively with the development of thermoregulatory capacity. Prolonged hypoxia has proinflammatory properties potentially underlying neurologic vulnerability, particularly with respect to the respiratory control system. Human populations that reside at altitude in the Himalayas, Andean altiplano, and Ethiopian highlands, however, exhibit a distinct composite of phenotypes, with similarities and differences in various physiological processes leading to increased hypoxia tolerance. The mechanisms that underlie enhanced tolerance can represent instances of acclimatization (phenotypic plasticity), or genetic adaptation (genetic assimilation of positive traits, or genetic compensation to mitigate maladaptive plastic responses to hypoxia). These phenomena are well described in the opening chapters of this section. What follows are chapters describing species in which the fetus, newborn, and/or adult are extremely hypoxia tolerant. These are species that thrive in hypoxic environments at altitude, in underground burrows, or while breathhold diving. These studies, and our growing knowledge of the phylogeny and ontogeny of differences in hypoxia tolerance, inform our understanding of the huge physiological shifts of the human neonatal transition and the dangers of perinatal hypoxia.

Part 2: Fetal hypoxia and neonatal transition

Satyan Lakshminrusimha

The current COVID-19 pandemic has highlighted the importance of maternal oxygenation during pregnancy. The morbidity and mortality of pregnant women with COVID-19 are

DOI: 10.1201/9780367494018-1

1

significantly higher than nonpregnant women. Several pregnant women with COVID-19 and hypoxemic respiratory failure have required extracorporeal membrane oxygenation (ECMO). While the placenta and fetal circulation protect the fetus from deleterious effects of mild maternal hypoxia, profound hypoxemia results in hypoxic fetoplacental vasoconstriction and deleterious effects on the fetus. Timely respiratory and cardiovascular support to correct maternal hypoxia is crucial to optimize fetal well-being.

Pulmonary transition at birth is truly a miracle! During fetal period, the placenta serves as the organ of gas exchange. All fetal organ systems are functional except the lungs. The fetal lungs are dormant and filled with liquid and has low blood flow, partly due to hypoxic pulmonary vasoconstriction. The fetus is relatively hypoxemic (compared to postnatal standards) but not hypoxic, as it efficiently delivers oxygen to its tissues with abundant cardiac output and high levels of fetal hemoglobin to compensate for low PaO_2. At birth, with the first cry, air enters the alveoli increasing PaO_2 resulting in a drop in pulmonary vascular resistance, switch in ductal shunt from right-to-left to left-to-right, and an 8–10-fold increase in pulmonary blood flow. Expiratory braking during crying and active absorption of lung liquid enables air to replace lung liquid in the alveoli.

As gas exchange shifts from placenta to the lungs at birth, the source of left ventricular preload changes from umbilical venous return shunting across the oval foramen to pulmonary venous return. This switch is gradual (with some much-needed overlap) while physiological cord clamping is "delayed" until respirations are established. Abrupt or immediate cord clamping soon after birth, prior to establishing neonatal respiration, can potentially lead to hypoxia and bradycardia as the newly born infant is deprived of both sources of oxygen from placenta and lungs. Physiological cord clamping is associated with better short-term and long-term outcomes.

Birth asphyxia, defined as failure to establish breathing at birth, accounts for 900,000 deaths every year, based on World Health Organization estimates, and is one of the leading causes of neonatal mortality. Ventilation of the lungs during resuscitation with the right concentration of oxygen is the key to minimizing morbidity and mortality from birth asphyxia. While 21% oxygen is adequate for most term infants for initial resuscitation, the optimal initial oxygen concentration in preterm infants is still an enigma. Chapters by eminent scientists covering these important topics are included in Part 2.

Part 3: Biology of hypoxic respiratory failure in the neonate

Steven H. Abman

Part 3 of this book addresses biologic mechanisms that contribute to hypoxic respiratory failure in sick newborns. At birth, the lung circulation rapidly responds to birth-related stimuli, including the sudden rise in alveolar PO_2 that leads to the fall in pulmonary vascular resistance and rise in pulmonary blood flow, which is essential for postnatal survival. PPHN, a key component of neonatal hypoxic respiratory failure, represents the failure of the lung circulation to undergo sufficient vasodilation, leading to profound hypoxemia due to marked right-to-left extrapulmonary shunting across the ductus arteriosus and foramen ovale. Past laboratory studies identified the critical role of the enhanced production of vital endothelium-derived vasodilators, such as

nitric oxide (NO) and prostacyclin (PgI_2), and reduced production of potent vasoconstrictors, especially endothelin-1 (ET-1) in mediating this dramatic transition of the pulmonary circulation. This past work led to the development of current pharmacologic interventions that are commonly used to treat neonatal pulmonary hypertension, including inhaled NO, phosphodiesterase type 5 inhibitors, diverse forms of synthetic PgI_2 analogs and ET-1 receptor inhibitors. Despite remarkable success in many settings, PPHN remains associated with substantial morbidity and mortality. In addition, growing recognition of the contribution of PPHN physiology to hypoxic respiratory failure in preterm infants has led to further challenges in how to best understand the underlying pathophysiology and optimal therapies in this fragile population. As a result, more work to better understand fundamental mechanisms through which prematurity, antenatal stress and postnatal injury impair pulmonary vascular, cardiac and respiratory function during the first weeks of life remains an important target for basic research.

In this section, chapters from outstanding investigators in the field of developmental lung biology, lung vascular disease and cardiac development, key signaling pathways that are altered in endothelial and smooth muscle cells by hypoxia, molecular biology of oxygen sensing and injury as related to the generation of reactive oxygen species, metabolic adaptations from fetal to neonatal life and novel epigenetic mechanisms of hypoxia-induced tissue injury are explored in great detail. Overall, this section provides exciting new leads that will yield important translational insights linking the science of vascular and cardiac function and disease with developmental biology, and ultimately, clinical care.

Part 4: Hypoxia and collateral damage

Po-Yin Cheung

Hypoxia is systemic and affects all organs and systems in the neonate with hypoxic respiratory failure.

"Oxygen Radical Disease of Neonatology", a term originally coined by Professor Ola Saugstad in 1988, remains one of the key concepts in the management of neonates with hypoxic respiratory failure. Reperfusion or reoxygenation injury remains the cornerstone of organ injury and complications. Indeed, oxygen may not be the silver bullet for hypoxia. Coming out of the *in utero* hypoxic environment, the relative postnatal hyperoxia and the interplay between oxygen and pathophysiological conditions of the neonate affect the developing respiratory system. As a defensive mechanism in the redistribution of blood flow during hypoxia, there are differential regional perfusion responses resulting in neuroprotection, intestinal and renal compromise. Tools for assessing organ perfusion and injury have been increasingly used in the clinical arena. The use of these tools improves the monitoring and management of perfusion deficits. Hypoxic-ischemic encephalopathy receives the most attention because of its significant acute and long-term neurodevelopmental consequences. While therapeutic hypothermia is the standard care for moderate or severe hypoxic-ischemic encephalopathy of term and near-term neonates, recent reports have fueled the discussion of its use in other populations. Further, adjunctive therapies are emerging to alleviate the cerebral injury. Understanding the pathogenetic course of cerebral injury including biochemical cascades and disruption of the blood-brain barrier helps develop therapeutic agents. The kidney is the first important organ that is affected by hypoxia. However, similar to the therapeutic agents for cerebral injury, clinical treatments cannot reverse, but are merely limited to the prevention of reno-tubular injury. While the renal injury may heal, the long-term sequelae in neonatal kidneys after hypoxia need further research. Systemic hypoxia causes a unique injury to the intestine with ischemia and necrosis. Hypoxic-ischemic intestinal injury has no clear association with inflammation or the dysbiosis that is typical for necrotizing enterocolitis, although the two diseases have similar clinical and histopathological presentations. An individualized therapeutic approach is the key in precision medicine. It is important to better understand clinical pharmacology in hypoxic neonates such that we can predict drug-related effects based on drug- and population-specific pharmacokinetics and pharmacodynamics. Little information is available regarding the interactions between drugs and therapeutic hypothermia. Some neonates with hypoxic respiratory failure will require surgeries and need special anesthetic considerations. The risk and management of intraoperative pulmonary hypertensive crisis require the evaluation of perioperative risk, evidence-based approaches to respiratory support and rationalized pathophysiology-driven anesthetic and hemodynamic management in these neonates. Taken together, collateral effects of hypoxia on the brain, intestine, kidneys and other systems are inter-related in the acute pathophysiology, intercurrent therapeutic states and long-term outcomes.

Part 5: Diagnosis and management of neonatal hypoxic respiratory failure

Patrick J. McNamara

Part 5 focuses on the approach to diagnosis and management of neonatal hypoxemic respiratory failure, which remains a major cause of both morbidity and mortality in many parts of the world. As highlighted in prior sections, the biology of the neonate, during the transitional period birth, is at higher risk of impairment in the normal postnatal fall in pulmonary vascular resistance – which may lead to impaired efficacy of oxygenation, suboptimal right ventricular function and poor systemic blood flow. One of the major challenges for clinicians relates to the fact that many forms of major congenital heart disease may have a similar presentation, which may lead to incorrect treatment choices and adverse patient outcomes. Therefore, immediate access to timely and comprehensive echocardiography is imperative to enable accurate diagnostic ascertainment and disease/physiology-specific interventions. Recent advances in echocardiography evaluation, and in particular the growth of neonatologist-led hemodynamic programs, have led to improvements in understanding of the relationship of pulmonary vascular resistance/pressure to right ventricular function, the interdependence between both ventricles and the downstream effects on both pulmonary and end-organ perfusion. The art of clinical care, and its relevance to management, is further emphasized through increased appreciation of the importance of mechanical ventilation strategies, optimization of functional residual capacity and the interaction between intrathoracic pressure, ventilation and hemodynamics. It is imperative that clinicians consider heart-lung interaction as a biological continuum that is an essential determinant of effective tissue oxygenation and carbon dioxide clearance. Traditionally, the terms "persistent fetal circulation" and "persistent pulmonary hypertension of the newborn" have been used to characterize this clinical syndrome where impaired efficacy of oxygenation is the dominant clinical feature. Several chapters in this section suggest that clinicians should classify the nature of pulmonary hypertension as "acute" or "chronic", which has both diagnostic and therapeutic relevance. In addition, both acute and chronic forms of pulmonary hypertension are distinguished by unique clinical phenotypes that influence the approach to monitoring and treatment choices. The importance of phenotypic characterization is best demonstrated in patients with congenital diaphragmatic hernia, where impaired oxygenation may relate to classic pulmonary arterial hypertension with impaired right heart performance or may relate to pulmonary venous hypertension secondary to a left ventricular phenotype. Timely access to comprehensive echocardiography facilitates enhanced diagnostic precision and the implementation of a disease-specific approach to treatment. Finally, acute pulmonary hypertension is an important consideration of hypoxemic respiratory failure in premature infants and adverse neonatal outcomes; however, timely diagnosis and early intervention with targeted pulmonary vasodilator therapy and heart function support may lead to improved outcomes.

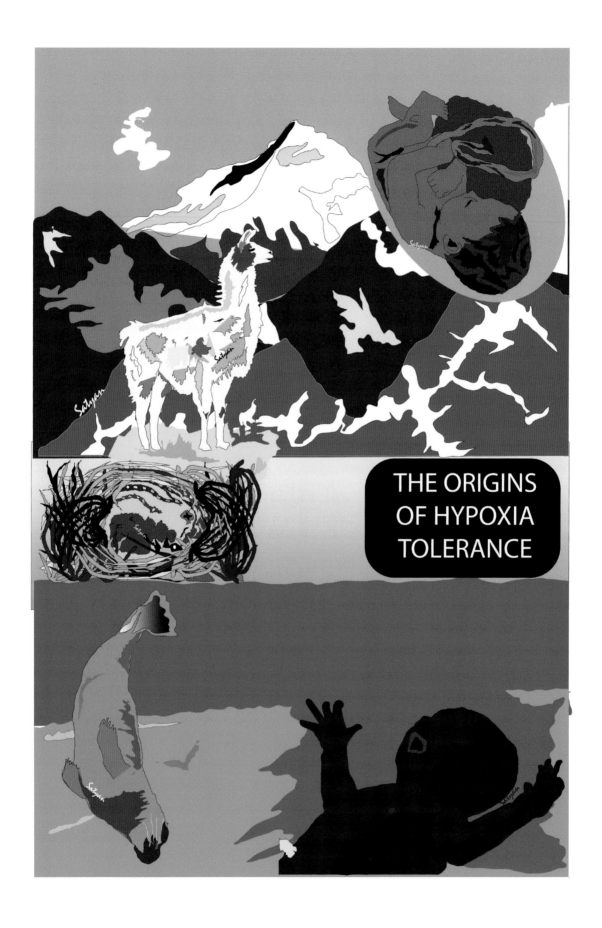

THE ORIGINS
OF HYPOXIA
TOLERANCE

Part 1
The Origins of Hypoxia Tolerance

Edited by William K. Milsom

THE HUMAN FETUS AND METABOLIC ADAPTATIONS TO HYPOXIA

Dominique Singer

Contents

Introduction

Perinatal hypoxia is one of the greatest, if not *the* greatest threat to human fetuses and newborns. Hypoxic-ischemic encephalopathy (HIE) can result in cerebral palsy and other life-long disabilities. Attempts to treat asphyxiated babies by induced hypothermia have proven to be fairly effective, yet complementary therapies to further mitigate or even repair HIE are still under investigation (1–3).

However, HIE would probably occur even more frequently if human fetuses and newborns were not able to protect themselves by a number of physiological mechanisms that show striking similarities with natural adaptation strategies to oxygen deficiency and food scarcity in the animal kingdom. A comparative physiological analysis of these adaptations may help to better understand both the progression of perinatal hypoxia and the diagnostic and therapeutic challenges of HIE.

Being born as a small endotherm – A delicate challenge

When looking for particularly hypoxia-tolerant creatures, one would actually expect anything but small endotherms. There are two main reasons for this.

Size relationship of metabolic rate

According to a common biological law, also known as Kleiber's rule (4), the specific basal metabolic rate (in watts per kilogram) is higher in small than in large animals (Figure 2.1a). The "allometric" (nonproportional) size relationship of metabolic rate is usually explained by the fact that small mammals (or birds) need a stronger "internal heater" to compensate for the higher heat losses caused by their relatively larger body surface area. However, a similar relationship applies to all living beings whether they

keep their body temperature constant or not. Hence, there must be a more fundamental explanation that probably involves the self-adjustment of energy requirements to supply conditions. Whatever may be the ultimate cause, the overall metabolic rule implies that small animals need more food and more oxygen per unit of body weight and should thus exhibit a worse tolerance to starvation and hypoxia than larger species. For mammalian neonates that also fall under this rule (the basal metabolic rate of a human term baby amounts to 2.0–2.5 Watts per kg compared to roughly 1 Watt per kg for adults), this would mean that they are inherently maladapted to the risks of undersupply and hypoxia simply because of their small body size (5–8).

Metabolic cost of temperature regulation

Mammals and birds are endothermic (warm-blooded) animals that maintain a higher gradient between body and ambient temperature than ectothermic (cold-blooded) organisms due to an elevated metabolic rate. The specific basal metabolic rate of mammals is 4(–10) times higher than the resting metabolic rate of reptiles of comparable body size. Endotherms are thus not only dependent on a continuous food supply, but they also exhibit a lower hypoxia tolerance than ectotherms that can often survive for long periods without any O_2 (and food) supply (9–11).

Furthermore, unlike ectotherms that usually tolerate larger thermal variations (poikilothermy), endothermic animals keep their body temperature constant (homeothermy). The cold defense reaction includes an increase in metabolic rate with decreasing ambient temperatures, which is steeper the smaller the body size and the larger the surface-to-volume ratio. In newborn mammals, heat is produced by nonshivering thermogenesis (NST) in the brown adipose tissue (BAT), which is based on an uncoupling of oxidative phosphorylation and thus accompanied by a high O_2 consumption rate. Thus, newborn babies experience

DOI: 10.1201/9780367494018-2

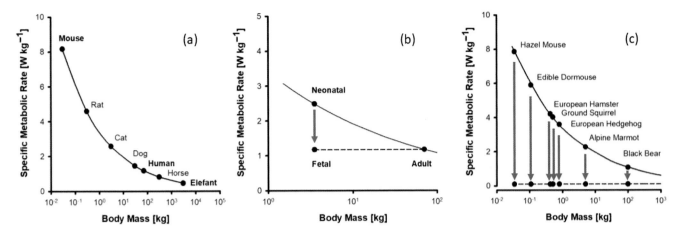

FIGURE 2.1 Metabolic size relationship as a target of perinatal and seasonal metabolic adaptations. (a) Following an overall biological rule ("mouse-to-elephant curve"), the specific metabolic rate increases with decreasing body mass. (b) The mammalian fetus, however, behaves more like an organ of its mother. The "disproportionately" low metabolic rate favors tissue oxygenation in spite of low intrauterine O_2 tensions. (c) A similar metabolic adaptation is found in hibernating mammals that exhibit a uniform minimal metabolic rate that equals the basal metabolic rate achieved by the largest mammals based on body size alone.

a higher thermometabolic stress than adults and are known to be at higher risk of hypothermia, due to the limits of thermoregulation being reached earlier (12–14).

All in all, small mammals have particularly high energy requirements both due to their small body size and thermoregulatory properties, making them particularly susceptible to conditions of undersupply. From this point of view, it is not surprising that over the some 150 million years of mammalian evolution, both the intrauterine development and – above all – the process of being born have been optimized by a number of self-protective mechanisms (15–17).

Being satisfied with little – The fetus as a euthermic hibernator

The intrauterine environment might be imagined as a Garden of Eden where everything is available in abundance. However, this is not the case. In particular with respect to O_2, the fetus has to cope with scarcity even under normal developmental conditions. The mean O_2 partial pressure in the fetal circulation amounts to 25–30 mmHg and thus corresponds to the arterial blood gas values that have been measured in extreme mountaineers climbing on the top of the world without additional oxygen ("Everest *in utero*"). The exceptionally low O_2 tension has previously been thought to reflect a worse gas exchange capacity of the placenta as compared to the lung. Meanwhile, it is assumed that (given the immaturity of O_2 free radical detoxification systems) Mother Nature deliberately put the mammalian fetus in a hypoxic compartment to prevent it from O_2 toxicity (18, 19).

Hematological adaptations to the low O_2 environment
Even though these ambient conditions are normal during intrauterine life (and should therefore be referred to as "low-oxygen" rather than as "hypoxic" conditions), the fetus has to compensate for the reduced pO_2 to cover its O_2 needs. As described in many physiological textbooks, this compensation primarily consists of two complementary hematological mechanisms.

Left shift of the O_2 dissociation curve
First, the well-known left shift of the O_2 dissociation curve of fetal hemoglobin (down to a half-saturation pressure of approximately

19 mmHg as opposed to approximately 28 mmHg in human adults). The markedly increased O_2 affinity results in the fact that at a pO_2 between 25 and 30 mmHg, the mean O_2 saturation in the fetal circulation amounts to 65–70% rather than 50% as would be expected, under comparable ambient conditions, in unacclimated adults.

Increase in hemoglobin concentration
Second, the increase in hemoglobin concentration (up to roughly 18–20 g/dl in term neonates as opposed to 13–15 g/dl in adults). This is a kind of high-altitude acclimatization responding to the fact that despite its higher O_2 affinity, the O_2 saturation of the fetal hemoglobin is still well below the almost 100% in oxygenated adult blood.

The two adaptive mechanisms ensure that the total O_2 content of fetal blood is in the order of adult blood which is often misinterpreted as if the low pO_2 in the fetal circulation was fully compensated. However, this is not true, since – independently of the amount of O_2 carried by the red cells – the driving force for the diffusion of gases is partial pressure. Hence, even the aforementioned adaptive responses cannot prevent the O_2 from being "pressed" into the fetal tissues under a much lower tension than in adults. This would inevitably affect tissue oxygenation if there were not another adaptive mechanism.

Metabolic adaptation to the low O_2 environment
The key to understanding this additional adaptation is Warburg's law (20), stating that the "critical depth" (of penetration of O_2 into tissue by diffusion) does not only depend on the partial pressure gradient from outside to inside but also on the rate at which O_2 is consumed by the tissue. The lower the O_2 consumption rate, the higher the penetration depth, or in other words: the adverse effect of a lowered partial pressure can be counteracted by a reduced tissue respiration rate.

This is the background for a widely underestimated self-protective mechanism to be found in mammalian fetuses, namely the suppression of the usual metabolic size relationship. In fact, the general rule that the specific metabolic rate increases with decreasing body mass ("mouse-to-elephant curve") seems to be somehow "switched off" during intrauterine life (Figure 2.1b). From a metabolic point of view, the mammalian fetus behaves more "like an organ of its mother," with the metabolic increase up to the level expected from body size occurring only after birth (6, 21–23).

The deviation from the usual metabolic size relationship was first described by Hasselbalch (24) in avian embryos and explained by the fact that if their energy turnover was as high as expected from their small body size, the diffusion capacity of the egg shell would not be high enough to cover the resulting O_2 demand (25). Unlike in avian embryos, metabolic measurements in mammalian fetuses are methodologically difficult and accordingly rare, starting from the first observations by Bohr (21, 26–30). Since then, it has been repeatedly shown that mammalian (including human) neonates still have a disproportionately low specific O_2 consumption rate immediately after birth, before rising more or less rapidly to the metabolic level appropriate to their own body size (22, 31–33). As was first observed by Brück (34) in his pivotal studies on the metabolism of human term and preterm neonates, and later confirmed by our own respirometric measurements (35), the earliest postnatal metabolic rates are remarkably independent of gestational age and birth weight and thus reflect the suppression of metabolic size relationship during intrauterine life.

Another indirect and often overlooked sign of intrauterine metabolic reduction in humans is heart rate. After a sharp increase in the first trimester, the fetal heart rate levels off at about 140 beats per minute, where it remains more or less unchanged until the expected date of birth (36). This is significantly lower than would be expected in adult mammals of comparable size, especially in the earlier stages of pregnancy (e.g. a 100 g mammal corresponding in body weight to a human fetus at 16 weeks of gestation would have a heart rate of around 400 beats per minute) (5, 37). Since the heart rate directly parallels the metabolic rate, the "inappropriately" low heart rate clearly reflects the metabolic suppression that adapts the human fetus to its low-oxygen habitat.

The protective effect of the reduced metabolic rate can be illustrated in marsupial mammals that are physiologically born in an extremely immature state and spend most of their fetal development in their mother's abdominal pouch. According to our own studies on *Monodelphis* neonates, tiny creatures of 100 mg weight and 1 cm length, these animals show no postnatal metabolic increase at all and maintain a metabolic level that in their case amounts to only 20% of what would be expected in an adult marsupial of comparable size (35). This has three major implications.

Favored gas exchange
First, it compensates for the scarce O_2 supply, which in their case is not due to an "insufficient" placenta, but to a very immature lung (38). As has been shown by Mortola and coworkers (39) in a slightly different marsupial species, a considerable part of the O_2 uptake in these animals during their first days of life occurs via skin respiration – which would be unimaginable without a unique combination of small size and disproportionately low metabolic rates (6).

Favored growth rate
Second, the low maintenance metabolism allows for a high growth efficiency despite a necessarily limited substrate supply. In the aforementioned marsupial species, an increase to 500% of birth weight within the first 10 days of life was observed, although neither their milk intake nor the caloric content of the milk was exceptionally high.

Favored temperature control
Third, both marsupial neonates and mammalian fetuses can "afford" the suppression of metabolic size relationship because they are passively thermostated, be it in the maternal abdominal pouch or in the womb, and therefore do not need a stronger "internal heater" to compensate for higher heat losses over their relatively larger body surface area. In the case of the mammalian fetus in particular, it could even be that with an appropriately high metabolic rate, the heat transport capacity of the placenta might not be sufficient to remove the excess heat from the amniotic cavity (28).

Remarkably, the intrauterine metabolic reduction is the only exception to the general metabolic size relationship apart from hibernating mammals that fall to a uniform minimum specific metabolic rate that corresponds to the specific basal metabolic rate of the very largest mammals and might thus reflect a common limit to metabolic reduction (Figure 2.1c) (40–42). This also applies to black bears that give birth to their offspring while in hibernation and thus provide a "missing link" between intrauterine and seasonal adaptations (43). Similar to fetuses, at least some hibernating mammals exhibit a decreased (venous) blood pO_2 (44, 45), suggesting that a low-oxygen atmosphere could be a common permissive factor of metabolic reduction both in the natural overwintering strategies and in the "euthermic hibernation" of mammalian fetuses.

Staying alive with even less – Oxyconforming responses of the feto-placental unit

Even though the fetus is already adapted to the low-oxygen atmosphere through hematological and metabolic adaptations, there is still a substantial adaptive reserve, in that a number of exogenous and endogenous conditions are tolerated without jeopardizing the pregnancy as a whole (46). This applies to high-altitude pregnancies, to food scarcity and famines, to pregnancy disorders with impaired placental perfusion, and to cases of severe fetal anemia. In terms of O_2 supply, a further reduction by approximately 50% (e.g. in highland pregnancies up to 4000–4500 m of altitude; or in fetal anemias down to 9–8 g/dl of serum hemoglobin) is usually tolerable without major adverse effects, except for a mild-to-moderate Intra-Uterine Growth Restriction (IUGR). This adaptive reserve is due to a coordinated response of the feto-placental unit that consists of two main factors.

Metabolic gatekeeper role of the placenta
Recent findings indicate that the placenta plays an important gatekeeper role in the allocation of energy flows. The basic premise here is that only 60% of the oxygen supplied to the feto-placental unit is passed on to the fetus, while 40% is consumed by the placental tissue itself. With reduced O_2 delivery, the placenta appears to reduce its own O_2 consumption in order to maintain fetal O_2 supply (Figure 2.2a). The metabolic reduction that is accompanied by a decrease in mitochondrial density impairs active transport and synthetic processes (thus resulting in a more or less pronounced IUGR), yet prevents the fetus from a critical O_2 deficit. It seems that maintaining adequate oxygenation has priority over unrestricted growth in intrauterine life (29, 30, 47, 48).

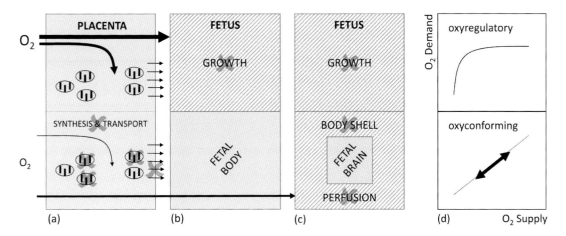

FIGURE 2.2 Self-protective responses of the feto-placental unit in mammals. (a) Since the placenta itself consumes up to 40% of the total O_2 supplied to the feto-placental unit, it can prevent the fetus from hypoxia by reducing its own metabolic rate. (b) The fetus is able to compensate for the resulting lack of substrate supply by "refraining" from growth in favor of maintenance metabolism. (c) A critical O_2 deficiency leads to a redistribution of blood flow from the body shell to the central organs (brain-sparing effect, diving reflex). (d) The gradual adjustment of metabolic demand to energy supply reflects an oxyconforming response that differs from the usual oxyregulatory behavior of mammalian tissues.

Metabolic programming of the fetus

The fact that the metabolic rate in mammalian fetuses is lower than expected from body size also means that the growth metabolism accounts for a relatively high proportion of the total energy turnover. This in turn offers the fetus the opportunity to adapt to an inadequate supply by "refraining" from growth (Figure 2.2b). Accordingly, IUGR that from a clinical perspective is usually considered as a pathological symptom of impaired supply, can be interpreted as a physiological adaptation that enables the fetus to survive a further shortage despite an already limited O_2, and substrate availability. The earlier the underlying metabolic changes start and the longer they last, the more the fetal organism is programmed to "low flame," meaning that even a normal supply of substrate acts as a surplus and thus promotes a metabolic syndrome later in life (49–51).

The placental decrease in O_2 consumption in response to decreasing O_2 supply, also referred to as hypoxic hypometabolism (52, 53), is an "oxyconforming" response that differs from the usual "oxyregulatory" behavior of mammalian tissues that tend to maintain their metabolic rate until final breakdown (Figure 2.2d). It has long been assumed that oxyconformism is confined to lower vertebrates (frogs) or even invertebrates (intertidal worms) that are able to adapt to changing supply conditions by adjusting their metabolic rate more flexibly (54, 55). Recent studies suggest that not only the placenta but also the fetus itself shows an oxyconforming behavior in that its own metabolic rate underlies some variations depending on the fluctuating O_2 tensions in the fetal circulation (30). This may reflect, among other things, the varying contribution of growth metabolism to the overall metabolic rate. However, it is also related to a redistribution of blood flow that the fetus exhibits in response to deteriorating O_2 supply conditions (brain-sparing effect), and that may be regarded as a precursor of the birth-related diving response (Figure 2.2c) (56, 57).

Surviving with a minimum – A deep dive through the birth canal

Whenever the fetus is at risk of suffering a severe O_2 deficiency during the birth process (58), a reaction occurs that is very well-known to the entire delivery room staff as a red flag: the so-called

dips or decelerations in the cardiotocographic (CTG) monitoring. They differ from the stress response an adult would show in the case of suffocation, namely an acceleration in heart rate and an increase in cardiac output to maintain an adequate O_2 supply to the tissues. Since this typical oxyregulatory response enables the organism to escape or fight a threatening situation, it has proven to be an obviously successful adult survival strategy in the course of evolution. Its major disadvantage, however, is that under the conditions of an already limited O_2 supply, the O_2 demand will increase even further. As the fetus completely relies on energy supply via the umbilical cord, any attempt to fight against the O_2 lack would be futile and would only lead to a reduced hypoxia tolerance due to the increased O_2 consumption rate. It is therefore reasonable from an evolutionary perspective that the fetus responds to an acute (perinatal) hypoxia with a different physiological reaction that is called the "diving response", by analogy to aquatic mammals (seals) that exhibit a similar pattern during longer periods of submersion (59–61). This comprises three main components.

Lowering heart rate

A cornerstone of the diving response in both aquatic mammals and mammalian fetuses is the gradual decrease in heart rate. Given that the myocardium, together with the brain, accounts for a significant proportion of total O_2 consumption in the fetal life, bradycardia per se makes a significant contribution to reducing energy requirements.

Redirecting blood flow

Since the slowed heart rate results in a reduced cardiac output, an adequate supply of the organism would no longer be possible if there were no redistribution of blood flow. That's why the diving reflex involves a centralization of the circulation in favor of the vital organs (heart, brain). The temporary reduction of peripheral perfusion leads to an accumulation of lactate in peripheral tissues and a subsequent washout after re-emergence. As pointed out by Scholander in a landmark paper (62), the post-diving lactate peak in seals is similar to the transient lactate increase that is observed in human neonates immediately after birth, and that, incidentally, makes it difficult to draw a clear line between a beneficial self-protective response and an actual perinatal asphyxia.

Holding breath

Not unlike at deep rest, all spontaneous fetal motor activity is also suppressed under stress, so as to avoid any unnecessary energy expenditure. This includes the intermittent respiratory movements the fetus is known to exhibit, just to prepare the diaphragm for its life-long activity. Only when a critical degree of hypoxia is reached, the apnea is interrupted by serial gasps that, if occurring in the birth canal, can lead to a meconium aspiration syndrome. Once the baby is born, the gasps provide the blood with a minimum of O_2, just enough to maintain the greatly slowed heart rate for a while ("autoresuscitation") (63–65).

As a whole, the diving response results in a slower consumption of the remaining O_2 reserves (that, both in fetuses and diving mammals, are elevated by a high hematocrit). The clinical appearance of a "depressed" neonate with apnea, bradycardia, and reduced peripheral perfusion actually corresponds to the full picture of the diving reflex. Just as in a seal taking a deep breath after re-emergence at the water surface, a rapid increase in the baby's APGAR values from the first to the fifth minute of life reflects a rapid recovery from a self-protective response (66, 67). In case of persisting hypoxia of any cause, the diving reflex will be maintained and completed by a suppression of thermogenesis in the O_2- and pH-sensitive BAT which, while preventing an adverse thermoregulatory increase in metabolic rate, increases the risk of inadvertent hypothermia (28, 52, 68, 69).

Summary and conclusions – The mammalian fetus as a paragon of coping with the lack

In summary, mammalian, including human, fetuses and newborns are equipped with a number of self-protective mechanisms that prevent them from the risks of intrauterine and perinatal life. Since the most important of these risks is a temporary lack of O_2 and nutrient supply, being in contrast to the particularly high metabolic demands of small endotherms, it is not surprising that these mechanisms are mainly based on a reduction in metabolic

rate. Most of them are known from adaptations to a predictable (e.g. seasonal) undersupply in the animal kingdom (53, 60, 70) suggesting that, vice versa, the perinatal period might even act as a common ontogenetic source of adaptive responses among mammals.

With regard to perinatal adaptation, it should be emphasized that the self-protective mechanisms are arranged in a cascade-like manner and exhaust themselves gradually (Figure 2.3). This means that the more of them have already been activated *in utero* (e.g., in a growth-restricted fetus), the fewer are left at birth. The cumulative protective benefit is only effective as long as the gap between supply and demand can be narrowed by reducing demand to an indispensable minimum. This also means that neonatal hypoxia tolerance is more a "resistance" than a "tolerance" in its strict sense, delaying the onset of critical hypoxia rather than attenuating the harmful effects of O_2 lack. In fact, there is little, if any, evidence that neonatal tissues really "tolerate" hypoxia better than adult ones do. Although lactate acidosis plays an important role in the assessment of perinatal asphyxia, an overall (enzymatic) increase in the anaerobic capacity, i.e. the ability to extract energy from lactic acid fermentation, has never been proven in neonatal tissues (71).

What is unique about placental, fetal, and neonatal tissues is their ability to "deliberately" reduce their metabolic rate in response to decreased energy supply – a capability often misinterpreted as a low metabolic trait. In adult mammals experiencing a gap between energy demand and supply, counter-regulatory responses (tachycardia) are initiated to compensate for the reduced supply (oxyregulatory behavior). If these are not successful, a "passive" breakdown in metabolic rate occurs – as if a light bulb goes out as soon as the battery is exhausted. An alternative way to respond to shortened supply is to "actively" reduce demand (oxyconforming behavior) – as if a light bulb is provisionally dimmed in view of the imminent exhaustion of the battery. The phenomenological similarity between active and passive reduction in energy consumption (the light bulb becomes darker) partly explains the clinical problems in determining the

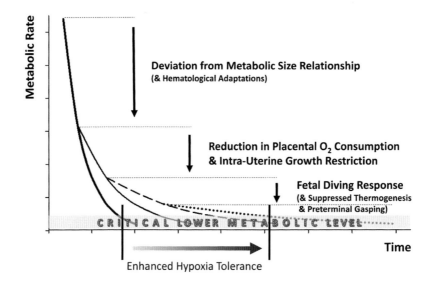

FIGURE 2.3 Cascade-like arrangement of self-protective mechanisms in mammalian fetuses and neonates. The declining curves represent the "passive" metabolic breakdown resulting from an imbalance between O_2 demand and supply. Whenever the metabolic rate falls below a critical lower limit, this results in irreversible damage. However, any "active" reduction in metabolic rate leads to a gradually slowed metabolic breakdown and an accordingly enhanced hypoxia tolerance (schematic view, arbitrary units).

boundaries between protective reactions and signs of damage in perinatal asphyxia.

Animal experiments on newborn mammals have revealed that their extra hypoxia tolerance is the more pronounced the smaller and more immature they are at birth (72, 73). In addition to a suppression of thermogenesis, a reduction of the metabolic rate at normal body temperature and thus a hypoxic hypometabolism was identified as the essential mechanism (15, 52, 74). Interestingly, however, this ability (obviously some kind of transient return to the fetal metabolic level) is lost more or less quickly, much in parallel with the postnatal increase in metabolic rate and its link to body size (23, 75). It may be that some of the natural adaptation strategies (e.g., hibernation) imply a temporary disabling of this link in a low-oxygen environment.

Finally, the optimization of the birth process over millions of years of mammalian evolution may explain the difficulties of finding effective treatments for HIE. It must be assumed that nature has left out nothing that could have contributed to reducing vulnerability. External cooling as an attempt to reduce the newborn's metabolic rate differs from the endogenous metabolic suppression occurring in natural adaptations. However, the latter is only effective as long as the hypoxic state persists. Should it eventually be possible to activate the "fetal hibernation gene" even after a hypoxic-ischemic event, this might be of huge benefit not only for asphyxiated neonates and adult stroke or cardiac arrest patients.

In the meantime, it is essential to make use of the time margins built into the birth process through a cascade of self-protective mechanisms. This offers the opportunity to identify perinatal risks in time and to avert them by taking appropriate obstetric and/or neonatological measures.

References

1. Shankaran S. Curr Opin Pediatr. 2015; 27:152–157.
2. Davidson JO, et al. Front Biosci. 2018; 23:2204–2226.
3. Gunn AJ, et al. Handb Clin Neurol. 2019; 162:217–237.
4. Kleiber M. *The fire of life: an introduction to animal energetics.* New York: Wiley; 1961.
5. Schmidt-Nielsen KC. Cambridge: Cambridge University Press; 1984.
6. Singer D. Respir Physiol Neurobiol. 2004; 141:215–228.
7. Singer D. Thermochim Acta. 2006; 446:20–28.
8. Bejan A, et al. *Design in nature.* New York: Anchor Books; 2012.
9. Belkin DA. Science. 1963; 139(3554):492–493.
10. Suarez RK, et al. Am J Physiol. 1989; 257:R1083–R1088.
11. Else PL, et al. Physiol Biochem Zool. 2004; 77:950–958.
12. Okken A, Koch J, eds. *Thermoregulation of sick and low birth weight neonates.* Berlin: Springer; 1995.
13. Agren J. *Fanaroff & Martin's neonatal-perinatal medicine: Diseases of the fetus and infant,* 10th. ed. Martin RJ, Fanaroff AA, Walsh MC, eds. Philadelphia: Elsevier Saunders; 2015. pp. 502–512.
14. Singer D, et al. *Innovations and frontiers in neonatology (Pediatr Adolesc Med, vol. 22);* Basel: Karger; 2020. pp. 95–111.
15. Mortola JP. Respir Physiol. 1999; 116:95–103.
16. Singer D. Comp Biochem Physiol A. 1999; 123:221–234.
17. Singer D. Anästhesiol Intensivmed Notfallmed Schmerzther. 2002; 37:441–460.
18. Ar A, et al. Israel J Zool. 1994; 40:307–326.
19. Reich B, et al. Dev Neurosci. 2016; 38:311–330.
20. Warburg O. Biochem Z. 1923; 142:317–333.
21. Rahn H. *A companion to animal physiology.* Taylor CR, Johansen K, Bolis L, eds. Cambridge: Cambridge University Press; 1982. pp. 124–137.
22. Wieser W. Respir Physiol. 1984; 55:1–9.
23. Singer D, et al. Comp Biochem Physiol A. 2007; 148:780–784.
24. Hasselbalch AK. Skand Arch Physiol. 1900; 10:353–402.
25. Paganelli CV, et al. In: *Respiration and metabolism of embryonic vertebrates.* Seymour RS, ed. Dordrecht: Dr W Junk Publishers; 1984. pp. 193–204.
26. Bohr C. Skand Arch Physiol. 1900; 10:413–424.
27. Dawes GS, et al. J Physiol. 1959; 146:295–315.
28. Schröder HJ, et al. Exp Physiol. 1997; 82:403–414.
29. Murray AJ. Placenta. 2012; 33:e16–e22.
30. Postigo L, et al. J Physiol. 2009; 587:693–708.
31. Hill JR, et al. J Physiol. 1965; 180:239–265.
32. Bauer K, et al. J Pediatr. 2003; 142:390–396.
33. Bauer J, et al. Am J Clin Nutr. 2009; 90:1517–1524.
34. Brück K. In: *Perinatal physiology,* 2nd. Stave U, ed. New York: Plenum; 1978. pp. 455–498.
35. Singer D. Thermochim Acta. 1998; 309:39–47.
36. DuBose TJ. Fertil Steril. 2009; 92:e57–e58.
37. Lindstedt SL, et al. Quart Rev Biol. 1981; 56:1–16.
38. Szdzuy K, et al. J Anat. 2008; 212:164–179.
39. Mortola JP. Nature. 1999; 397:660.
40. Geiser F. J Comp Physiol. 1988; 158B:25–37.
41. Singer D, et al. In: *Surviving hypoxia: mechanisms of control and adaptation.* Hochachka PW, Lutz PL, Sick T et al., eds. Boca Raton FL: CRC Press; 1993. pp. 447–458.
42. Heldmaier G, et al. Respir Physiol Neurobiol. 2004; 141:317–329.
43. Tøien, et al. Science. 2011; 331:906–909.
44. Musacchia XJ, et al. Am J Physiol. 1971; 221:128–130.
45. Kevsbech IG, et al. J Comp Physiol B. 2017; 187:847–856.
46. Bennet L. J Physiol. 2017; 595:1865–1881.
47. Carter AM. Placenta. 2000; 21(Suppl A):S31–S37.
48. Schneider H. Placenta. 2000; 21(Suppl A):S38–S44.
49. Godfrey KM, et al. Public Health Nutr. 2001; 4:611–624.
50. Rinaudo P, et al. Annu Rev Physiol. 2012; 74:107–130.
51. Myers DA, et al. Adv Exp Med Biol. 2014; 814:147–157.
52. Mortola JP. Respir Physiol Neurobiol. 2004; 141:345–356.
53. Gorr TA. Acta Physiol. 2017; 219:409–440.
54. Boutilier RG, et al. J Exp Biol. 1997; 200:387–400.
55. Buchner T, et al. Comp Biochem Physiol B. 2001; 129:109–120.
56. Jensen A, et al. Eur J Obstet Gynecol Reprod Biol. 1999; 84:155–172.
57. Cohen E, et al. Neonatology. 2015; 108:269–276.
58. Turner JM, et al. Am J Obstet Gynecol. 2020; 222:17–26.
59. Elsner R, et al. Monogr Physiol Soc. 1983; 40:1–168.
60. Hill RW, et al. *Animal physiology.* Sunderland (Mass): Sinauer; 2004.
61. Panneton WM. Physiology. 2013; 28:284–297.
62. Scholander PF. Sci Am. 1963; 209:92–106.
63. Sanocka UM, et al. J Appl Physiol. 1992; 73:749–753.
64. Fewell JE. Respir Physiol Neurobiol. 2005; 149:243–255.
65. Manole MD, et al. Pediatr Res. 2006; 60:174–179.
66. Casey BM, et al. N Engl J Med. 2001; 344:467–471.
67. Iliodromiti S, et al. Lancet. 2014; 384:1749–1755.
68. Malan A, et al. J Comp Physiol B. 1988; 158:487–493.
69. Jayasinghe D. Neonatology. 2015; 107:220–223.
70. Larson J, et al. J Exp Biol. 2014; 217:1024–1039.
71. Jones CT, et al. Physiol Rev. 1985; 65:357–430.
72. Himwich HE, et al. Am J Physiol. 1941; 133:327–339.
73. Lutz PL, et al. Comp Biochem Physiol B Biochem Mol Biol. 1996; 113:3–13.
74. Rohlicek CV, et al. J Appl Physiol. 1998; 84:763–768.
75. Mourek J. Physiol Bohemoslov. 1959; 8:106–111.

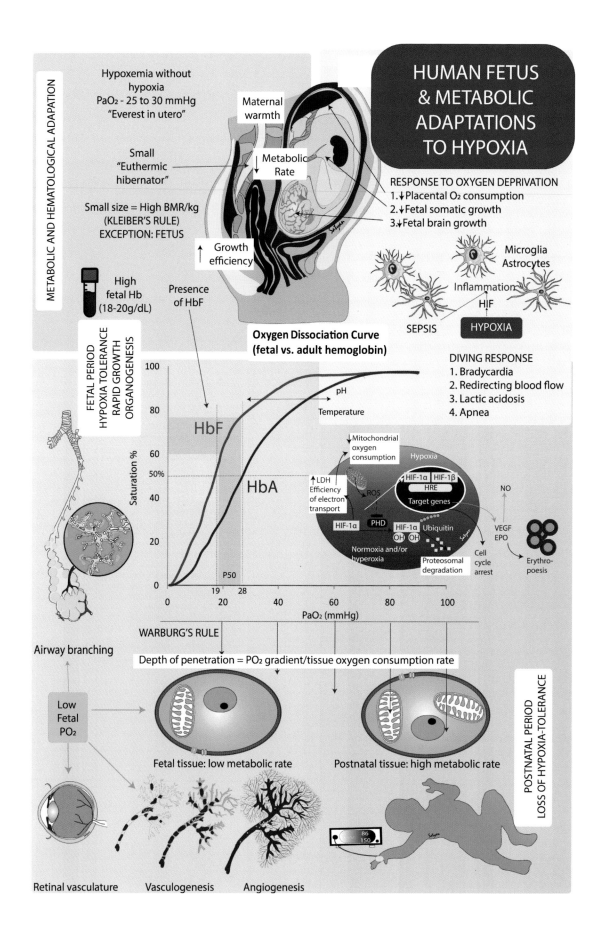

HUMAN FETUS & METABOLIC ADAPTATIONS TO HYPOXIA

METABOLIC AND HEMATOLOGICAL ADAPTATION

Hypoxemia without hypoxia
PaO₂ - 25 to 30 mmHg
"Everest in utero"

Maternal warmth

Small "Euthermic hibernator"

↓ Metabolic Rate

Small size = High BMR/kg
(KLEIBER'S RULE)
EXCEPTION: FETUS

↑ Growth efficiency

High fetal Hb (18-20g/dL)

Presence of HbF

RESPONSE TO OXYGEN DEPRIVATION
1. ↓Placental O₂ consumption
2. ↓Fetal somatic growth
3. ↓Fetal brain growth

Microglia Astrocytes

Inflammation

HIF

SEPSIS   HYPOXIA

FETAL PERIOD HYPOXIA TOLERANCE RAPID GROWTH ORGANOGENESIS

Oxygen Dissociation Curve (fetal vs. adult hemoglobin)

DIVING RESPONSE
1. Bradycardia
2. Redirecting blood flow
3. Lactic acidosis
4. Apnea

HbF

HbA

pH
Temperature

Saturation %
100
80
60
50%
40
20
0

P50

0   19 28   40   60   80   100
        20
PaO₂ (mmHg)

↓Mitochondrial oxygen consumption

Hypoxia

↑LDH Efficiency of electron transport

ROS

HIF-1α HIF-1β
HRE
Target genes

HIF-1α   PHD   HIF-1α
OH OH   Ubiquitin

Normoxia and/or hyperoxia

Proteosomal degradation

Cell cycle arrest

NO

VEGF
EPO

Erythro-poesis

WARBURG'S RULE

Depth of penetration = PO₂ gradient/tissue oxygen consumption rate

Airway branching

Low Fetal PO₂

Fetal tissue: low metabolic rate

Postnatal tissue: high metabolic rate

POSTNATAL PERIOD LOSS OF HYPOXIA-TOLERANCE

86
150

Retinal vasculature   Vasculogenesis   Angiogenesis

HYPOXIA AS A NEUROINFLAMMATORY STIMULUS DURING DEVELOPMENT

Peter M. MacFarlane and Allison S. Osborne

Contents

Fetal "hypoxia" as a stimulus for development

The fetal environment is relatively hypoxemic compared to the extra-uterine air-breathing one, and the "Oxygen Cascade" describes the O_2 gradients and associated transport mechanisms from the atmosphere to mitochondria (1). The atmospheric partial pressure of O_2 (PO_2) at sea level, which is perceived postnatally as "normoxia," is ~160 mmHg. The PO_2 of the umbilical artery that returns fetal blood to the placenta is ~40 mmHg and the fetal arterial PO_2 (PaO_2) reaches ~30 mmHg (2). The placental environment, therefore, is classically categorized as relatively hypoxic from an atmospheric air-breathing standpoint. However, it is a necessary "normoxic" state for the fetus especially since O_2 supply to the tissue is adequate and does not necessitate anaerobic metabolic pathways to support energy demands. The O_2 demand of the fetus is low compared to the newborn infant primarily because two significant energy-demanding processes are minimal – thermogenesis is low because it is provided maternally, and the infrequent fetal breathing movements also minimize energy costs. Growth and development comprise the predominant energy demands of the fetus, and the intrinsic O_2 levels comprise a necessary stimulus to guide appropriate development. The "hypoxic" embryonic environment stimulates trophoblast cell differentiation and placentation during early pregnancy, while in later stages of pregnancy, the low-O_2 tensions promote organ development including airway branching, lung morphogenesis, and angiogenesis (3, 4). Cellular (adaptive) responses to hypoxia are largely modulated by transcriptional activity involving hypoxia-inducible factor signaling (5). However, there are of course limits below which abnormally low-O_2 availability (e.g. severity of hypoxia) can have unfortunate consequences for the developing organism and the vulnerability to hypoxia is age- and tissue-specific. Given the susceptibility of exposure to hypoxic insults during development, in this chapter, we highlight the pro-inflammatory properties of hypoxia and the ways in which it can affect various elements of the respiratory neural control system during development.

Inflammation

Inflammation is a physiological response of the immune system triggered by a wide variety of insults including injury, pathogens, and toxins, and even excessive or deficient O_2 exposure (6). Both infectious and noninfectious insults activate immune cells that initiate inflammatory signaling pathways; these responses are intended to be beneficial through the removal of harmful material and activation of the healing process (7). On the other hand, uncontrolled or chronic inflammatory responses can have inadvertent effects and, therefore, there are both benefits and consequences associated with immune system activation (8). Abnormalities in inflammatory responses have been proposed in autism spectrum disorders (9), fragile X syndrome (10), sudden infant death syndrome (SIDS), and fetal inflammatory syndrome (11, 12). Responses are also vastly diverse and can vary by location (e.g. cell/tissue-specific, peripheral [systemic], central [CNS]), duration, age, and nature of the insult or pathogen. Although immune and inflammatory activation mechanisms are complex, a simplified characterization could generally be categorized as a response that involves activation of immune cells (peripherally – leukocyte recruitment; centrally – microglia, astrocytes) and/or release of pro-inflammatory cytokines/chemokines (6). While the profile of cytokine/chemokine responses are also complex, increased expression, synthesis, and release of pro-inflammatory cytokines IL-1β, IL-6, and TNFα are commonly recognized.

Inflammatory responses can also involve increased (transcriptional) cellular signaling of MAP kinases, NF-kB, JAK, and STAT pathways, but discussion of the complexities of these responses are beyond the scope of this chapter. Changes in endogenous O_2 levels (particularly hypoxia) can also activate immune responses leading to inflammation. In this context, the severity/intensity, duration (acute, chronic), and pattern (continuous/sustained, intermittent/recurrent) of O_2 exposure can be expected to determine the characteristics of the immune/inflammatory response. The effect of hypoxia in the context of an inflammatory stimulus can impact individuals of all ages particularly the fetus and developing neonate.

DOI: 10.1201/9780367494018-3

Hypoxia as an inflammatory stimulus

A variety of clinical scenarios are associated with fetal hypoxia including umbilical cord compression, pre-eclampsia, maternal anemia, substance abuse, multiple pregnancies, chorioamnionitis, gestational diabetes, and sleep-disordered breathing (13). The fetus is fairly well-equipped with various physiological adaptations to defend against excessive or inadvertent hypoxia. The higher fetal hemoglobin affinity, ability to shunt blood preferentially to vulnerable organs, bradycardia, and implementation of hypoxic-hypometabolism are important defense mechanisms to avoid ischemic injury, most of which are largely lost postnatally. However, there are limits to the functional benefits of these hypoxia defense strategies especially with prolonged/chronic exposure. The concept of fetal origins of adult disease has been postulated for several decades (14) and a large body of evidence has arisen from studies focused on the effects of fetal nutritional compromise and stress. More recent studies have shed light on developmental reprogramming following fetal hypoxia, which can lead to cardiovascular and metabolic susceptibility later in postnatal life (15). Delineating the basic mechanisms has been challenging, but emerging evidence has revealed pro-inflammatory properties of hypoxia at multiple ages. In adults suffering from mountain sickness, increased serum levels of IL-6, IL-6 receptor, and C-reactive protein are some markers of inflammation (16) in association with physiological effects of altitude hypoxia including vascular leakage, pulmonary, and cerebral edema (17, 18). Hypoxia can also amplify the innate immune response to invading pathogens by recruiting adaptive immune cells; inflammatory pathologies in which tissue hypoxia has been documented include inflammatory bowel disease, ischemia, cancer, obesity, and arthritis (19).

However, rather than hypoxia manifesting as a consequence of inflamed tissue, it can also activate inflammatory responses through O_2-sensitive signaling pathways such as hypoxia-inducible factor (HIF) in a variety of immune cell types (20). Microglia and astrocytes are the main CNS inflammatory mediators and are responsive to hypoxia (21). They are the resident immune cells of the CNS; their inflammatory role is complex and has adverse effects on the respiratory neural control system, particularly during development (discussed in more detail later). Microglial activation increases microglia motility by releasing cytokines and chemokines, which also play a role in the removal of cellular debris and phagocytosis of synapses as well as modulation of neurotransmitters critically involved in respiratory neuron excitability (22). Previous studies have demonstrated increased microglia expression in specific brainstem cardiorespiratory control regions following neonatal hypoxia, resulting in altered neurotransmitter expression and respiratory control dysfunction (23). Hypoxia has similar effects on various brain autonomic regions in adult rats leading to increased inflammatory mediators IL-1β, IL-6, MMP9, and TNFα (24). In neonatal mice, a transient anoxic event was sufficient to induce microsomal prostaglandin E synthase-1 (mPGES-1) activity (25). In the same study, the C-reactive protein was correlated with elevated PGE2 in cerebral spinal fluid, which was associated with increased apnea frequency. Finally, *in utero*, fetal brain sparing in which cardiovascular responses to hypoxia include increased carotid (i.e. brain) blood flow relative to peripheral regions (e.g. hindlimbs) is a mechanism intended to protect the CNS from hypoxic injury (13). The long-term impact of this response, however, manifests as asymmetrical growth restriction, small for gestational age,

and disproportional head/body size (26–28). Of interest is that the carotid body chemoreceptors play an important role in this fetal response to hypoxia, since it is largely blunted following carotid body denervation (29). The effects of hypoxia and immunosensing capabilities of the carotid body are discussed later. Physiologically, hypoxia during development manifests in many forms and the subsequent inflammatory response can vary with age and as a function of hypoxia (e.g. acute, chronic sustained [CSH], and intermittent hypoxia [CIH]).

Effects of pro-inflammatory mediators on respiratory control

Following birth, the increase in arterial PO_2 has a profound effect on the respiratory control system. The rapid oxygenation leads to resetting of the O_2-sensing properties of carotid bodies, the primary peripheral chemoreceptors responsible for initiating the ventilatory defense response to hypoxemia, or HVR (an index of respiratory control [dys]function, pertaining to the capacity to mount an increase in minute ventilation to defend against hypoxemia). The respiratory system rapidly adapts to the postnatal environment, and over several days (animal studies, see Bavis (30) for a review), or weeks (human infants), the HVR then becomes more robust and begins to mature (31), although the HVR is blunted in preterm infants (32). A similar phenomenon probably explains the blunted HVR in infants born at high altitude (33). In rodents, chronic postnatal hypoxia blunts the HVR and delays its maturation largely through a disruption in the resetting of carotid body O_2 sensitivity (34–36) and impairment of carotid body growth and development. Since hypoxia has pro-inflammatory properties resulting in increased expression of various cytokines such as IL-1β, IL-6, and TNFα in multiple brain regions, it is pertinent to discuss the effects of inflammation on the peripheral and central neural circuitry controlling breathing.

Hypoxia, inflammation, and breathing

Two of the most prominent examples in which IH stimulates an inflammatory response is sleep apnea (adolescents and adults) and apnea of prematurity (preterm infants) (20, 37). IH is a distinctly different stimulus than chronic-sustained hypoxia because of the repetitive reoxygenation and, therefore, IH likely involves a combination of both an inflammatory and oxidative stress response. In preterm infants, the incidence of IH events commonly associated with apnea of prematurity increases over the first 2 postnatal weeks (38), which has also been associated with increased serum oxidative stress markers (39). In the *in vitro* brainstem slice preparation of neonatal rats, IH-induced increases in respiratory rhythmic activity were attenuated by the microglia inhibitor minocycline, which implies an inflammatory-mediated stimulation of breathing (40). In a rat model of CIH exposure, blood cytokine levels were elevated in both serum and brain (specifically brainstem) (41). In pregnant women, IH occurs more frequently, which can lead to developmental disturbances in fetal somatic growth leading to reduced birthweight (42) as well as preterm delivery, NICU admissions, and intrauterine growth restrictions (43). Pregnant rats exposed to CIH caused impairments in ventilatory defense responses to acute hypoxic challenge in their offspring (44). In contrast, early postnatal CIH enhances the HVR (45, 46). Also of interest is that gestational IH increases susceptibility of the offspring to subsequent inflammatory insults (47) suggesting reprogramming of fetal immune responses.

The carotid body chemoreceptors contain specialized cells to detect changes in arterial oxygenation (both hypoxia and hyperoxia) (48). Type I glomus cells contain the O_2-sensing machinery that results in the release of various neurotransmitters as part of the afferent hypoxemic stimulus that gets transmitted into brainstem respiratory control regions, specifically the nucleus tractus solitarius (nTS). Peripheral hypoxic signals are received in nTS via the vagus nerve where the inputs are integrated and transmitted to other brainstem regions to stimulate an increase in minute ventilation (i.e. the HVR) (48). Type II cells of the carotid body are sustentacular supportive cells and resemble glial cells, which could imply the carotid body itself has inflammatory responsive capabilities. Many of these components involved in respiratory control have demonstrated sensitivity to inflammatory cytokines/chemokines and, therefore, result in a functional effect on respiratory output. IL-1β administration decreased respiratory frequency, hypoxic gasping, and autoresuscitation, a mechanism related to activation of prostaglandin E2 (PGE2) pathways (25). PGE2 administration to neonatal rats resulted in unstable breathing and increased sigh-related apneas (49). In the latter case, these effects could be prevented by pre-treatment with caffeine and an adenosine receptor antagonist. Caffeine has anti-inflammatory properties and is widely used clinically in preterm infants to mitigate apnea (50). Intraperitoneal injection of IL-1β decreased respiration in neonatal mice and also worsened anoxic survival (25). IL-1β also attenuated the ventilatory defense response to acute hypercapnic challenge in neonatal mice (51), whereas PGE2 depressed breathing in movements in several species including humans (25, 52, 53). The effects of individual inflammatory elements on breathing could be mediated at multiple sites of the respiratory control system.

Sensitivity of carotid body chemoreceptors to inflammatory mediators

The presence of the glial-like sustentacular cells of the carotid body makes it a promising candidate for having immunosensing properties (54). Chronic hypoxia upregulates expression of proinflammatory cytokines in the adult carotid body. As little as 3 days of hypoxia (10% FIO_2) increased IL-1β, IL-6, TNFαR1, and their cytokines in the carotid body and some were localized to glomus cells (55). Further, exogenous application of bath-applied IL-1β, IL-6, and TNFα to dissociated glomus cells enhanced the hypoxic-induced intracellular calcium response (55, 56), whereas IL-1β administration caused glomus cell depolarization (57). In contrast, TNFα application decreased carotid body sensitivity to acute hypoxia (54), suggesting different cytokines/chemokines could have differential effects on carotid body excitation, which could depend on interactions with other stimuli. CIH-induced increases in carotid body sensory activity were associated with increased TNFα and IL-1β (58, 59). However, although ibuprofen treatment had anti-inflammatory effects, it failed to decrease the augmented sensory responses, suggesting mechanisms underlying carotid body potentiation might not necessarily be linked to increased inflammatory expression. *In vivo* studies on anesthetized adult rats also showed exogenous/topical application of IL-1β to the carotid body increased carotid sinus nerve activity, which was blocked with an IL-1 receptor antagonist (57). Similarly, topical application of LPS to the carotid body also caused tachypnea in anesthetized rats (54). Collectively, these data support the immunosensing capabilities of the carotid body both under generalized inflammatory environments and following hypoxia (60).

Sensitivity of brainstem respiratory neurons to inflammatory mediators

Hypoxia and various pro-inflammatory cytokines/chemokines also affect brainstem respiratory neural control regions. IL-1β injections into the fourth ventricle increased c-Fos activity in tyrosine hydroxylase-expressing neurons of the nTS, the brainstem integrative site of vagal (and carotid body) afferent inputs (61). Similarly, in a neonatal rat model of sepsis, nTS neuron excitability was increased (62). CSH increased the excitability of nTS neurons, which was suspected to involve a disturbance in astrocyte-neuron interactions (63). Neonatal rats exposed to CSH followed by CIH had increased spontaneous bursting of nTS neurons (64), although neonatal CIH alone depressed nTS neuron activity through a mechanism related to reduced numbers of active synapse (65). While the reduced activity of nTS neurons could translate into a depressant effect on breathing, increased excitability could be a compensatory response to reduced carotid body inputs, or a form of over-compensation (64). Increased excitation of brainstem neurons could also reflect loss of efficient neurotransmission and, therefore, an inability to respond to hypoxia resulting from excessive glutamate release and cytotoxicity (66). PGE2 administration, which binds to EP3 receptors, decreased respiratory rhythm generation and increased apnea in brainstem spinal cord preparation of neonatal mice (25). Acute hypoxia has direct effects on the activity of preBotzinger (preBotC) neurons, a pre-motor respiratory nucleus critical for generating inspiratory rhythm. The initial responses of a single cell PreBotC neuron to acute hypoxia reflects the biphasic ventilatory response of newborns, comprising an initial increase in inspiratory bursting, followed by a rapid decline over several minutes (67). However, *in vivo* neonatal CIH increases irregularity of respiratory rhythm of these same neurons (68) and enhances respiratory frequency following *in vitro* IH, which was attenuated by microglial inhibitors (40). Overall, there is evidence demonstrating pro-inflammatory effects on excitability of neurons in both central and peripheral respiratory control regions.

Peripheral-to-central inflammatory transmission

Immunoresponsive cells including macrophages, dendritic cells, and B cells located in the spleen and lymphatic system are some of the "first responders" to peripheral detection of foreign or pro-inflammatory challenges (69). A large portion of the immune response includes cell proliferation and secretion of pro-inflammatory cytokines often leading to a large-scale, system-wide inflammatory cascade. There are several proposed mechanisms by which the peripheral pro-inflammatory response can be transmitted to the CNS including activation of endothelial cells, leading to direct release of other cytokines into the CNS. Cytokines acting indirectly across the blood-brain barrier include circulating IL-1β activation of IL-1 receptors located on vascular endothelial cells of the BBB, leading to increased COX-2 and microsomal PGE1 activity (25, 70).

More recently, the novel concept of localized peripheral CNS inflammatory responses in regions that receive afferent/peripheral nerve inputs has gained traction. Effects on peripheral nerves and associated tissue can transmit afferent signals to corresponding brain regions that initiate localized CNS inflammatory responses. How this takes place is unknown, but could involve direct transport of peripheral signals (e.g. cellular proteins or content), using the nerve as a physical conduit into the CNS, or through modification of electrical activity (sensory denervation or increased excitation). From a respiratory control standpoint, modulation of brainstem inflammation via the afferent origins of the vagus nerve is a prominent example. Intravenous administration of LPS increased c-FOS expression in the nTS, which was blunted following ipsilateral cervical vagotomy (71). Loss or diminished peripheral inputs can also cause localized CNS effects. Unilateral nodose ganglionectomy increased OX-42 expression in the ipsilateral, but not contralateral, side of the NTS, DMNV, and nucleus ambiguous (NA), which was prevented with the microglia inhibitor minocycline (72). The localized response on the ipsilateral side adds further support for a CNS method of inflammatory responsiveness via alterations in peripheral inputs. This concept offers novel avenues to explore therapeutic targets using compounds (or technology, e.g. nerve stimulation) that aren't required to cross the BBB, which can often have otherwise unintended nonspecific effects.

Sepsis and other pro-inflammatory insults

Common causes of neonatal inflammation include infection from sepsis, pneumonia, and meningitis. Sepsis and associated irreversible organ dysfunction are the major contributing factor in infant morbidity and mortality, particularly in preterm infant populations.

Neonatal infections account for ~1/3 of infant deaths (73) and increase apnea in preterm infants. *In utero*, chorioamnionitis is a common cause of prematurity, and neonatal infections are associated with meningitis, intraventricular hemorrhage, and white matter damage including periventricular leukomalacia (74). These conditions, in turn, are associated with long-term neurodevelopmental impairments including cerebral palsy (75, 76). LPS is commonly used experimentally as a potent pro-inflammatory/endotoxic insult and has also been used to mimic sepsis (54). It is a glycolipid portion of gram-negative bacterial surface molecule that initiates a potent inflammatory response largely via activation of toll-like receptors. In adult cats, LPS infusion caused tachypnea, tachycardia, and hypotension, although the effects on ventilation were absent following carotid body denervation (54). LPS also increased basal frequency of carotid body discharge suggesting an excitatory effect even in the absence of hypoxia (54). LPS application to the *in vitro* brainstem spinal cord preparation of ~2-day-old rats decreased respiratory burst frequency, but the magnitude of the depressant effect of LPS was reduced in rats preconditioned with gestational IH, a model aimed to mimic maternal IH associated with sleep apnea in pregnancy (47).

The possibility that *in utero* insults can re-program CNS inflammatory processes in a way that modifies subsequent (e.g. postnatal) challenges is largely under-investigated, yet likely has fundamentally important implications for infant mortality and morbidity. More recent studies have begun to shed light on inflammatory responses to substance of abuse. Animal studies have demonstrated increased CNS cytokine expression and glial activation/neuroinflammation following prenatal exposure to opioids (77) and alcohol (78) and postnatally to nicotine (79).

Critical windows of vulnerability to inflammatory insults

The terms critical window of plasticity and critical period of vulnerability refer to time periods of heightened sensitivity to environment insults or challenges. However, during a critical period

of vulnerability, the risk/outcome associated with an environmental challenge may be loss of homeostasis, injury, or death rather than the induction of phenotypic or adaptive plasticity, which would normally be intended to be beneficial (80). There are windows of development that are revealed by natural changes in respiratory control. The HVR doubles in magnitude between P10 and P15 (81), despite a transient loss of an effective HVR on day P13 (82). Such large swings in respiratory control capabilities coincide with a time of rapid and in some cases transient changes in brainstem neurochemistry (83–86). For example, glutamate, GABA, glycine, and 5-HT receptor expression change dramatically in brainstem cardio-respiratory control regions during the second week of life in the rat (~P12–P13) (83, 87). Similar unique and transient changes in various components of the ECM also take place during postnatal development (88). An extensive discussion on the role of the ECM in brain development is beyond the scope of this chapter; however, various ECM components interact with microglia and in some cases also comprise important inflammatory responses leading to altered neurotransmitter expression (e.g. 5-HT). Constitutive expression of TNFα and iNOS mRNA increases transiently at P10 whereas TLR4 increases at ~3 weeks of age in brainstem (89). Similarly, there is a transient reduction in brain metabolites during acute hypoxia that occur in 9- to 13-day-old rats (90), suggesting key neurodevelopmental events related to brain energy metabolism. However, these changes appear to represent necessary events required for architectural organization for appropriate brainstem development. Such critical periods also define a time when developmental plasticity can be elicited, although they can also comprise transient periods during which the organism is particularly vulnerable to environmental insults (80).

This is especially the case with respect to pro-inflammatory challenges including prolonged (days) hypoxia and acute LPS exposure. CSH during these key neurochemical adjustments increased microglia expression and decreased 5-HT immunoreactivity in two distinct brainstem cardio-respiratory control regions, the nTS, and DMNV (23). These effects of CSH were associated with an unexplained high mortality that was not observed in younger or older rats exposed to CSH (23, 91) and could be prevented with the microglia inhibitor minocycline. These data indicate that the heightened vulnerability during the critical window of development may involve a microglia-mediated disruption to brainstem neurochemical development. Similarly, LPS had a similar lethal effect during the same critical window of development (89). LPS administration to neonatal rats close to the time point of these neurochemical adjustments also caused a uniquely elevated degree of mortality. In this case, the mortality could be predicted in rats by prior assessment of their HVR, which offers some insight into the association between the lethality of inflammatory insults and disturbances in respiratory control. How these windows of development compare to humans is not clear, although it should be noted that there are multiple windows of postnatal vulnerability to pro-inflammatory insults, especially surrounding birth.

Vulnerability in the fetal-neonatal transition – Postnatal loss of hypoxia tolerance

With normal transition to extrauterine life, lung fluid clears and the newborn's first breaths begin to establish the lung's functional residual capacity, concurrent with a rapid drop in pulmonary vascular resistance (PVR) and increase in pulmonary blood flow. Clamping of the umbilical cord removes the low-resistance placenta from the circuit of systemic blood flow and increases systemic blood pressure. Together with the drop in PVR, this decreases the right-to-left shunt across the ductus arteriosus, which further increases the PaO_2 and stimulates closure of the ductus. Finally, the other physiologic right-to-left shunt (the foramen ovale) closes as pulmonary blood flow increases and left atrial pressure exceeds the right side. PaO_2 rises quickly to ~35–40 mmHg within a few minutes of birth, increasing to ~60–65 mmHg within an hour. These physiological adjustments associated with birth promote postnatal viability in an O_2-rich air-breathing environment.

While the low fetal O_2 levels provide a necessary stimulus to encourage normal growth, there is also an apparent and unexplained loss of tolerance to hypoxia immediately following birth. Rats born into hypoxia, which would in part mimic a postnatal continuation of fetal hypoxia, resulted in unexplained mortality (92). The mortality occurred precipitously at ~2 weeks of age, but not when initiation of hypoxia was delayed for a few days after birth. This could imply that the postnatal hypoxia intolerance is initiated by events immediately surrounding, or directly associated with birth (93). While the underlying mechanisms of loss of hypoxia tolerance are speculative, the mechanisms may be O_2-sensitive, since being born into hypoxia would have eliminated the sudden hyperoxic stimulus. One consequence of birthing into hypoxia is the resultant delay in normal postnatal processes including resetting of carotid body hypoxia sensing (36). Carotid body denervation can be lethal, especially in neonates (94), suggesting that carotid body activity may provide necessary inputs into brainstem cardiorespiratory control regions (95). Whether postnatal hypoxia-induced inflammation of the carotid bodies plays a role in the vulnerability could be speculated; although at a minimum, these data suggest early postnatal survival is critically dependent on peripheral carotid bodies (96).

The postnatal hypoxia intolerance is also true for preterm infants, which are prematurely expelled from their hypoxic *in-utero* environment. A meta-analysis combined data from five clinical trials that randomized preterm infants into either a low target range of baseline arterial O_2 saturation (85–89%) (i.e. mimicking very mild CSH) or a higher range (91–95%) starting within 24 hours of birth (97). One unexpected and concerning finding was a higher mortality rate in the *low* target (ie. relatively hypoxic) group compared to the *high* target group of infants. However, within the low target group of infants, there was an increased risk of death in infants who received the low oxygen <6 hours after birth, which was not seen in infants who received low oxygen >6 hours after birth (97). These data add further support to the concept of a postnatal loss of hypoxia tolerance, particularly when it occurs closer to the time of birth.

Conclusions

Overall, antenatal hypoxia exposure manifests in many forms, patterns, and severities, which can depend on associated clinical or pathological conditions. Hypoxia clearly has pro-inflammatory properties affecting both peripheral and central mechanisms of respiratory neural control. An understanding of the mechanistic basis for the vulnerabilities associated with hypoxia exposure, particularly during critical windows of development, may help to tease out underlying features associated with postnatal loss of hypoxia tolerance. Key breakthroughs in these areas will be instrumental in advancing the clinical care of (particularly) preterm infants.

Acknowledgments

Supported by grants from US National Institutes of Health R01 HL056470 and R01 HL138402.

References

1. Weibel ER, et al. Respir Physiol. 1981; 44(1):151–164.
2. Meschia G In: *Maternal-fetal medicine: principles and practice.* Creasy R, ed; Philadelphia: Saunders; 1989.
3. Soares M, et al. Birth Defects Res. 2017; 109(17):1309–1329.
4. Gebb SA. Adv Exp Med Biol. 2003; 543:117–125.
5. Semenza GL. Wiley Interdiscip Rev Syst Biol Med. 2010; 2(3):336–361.
6. Chen L, et al. Oncotarget. 2017; 9(6):7204–7218.
7. Nathan C, et al. Cell. 2010 Mar 19; 140(6):871–882.
8. Chertov O, et al. Immunol Rev. 2000; 177:68–78.
9. Mitchell RH, et al. J Am Acad Child Adolesc Psychiatry. 2014; 53(3):274–296.
10. Higashimori H, et al. Hum Mol Genet. 2013; 22(10):2041–2054.
11. Vennemann MM, et al. Int J Legal Med. 2012; 126(2):279–284.
12. Ferrante L, et al. Hum Immunol. 2008; 69(6):368–373.
13. Giussani DA. J Physiol. 2016; 594(5):1215–1230.
14. Barker DJ. J Int Med. 2007; 261(5):412–417.
15. Giussani DA, et al. J Dev Orig Health Dis. 2013; 4(5):328–337.
16. Hartmann G, et al. Cytokine. 2000; 12(3):246–252.
17. Semenza GL. Science. 2007; 318(5847):62–64.
18. Hackett PH, et al. N Engl J Med. 2001; 345(2):107–114.
19 Eltzschig HK, et al. N Engl J Med. 2011; 361(7):656–665.
20. Taylor CT, et al. J Clin Invest. 2016; 126(10):3716–3724.
21. Bilbo S, et al. Front Behav Neurosci. 2009; 3:14.
22. Bilbo SD, et al. Front Neuroendocrinol. 2012; 33(3):267–286.
23. MacFarlane PM, et al. J Physiol. 2016; 594(11):3079–3094.
24. Silva TM, et al. Exp Physiol. 2018; 103(6):884–895.
25. Hofstetter AO, et al. Proc Natl Acad Sci USA. 2007; 104(23):9894–9899.
26. Soria R, et al. Pediatr Res. 2013; 74(6):633–638.
27. Halliday HL. Best Pract Res Clin Obstet Gynaecol. 2009; 23(6):871–880.
28. McMillen IC, et al. Reproduction. 2001; 122(2):195–204.
29. Giussani DA, et al. J Physiol. 1993; 461:431–449.
30. Bavis RW. Respir Physiol Neurobiol. 2005; 149(1–3):287–299.
31. Williams BA, et al. J Physiol. 1991; 442:81–90.
32. Gerhardt T, et al. Pediatrics. 1984; 74(1):58–62.
33. Gamboa A, et al. J Appl Physiol (1985). 2003; 94(3):1255–1256.
34. Eden GJ, et al. J Physiol. 1987; 392:11–19.
35. Eden GJ, et al. J Physiol. 1987; 392:1–9.
36. Sterni LM, et al. Am J Physiol. 1999; 277(3 Pt 1):L645–L652.
37. Ryan S, et al. Circulation. 2005; 112(17):2660–2667.
38. Di Fiore JM, et al. J Pediatr. 2012; 161(6):1047–1052.
39. Shah VP, et al. Neonatology. 2020:1–7.
40. Camacho-Hernández NP, et al. Respir Physiol Neurobiol. 2019; 265:9–18.
41. Snyder B, et al. Physiological Reports. 2017; 5(9):e13258.
42. Loube DI, et al. Chest. 1996; 109(4):885–889.
43. Ding XX, et al. Sleep Breath. 2014; 18(4):703–713.
44. Gozal D, et al. Am J Respir Crit Care Med. 2003; 167(11):1540–1547.
45. Reeves SR, et al. Pediatr Res. 2006; 60(6):680–686.
46. Julien CA, et al. Respir Physiol Neurobiol. 2011; 177(3):301–312.
47. Johnson SM, et al. Respir Physiol Neurobiol. 2018; 256:128–142.
48. Feldman JL, et al. Annu Rev Neurosci. 2003; 26:239–266.
49. Mitchell LJ, et al. Am J Physiol Regul Integr Comp Physiol. 2020; 319(2):R233–R242.
50. Abu-Shaweesh JM, et al. Semin Fetal Neonatal Med. 2017; 22(5):342–347.
51. Siljehav V, et al. J Appl Physiol (1985). 2014; 117(9):1027–1036.
52. Kitterman JA, et al. J Appl Physiol Respir Environ Exerc Physiol. 1983; 54(3):687–692.
53. Taylor TC, et al. Am J Physiol Regul Integr Comp Physiol. 2000; 278(6):R1460–R1473.
54. Zapata P, et al. Respir Physiol Neurobiol. 2011; 178(3):370–374.
55. Lam SY, et al. Histochem Cell Biol. 2008; 130(3):549–559.
56. Fan J, et al. J Neurosci Res. 2009; 87(12):2757–2762.
57. Shu HF, et al. Eur J Neurosci. 2007; 25(12):3638–3647.
58. Rio D, et al. Adv Exp Med Biol. 2012; 758:199–205.
59. Del Rio R, et al. Eur Respir J. 2012; 39(6):1492–1500.
60. Gauda EB, et al. Respir Physiol Neurobiol. 2013; 185(1):120–131.
61. DeBoer MD, et al. Peptides. 2009; 30(2):210–218.
62. Eftekhari G, et al. Shock. 2020; 54(2):265–271.
63. Accorsi-Mendonça D, et al. J Neurosci. 2015; 35(17):6903–6917.
64. Mayer CA, et al. Respiratory physiology & neurobiology. 2015; 205:28–36.
65. Almado CE, et al. J Neurosci. 2012; 32(47):16736–46.
66. Zhang W, et al. Am J Physiol Regul Integr Comp Physiol. 2008; 295(5):R1555–R1562.
67. Garcia AJ 3rd, et al. Respir Physiol Neurobiol. 2019; 270:103259.
68. Garcia AJ 3rd, et al. Front Neuroscience. 2016; 10:4.
69. Chaplin DD. J Allergy Clin Immunol. 2010; 125(2 Suppl 2):S3–S23.
70. Ek M, et al. Nature. 2001; 410(6827):430–431.

71. Hermann GE, et al. Am J Physiol Regul Integr Comp Physiol. 2001; 280(1):R289–R299.
72. Roulston CL, et al. Neuroscience. 2005; 135(4):1241–1253.
73. Black RE, et al. Lancet. 2010; 375(9730):1969–1987.
74. Dammann O, et al. Ment Retard Dev Disabil Res Rev. 2002; 8(1):46–50.
75. Heep A, et al. Arch Dis Child Fetal Neonatal Ed. 2003; 88(6):F501–F504.
76. Moscuzza F, et al. Gynecol Endocrinol. 2011; 27(5):319–323.
77. Jantzie LL, et al. Brain Behav Immun. 2020; 84:45–58.
78. Noor S, et al. Front Immunol. 2018; 9:1107.
79. Peixoto TC, et al. Neuroscience. 2019; 418:69–81.
80. Bavis RW, et al. Exp Neurol. 2017 Jan; 287(Pt 2):176–191.
81. Ohtake PJ, et al. Am J Respir Crit Care Med. 2000; 162(3 Pt 1):1140–1147.
82. Liu Q, et al. J Appl Physiol. 2009; 106(4):1212–1222.
83. Liu Q, et al. J Appl Physiol. 2002; 92(3):923–934.
84. Liu Q, et al. J Appl Physiol. 2005; 98(4):1442–1457.
85. Liu Q, et al. Neuroscience. 2010; 165(1):61–78.
86. Wong-Riley MT, et al. Respir Physiol Neurobiol. 2005; 149(1-3):83–98.
87. Liu Q, et al. J Comp Neurol. 2010; 518(7):1082–1097.
88. Stryker C, et al. Am J Physiol Regul Integr Comp Physiol. 2018; 314(2):R216–R227.
89. Rourke KS, et al. Respir Physiol Neurobiol. 2016; 232:26–34.
90. Jensen F, et al. Brain Res Dev Brain Res. 1993; 73(1):99–105.
91. Mayer CA, et al. J Appl Physiol (1985). 2014; 116(5):514–521.
92. Mortola JP *Respiratory physiology of newborn mammals.* Baltimore, MD: Johns Hopkins University Press; 2001. 334 p.
93. Mitchell L, et al. Respir Physiol Neurobiol. 2020; 273:103318.
94. Serra A, et al. J Appl Physiol (1985). 2001; 91(3):1298–1306.
95. MacFarlane PM, et al. Respir Physiol Neurobiol. 2013; 185(1):170–176.
96. Donnelly DF, et al. J Appl Physiol (1985). 1990 Mar; 68(3):1048–1052.
97. Askie LM, et al. JAMA. 2018; 319(21):2190–2201.

HUMAN ADAPTATIONS TO HIGH ALTITUDE

Tatum Simonson

Contents

Introduction

Populations have resided in the Himalayas, Andean Altiplano, and Ethiopian highlands for hundreds of generations. Present-day highlanders on each continent exhibit a distinct composite of phenotypes, with similarities and differences noted in various physiological assessments, including but not limited to hematological parameters, ventilatory control, and birth weight. In addition to these physiological assessments, recent large-sale genomic efforts aim to understand how genetic factors contribute to such different responses despite comparable environmental stresses. Investigation into -omic-level signatures (e.g. epigenomics, transcriptomics, proteomics, and metabolomics) provides an additional layer of information regarding the genetic pathways involved in responses to hypoxia and promising insights into generational as well as short-term pathway responses to hypoxia.

The term adaptation, specifically in reference to highland populations, is distinct from more immediate changes that may occur in response to an environmental challenge over a relatively brief period of time (i.e. acclimatization). In highland populations, adaptations have occurred by means of increased survival and/or ability to reproduce (1, 2). Genome-wide scans of selection, which search for outlier adaptive patterns in the genome, are especially powerful given the strong selective pressure imposed by hypoxia over thousands of years and provide important clues to human adaptations to high altitude (1).

The thousands of years that populations have lived at altitude provide sufficient time for selection to occur and for the frequency of adaptive alleles to increase in the population. The Tibetan highlands have been occupied for 30,000 and possibly 40,000 years (3), more than double the amount of time populations have resided in the Andes (~12,000 to 14,000 years ago) (4) with notable European contribution to the gene pool nearly 500 years ago (5). While the history of various Ethiopian populations at high altitude involves migrations into and out of the highland regions throughout the past 70,000 years, more recent migrations are noted as recent as 500 years ago (6–9). The number of generations a population has spent at altitude is important to consider in studies of adaptation as distinct evolutionary histories, and ensuing phenotypes, have been uniquely shaped in each population.

Phenotypic differences among highland populations

One of the most extensively examined traits among highlanders is hemoglobin concentration, which varies markedly between Tibetan and Andean populations (10). Tibetans' relatively lower hemoglobin concentration at high altitude (comparable to values observed at sea level) is associated with greater exercise capacity (11) and reproductive success (12). Some Ethiopian populations also exhibit relatively lower hemoglobin concentrations at high altitude (13–15), although additional associations remain to be determined. Lower hemoglobin concentration in Tibetans has been attributed to a reduced erythropoietic response to hypoxemia. However, hemoglobin mass is elevated in Sherpa compared to lowlanders, and Sherpa has a larger plasma volume and comparable total blood volume at a lower hemoglobin concentration relative to Andeans, which may minimize high-viscosity-related damage of microcirculatory blood flow (16).

Increased hemoglobin-oxygen-binding affinity has been noted among various high-altitude species, and may provide benefit at altitude through an improved rate of oxygen equilibration across the alveolar-capillary barrier. While many studies provide varying conclusions among highland populations examined, recent studies in Andeans (17) and Tibetans (18) indicate that these populations exhibit a reduced P_{50} at high altitude.

Another hallmark difference between populations is in resting ventilation, which is higher in many Tibetans compared to Aymara Andeans as is the hypoxic ventilatory responses (HVR), which varies much more in Tibetans relative to minimal responses observed among Andeans (19). However, most studies report that arterial oxygen saturation is lowest among Himalayan highlanders, slightly higher in Andeans, and highest in Amhara Ethiopians (19, 20). Tibetan infants, relative to Han Chinese or Andean infants, have higher oxygen saturation, which is hypothesized to underlie susceptibility to high altitude pulmonary hypertension and chronic mountain sickness in Andeans (21). The potential for hypoxia's long-term effects are also noted among individuals with excessive erythrocytosis, who were more likely to have been born to mothers with hypertension and perinatal hypoxia (22).

DOI: 10.1201/9780367494018-4

Recent studies suggest that the effects of hypoxia during pregnancy are proportional to the hypoxia severity (23), and at altitudes greater than 2500 meters, birth weights generally decrease (24–28). Reproductive success and infant survival are crucial components of transgenerational adaptation in highlanders. Compared to individuals of lowland ancestry at high altitude, Tibetans and Andeans exhibit increased common iliac blood flow into uterine arteries and less intrauterine growth restriction during pregnancy with Tibetans tending to have less pre- and postnatal mortality (29–33). Birth weights are also higher among Tibetan and Andean babies (34). It appears that adverse reproductive effects are lessened among highlander groups who have resided at high altitude for many generations, suggesting a genetic basis for these differences (31).

The prevalence of chronic mountain sickness (CMS), characterized by excessive erythrocytosis, hypoxemia, and in some cases pulmonary hypertension and possible development of cor pulmonale and congestive heart failure, varies across populations resident more than 2500 m above sea level. While Tibetans appear to be at lower risk of developing CMS, it is more common in Andeans and noted in nearly 30% of men more than 60 years of age (34–35). Research in Ethiopian highlanders is limited. CMS is also noted among Han Chinese who have moved to high altitude (36) and residents of Leadville, CO, in the United States (37). Population differences in susceptibility to CMS may be attributed to genetic, epigenetic, and environmental factors.

Various reviews regarding physiological traits exhibited by highland populations are available and provide insight into remaining questions in this field (2, 14, 20, 38, 39). Integration of key phenotype information, longitudinal outcomes, and the genetic and molecular basis of adaptation within and across Tibetan, Andean, and Ethiopian populations will be necessary to address the complexities of human adaptation to altitude (Figure 4.1).

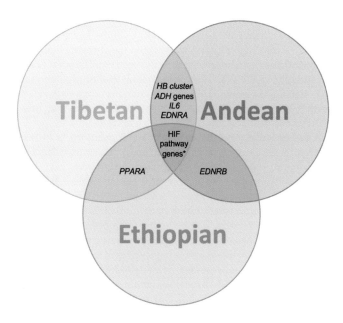

FIGURE 4.1 Genomic signatures of adaptation identified in more than one continental highland population. Gene names provided for findings reported in genomic studies of Tibetan, Andean, and Ethiopian populations. *HIF pathway genes include *EPAS1* in all three populations, *EGLN1* in Tibetans, and *BHLHE41* in Ethiopians.

Evidence for genetic adaptations to high altitude

Recent advances in genomics provide opportunities to examine thousands to millions of genetic markers at once, providing important information about adaptive genetic signatures in highland populations. Microarrays, which provide information about variable sites scattered throughout the entire genome, as well as exome and whole genome sequence analyses, which provide information about protein coding and both coding and noncoding sites, respectively, have been utilized over the past decade to pinpoint key genetic targets for high-altitude adaptation. In addition to these genomic tools, other -omics techniques (epigenomics, transcriptomics, metabolomics, proteomics) have become increasingly accessible and provide important complementary information to genomic and physiological data from these populations.

Genetic signatures of adaptation may be detected by examining patterns of variation within a collection of genomes from a population exposed to strong selective pressures. Many tests of selection search for outlier signals exhibiting reduced genetic diversity. This reduction in variation results from beneficial genetic variant(s), and surrounding linked genetic markers, increasing rapidly in the population over hundreds of generations as they provide an advantage for survival (20). Extreme or even subtle allele frequency differences in highland genomes relative to lowland populations may also be used to identify potentially adaptive genetic markers. These approaches, based on patterns in genomic regions or specific sites, may also be examined in combination; such a technique was recently applied to whole genome sequence data from Tibetans (40).

One of the key genetic pathways identified within regions exhibiting a signal of positive selection in multigenerational highland populations is the hypoxia-inducible factor (HIF) pathway. HIFs are transcription factors that bind to specific DNA sequences and regulate the expression of messenger RNA that encodes for hypoxia-response proteins. There are three isoforms of HIF with HIF-1α, HIF-2α, and HIF-3α subunits that form a heterodimer with a constitutively expressed HIF-β subunit. HIF-1α and HIF-2α have distinct patterns of expression with tissue- and temporal-specific effects (41, 42), although HIF-3α activity is not as well characterized. During conditions of normoxia, the α subunits are targeted for degradation via oxygen-dependent prolyl hydroxylase domain (PHD) proteins (PHD-1, PHD-2, PHD-3) and ubiquitination that occurs through interaction with the von Hippel-Lindau (VHL). HIFs play various roles in response to cellular hypoxia (43) that involve thousands of downstream genes involved in erythropoiesis, angiogenesis, metabolic pathways, vasomotor tone, cell proliferation, and survival (42). Most oxygen-dependent species utilize this important pathway.

Genomic studies of high-altitude populations provide important insight into key hypoxia-response genes as well as non-HIF-associated pathways important for long-term adaptation. Cross-population comparisons further highlight potential mechanisms of adaptation that underlie distinct physiological aspects of adaptation. While various genetic pathways and, in some cases, specific genes have been identified in more than one continental highland population, the precise putatively adaptive variants remain to be identified with the exception of only a few cases. Additional studies will be necessary to determine the functional relevance of adaptive signals reported thus far and determine whether the specific variants are associated with key phenotypes, as reported in many studies of Tibetan adaptation thus far (2, 20, 44).

Genetic adaptation in Tibetan highlanders

Some of the strongest evidence for adaptation in Tibetans is based on assessments of genotype-phenotype relationships between putatively adaptive markers and unique physiological traits exhibited by Tibetans. Using microarray analyses of nearly one million genetic markers, in 2010 Simonson et al. conducted within and across-population (comparing Han Chinese and Tibetan populations) tests of selection (45). The list of adaptive candidate genes identified in this analysis was compared to an *a priori* list of candidate genes based on known function in hypoxia-related pathways (45). Two HIF pathway genes, *EPAS1* which encodes HIF-2α, and *EGLN1* which encodes prolyl hydroxylase PHD2, were identified among the top ten genes reported, and adaptive copies of *EGLN1* and *PPARA* gene candidates were associated with relatively lower hemoglobin concentration. These genes were also associated with metabolic parameters in Tibetans (46), and *PPARA* was associated with metabolic alterations in skeletal muscle of Sherpa (47, 48). The top candidate gene *HMOX2* reported by Simonson et al. (45) was also associated with hemoglobin concentration in an analysis of data from 1250 Tibetan men (49).

Based on analysis of exome sequence data from 50 Tibetans, Yi et al. in 2010 identified variants in the *EPAS1* gene that were highly differentiated between Tibetans and Han Chinese (50). A single variant, which differed by 78% frequency between the two populations, was associated with hemoglobin concentration in Tibetans. Many of the same genes (e.g. *EPAS1*, *EGLN1*, the hemoglobin gene cluster, *PKLR*, and *HFE*) were reported by both Simonson et al. (45) and Yi et al. (50), despite the use of different techniques (20).

In an effort to identify major differences in allele frequencies between Han Chinese and Tibetans, Beall et al. analyzed data from approximately 500,000 SNPs and found eight variants close to the *EPAS1* gene that were highly differentiated and further associated with hemoglobin concentration in Tibetans (51). The findings of these three studies, which were the first to provide phenotypic associations with adaptive genetic factors in Tibetans, were replicated in numerous subsequent analyses (2, 20, 39). Given that HIFs regulate hundreds to thousands of genes and pathways, these findings provide a glimpse into the complexity of genetic adaptation to high altitude. In addition, hundreds of distinct putatively adaptive genes have been identified across studies, including HIF and non-HIF pathway genes. Efforts to systematically investigate the overlap of these signatures across studies will provide important insight for prioritization in future studies.

Each highland population's evolutionary history, which impacts present-day physiology, is distinct, and recent findings based on comparisons of Tibetan and archaic genomes illustrate this important point. Increased technological advancements have provided opportunity to sequence ancient DNA samples from populations no longer living, including Neanderthals and Denisovans who were contemporaries of modern humans until tens of thousands of years ago. Genetic material from these populations is, however, still present in the genomes of extant modern humans. Genetic variants in the *EPAS1* gene region in Tibetans, noted as one of the strongest adaptive signatures in Tibetans, is most similar to Denisovan DNA compared to DNA of other human populations (40, 52). Therefore, archaic genetic admixture provided variation that helped Tibetans to adapt to the high-altitude environment. This finding highlights the importance of understanding distinct population histories, and unique genetic backgrounds, in studies of genetic adaptation to high altitude.

Genetic adaptation in Andean highlanders

While fewer genomic studies have been completed in Andeans relatives Tibetans, various high-altitude candidate genes in this population have been identified and, in few cases, replicated in independent studies. The first genome-wide analysis was based on nearly a half million SNPs examined in Aymara and Quechua Andeans (53), which was followed by subsequent analysis comparing Andean and Tibetan populations that concluded genomic adaptation was dissimilar, although an exception was noted at the *EGLN1* gene that appeared to have different haplotype structure in Andeans and Tibetans (54). Sequence analysis of this region revealed that while both Andeans and Tibetans exhibit an adaptive signal at this locus, the putatively adaptive variants identified in Tibetans were absent or found at low frequency in Andeans (55). Among the genes originally identified by Bigham et al., *EDNRA* (endothelin receptor type A) and *PRKAA1* (protein kinase AMP-activated catalytic subunit alpha 1) were found to be associated with birthweight, and *PRKAA1* with metabolic homeostasis (56).

Additional analyses suggest genes related to cardiac function have been important for adaptive processes in Andeans. Genes identified in larger genome-wide SNP analyses identified *VEGFB*, which encodes vascular endothelial growth factor B and *ELTD1*, the adhesion G protein-coupled receptor L4 (57). Low-coverage whole genome sequencing revealed signals of positive selection at *BRINP3* (BMP/retinoic acid inducible neural specific 3), *NOS2* (nitric oxide synthase 2), and *TBX5* (T-box transcription factor 5) loci (58). Another whole genome sequence analysis, based on 10 individuals with and 10 without CMS, identified *SENP1* (SUMO specific peptidase 1) and *ANP32D* (acidic nuclear phosphoprotein 32 family member D) as top targets for adaptation (59). Decreased levels of these genes were detected in Andeans without CMS and decreased expression in a *Drosophila* genetic model was associated with greater survival under conditions of hypoxia (59). Additional studies based on SNP microarray analysis indicate *FAM213A* (peroxiredoxin like 2A) and *SFTPD* (surfactant protein D) are also strong targets of selection in Andeans (60). Whole genome sequence analysis based on highland Argentinians and lowland Native Americans also revealed an adaptive signature at the *EPAS1* locus previously identified as a top candidate gene in Tibetans, and *GPR126* (adhesion G protein-coupled receptor G6). Several additional genes reported in these studies have since been reported as adaptive in other Andean populations or identified in Tibetans (e.g., the B hemoglobin locus and *EDNRA*) (20), as well as *IL6* (interleukin 6), *ALDH2* (aldehyde dehydrogenase 2 family member), and alcohol dehydrogenase genes, among others, including *EPAS1* (61).

Genetic adaptation in Ethiopian highland populations

Fewer physiological and genomic studies have been completed in highland Ethiopian populations. Populations have resided in the Ethiopian highlands for more than 70,000 years (6), although people likely moved in and out of high-altitude areas, with a permanent settlement (at 4200 m) recently dated to 31,000–47,000 years ago (62). While the genomic findings thus far suggest involvement of the HIF pathway in Ethiopian adaptation (63), which is similar to various reports in Tibetans and Andeans, other distinct adaptive pathways have been reported (2, 8, 20).

Some of the putatively adapted gene regions identified in Ethiopians are associated with hemoglobin concentration. For example, *THRB* (thyroid hormone receptor beta) and the gene regions of *PPARA* and *EPAS1* are reported as adaptive targets of selection and/or associated with hemoglobin concentration (45, 50, 51) in Tibetans, are also associated with this phenotype in Amhara Ethiopians (8). Another HIF pathway gene *BHLHE41* (basic helix-loop-helix family member E41) is also a top selection candidate identified across three Ethiopian populations (Amhara, Oromo, and Tigray Ethiopians) (9).

Other genes not associated with phenotypes but previously identified in other highland population include *EDNRB* (endothelial receptor B) identified in Amhara Ethiopians as well as in Andeans (54), while *EDNRA*, within the same gene family, is also a selection candidate gene in Tibetans (45). In a mouse model, decreased expression of *EDNRB* is associated with hypoxia tolerance (64).

Others non-hypoxia-associated genes identified thus far in Amhara Ethiopians include *VAV3* (vav guanine nucleotide exchange factor 3) and *RORA* (RAR-related orphan receptor A) (8). Adaptive targets of a regions in chromosome 19 in Oromo and Simen Ethiopians include *CIC* (capicua transcriptional repressor), *LIPE* (lipase E hormone-sensitive type), and *PAFAH1B3* (platelet-activating factor acetylhydrolase 1b catalytic subunit 2), and appear to afford tolerance to hypoxia in a *Drosophila* model (64).

Cross-population and cross-species insights into adaptive genetic factors

Many studies of genetic adaptation in humans have converged on HIF pathway genes as top candidates of selection. In many cases, it appears that key distinct pathway genes, and in some cases, the same genes may underlie adaptation. Various studies have searched the genomes of other high-altitude species and identified overlapping targets of selection related to various conditions of environmental hypoxia (65). Although there is major overlap in genetic pathways highlighted thus far (i.e. the hemoglobin gene cluster, associated with blood-oxygen affinity, HIF pathway genes such as *EPAS1* and *EGLN1*), different variants with putatively distinct functions are most commonly reported as targets of selection (65).

The genes mentioned in this chapter by no means provide a comprehensive list of candidates to compare, as many studies based on human genomic data thus far highlight only prioritized sets within regions of the genome exhibiting an adaptative signal and/or report hundreds of genes or subsets of the genes that meet criteria established by the authors of the study. In addition, various analytical approaches may be employed across studies, sampling strategies may vary, and adaptive signals may be detected or not based on individual or population histories within a region. Efforts to more fully capture genomic information across geographical regions and to perform standardize analyses will provide greater insight into individual variation needed to fully appreciate unique and shared signatures of adaptation in humans.

Functional insights into genetic adaptation

While thousands of high-altitude selection candidate genes and gene regions have been reported, the functional variant(s) underlying adaptation largely remain to be determined. Some progress has been made for the *EGLN1* gene, which encodes PHD2, a top target of selection in Tibetans. One variant in the first exon

(Asp4Glu, Cys127Ser) exhibits a gain of function (a lower Km for oxygen) and is associated with increased HIF degradation in hypoxia and potential erythroid progenitor proliferation disruption (66). Additional reports suggest a loss-of-function role via defective binding of co-chaperone p23 and increased HIF activity (67, 68). In addition to this protein-coding change, variation within the first intron of *EGLN1* was associated with increased expression and high-altitude pulmonary edema (HAPE) in a population from India (69).

Increased availability of whole genome sequence data indicate that regions of the genome with heterochromatic marks, DNA methylations sites, and non-coding variants are crucial for adaptation [e.g. in Andeans (59) and Tibetans (40)]. Genetic factors that influence patterns of gene expression provide mechanisms for variation across tissues and/or stages of development in contrast to variants that impact protein function, resulting in uniform alterations across all cells. These fine-tuned, context-specific changes could underlie important molecular mechanisms of adaptation including key changes in hypoxia-related or hypoxia-independent pathways.

In addition to progress regarding whole genome sequence analysis, insights have been more recently obtained using complementary -omics strategies, such as transcriptomics, epigenomics, metabolomics, and proteomics. Given various -omics factors may be impacted by environmental cues, this is an important and active area of study. For example, variation in DNA methylation may impact gene expression, although limited data are currently available for populations resident at high altitude. A study of saliva samples from Oromo Ethiopians at high and low altitudes showed distinct patterns of CpG methylation at four sites (7). Based on a limited study of Andeans with and without excessive erythrocytosis, differential methylation was identified within the *EGLN1*gene (70, 71). A more recent study showed that the number of years spent living at high altitude was associated with decreased DNA methylation at the promoter region of *EPAS1*, and higher levels at *LINE-1* that also correlated with altitude at birth, based on epigenetic analyses of Quechua individuals living at high versus low altitude in Peru (72).

Additional genomic and -omics studies that integrate information with physiological findings and functional analyses of precise variants will provide greater insight into the adaptive landscape of highland populations. Candidate variants, prioritized based on identification as targets of positive selection and, in some cases, phenotype associations, may be evaluated through gene-editing techniques in various cell lines and under varying physiological conditions (73). Such studies may yield important insight into causality and further understanding of ancestry-specific responses to hypoxia relevant in the contexts of health and disease.

References

1. Simonson TS. High Alt Med Biol. 2015; 16(2):125–137.
2. Moore LG. J Appl Physiol. 2017; 123:1371–1385.
3. Zhang XL, et.al. Science. 2018; 362(6418):1049–1051.
4. Rademaker K, et.al. Science. 2014; 346(6208):466–469.
5. Cook ND. *Born to die: disease and New World conquest, 1492-1650*. Cambridge, NY: Cambridge University Press; 1998. p. 268.
6. Hassen M. *The Oromo of Ethiopia: a history, 1570–1860*. Trenton, NJ: Red Sea Press; 1990.
7. Alkorta-Aranburu G, et al. PLoS Genet. 2012; 8:e1003110.
8. Scheinfeldt LB, et.al. Genome Biol. 2012; 13:R1.
9. Huerta-Sánchez E, et.al. Mol Biol Evol. 2013; 30:1877–1888.
10. Beall CM. Proc Natl Acad Sci USA. 2007; 104:8655–8660.
11. Simonson TS, et al. J Physiol. 2015; 593:3207–3218.
12. Jeong C, et al. Nat Commun. 2014; 5:3281.

13. Beall CM, et al. Proc Natl Acad Sci USA. 2002; 99:17215–17218.
14. Beall CM. Integr Comp Biol. 2006; 46:18–24.
15. Cheong HI, et al. Am J Physiol Lung Cell Mol Physiol. 2017; 312:L172–L177.
16. Stembridge M, et al. Proc Natl Acad Sci USA. 2019; 116:16177–16179.
17. Balaban DY, et al. Respir Physiol Neurobiol. 2013; 186:45–52.
18. Simonson TS, et al. Exp Physiol. 2014; 99:1624–1635.
19. Beall CM. Hum Biol. 2000; 72:201–228.
20. Simonson TS. High Alt Med Biol. 2015b; 16:125–137.
21. Niermeyer S, et al. Pulm Circ. 2015; 5:48–62.
22. Julian CG, et al. Am J Physiol Heart Circ Physiol. 2015; 309:H565–H573.
23. Jang EA, et al. Front Physiol. 2015; 6:176.
24. Jensen GM, et al. Am J Public Health. 1997; 87:1003–1007.
25. Krampl E, et al. Ultrasound Obstet Gynecol. 2000; 16:9–18.
26. Giussani DA, et al. J Dev Orig Health Dis. 2013; 4:328–337.
27. Giussani DA, et al. Pediatr Res. 2001; 49:490–494.
28. Levine LD, et al. Am J Obstet Gynecol. 2015; 212:210 e211–218.
29. Zamudio S, et al. Am J Phys Anthropol. 1993; 91:215–224.
30. Moore LG, et al. Am J Phys Anthropol. 1998; Suppl 27:25–64.
31. Moore LG. High Alt Med Biol. 2001; 2:257.–279.
32. Moore LG, et al. Am J Hum Biol. 2001; 13:635–644.
33. Tripathy V, et al. Am J Hum Biol. 2005; 17:442–450.
34. Monge C, et al. N Engl J Med. 1989; 321(18):1271.
35. Villafuerte FC, et al. High Alt Med Biol. 2016; 17:61–69.
36. Jiang C, et al. BMC Public Health. 2014; 14:701.
37. Asmus IV. In: *Health and behavioral sciences*. Denver, CO: University of Colorado; 2002.
38. Gilbert-Kawai ET, et al. Physiology. 2014; 29:388–402.
39. Bhandari S, et al. Front Physiol. 2019; 10:1116.
40. Hu H, et al. PLoS Genet. 2017; 13:e1006675.
41. Hu CJ, et al. Mol Cell Biol. 2003; 23:9361–9374.
42. Semenza GL. Ann Rev Genomics Hum Genet. 2020; 21:183–204.
43. Samanta D, et al. Wiley Interdiscip Rev Syst Biol Med. 2017; 9(4):10.1002/wsbm.1382.
44. Azad P, et al. J Mol Med (Berl). 2017; 95:1269–1282.
45. Simonson TS, et al. Science. 2010; 329:72–75.
46. Ge R-L, et al. Mol Genet Metab. 2012; 106:244–247.
47. Horscroft JA, et al. Proc Natl Acad Sci USA. 2017; 114(24):6382–6387.
48. O'Brien KA, et al. Curr Opin Endocr Metab Res. 2019; 11:33–41.
49. Yang D, et al. Hum Mutat. 2016; 37:216–223.
50. Yi X, et al. Science. 2010; 329:75–78.
51. Beall CM, et al. Proc Natl Acad Sci USA. 2010; 107:11459–11464.
52. Huerta-Sánchez E, et al. Nature. 2014; 512:194–197.
53. Bigham AW, et al. Hum Genomics. 2009; 4:79–90.
54. Bigham A, et al. PLoS Genet. 2010; 6:e1001116.
55. Heinrich EC, et al. Ann Hum Genet. 2019; 83:171–176.
56. Bigham AW, et al. Physiol Genomics. 2014; 46:687–697.
57. Eichstaedt CA, et al. PloS one. 2014; 9(3):e93314
58. Crawford JE, et al. Am J Hum Genet. 2017; 101:752–767.
59. Zhou D, et al. Am J Hum Genet. 2013; 93:452–462.
60. Valverde G, et al. PLoS One. 2015; 10(5):e0125444
61. Foll M, et al. Am J Hum Genet. 2014; 95:394–407.
62. Ossendorf G, et al. Science. 2019; 365:583–587.
63. Bigham AW, et al. Genes Dev. 2014; 28:2189–2204.
64. Udpa N, et al. Genome Biol. 2014; 15:R36.
65. Pamenter ME, et al. Front Genet. 2020; 11:743.
66. Lorenzo FR, et al. Nat Genet. 2014; 46:951–956.
67. Song D, et al. J Biol Chem. 2014; 289:14656–14665.
68. Song D, et al. Proc Natl Acad Sci USA. 2020; 117:12230–12238.
69. Aggarwal S, et al. Proc Natl Acad Sci. 2010; 107:18961–18966.
70. Julian CG. J Appl Physiol. 2017; 123:1362–1370.
71. Julian CG. Front Physiol. 2019; 10:1397.
72. Childebayeva A, et al. Epigenetics. 2019; 14:1–15.
73. Hall JE, et al. Front Genet. 2020; 11:471.

FETAL LLAMA ADAPTATION TO ALTITUDE IN THE ANDEAN ALTIPLANO

Aníbal J. Llanos, Germán Ebensperger, Emilio A. Herrera,
Roberto V. Reyes and María Serón-Ferré

Contents

Introduction

Aquí la hebra dorada salió de la vicuña
a vestir los amores, los túmulos, las madres,
el rey, las oraciones, los guerreros

(The fleece of the vicuña was carded here
to clothe men's love in gold, their tombs and mothers,
the king, the prayers, the warriors)

"The Heights of Macchu Picchu," Pablo Neruda
(translated by Nathaniel Tarn)

High on the Andes, the whole Altiplano is immersed in thin atmospheric air, but despite of the latter, it sustains a good number of animals, including the llama (*Lama glama*), a member of the Camelidae family, presently residing over 4000 m above sea level. The llama's journey began about 2 million years ago, as the llama North American ancestor climbed and dived onto the Andes' atmospheric ocean of the *Alto Andino* (1). Between 7000 and 6000 years ago, the llama and the alpaca became domesticated by the Amerindians in today's Peruvian Andes (2), the guanaco being the ancestor of the llama and the vicuña of the alpaca (3).

The adult llama

The adult llama displays important physiological adaptations permitting it to thrive at altitudes over 4000 m. Some traits may be the expression of genetic changes since they persist after many generations of residing at lowlands. Among them are a low P50 (4, 5), small elliptical red cells with a slight increase in blood hemoglobin content (6, 7), and decreased expression of the carbonic anhydrase II isozyme (CA II) (8), permitting better O_2 extraction by the tissues (9). More recently, it has been found that alpacas hold an archaic helix-loop-helix deletion in the HIF-1 alpha protein, which could be reducing the hypoxic responses at high altitudes (10), since HIFs could produce maladaptation to chronic hypoxia, inducing polycythemia and pulmonary arterial hypertension (11). In this regard, a notable physiological attribute of the highland llama is an arterial pulmonary pressure like lowland llamas, without remodeling of pulmonary vessels (12), and a lesser pulmonary pressure increase to acute hypoxia than sheep at low altitude (13). Conversely, the high muscle myoglobin concentration and lactic dehydrogenase activity present in highland llamas

disappear at lowland, indicating that they were acclimatization instead of adaptation (14).

The fetal llama

Species survival requires the ability to produce kin. To describe fetal oxygenation in the womb, Professor Joseph Barcroft coined his famous phrase summarized as *Everest in utero* (15, 16). At lowland, the umbilical vein has the highest fetal PO_2 (30 mmHg), two-thirds lower than the maternal aortic PO_2. Barcroft's metaphor is apt, as years later, at the summit of Mount Everest, at 8848 m of altitude, Christopher Pizzo's alveolar gas PO_2 was 28 mmHg (17). Nonetheless, the natural habitat of the maternal and fetal llama is 4000 m. We measured PO_2 in fetal and maternal llamas at 4400 m above sea level, and the values dropped from 21 mmHg at sea level to 15 mmHg at 4400 m (18), while in the maternal llama, PO_2 went from 98 to 44 mmHg at 4400 m (Llanos, unpublished data). Consequently, in Andean pregnancies, we were witnessing hypoxia inside hypoxia, exceeding Professor Barcroft's description.

In this chapter, we describe three rather unknown features, paramount in determining the ability of the fetal and neonatal llamas to thrive in the high-altitude plateau. First, the fetal llama has an augmented function of the α-adrenergic receptors to sustain cardiovascular function. Second, the fetal llama has mechanisms that allow the brain to withstand hypoxia. Third, the neonatal llama lung has increased production of carbon monoxide (CO), a mechanism preventing neonatal pulmonary high-altitude arterial hypertension. A brief description of these notable changes gives a glimpse of how the fetal and neonatal llama cope with the high-altitude hypoxia of the *Alto Andino*.

The fetal llama cardiovascular system and adrenergic mechanisms

We assessed fetal cardiovascular function in our model of a chronically catheterized fetal llama at Santiago (580 m) (19), by comparing values with fetal sheep at similar gestational ages. The fetal and neonatal sheep are the "gold standard," since most of the perinatal research with results translated to humans took place in this species. Our comparative studies detected differences between fetal llama and fetal sheep, already in a situation of normoxia, at which PO_2 levels were rather similar in both species. Nevertheless, the fetal llama systemic arterial pressure,

DOI: 10.1201/9780367494018-5

cardiac output, and organ blood flows were lower than in fetal sheep, together with a higher total vascular resistance pointing to important differences between both species (19–21).

These differences are further highlighted when fetal llamas are exposed to an episode of acute hypoxia, as described here. We studied the fetal llama cardiovascular responses to acute hypoxia extensively (18, 20, 22–26). Our results showed that in fetal llama at 0.6- to 0.7-gestation, at lowland, acute hypoxia elicited a rise in mean arterial pressure, a short-lived bradycardia (23), and a redistribution of blood flow towards to heart and adrenals glands, but oddly not to the brain (22, 25). The latter is a feature not observed in the fetal sheep or in any other mammalian species exposed to acute hypoxia. Another notable finding was the considerable peripheral vasoconstriction produced by hypoxia, exemplified by a femoral resistance almost fivefold greater than that of fetal sheep at the same gestational age (23, 27, 28).

The mechanisms mediating the fetal cardiovascular responses to acute hypoxia involve neural (chemoreflex), endocrine, and vasoactive local molecules, such as NO, CO, endothelin, and others (28). A potent carotid chemoreflex mediates cardiovascular responses to hypoxia in the fetal sheep. Surprisingly, and in marked contrast to the fetal sheep, we found that the chemoreflex plays a minor role in the fetal llama. Bilateral carotid body denervation did not change the substantial femoral vascular vasoconstriction induced by hypoxia (23). However, the chemoreflex may trigger other mechanisms, such as fetal llama adrenocortical responses to hypoxia, since carotid body denervation abolished cortisol increase, despite maintaining plasma ACTH (29). In contrast, the rise in plasma cortisol ensued, but more slowly than controls in fetal sheep (23). Therefore, in the fetal llama, the neural input is a principal regulator for the adrenal cortex.

Given the limited cardiovascular effect of the chemoreflex, we next addressed the role of endocrine and local mechanisms in regulating peripheral vascular response to hypoxia in the fetal llama (23, 30).

The fetal llama has a greater basal concentration of plasma catecholamines than the fetal sheep, revealing an important basal sympathetic tone (31, 32). Hypoxia induced a norepinephrine (NE) surge that was more important than that of epinephrine (E) (32), associated with increases of neuropeptide Y (NPY) and vasopressin, but no changes in angiotensin II (18). Neuropeptide Y is colocalized and cosecreted with catecholamines (33). Further, fetal sheep treated with exogenous NPY mimic the vasoconstriction produced by hypoxia. Due to this notable vasoconstriction effect and the high NPY levels attained in fetal llama hypoxia, NPY could be participating in the potent vasoconstriction observed in the fetal llama (34).

To dissect the role of some hormones and local factors in the intense vasoconstriction experienced in hypoxia by the fetal llama, we administered the respective endothelin (ET), arginine vasopressin (AVP), and alpha-adrenergic receptors antagonists.

Endothelin-1 acts through its receptors ETA and ETB located in the vascular smooth muscle. ET-1 contributed to the augment of peripheral resistance in the fetal llama under acute hypoxia, since the infusion of an ETA receptor blocker, BQ123, precluded the rise of femoral vascular resistance without modifying the basal femoral tone (26). In contrast, when vasopressin V1 receptor antagonist was administered in normoxia, it decreased fetal femoral vascular resistance, increasing the blood flow, but did not alter cardiovascular variables during acute hypoxia (24, 35). Additionally, vasopressin could also act on the renal V2 receptor,

reabsorbing a great deal of water, explaining the high osmolality found in the fetal llama urine (36).

Administration of phentolamine (alpha-1- and alpha-2-adrenergic receptor antagonist) during normoxia had major effects, eliciting systemic hypotension and tachycardia, with a reduction in vascular resistance, and rising blood flow in carotid and femoral territories. Furthermore, it elicited dramatic effects when the fetal llamas were submitted to acute hypoxia, inducing a rapid and pronounced systemic hypotension, paralleled with marked bradycardia plus deterioration of all the measured cardiovascular variables, that led all six fetuses to cardiovascular collapse and death. The continent (the vessels' territory) was greater than the content (the blood), producing the collapse. To identify which of the two alpha-adrenergic receptors brought this dramatic result, we repeated the experiments using the more specific alpha-1-adrenergic receptor antagonist, prazosin, finding a similar outcome. In contrast, administration of yohimbine, an alpha-2-adrenergic receptor antagonist, showed no cardiovascular effects either in normoxia or in hypoxia (26). Therefore, the alpha-1-adrenergic receptor function appears to be the fundamental mediator in the vasoconstrictor response to hypoxia in the fetal llama. This outcome was in marked contrast to what is observed in the fetal sheep with hypoxia, in which alpha-adrenergic receptor blockade also abolished femoral vasoconstriction; and only when hypoxia was accompanied with carotid sinus nerve section the fetal sheep did not survive (27). Thus, in lowland species such as sheep, two mechanisms are important for fetal survival during acute hypoxia: alpha-adrenergic function and carotid chemoreflexes. For fetal llamas, only alpha-1-adrenergic mechanisms are fundamental to cope with acute hypoxia.

The importance of the fetal alpha-1-adrenergic mechanisms during chronic hypoxia is further highlighted in fetal sheep made chronically hypoxic by placental embolization (37), and in chronically hypoxic fetal sheep at 3600 m (Llanos, unpublished data). In both situations, administration of phentolamine during a superimposed episode of acute hypoxia produced cardiovascular collapse and death, as in the fetal llama.

Thus, fetal chronic hypoxia in lowland species, or evolutionary chronic hypoxia in highland species at near sea level, amplifies the contribution of the alpha-adrenergic system in the defense against episodes of acute hypoxia.

These findings are critical on clinical grounds, since administration of alpha-adrenergic blockers to pregnant mothers, either at high altitudes where more than 140 million people live (38) or in pregnancies complicated with chronic fetal hypoxia at lowlands, would block in the fetus, the meaningful alpha-adrenergic compensation during chronic hypoxia leads to a poor outcome.

The intensity of the peripheral vasoconstriction in the hypoxic fetal llama has a robust counterpart of vasodilators at the vascular level. Indeed, local endothelial NO production has a vital role in maintaining basal blood flow literally in all local circulations (cerebral, carotid, heart, adrenal and femoral vascular beds) in normoxia, and it lessens the robust vasoconstrictor influence on these beds during acute hypoxia as demonstrated by L-NAME blockade of NO synthesis (26, 39).

These results show an essential role of NO signaling in the preservation of a dilator tone in the cerebral and femoral circulations, lessening the strong vasoconstrictor influences upon these territories during acute hypoxia in the fetal llama. Additionally, these experiments show that NO plays a central role in augmenting the heart blood flow in acute hypoxia in this species (26, 39). Furthermore in hypoxia, L-NAME did not affect the rise in fetal plasma ACTH but precluded the increments in adrenal blood flow and cortisol and adrenaline concentrations in the fetal llama. In contrast, L-NAME further augmented the fetal plasma noradrenaline. All these data support a regulatory role of NO on adrenal blood flow and function in the fetal llama (32).

The pronounced intensity of the peripheral vasoconstriction response to cope with acute hypoxia in the fetal llama opens an important question about its adaptive function(s). Certainly, we do not have the answers, but we can speculate. First, reducing the blood flow and O_2 supply to several organs and reducing the O_2 consumption and temperature could induce a hypometabolic adaptation of these organs. Second, it permits redirection of the blood flow and O_2 supply toward the vital organs, in this case, heart and adrenal glands. The brain blood flow did not increase with hypoxia but showed certain degree of hypometabolism, as we will discuss later. Third, reducing the blood flow and O_2 supply to several organs may trigger the release of molecules that may produce ischemic preconditioning in the brain, heart, adrenals, in the tributary organ of the constricted artery, or in the whole body (40). In this regard, alpha-1-adrenergic receptors are involved in adult heart preconditioning and may do so in fetal llama heart as well in other organs (41).

Hypoxia tolerance and the llama brain

An outstanding difference between fetal llama and sheep responses to hypoxia resides in the brain. During an episode of acute hypoxia in the fetal sheep at 0.85 gestation, cerebral vascular resistance decreases, enhancing blood flow threefold to all regions of the brain. This preserves brain oxygen supply and maintains oxygen consumption until ascending aortic blood oxygen content fall to approximately 2.2 ml/dl. Below this threshold, the brain oxygen consumption begins to fall (21, 42–44).

In the fetal llama, the response was utterly different. Acute hypoxia in the fetal llama neither changes cerebral vascular resistance nor cerebral blood flow (20, 22, 23, 25). As carotid vascular resistance and carotid blood flow remain unaltered (23, 24), the cerebral oxygen delivery was reduced (23), whereas cerebral oxygen extraction was maintained, reducing cerebral oxygen consumption in the acutely hypoxic fetal llama. In marked contrast with the sheep, the electrocorticogram flattened under this episode of acute hypoxia, but seizure activity did not take place (25). Analyzing the data more in detail, the total brain, cerebellum, and pons did not modify the vascular resistance or blood flow, while the medulla had a reduction in vascular resistance and a rise in blood flow during acute hypoxia in the fetal llama (25). The preferential redistribution of blood flow within the fetal llama brain to the medulla suggests that this area is important in cardiovascular control during hypoxia in this species.

A fundamental question is which are the mechanisms used by the fetal llama to prevent the hypoxic neural injury? As mentioned, the electrocorticogram flattened under the episode of acute hypoxia, but seizure activity did not take place (25). This result suggested the absence of hypoxic damage by an adaptive brain hypometabolism. We look for further evidence by submitting the fetal llama to an extended episode of hypoxia, lasting 24 hours, determining brain temperature, Na^+ channel density, and Na-K-ATPase activity. Furthermore, we looked at the poly ADP-ribose polymerase (PARP) protein degradation, as an index of cell death in the brain cortex. We found a fall of 0.56°C in the brain cortex temperature, along with a 51% decrease in Na-K-ATPase activity and a 44% drop in protein level of NaV1.1, a voltage-gated sodium channel. Additionally, there was a little production of

lactate by the fetal llama brain and absence of PARP protein degradation. All these findings support the hypothesis that the fetal llama responded with brain hypometabolism to cope with an episode of prolonged hypoxia (45). The hypometabolic responses and hypoxia tolerance have been described in a wide range of species that, for limitation of space, are not possible to describe.

The strategy of hypoxic hypometabolism found in the fetal llama brain is an effective adaptation to dwell amidst the thin air milieu of the *Alto Andino*. Whether this is present in other fetal tissues needs to be investigated.

The newborn llama pulmonary circulation

To emerge from the womb "into this breathing world" (Shakespeare, Richard the Third) is one of the most dramatic events in the life of the individual, since the neonate in barely 2–3 minutes establishes its complete pulmonary function, including the pulmonary circulation. The latter strikingly changes from constricted fetal pulmonary to neonatal dilated vessels accommodating ten times more blood flow than before (46). A necessary condition is a rapid fall of pulmonary vascular resistance, and failure to do so results in pulmonary hypertension in the newborn. In the Altiplano, the llama neonate rapidly establishes an efficient pulmonary circulation without pulmonary hypertension, in contrast, the neonatal lambs end with different degrees of hypoxic pulmonary hypertension (47).

Neonatal llama systemic circulation maintains some features already present *in utero*, like a femoral vasoconstriction 3.6 times greater than in newborn sheep, in response to acute hypoxia at low altitude. This is mediated by an enhanced peripheral vasoconstrictor sensitivity to norepinephrine and femoral vascular bed expression of alpha-1B-adrenergic instead of alpha-1A- adrenergic receptor. The latter, less sensitive to adrenergic agonists, is more abundant in the femoral circulation of the newborn sheep (48). Thus, the fetal and newborn llama alpha-adrenergic tone may be paramount to withstand the harsh life at the Andean plateau.

Regarding the pulmonary circulation, the increase of mean arterial pulmonary pressure (mPAP) in newborn llamas has a biphasic shape during acute hypoxia, suggesting changes in vasoconstrictors and vasodilators functions along the course of hypoxia. The newborn llama at high altitude have a lower rise in mPAP than newborn llama at lowlands, suggesting increased vasodilator mechanisms in the former. In contrast, the high-altitude newborn sheep, already with a higher basal mPAP, augmented mPAP further than low-altitude newborn sheep and did not have the biphasic response observed in the newborn llama (49, 50).

At least two mechanisms determine the lack of pulmonary artery hypertension and pulmonary vascular remodeling in highland newborn llama. One of them is the hemoxygenase-carbon monoxide pathway (HO−CO). Hemoxygenases 1 and 2 (HO1 and HO2), found in vessels, degrade the heme group producing equimolar amounts of CO, Fe^{2+}, and biliverdin. Fe^{2+} rapidly combines with ferritin, while biliverdin generates bilirubin. Importantly, CO has vasodilator, anti-inflammatory and antiproliferative properties, whereas biliverdin, bilirubin, and ferritin have antioxidant properties (30). Chronically administered inhaled CO reduces pulmonary hypertension in rodents submitted to chronic hypoxia, while CO administered acutely diminishes pulmonary resistance in hypoxic adult sheep (13, 51). CO induces vasodilatation through activation of sGC and BK_{Ca} potassium channels, increasing the smooth muscle cGMP and hyperpolarizing the cell membrane, respectively. Additionally, it decreases smooth muscle proliferation (52). High-altitude newborn llamas have augmented

HO1 and HO2 protein expression and a pulmonary CO production almost sevenfold higher than high-altitude newborn sheep (30, 52, 53). Altogether, these data indicate that HO−CO signaling is a crucial player in preventing the occurrence of pulmonary hypertension in the newborn llama at the *Alto Andino*.

The second mechanism regulating pulmonary vasodilation is nitric oxide (NO). We studied the role of NO in mPAP regulation in lowland and highland newborn llama and newborn sheep, basally and under an episode of acute hypoxia, by blocking NO synthesis with L-NAME. These experiments showed that basally the NO role is limited in lowland and highland newborn llamas. However, it is important in both during acute hypoxia. In contrast, in newborn sheep, NO plays an important basal role in maintaining mPAP in pulmonary normotensive lowland and pulmonary hypertensive highland sheep. In the latter, NO is maximally stimulated, as mPAP does not increase further with an acute hypoxia challenge. Thus, NO does not suffice for compensating the pulmonary hypertension suffered by newborn sheep in the *Andean* plateau (49, 50). Basal NOS activity, eNOS, and soluble guanylyl cyclase (sGC) protein expression in lung tissue were consistent with L-NAME findings. As expected, eNOS activity and protein were much higher in lowland and highland newborn sheep than in newborn llama (53).

However, differences between newborn sheep and newborn llama were found for other proteins. The highland newborn llama lung has a lower expression of the vasoconstrictor Rho-associated kinase 2 (ROCK 2) and phospho-serine19 myosin light chain than lowland newborn llama, thus favoring vasodilation in the pulmonary circulation at high altitude (49). Finally, highland and lowland newborn llama had an exceptionally low asymmetric dimethylarginine (ADMA) and homocysteine plasma concentrations, and a low arginase type II activity in lung parenchyma. ADMA and homocysteine are inhibitors of NOS while arginase hydrolyzes arginine is the main substrate for NO production. In contrast, both groups of newborn sheep had significantly higher plasma concentrations of ADMA and homocysteine, and ten times more lung arginase II activity than newborn llamas (54). Plasma ADMA and homocysteine increase in adult pulmonary hypertension (55). Thus, modest arginase activity and low concentrations of ADMA and homocysteine in the newborn llama constitute new and interesting mechanisms of pulmonary adaptation to deal with chronic hypoxia.

After finishing to describe and discuss these notable traits found in the fetal and neonatal llamas, we just adapted a phrase coined by 19th century French physiologist Claude Bernard: "No matter how far the Lama glama wanders at sea level it will always carry the Altiplano in its milieu intérieur."

Acknowledgments

Supported by grant 1040647, FONDECYT, Chile.

References

1. Stanley H, et al. Proc Biol Sci. 1994; 256(1345):1–6.
2. Wheeler JC. Biol J Linn Soc. 1995; 54(3):271–295.
3. Kadwell M, et al. Proc Biol Sci. 2001; 268(1485):2575–2584.
4. Meschia G, et al. Exp Physiol. 1960; 45(3):284–291.
5. Moraga F, et al. Comp Biochem Physiol A Physiol. 1996; 115(2):111–115.
6. Sanhueza E, et al. Pediatr Res. 1992; 32(6):737.
7. Reynafarje C, et al. J Appl Physiol. 1968; 24(1):97–98.
8. Yang H, et al. Biochem Genet. 2000; 38(7–8):241–252.
9. Banchero N, et al. Respir Physiol. 1971; 13(1):102–115.
10. Moraga FA, et al. J Health Med Sci. 2020; 6(2):97–106.
11. Prabhakar NR, et al. Physiol Rev. 2012; 92(3):967–1003.
12. Harris P, et al. Thorax. 1982; 37(1):38–45.
13. Nachar R, et al. High Alt Med Biol. 2001; 2(3):377–385.
14. Reynafarje C, et al. J Appl Physiol. 1975; 38(5):806–810.
15. Barcroft J, et al. J Physiol. 1933; 77(2):194–206.
16. Allison BJ, et al. J Physiol. 2016; 594(5):1247–1264.
17. West JB. Science. 1984; 223(4638):784–788.
18. Llanos AJ, et al. High Alt Med Biol. 2003; 4(2):193–202.
19. Benavides CE, et al. Respir Physiol. 1989; 75:327–334.
20. Llanos A, et al. Comp Biochem Physiol. 1998; 119(3):705–709.
21. Perez R, et al. Am J Physiol Regul Integr Comp Physiol. 1989; 256:R1011–R1018.
22. Llanos AJ, et al. Reprod Fertil Dev. 1995; 7(3):549–552.
23. Giussani DA, et al. Am J Physiol. 1996; 271:R73–R83.
24. Giussani DA, et al. J Physiol. 1999; 515(Pt 1):233–241.
25. Llanos AJ, et al. J Physiol. 2002; 538(3):975–983.
26. Llanos AJ, et al. Respir Physiol Neurobiol. 2007; 158(2–3):298–306.
27. Giussani DA, et al. J Physiol. 1993; 461:431–449.
28. Giussani DA, et al. J Physiol. 1994; 477:81–87.
29. Riquelme RA, et al. Endocrinology. 1998; 139:2564–2570.
30. Reyes RV, et al. J Appl Physiol. 2020; 129:152–161.
31. Jones CT, et al. J Physiol. 1975; 285(1):381–393.
32. Riquelme RA, et al. J Physiol. 2002; 544(1):267–276.
33. Fletcher AJW, et al. Endocrinology. 2000; 141(11):3976–3982.
34. Sanhueza EM, et al. J Physiol. 2003; 546(3):891–901.
35. Herrera EA, et al. High Alt Med Biol. 2000; 1(3):175–184.
36. Wintour EM, et al. Reprod Fertil Dev. 1995; 7:1311–1319.
37. Block BS, et al. Am J Obstet Gynecol. 1984; 148(7):878–885.
38. Moore LG, et al. Am J Phys Anthropol. 1998; 107(Suppl 27):25–64.
39. Sanhueza EM, et al. Am J Physiol Regul Integr Comp Physiol. 2005; 289(3):R776–R783.
40. Perez-Pinzon MA. Comp Biochem Physiol Part A. 2007; 147:291–299.
41. Jensen BC, et al. J Cardiovasc Pharmacol. 2014; 63(4):291–301.
42. Field DR, et al. J Dev Physiol. 1990; 14:131–137.
43. Jones MD, et al. J Appl Physiol. 1977; 43:1080–1084.
44. Richardson BS, et al. J Dev Physiol. 1989; 11(1):37–43.
45. Ebensperger G, et al. J Physiol. 2005; 567:963–975.
46. Rudolph AM. Ann Rev Physiol.1979; 41:383–395.
47. Herrera EA, et al. Am J Physiol Regul Integr Comp Physiol. 2007; 292:R2234–R2240.
48. Moraga FA, et al. Am J Physiol Regul Integr Comp Physiol. 2011; 301(4):R1153–R1160.
49. Reyes RV, et al. J Physiol. 2018; 596:5907–5923.
50. Herrera EA, et al. Nitric Oxide. 2019; 89:71–80.
51. Zuckerbraun BS, et al. J Exp Med. 2006; 203:2109–2119.
52. Llanos AJ, et al. Respir Physiol Neurobiol. 2012; 184:186–191.
53. Herrera EA, et al. Cardiovasc Res. 2008; 77:197–201.
54. López V, et al. Front Physiol. 2018; 9:606.
55. Arrigoni FI, et al. Circulation. 2003; 107:1195–1201.

NEONATES OF BURROWING AND HIBERNATING MAMMALS

Metabolic and Respiratory Adaptations to Hypoxia

Yvonne A. Dzal and William K. Milsom

Contents

Introduction

In this review, we explore the different hypoxic ventilatory and metabolic responses employed by neonates and adults of species of small mammals, which may underlie differences in their resistance to hypoxic respiratory failure. In the process, we address *the hibernator as neonate* hypothesis: *are hibernators just big babies?* Neonatal mammals exhibit several physiological differences from their adult counterparts. Interestingly, there are striking parallels in physiological traits between neonatal mammals and adults of species capable of hibernation (1–3) (Table 6.1). These similarities are numerous and not likely confined to just the traits listed in Table 6.1. Nevertheless, this extensive list of similarities has given rise to the hypothesis that the ability of heterothermic mammals to hibernate has evolved from the retention of neonatal traits and that the genetic potential for heterothermy is expressed, to some extent, in all neonatal mammals (2).

Among the striking parallels between neonatal mammals and adult hibernators is their remarkable tolerance to low environmental O_2 (i.e. hypoxia). While most adult mammals are not hypoxia tolerant, hibernating mammals are exceptional in this regard (4–7) (Figure 6.1A). This was beautifully demonstrated in the pioneering study of Hiestand et al. (4), in which survival times were measured in several species of adult mammals exposed to extremely low levels of environmental O_2 (2.8% O_2; Figure 6.1A). Nonhibernators did quite poorly, with no species surviving more than 3 minutes (Figure 6.1A). Hibernators, however, survived significantly longer than nonhibernators, with some species surviving 2.8% O_2 for over 3 hours (4) (Figure 6.1A).

While adult hibernators are far more hypoxia tolerant than adult nonhibernators, as neonates, both groups are more tolerant of hypoxia than their adult counterparts (8–19) (Figure 6.1B). Thus, postnatal changes occur in hypoxia tolerance of both hibernators and nonhibernators, but the changes are greater in nonhibernating species (Figure 6.1B).

The basis of neonatal hypoxia tolerance and the postnatal changes that occur in different species have, thus far, attracted little attention. In this chapter, we focus on recent research on hibernating species to identify the physiological strategies

different mammals use to combat low environmental O_2 and how these physiological strategies change with postnatal development. The similarities and differences between species highlight the unity and the diversity of evolutionary strategies for coping with O_2 deprivation and allow us to examine the extent to which species that hibernate retain strategies common to mammalian neonates.

TABLE 6.1 Diversity of Physiological Traits Common to Hibernating Mammals That May Have Originated from the Retention of Neonatal Traits

PHYSIOLOGICAL TRAITS
VENTILATORY SPECIALIZATIONS
high tolerance to hypoxia, ischemia, & asphyxia
greater reliance on vagal feedback for breathing
pulmonary surfactant composition with a wide thermal range
METABOLIC SPECIALIZATIONS
low mass specific resting metabolic rate
controlled & extreme reductions in body temperature
ability to autoresusicate from hypothermic respiratory arrest
ability to use brown adipose tissue for non-shivering thermogenesis
metabolism fuelled primarily through fat
CARDIAC & CIRCULATORY SPECIALIZATIONS
enhanced O_2 carrying capacity of hemoglobin
elevated hematocrit
low arterial O_2 tension and high arterial O_2 tension
reduced cardiac sympathetic innervation
resistance to ventricular fibrillation in hypothermia
ENDOCRINE, CELLULAR, & MOLECULAR SPECIALIZATIONS
extreme neural plasticity & neuroprotection from insults
high levels of molecular chaperones & heat shock proteins
low levels of thyroid & growth hormone
downregulation in insulin-like growth factor

Source: Data from (4, 7, 12–14, 22, 23, 34, 50, 56, 72–91).

DOI: 10.1201/9780367494018-6

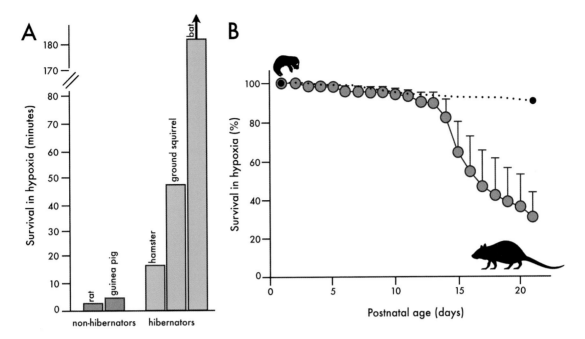

FIGURE 6.1 Hibernators are more hypoxia tolerant than nonhibernators. (A) Survival time in hypoxia of adult nonhibernators and hibernators exposed to extremely low levels of hypoxia (2.8% O_2); modified from (4). (B) Postnatal changes in the survival of nonhibernators (circles) [data from (36)] and predicted trend for hibernators (dotted line) exposed to mild hypoxia (11.8% O_2) from birth.

Physiological responses to hypoxia in adult mammals

When mammals are exposed to low O_2 environments, their immediate compensatory response is to hyperventilate (20, 21). Exposure to hypoxia, particularly in small mammals, produces two opposing effects on the drive to breathe, reflecting a balance between: (1) an increase in chemosensitive drive, due to the stimulation of the peripheral chemoreceptors and (2) a reduced metabolic drive, linked to the depression of body temperature and O_2 consumption rate (20–22). Thus, hyperventilation in hypoxia may occur either through an increase in ventilation (i.e. the hypoxic ventilatory response) (20), a decrease in metabolic demand (i.e. the hypoxic metabolic response) (23), or both.

The immediate hypoxic response is typically not sustained. Most mammals studied to date elicit a well-documented biphasic ventilatory response in hypoxia (20–21). This is particularly true of small mammals (24). The first phase of the hypoxic ventilatory response is an immediate increase in ventilation within one breath of a change in arterial O_2 levels, mediated by the stimulation of the peripheral chemoreceptors (20–22, 25, 26). The second phase of the ventilatory response begins with a slow decline in ventilation to a steady lower level. This is mediated by: (1) central mechanisms, such as the reduction in the thermoregulatory set-point — the temperature at which body temperature is regulated, accompanied by a fall in metabolism (26–30); as well as (2) peripheral mechanisms — due to the time dependent decline in the sensitivity of the carotid bodies to hypoxic stimuli (26, 31–33).

If metabolic rate is to be maintained in hypoxia, then any fall in ventilation must be accompanied by an increase in pulmonary O_2 extraction and would result in a decrease in the ventilatory equivalent or air convection requirement (the ratio of ventilation/metabolism) (23, 34–37). Given that the O_2 content of each breath is progressively reduced in hypoxia extracting more O_2 per breath is not sustainable. On the other hand, if metabolism is

reduced, then the ventilatory equivalent may remain constant or even increase, while pulmonary O_2 extraction remains the same or even decreases with decreasing levels of inspired O_2. Thus, one of the primary characteristics of hypoxia tolerance is rebalancing O_2 demand with O_2 supply (6, 38–40). This remarkable resilience to O_2 deprivation is achieved through controlled, yet fully reversible, reductions in O_2-demanding processes such as thermoregulation, excitatory neurotransmitter release, and ion permeability (channel arrest and action potential spike arrest) (7, 8, 41). Although it is possible that the hypoxia-induced reduction in O_2 demand is a passive response due to a lack of O_2 supply, a large body of evidence has accumulated in support of the hypothesis that the hypoxic metabolic response is a regulated and reversible oxy-conforming mode of O_2 uptake; i.e. it is controlled metabolic suppression and *NOT* hypometabolism (an oft misused term) (42–47).

Although the biphasic ventilatory response to hypoxia is typical of mammals, the relative contributions of different components of the response (the components of the Fick equation for pulmonary exchange; changes in metabolic rate, ventilation, and pulmonary O_2 extraction) can vary depending on many factors, both within and between species. These factors include the level of hypoxia, chemoreceptor sensitivity, levels of CO_2, pH, time course of hypoxic exposure, pattern of repeated exposure, O_2 consumption rate, body temperature, and developmental stage (20–22).

We now take a look at the strategies employed by neonates of hibernating and nonhibernating species. Unlike adults of nonhibernating species, adults of species capable of hibernating are capable of extreme reductions in metabolism, body temperature, heart rate, and ventilation. We examine the extent to which the neonates of rodents ranging in their degree of heterothermic expression (homeotherm: rats, facultative heterotherms: mice and hamsters, and obligate heterotherms: ground squirrels) differ in the balance of metabolic suppression and increased ventilation employed under hypoxic conditions.

Metabolic and respiratory responses to hypoxia in neonatal rodents

The mass-specific metabolic rates of rodent neonates are similar to those of their mothers, which are extremely low for a mammal of their size. It is only as rodents grow and develop the adult capacity for thermogenesis that their mass-specific metabolic rates rise to allometrically predicted levels (3). For neonates of altricial species, this can take several weeks. At birth, their primary response to reduced O_2 availability is to reduce O_2 demand (14, 16, 19, 36, 48). With exposure to progressive hypoxia, neonates of species with varying degrees of heterothermy all respond in a similar fashion, with decreases in O_2 consumption rates. For the species shown in Figure 6.2A, decreases range from 35 to 50% when exposed to a 9% O_2 gas mixture. Accompanying these large falls in O_2 demand are modest increases in ventilation (40 to 100% for the species in Figure 6.2A). In general, the increases in ventilation have been reported to vary in an inverse manner with the falls in metabolic rate (24, 49–51). These hypoxia-induced increases in ventilation are primarily the result of increases in breathing frequency, as tidal volume either increases slightly, decreases, or remains constant (24).

The balance between changes in ventilation and changes in O_2 consumption is reflected in the ventilatory equivalent (the ratio of ventilation/O_2 consumption rate). Under normoxic conditions, changes in O_2 consumption rate (such as during exercise) are matched by changes in ventilation and the ratio remains relatively constant. This is not the case in hypoxia, as the amount of O_2 in each breath decreases. Whether the response to hypoxia is an increase in ventilation or a fall in O_2 consumption rates, the ratio between the two will increase and the % change in this ratio will reflect the % change in the O_2 composition of the inspired gas. If the amount of O_2 extracted from each breath were to remain constant, for animals breathing 9% O_2 the ventilatory equivalent should increase by 133% (as indicated by the dotted line in Figure 6.2). As described by the Fick equation [O_2 consumption rate = total ventilation × (fraction of O_2 in inspired air – fraction of O_2 in expired air)], any difference in these ratios from 133% must be due to changes in the amount of O_2 extracted from the lung with each breath. The neonates of the species shown in Figure 6.2 when breathing 9% O_2 exhibit increases ranging from 108 to 307% spanning the ratio of the change in O_2 content of inspired gas (133%) required to match O_2 supply and demand based on changes in O_2 consumption rate and ventilation alone. The highest value is for the rat and reflects a significant decrease in pulmonary O_2 extraction. The lowest value is in the mouse and reflects an increase in pulmonary O_2 extraction. Pulmonary O_2 extraction remains relatively constant in hamsters and ground squirrels (Figure 6.2A). The differences seen in pulmonary O_2 extraction in the different species could reflect species differences in lung morphology, lung perfusion, or the carrying capacity of the blood. The greater hemoglobin concentration and hemoglobin-O_2 affinity of neonatal rodents undoubtedly contribute to their reported blunted hypoxic ventilatory responses (52). On the one hand, this indicates that hibernators maintain a greater diffusion gradient for O_2 uptake at the lung. On the other hand, it indicates that the differences in the magnitude of the ventilatory responses seen in the different species are largely due to the differences in pulmonary O_2 extraction and not to differences in O_2 chemosensitivity.

Given the poor thermogenic capacity of neonatal rodents, their body temperatures approximate ambient temperature when held in isolation. Thus, there is little scope for body temperature to fall in hypoxia (24) (Figure 6.2A). In adult mammals, it appears that the fall in O_2 consumption rates in hypoxia are the result of resetting the thermoregulatory set-point for body temperature regulation to a lower level, leading to an inhibition of both shivering, and nonshivering thermogenesis (42, 48, 53, 54), as well as an increase in heat dissipation until body temperature falls to the new set point (47). The reduction in O_2 consumption rate in neonates, however, occurs despite little or no fall in body temperature (Figure 6.2A). Whether this body temperature independent fall in O_2 consumption rate is due to O_2 limitation or active suppression by some other means is not yet known. Because of the lack of thermogenic capacity, cooling cannot be used to determine whether metabolism can be elevated further, and whether this hypoxia-induced reduction in O_2 consumption rate is in fact controlled.

In summary, neonates of all rodent species, whether hibernating or nonhibernating primarily respond to reduced O_2 availability in hypoxia with modest increases in ventilation and in pulmonary O_2 extraction, and large decreases in their need for O_2 by decreasing metabolism. It is not clear whether their ventilatory responses are inadequate and the fall in metabolism is due to limited O_2 availability, or whether this is an orchestrated reduction in metabolism that is not quite sufficient to accommodate the reduced O_2 supply resulting in modest increases in ventilation and in pulmonary O_2 extraction. Metabolic suppression in response to low O_2 conditions becomes disadvantageous when hypoxic conditions persist. In the developing rodent, prolonged O_2 consumption rate suppression inhibits tissue and organ growth, tissue differentiation, and cell repair (55).

Metabolic and respiratory responses to hypoxia in adult rodents
Effects of progressive hypoxia within the thermoneutral zone

Similar to neonatal rodents, adult rodents also respond to hypoxia by reducing O_2 consumption rates, to some extent. The magnitude of this reduction has been shown to be size dependent, being greater in smaller mammals (24). The magnitude of the hypoxic metabolic response has also been shown to be greater in adult hibernators than in adult nonhibernators (23, 56), although the extent of this difference is temperature dependent (see next section). The species of rodents shown in Figure 6.2B are all relatively small (i.e. less than a kilogram); and exhibit significant falls in O_2 consumption rate when inspiring 9% O_2. The decreases in O_2 consumption rates of hibernating species within their thermoneutral zones are marginally (but not significantly) greater than in the non-hibernating rat. The magnitude of these reductions in O_2 consumption rates, however, are also significantly reduced compared to the reductions seen in the neonates of the same species (Figure 6.2A, B).

As mentioned above, the hypoxic metabolic response in adult mammals appears to initially be mediated by a reduction in the thermoregulatory set-point, accompanied by a fall in metabolism (26-30). If exposure to hypoxia is prolonged, there is a time-dependent decline in the sensitivity of the carotid bodies to hypoxic stimuli (26, 31–33). Thus, in adult rats, it has been shown that there are time domains to the hypoxic metabolic response, that the immediate suppression of metabolism in hypoxia is not sustained, and that the magnitude of the hypoxic metabolic response decreases over time in an ambient temperature-dependent fashion (57, 58). To our knowledge, this has not been examined in other species.

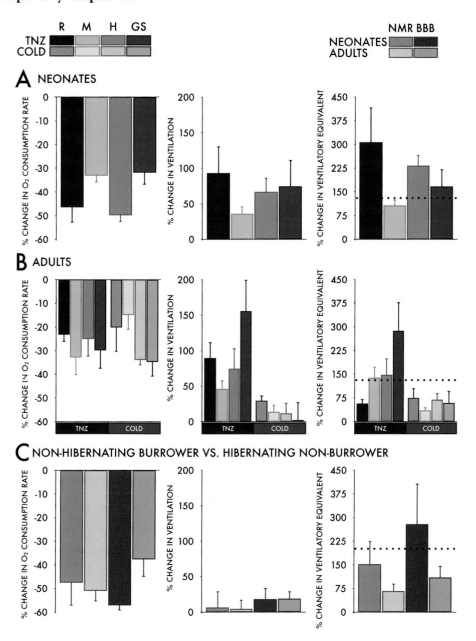

FIGURE 6.2 Hibernators do not match O_2 supply with O_2 demand through the retention of neonatal traits, but the two most hypoxia-tolerant mammals, naked mole rats, and big brown bats may. Changes in O_2 consumption rate, ventilation, and ventilatory equivalent of (A) neonate and (B) adult rodents, following progressive hypoxia (9% O_2), represented as percent change from normoxic values at ambient temperature within their thermoneutral zone (TNZ; dark solid bars), and in the cold (15°C; light transparent bars). Data presented in order of heterothermic expression, with the least heterothermic rodent, the rat (red bars [R]; *Rattus norvegicus*), farthest to the left, the most heterothermic rodent, the ground squirrel (blue bars [GS]; *Ictidomys tridecemlineatus*) farthest to the right, and the facultative heterotherms, the mouse (yellow bars [M]; *Mus musculus*) and hamster (green bars [H]; *Mesocricetus auratus*) in between. (C) changes in O_2 consumption rate, ventilation, and ventilatory equivalent of a burrowing nonhibernator (pink bars; naked mole rat [NMR]; *Heterocephalus glaber*) and a nonburrowing hibernator (purple bars; big brown bat [BBB]; *Eptesicus fucus*) following progressive hypoxia (7% O_2), as percent-change from normoxic values at ambient temperature within their thermoneutral zone; neonates = darker solid bars, adults = lighter transparent bars. In ventilatory equivalent graphs, dotted lines = amount the ventilatory equivalent should increase to match O_2 demand and O_2 supply in hypoxia, if the O_2 extracted from each breath remained constant.

With only modest decreases in metabolic rate in hypoxia, increases in ventilation are essential to match O_2 supply and demand. Thus, typical of most adult mammals, hibernating and nonhibernating rodents significantly increase ventilation when exposed to progressive hypoxia (Figure 6.2B). Interestingly, the relative increases in ventilation in hypoxia in the adult rodents in Figure 6.2B are similar

to those of their neonates with the exception of the ground squirrel where the relative increase has doubled when exposed to 9% O_2. Strong ventilatory responses to hypoxia have consistently been shown in multiple ground squirrel species during their active season (24, 51, 56, 59–62) (Figure 6.2B). As in neonates, the hypoxia-mediated increase in ventilation in most adult mammals is achieved mainly through an increase in breathing frequency; changes in tidal volume are variable. Generally, increases in breathing frequency prevail in moderate hypoxia, while an increase in tidal volume appears at more severe levels of hypoxia (24, 61, 62).

Thus, compared to their neonatal counterparts, the adult rodents have a reduced hypoxic metabolic response but a similar relative increase in their hypoxic ventilatory response. The ventilatory equivalent increases two- to threefold in adults of all species. There is a progressive increase in the ventilatory equivalent from the homeothermic rat (57%) to the facultative heterotherms (138–148%) to the obligate heterotherm, the ground squirrel (287%). This represents a relative hypoventilation in the rat and a relative hyperventilation in the ground squirrel that may potentially contribute to the differences in hypoxia tolerance seen in the adults of these species.

Effects of progressive hypoxia in the cold

Ambient temperature plays a pervasive role in determining the magnitude of the hypoxic metabolic response. The hypoxic metabolic response has been shown to be more pronounced at ambient temperatures below the thermoneutral zone (23, 42, 51, 53, 63, 64). The magnitude of the hypoxic metabolic response at colder temperatures has also been shown to be greater in adult hibernators than nonhibernators (23, 56). For example, when exposed to 10% O_2 adult homeothermic rats reduced O_2 consumption by 20% from normoxic values (56), whereas adult heterothermic mice and hamsters reduced O_2 consumption by 30 and 50%, respectively (56). Figure 6.2B illustrates the extent to which exposure to cold (15°C) alters the hypoxic metabolic response in several rodent species. Compared to the fall in O_2 consumption rates in hypoxia at thermoneutrality, the fall in O_2 consumption rate in hypoxia in the cold is roughly the same in the rat, less in the mouse but greater in the hamster and ground squirrel. The cold exposure, however, greatly attenuates the hypoxic ventilatory response in all species. With the exception of the mouse in this example, the magnitude of the hypoxic ventilatory response was inversely proportionate to the magnitude of the hypoxic metabolic response (Figure 6.2B).

Given the changes that occur in ventilation and O_2 consumption rates, the ventilatory equivalent of the various rodent species breathing 9% O_2 in the cold is only roughly twice that seen under normoxic conditions (Figure 6.2B). Adult rodents in the cold breathe less for each volume of O_2 they consume (their ventilatory requirement is reduced). The modest increase in ventilation relative to O_2 consumption while breathing a gas with only 9% O_2 indicates that an increased amount of O_2 is extracted from each breath. These increases range from 40 to 90%. The increase in lung O_2 extraction in the cold could be due to a combination of factors, such as a longer resident time of inspired air in the lungs due to a lower breathing frequency and greater tidal volume, increased hemoglobin-O_2 affinity, or changes in ventilation/ perfusion. This could underlie the attenuation of the hypoxic ventilatory response in the cold as could other factors that are sensitive to temperature, such as a decrease in the responsiveness of chemoreceptors (65, 66), and an increase in the release of inhibitory neurotransmitters (67). Regardless of mechanism, the reduced hypoxic ventilatory response in the cold may represent a beneficial adaptation, since increased ventilation is an energetically expensive response to hypoxia.

What causes this temperature-dependent switch in strategies remains unknown but there appears to be a correlation between the increased drop in O_2 consumption rate and the reduction in

the hypoxic ventilatory response in the cold (Figure 6.2B). The reductions in the hypoxic ventilatory response are in turn correlated with increases in pulmonary O_2 extraction.

Metabolic and respiratory responses to hypoxia in adult naked mole rats and big brown bats

Most hibernators inhabit underground burrows, living the majority of their lives in low O_2 environments (6–14% O_2) (68, 69). It is thus conceivable that the enhanced hypoxia tolerance reported in hibernating mammals is the result of their burrowing lifestyle and not the ability to hibernate, per se. Among mammals, naked mole rats (*Heterocephalus glaber*; a burrowing nonhibernator) and big brown bats (*Eptesicus fuscus*; a non-burrowing hibernator) are the most hypoxia tolerant. Indeed, both naked mole rats and big brown bats can withstand prolonged exposures (>3 hours) to severe hypoxia (3% O_2) (4, 70, 71).

We have recently measured the metabolic and ventilatory responses to progressive hypoxia in neonates and adults of both of these species. The neonates when exposed to 7% O_2 reduce O_2 consumption rates by 50 to 60% and increase ventilation by only 7 to 18% (Figure 6.2C), a pattern similar to that seen in neonatal rodents. What is unique in these species is the extent of the hypoxic metabolic response and that this pattern is retained in the adults, it does not change through development. The ventilatory equivalents, however, do change. They are lower in the adults than the neonates associated with increases in relative pulmonary O_2 extraction (Figure 6.2C).

Conclusion: Are hibernators just big babies?

Throughout this chapter, we question whether differences in the hypoxia tolerance of adult hibernators and nonhibernators reflect developmental changes in the way O_2 supply and demand are matched in hypoxia and whether it is due to retention of the hypoxia tolerance typical of neonates. Additionally, we compare the strategies employed to match O_2 supply and demand in hypoxia in two of the most hypoxia-tolerant mammals, a burrowing nonhibernator (naked mole rat), and a nonburrowing hibernator (big brown bat) to determine whether the enhanced hypoxia tolerance of hibernating mammals is due to a burrowing lifestyle, or the ability to hibernate.

We find that the enhanced hypoxia tolerance reported in rodent neonates is primarily due to hypoxic metabolic suppression accompanied by modest increases in ventilation, such that the relative amount of O_2 extracted from each breath remains roughly the same. This appears to be characteristic of all rodent neonates (Figure 6.2A). We find that the enhanced hypoxia tolerance of adults of hibernating mammals is not simply due to the retention of neonatal traits. While in their thermoneutral zone, the metabolic suppression is not as great in adults as in neonates in all species (Figure 6.2A, B) and the increases in ventilation are accompanied by increases in the relative amount of O_2 extracted from each breath (Figure 6.2A, B). There is a progressive increase in the ventilatory equivalent with increasing heterothermic capacity that represents a relative increase in the matching of ventilation to metabolism in the heterothermic species (Figure 6.2A, B). Adult hibernators show a greater reduction in metabolic rate in the cold, accompanied by a large reduction in ventilation, thus, behaving more like neonates but only when exposed to hypoxia in the cold (Figure 6.2A, B). The large reduction in the hypoxic ventilatory response in the cold, however, was common to all species (Figure 6.2B). Finally, the neonates of the naked mole rat and the big brown bat, the two most hypoxia-tolerant mammalian species, exhibited the greatest reductions in metabolic rate, very modest increases in ventilation, and large increases in the relative amount of O_2 extracted from each breath, compared to all other mammals investigated in this review (Figure 6.2). These characteristics were retained by the adults of these species (Figure 6.2C). Thus, while the data do not lend support for the hibernator as a neonate hypothesis, they do suggest that hypoxia tolerance in many species arises through the retention of neonatal characteristics. We note that the link between neonatal responses to hypoxia and hypoxia tolerance is shared by adults of burrowing hibernators, a nonburrowing hibernator and a burrowing nonhibernator. This indicates that neonatal hypoxic responses have been retained in adults of mammals of several different taxa. We also note that although bats are nonburrowers, like the burrowing species they occupy habitats that are relatively safe from predators, and that metabolic suppression as a strategy for enhancing hypoxia tolerance may not be an option for more vulnerable species.

Acknowledgments

This research was funded by a Liber Ero Postdoctoral Fellowship and a University of British Columbia Four Year Doctoral Fellowship (YAD) and the NSERC of Canada (WKM).

Literature cited

1. Ar A. In: Dejours P, ed. *Comparative physiology of environmental adaptations.* Basel, Switzerland: Karger Publishers; 1987. p.208–21.
2. Harris M, et al. In: Barnes B, Carey H, eds. *Twelfth International hibernation symposium. Life in the cold: evolution, mechanisms, adaptation, and application.* Fairbanks, Alaska: Institute of Arctic Biology; 2004. p.41–50.
3. Singer D In: Dakshinamurti S, ed. *Hypoxic respiratory failure in the newborn – From origins to clinical management.* Boca Raton FL: CRC Press, Taylor & Francis; 2021.
4. Hiestand WA, et al. Physiol Zool. 1950; 23:264–8.
5. Bullard RW, et al. In: Lyman CP, Dawe AR, eds. *Mammalian hibernation.* Cambridge, Massachusetts: Bulletin of the Museum of Comparative Zoology at Harvard College; 1960. p.321–35.
6. Boutilier RG. J Exp Biol2001; 204:3171–81.
7. Drew KL, et al. J Exp Biol. 2004; 207:3155–62.
8. Avery RC, et al. Exp Biol Med. 1932; 29(9):1184–6.
9. Kabat H. Am J Physiol1940; 130:588–99.
10. Fazekas JF, et al. Am J Physiol. 1941; 134:281–7.
11. Glass HG, et al. Am J Physiol. 1944; 140(5):609–15.
12. Adolph E. Am J Physiol1948; 155:366–77.
13. Hiestand WA, et al. Physiol Zool. 1953; 26:167–73.
14. Adolph EF. Respir Physiol1969; 7:356–68.
15. Scremin AM, et al. Stroke. 1980; 11(5):548–52.
16. Singer D. Comp Biochem Physiol A Mol Integr Physiol. 1999; 123(3):221–34.
17. Hill RW. In: *Life in the cold.* Heldmaier G, Klingenspor M, eds. Berlin, Germany: Springer; 2000. p. 199–205.
18. Singer D, et al. Comp Biochem Physiol A Mol Integr Physiol. 2007; 148(4):780–4.
19. Fong AY. Respir Physiol Neurobiol. 2010; 174:146–55.
20. Powell FL, et al. Respir Physiol. 1998; 112(2):123–34.
21. Pamenter ME, et al. Compr Physiol. 2016; 6(3):1345–85.
22. Dzal YA, et al. Respir Physiol & Neurobiol. 2020; 272:103313.
23. Barros RC, et al. J Appl Physiol. 2001; 91:603–12.
24. Mortola JP, et al. Respir Physiol. 1989; 78(1):31–43.
25. Eldridge FL, et al. In: Bethesda MD, ed. *Handbook of physiology. The respiratory system. Control of breathing.* Vol. 2. Rockville, Maryland: American Physiological Society; 1986. p. 93–114.
26. Bisgard GE, et al. In: Dempsey JA, Pack AI, eds. *Regulation of breathing.* New York, NY: Marcel Dekker; 1995. p. 617–68.
27. Martin-Body RL, et al. Respir Physiol. 1988; 71:25–32.
28. Clark DJ, et al. Can J Physiol Pharm. 1996; 74:331–6.
29. Gautier H. J Appl Physiol1996; 81:521–7.
30. Madden CJ, et al. J Physiol. 2005; 566:559–73.
31. Zhou A, et al. J Neurosci. 1997; 17:5349–56.
32. Gozal D, et al. Respir Physiol. 2000; 121:209–21.
33. Cummings KJ, et al. Am J Physiol. 2005; 288:1571–80.
34. Osborne S, et al. Respir Physiol. 1993; 92:305–18.
35. Saiki C, et al. J Physiol. 1996; 491:261–9.
36. Mortola JP. Respir Physiol Neurobiol. 2004; 141(3):345–56.
37. Dzal YA, et al. Front Physiol. 2019; 10:106.
38. Hochachka PW, et al. Proc Natl Acad Sci USA. 1996; 93(18):9493–8.
39. Lutz PL, et al. J Exp Biol. 2004; 207(18):3141–7.
40. Gorr TA. Acta Physiol. 2017; 219(2):409–40.
41. Larson J, et al. J Exp Biol. 2014; 217(7):1024–39.
42. Hill JR. J Physiol. 1959; 149:346.–73.
43. Sidi D, et al. Am J Physiol Heart Circ Physiol. 1983; 245(4):674–82.
44. Fahey JT, et al. Pediatr Res. 1989; 26(3):180–7.
45. Frappell PB, et al. Respir Physiol. 1991; 86:115–24.
46. Steiner AA, et al. Annu Rev Physiol. 2002; 64:263–88.
47. Tattersall GJ, et al. J Physiol. 2009; 587(21):5259–74.
48. Mortola JP. Respir Physiol. 1999; 116:95–103.
49. Adolph EF, et al. J Appl Physiol. 1960; 15:1075–86.
50. Mortola JP. Respir Physiol. 1991; 85:305–17.
51. Dzal YA, et al. Effects of hypoxia on the respiratory and metabolic responses to progressive cooling in newborn rodents that range in heterothermic expression. Exp Physiol. In publication; EP-RP-2020-08908.
52. Hardison RC. Cold Spring Harb Perspect Med. 2012; 2(12):a011627.
53. Mortola JP, et al. In: Dempsey JA, Pack AI, eds. *Regulation of breathing,* 2nd ed., New York, NY: Marcel Dekker; 1995. p. 1011–1064.
54. Morrison SF, et al. Ann Rev Physiol. 2019; 81:285–308.
55. Frappell PB, et al. J Appl Physiol. 1994; 77(6):2748–52.
56. Frappell PB, et al. Am J Physiol. 1992; 262:1040–6.
57. Bishop B, et al. Am J Physiol. 2001; 280:1190–6.
58. Mortola JP, et al. J Appl Physiol. 2000; 88:365–8.
59. Cragg PA, et al. J Physiol. 1983; 341:477–93.
60. Holloway DA, et al. Comp Biochem Physiol A. 1984; 77:267–73.
61. Walker BR, et al. J Appl Physiol. 1985; 59:1955–60.
62. McArthur MD, et al. Physiol Zool. 1991; 64(4):921–39.
63. Saiki C, et al. J Appl Physiol. 1994; 76(4):1594–9.
64. Mortola JP, et al. Compr Physiol. 2011; 1:1679–1709.
65. McQueen DS, et al. J Neurophysiol. 1974; 37:1287–96.
66. Alcayaga J, et al. Brain Res. 1993; 600:103–11.
67. Waters KA, et al. Respir Physiol Neurobiol. 2003; 136:115–129.
68. Arieli R. Comp Biochem Physiol A Mol Integr Physiol. 1979; 63(4):569–75.
69. Nevo E. Annu Rev Ecol Syst. 1979; 10(1):269–308.
70. Larson J, et al. Neuroreport. 2009; 20:1634–7.
71. Nathaniel TI, et al. Int J Dev Neurosci. 2012; 30(6):539–44.
72. Donnelly DF. Respir Physiol Neurobiol. 2005; 149(1-3):191–9.
73. Webb CL, et al. J Comp Physiol B 2017; 187(5-6):793–802.
74. Bernhard W, et al. Am J Respir Cell Mol Biol. 2001; 25(6):725–31.
75. Suri LN, et al. Biochim Biophys Acta. 2012; 1818(7):1581–9.
76. Snapp BD, et al. Physiol Zool. 1981; 54(3):297–307.
77. Mortola JP, et al. Respir Physiol. 1998; 113:213–22.
78. Staples JF. Compr Physiol. 2016; 6:737–71.
79. Tattersall GL, et al. Respir Physiol Neurobiol. 2003; 137:29–40.
80. Smith RE, et al. Science. 1963; 140(3563):199–200.
81. Cannon B, et al. Physiol Rev. 2004; 84(1):277–359.
82. Buck MJ, et al. Physiol Genomics. 2002; 8(1):5–13.
83. Maginniss LA, et al. Respir Physiol. 1994; 95:195–208.
84. Mortola JP. *Respiratory physiology of newborn mammals: a comparative perspective.* Baltimore, MD: John Hopkins University Press; 2001.
85. Neilsen KC, et al. Acta Physiol. 1968; 74:1–16.
86. Kralios FA, et al. Reprod, Fertil Dev. 1996; 8(1):49–60.
87. Zhou F, et al. Am J Physiol. 2001; 158(6):2145–51.
88. D'Souza SM, et al. Cell Stress Chaperon. 1998; 3(3):188–99.
89. Carey HV, et al. Am Zool. 1999; 39(6):825–35.
90. Frare C, et al. Mol Cell Endocrinol. 2020; 11054.
91. Davies KT, et al. Gene. 2014; 549(2):228–36.

DIVING RESPONSE AND HYPOXIA IN DEEP SEA MAMMALS

Allyson Hindle

Contents

Introduction

The developmental timing of human hypoxia tolerance creates a dichotomy between the fetus and the adult; the human fetus can withstand hypoxia but the adult cannot. This is the case in many mammals, prompting the question of whether fetal hypoxia tolerance derives from evolutionarily conserved mechanisms? If so, a better understanding of the physiological and metabolic elements of mammalian hypoxia tolerance might be found in the successful strategies of innately hypoxia-tolerant mammals. Diving mammals stand out in this regard, routinely experiencing acute hypoxic apnea during submergence, and eupneustic normoxia at each surface interval. Many species of seals and whales embark on extended breath-holds well beyond the bounds of human capabilities, with dives lasting minutes to hours that descend to crushing depths. Contrary to humans, the adult marine mammal retains or even improves its hypoxia tolerance compared to the fetus; this natural model system provides an opportunity to examine and understand the components of physiological tolerance to acute hypoxia. This chapter discusses the adult elite-diving physiology of marine mammals, along with what is known of fetal marine mammal physiology.

Diving mammals fall into three distinct lineages: Dolphins and whales; seals, sea lions, and walruses; and manatees and dugongs. While some of the most elite diving species are also the best studied, research into the physiological specializations of each lineage is incomplete. Therefore, it is not always possible to identify whether a particular feature associated with hypoxia tolerance is generalizable and conserved across marine mammals, or whether it represents a species- or lineage-specific specialization. Consistently, a central element in the ability of marine mammals to withstand periods of oxygen deprivation is their enhanced body oxygen stores (1). These stores exist primarily in blood and muscle (Figure 7.1), through high concentrations of respiratory pigments, as well as an approximate doubling of blood volume in the seal, for example (14% body mass), compared to the human (7% body mass). The Antarctic Weddell seal was also the model in which the role of a large, contractile spleen as a source of oxygenated red blood cells that could be injected into the blood during diving was identified (2). Splenic storage of oxygenated red blood cells has been estimated at 20L in the Weddell seal (2). Yet, despite an ability to stave off oxygen depletion with large internal oxygen stores, marine mammals still experience and withstand impressive hypoxemia. Measurements of arterial blood gas tensions reveal that Weddell seals deplete oxygen to 12.8 mmHg during diving, with arterial saturations dropping to 28% (3). Elephant seals exhaust nearly all of their available blood oxygen during dives at sea with venous blood oxygen tensions declining to 2 mmHg (4).

Cardiovascular changes and blood flow redistribution during prolonged apnea

Diving mammals rely on a suite of cardiovascular adjustments to reduce cardiac output, which lowers overall oxygen consumption and extends submergence capability. The best-studied indicator of this response is profound bradycardia that occurs with apnea and facial immersion, initiated by trigeminal afferents and mediated by the vagus nerve (5). This neurally regulated dive response is present in all air-breathing vertebrates, including humans, generally producing 15–40% heart rate reduction (6). Adult human heart rates can decline below 20 beats/min in some extreme cases of submergence (7, 8); however, the marine mammal cardiovascular dive response is highly elaborated, with instantaneous heart rates reaching 3 beats per minute in diving elephant seals (9), and 2 beats per minute in the world's largest animal, the blue whale (10).

Another hallmark of the dive response is the development of sympathetically mediated peripheral vasoconstriction (11). This has the effect of centralizing blood volume, retaining available oxygenated blood for organs such as the brain and heart (12), which are presumed to be more critically dependent on aerobic metabolism. At the same time, increased peripheral vascular resistance reduces blood flow and therefore oxygen delivery to visceral and distal tissues, which lowers whole-body metabolic requirements. Vasoconstriction also has a counterbalancing effect to maintain stable central arterial pressure over a wide range of heart rate and cardiac output (13). Anatomically, seals have an extremely large and compliant vena cava, which is key to centralizing blood volume without knock-on effects to blood pressure (14). Adult humans are capable of similar cardiovascular responses during a facial immersion/exercise protocol; however, the overall response (primarily the degree of bradycardia) is insufficiently intense to prevent systemic hypertension arising from peripheral vascular constriction (15).

Diving is, therefore, controlled by activation of both the parasympathetic and sympathetic nervous systems to maintain bradycardia and peripheral vasoconstriction, respectively (5). Yet, there is also evidence of tissue-specific management of perfusion during submergence. Notably, the pregnant Weddell seal maintains perfusion to her placenta and uterus during diving (16), while the nonpregnant seal does not (12). Despite these tissue-specific differences, the role of local vasoregulators to fine-tune

DOI: 10.1201/9780367494018-7

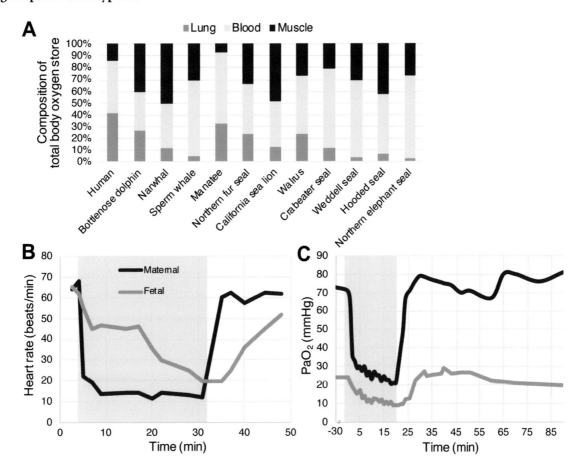

FIGURE 7.1 Oxygenation and heart rate in diving mammals. (A) The distribution of body oxygen stores in humans compared to marine mammals. The percentage of the body oxygen store present in the lungs, blood, and skeletal muscle is presented for three odontocete whales, manatee, and a range of pinnipeds. Consistently, it is apparent that the deepest diving species within a particular group (sperm whale, weddell, hooded, and northern elephant seals) have the smallest percent of the body oxygen store contained in the lungs. Composition of total body oxygen stores plotted from Ponganis and Williams (52), based on references therein. (B) Simultaneous recordings of maternal and fetal heart rates in a weddell seal. The gray-shaded area indicates an experimental dive, elicited by asphyxia. Fetal bradycardia occurs during breath-hold; however, its decline and recovery occur gradually, relative to the rapid changes in heart rate occurring in the adult female. (Replotted from Elsner et al. (43). Used with permission: The Yale Journal of Biology and Medicine.) (C) Maternal and fetal (lower) arterial oxygen tension (PaO$_2$, mmHg) during a simulated dive. [Replotted from Liggins et al. (16)].

perfusion in diving mammals appears dampened, compared to terrestrial species. A critical difference between aquatic and terrestrial mammals is their avoidance of hypoxic vasodilation, despite globally declining oxygen stores during submergence. Marine mammals must avoid hypoxia-induced vasodilation to maintain a centralized blood volume and to defend mean arterial pressure during periods of dramatically reduced cardiac output. Moreover, diving mammals may have reduced biochemical responses to local vasodilatory substances that would typically provoke hypoxic vasodilation in peripheral tissues. One such example is nitric oxide (NO); this gasotransmitter is implicated in vasodilation through the NO-cGMP signal transduction pathway in response to hypoxia in terrestrial mammals. This pathway has been investigated in Weddell seals, which appear to have low to no nitric oxide in their exhaled breath (17), and a dampening of a key NO-responsive enzyme in the signal transduction pathway (18). Reduction of control through local vasoactive substances could prevent detrimental hypoxic vasodilation in marine mammals and maintain the high peripheral vascular resistance necessary to withstand low cardiac output.

Structural and functional mechanisms for cerebral hypoxia tolerance

The human brain is our most hypoxia sensitive tissue, tolerating only a few minutes of oxygen deprivation. The marine mammals' brain, by contrast, endures acute hypoxia during diving along with all tissues. While studies of tissue-specific blood flow distribution in seals indicate that the proportion of cardiac output perfusing the brain is relatively increased during submergence compared to visceral organs (12), very low arterial O$_2$ saturations observed even in routine dives [SaO$_2$ = 28% in Weddell seals (19), SaO$_2$ = 8% in northern elephant seals (4)] indicate substantial whole-body hypoxia. However, the brain of diving mammals does mitigate hypoxia to some degree. Relatively improved cerebral perfusion (12, 20) combines with enhanced cerebral capillary densities and reduced mean capillary distances (21), allowing marine mammals to sustain cerebral O$_2$ delivery through reduced diffusion gradients and thereby maximize O$_2$ delivery to the diving brain. Increasing arterial pCO$_2$ that develops during long dives (19) would also benefit perfusion of the brain by promoting cerebral vasodilation. Not only may marine mammals experience high $PaCO_2$ on account of extended breath-holding, but hypercapnia appears to be a more effective cerebral vasodilator in some species (sea otters and sea lions) compared to mice (22).

The brain does not benefit from enhanced internal oxygen stores, such as those provided by hemoglobin in the blood or myoglobin in skeletal muscles and heart. Instead, diving mammals appear to capitalize on specializations in noncirculating globins (neuroglobin and cytoglobin) to facilitate the transfer and diffusion of oxygen from circulating hemoglobin and into neural tissues in hypoxia. The concentration and localization of neuroglobin differs between species. Minke whales and harbor porpoise brains express 4–15× more neuroglobin mRNA than do hooded or harp seals or terrestrial mammals examined (23). Neuroglobin content may reflect physiological trade-offs between O_2 storage and O_2 delivery in divers. Long-duration, deep-diving marine mammals (for example, pilot whales) prioritize O_2 storage through enhanced blood hemoglobin content (22). It has been suggested that fast-swimming marine mammals instead prioritize O_2 transfer to the brain via elevated neuroglobin (22). The presence of O_2-binding globin proteins in the form of neuroglobin versus hemoglobin improves cerebral oxygenation in hypoxia while avoiding a trade-off that high blood viscosity due to high hemoglobin could compromise exercise performance. Seals are generally considered slow-swimming, deep divers, and demonstrate high blood O_2 stores (Figure 7.1).

In addition to the specializations that enhance brain O_2 supply, both the intact brain and neurons in brain slices of marine mammals remain viable in hypoxia. Normal EEG activity is maintained in the hypoxic Weddell seal brain to a pO_2 of 10mmHg (24). Seal neurons resist experimental hypoxia, aglycemia, and the presence of lactate, whereas mouse neurons do not (25), suggesting innate biochemical differences that support diving. The mammalian brain typically relies on oxidative phosphorylation to meet its energetic demand, fueled by glucose or ketone bodies delivered through the circulation. Seal neurons have 3X more glycogen than the neurons of mice, indicating a larger internal energy reserve that could be protective in hypoxia (25). Further, in terrestrial mammals, the oxidative machinery is localized to neurons, with an astrocyte-neuron lactate shuttle supplementing neuronal fuel from circulating glucose with pyruvate oxidized from lactate produced by glycolysis in astrocytes. In seals, the localization of these metabolic processes is reversed; neurons are better able to metabolize lactate and oxidative phosphorylation is instead enriched in astrocytes (26). Concordantly, cytochrome c is also localized to astrocytes in the seal brain (26). As a result of this metabolic rewiring, astrocyte-derived lactate appears to be the preferred source of pyruvate for hooded seal neurons (26) and contributes to tolerance of low O_2 and rising blood lactate during diving. Transcriptome analysis of seal and whale brain tissue also indicates high baseline levels of proteins expected to play a role in neuroprotection, including clusterin (a chaperone), S100B (a calcium binding stress protein) (27), and protection from redox stress (28).

One final neuroprotective strategy that may be employed in marine mammals to withstand hypoxia is brain cooling. Freely diving Weddell seals in icy Antarctic waters may experience a decline in central body temperature (measured via a thermistor in the dorsal aorta) of several degrees (29), and cranial skin surface temperatures may reach $-1.9°C$ (30). Marine mammals dissipate heat from their highly insulated bodies via arteriovenous anastomoses in the skin. In Arctic seals (e.g. hooded and harp seals), the primary location of these AV shunts is associated with the brachial artery in the foreflippers, which returns blood cooled by the surrounding environment directly to the heart (31). Brain temperatures of hooded and harp seals diving in cold water can decline $1–2.5°C$ (31). Cooling rates increased throughout these experimental dives, corresponding to maximum cerebral hypoxia; however, cooling could be detected prior to the commencement of diving, indicating that body cooling is centrally controlled, similar to the other elements of the cardiovascular dive response (31).

Myocardial and pulmonary vascular protection from hypoxia

Bradycardia along with peripheral vasoconstriction plays a critical role in redistributing blood during diving and limiting perfusion to select tissues. An additional outcome of strong submergence bradycardia in marine mammals is that a decreased cardiac output reduces the workload of the heart, decreasing cardiac metabolic demand during the hypoxic period. Microsphere studies of simulated dives indicate that myocardial perfusion in seals is maintained as a relative proportion of total cardiac output during submergence (12), although absolute cardiac output and therefore flow through the coronary arteries is dramatically reduced. Indeed, the seal heart experiences pulsatile coronary flow during submergence (32).

Control of the myocardial vasculature of the seal heart appears to differ from other mammals. Contrary to the human heart, seal coronary conduit arteries lack sympathetic innervation (33). Instead, only the coronary resistance arteries are innervated. Myocardial vasculature tone is controlled by acetylcholine via vagal innervation (33). Control by the vagus nerve likely matches the timing of adjustments to myocardial vasomotor tone with the onset of submergence bradycardia. The seal heart has high anaerobic potential relative to terrestrial mammals, with high internal glycogen stores (34), as well as a shift in metabolic enzymes, including high lactate dehydrogenase (35). These metabolic features enable the seal heart to sustain periods of coronary artery occlusion (10–45 sec) without harm (32).

There are also key differences in regulation of the pulmonary vasculature between adult humans and marine mammals. Free-diving humans rely on O_2 stored in the lung for breath-holding. By contrast, lung O_2 storage in marine mammals widely varies, with most deep diving species having a relatively small lung O_2 store (Figure 7.1). This is largely because the high pressures encountered at deep depths make stored gases a liability. High solubility of nitrogen and oxygen at depth, with ongoing exposure over repeated dives, could lead to oxygen toxicity in the CNS or to diseases of nitrogen solubility such as nitrogen narcosis or decompression sickness. Many deep divers, therefore, reduce stored oxygen in the lungs by either exhaling before submergence and/or through lung collapse at depth. Deep divers have a highly compliant chest cavity as well as anatomical modifications of the trachea that allow chest compression without trapping gases in the alveoli, and subsequent re-expansion without harm. Lung collapse at depth forces air from the lungs into the noncompressible bronchi and trachea, where gas exchange cannot occur. This limits the potential for high-pressure conditions to manifest, but removes the lung as a potential oxygen store during diving.

The completely collapsed lung creates a 100% pulmonary AV shunt, and graded responses may occur at moderate depths. In seals and sea lions diving to 100 m in a compression chamber, the pulmonary shunts ranged from 8.4% at the surface to up to 70% at the bottom of a simulated dive (36). Lung collapse limits or eliminates the metabolic O_2 consumption from the lung tissue itself, but produces acute ischemic and hypoxic conditions in the deep-diving pulmonary vasculature. Pulmonary arterial pressures of harbor seals consistently fall to the level of right atrial pressure during diving, suggesting that pulmonary blood flow ceases between heartbeats (37). Interestingly, these declines in diastolic pulmonary artery pressures occurred in simulated dives that were performed at both atmospheric pressure (mimicking a shallow/surface dive) and under compression (mimicking a deep dive) suggesting that reduced cardiac output during submergence is as important as high pressure in reducing pulmonary perfusion and developing pulmonary shunts.

The mammalian pulmonary vasculature typically responds to hypoxia by hypoxic pulmonary vasoconstriction (HPV). Constriction of local branches of the pulmonary artery distributes blood away from hypoxic alveoli, minimizing intrapulmonary shunting and better matching ventilation to perfusion. Chronic HPV is maladaptive, producing pulmonary hypertension, right heart hypertrophy, and ultimately heart failure. Despite repeated hypoxic exposure associated with a lifetime of breath-hold diving, marine mammals do not display a baseline pulmonary hypertension (37). Further, HPV does not develop during episodes of sleep apnea in elephant seals (38). A study of isolated pulmonary arteries of sea lions revealed that these marine mammals lack an acute HPV response. Rather than HPV, sea lion pulmonary arterial resistance vessels dilate under in vitro hypoxic conditions (39). The gasotransmitter hydrogen sulfide has been proposed as a novel oxygen sensor, which is endogenously produced in hypoxic conditions, and facilitates vasodilation in sea lion pulmonary arterial rings, but not in the same arterial preparations of terrestrial mammals.

Physiology of fetal hypoxia in deep sea diving species: Comparison with human fetal physiology

Pregnant females are among the most prolific of marine mammal divers. These females must continue to forage, gaining energy to support pregnancy and also to prepare for the energetic demands of the lactation period, in which many species of marine mammal will fast, forgoing foraging trips to remain with their newborn. Although elephant seal females reduce diving after week 17 of gestation, presumably in response to increase demands for oxygen from the fetus (40), pregnant Weddell seals are the most accomplished divers of their species, having the longest recorded dive times late in gestation (41, 42).

Blood flow through the seal uterine artery remains unchanged or only slightly diminished during simulated diving (43). Placental mammals rely on a high O_2 affinity of fetal blood to draw O_2 from placental vasculature to meet metabolic needs. This is especially necessary in the diving mammal, as maternal O_2 content declines during submergence. Similar to humans, seal fetal hemoglobin has a higher O_2 binding affinity compared to the adult of its species (44, 45). This is due to an increased amount of 2,3-DPG in the fetal circulation (45). Contrary to humans, fetal seals do not appear to express fetal-type hemoglobins, although confirmatory

sequencing has not been performed. Despite blood biochemistry that facilitates O_2 uptake to the fetus across the placenta in marine mammals, the intense hypoxemia experienced by the diving female indicates that the fetus also experiences significant episodes of hypoxia, even late in development (16). Fetal O_2 declines alongside the female (Figure 7.1B), and blood pH declines in parallel (16). Due to a faster rate of decline in arterial oxygen tension in the female compared to the fetal Weddell seal, the fetal-maternal gradient for O_2 transfer also declines, from 47 Torr prior to diving to 14 Torr at the end of the dive (16).

The fetal marine mammal also experiences dive bradycardia, and presumably other similar cardiovascular adjustments to the diving female. Heart rate of the fetal Weddell seal declines from ~80 to ~45 beats/min during a 15-min, unrestrained dive under the Antarctic sea ice (29). The lowest fetal heart rate observed during unrestrained diving was 40 beats/min at the end of the a 37-min dive; in comparison, the maternal heart rate at this time was 30 beats/min (29). These adjustments would serve to lower tissue oxygen consumption, specifically cardiac metabolic demand during these hypoxic episodes. A difference between the adult and the fetus, however, may occur in the control of bradycardia. In the adult, the onset of bradycardia and the dive response are initiated by neuro-cortical processes and is subsequently modulated by chemoreceptors detecting O_2, CO_2, or pH. The intensity of bradycardia is affected by several behavioral factors including dive duration, with longer dives associated with lower heart rates (9). This association has been noted in many species of freely diving marine mammal, but does not occur in forced dives or trained dives, for which the animal does not know how long the dive will be prior to submersion; in these cases, a maximal cardiovascular dive response develops (46, 47). Moreover, decerebrate divers (muskrats, ducks) are able to evoke a dive response upon submergence (48, 49), but lack the fine-scale control of bradycardia that associates this metric with dive duration (50). This indicates an important role for central, cerebral modulation of the dive response (51). The fetus would not benefit from any foreknowledge of the upcoming dive, thus fetal bradycardia must rely on chemoreceptor input. The result is a fetal dive response that lags behind the response of the female, steadily declining throughout the dive, compared to the female, whose heart rate reaches its minimum within minutes of submersion (Figure 7.1B).

References

1. Ponganis PJ, et al., J Exp Biol. 2011; 214(20):3325–39.
2. Hurford WE, et al., J Appl Physiol. 1996; 80(1):298–306.
3. Qvist J, et al., J Appl Physiol. 1986; 61(4):1560–1569.
4. Meir JU, et al., Am J Physiol Regul Integr Comp Physiol. 2009; 297(4):R927–R939.
5. Ponganis PJ, et al., J Exp Biol. 2017; 220(8):1372–81.
6. Alboni P, et al., J Cardiovasc Med. 2011; 12(6):422–7.
7. Arnold R. Undersea Biomed Res. 1985; 12(2):183–90.
8. Paulev PE, et al., Jpn J Physiol. 1990; 40(5):701–12.
9. Andrews RD, et al., J Exp Biol. 1997; 200(15):2083–95.
10. Goldbogen J, et al., Proc Natl Acad Sci USA. 2019; 116(50):25329–25332.
11. Panneton WM. Physiology. 2013; 28(5):284–97.
12. Zapol WM, et al., J Appl Physiol. 1979; 47(5):968–73.
13. Irving L, et al., Am J Physiol. 1942; 135(3):557–566.
14. Blix AS. J Exp Biol. 2011; 214(21):3507–10.
15. Bjertnaes L, et al., Acta Physiol Scand. 1984; 120(4):605–12.
16. Liggins GC, et al., J Appl Physiol. 1980; 49(3):424–30.
17. Falke K, et al., Respir Physiol Neurobiol. 2008; 162(1):85–92.
18. Hindle AG, et al., Am J Physiol Regul Integr Comp Physiol. 2019; 316(6):R704–R715.
19. Qvist J, et al., J Appl Physiol. 1986; 61(4):1560–9.
20. Hindle AG, et al., Am J Physiol Regul Integr Comp Physiol. 2019; 316(6):R704–R715.
21. Kerem D, et al., Resp Physiol. 1973; 19(2):188–200.
22. Williams TM, et al., Proc R Soc B: Biol Sci. 2008; 275(1636):751–8.
23. Schneuer M, et al., Neuroscience. 2012; 223:35–44.
24. Elsner R, et al., Resp Physiol. 1970; 9(2):287–97.
25. Damal N, et al., Neuroscience. 2014; 275:374–83.

26. Mitz S, et al., Neuroscience. 2009; 163(2):552–60.
27. Fabrizius A, et al., BMC Genomics. 2016; 17(1):583.
28. Krüger A, et al., Comp Biochem Physiol A: Mol Integr Physiol. 2020; 240:110593.
29. Hill RD, et al., Am J Physiol. 1987; 253(2 Pt 2):R344–R351.
30. Hindle AG, et al., Anim Biotelem. 2015; 3(1):1.
31. Blix AS, et al., J Exp Biol. 2010; 213(15):2610–6.
32. Elsner R, et al., Am J Physiol Heart Circ Physiol. 1985; 249(6):H1119–H1126.
33. Elsner R, et al., Comp Biochem Physiol A: Mol Integr Physiol. 1998; 119(4):1019–25.
34. Kerem D, et al., Comp Biochem Physiol A: Mol Integr Physiol. 1973; 45(3):731–6.
35. Fuson AL, et al., J Exp Biol. 2003; 206(22):4139–54.
36. Kooyman G, et al. Physiol Zool. 1982; 55(1):105–11.
37. Sinnett E, et al. J Appl Physiol. 1978; 45(5):718–27.
38. Ponganis P, et al., Comp Biochem Physiol A: Mol Integr Physiol. 2006; 145(1):123–30.
39. Olson KR, et al., Am J Physiol Regul Integr Comp Physiol. 2010; 298(1):R51–R60.
40. Hückstädt LA, et al., Biol Lett. 2018; 14(2):20170722.
41. Kooyman GL. Science. 1966; 151(3717):1553–4.
42. Shero MR, et al., Ecol Evol. 2018; 8(23):11857–74.
43. Elsner R, et al., Yale J Biol Med. 1969; 42(3–4):202.
44. Lenfant C, et al. Am J Physiol. 1969; 216(6):1595–7.
45. Qvist J, et al., J Appl Physiol. 1981; 50(5):999–1005.
46. Jobsis PD, et al., J Exp Biol. 2001; 204(22):3877–85.
47. Kanwisher JW, et al., Science. 1981; 211(4483):717–9.
48. Andersen HT. Acta Physiol Scand. 1963; 58(2):263–73.
49. Drummond P, et al., J Physiol. 1979; 290(2):253–71.
50. McCulloch PF, et al., Physiol Zool. 1990; 63(6):1098–1117.
51. Blix AS. J Exp Biol. 2018; 221(12):jeb182972.
52. Ponganis PJ, Williams CL. In: *Marine mammal physiology: requisites for ocean living.* Castellini MA, Mellish J, eds. Boca Raton, FL: CRC Press; 2015. p. 29–46.

THE PHYLOGENY AND ONTOGENY OF CARDIORESPIRATORY COUPLING IN VERTEBRATES AND ITS RELEVANCE TO NONINVASIVE MONITORING OF THE HUMAN FETUS

Edwin W. Taylor and Harry Gee

Contents

Introduction

This chapter begins with a brief account of our current knowledge of the control of heart rate f_H and its variability heart rate variability (HRV) in mammals, then provides a synopsis of the phylogeny of control of the HRV in nonmammalian vertebrates, based on an update of previous detailed reviews (1–3). The ease of access to embryos of the oviparous amphibians, reptiles, and birds is enabling us to improve our understanding of the embryonic development and possible evolution of central control of cardiorespiratory interactions, informing our knowledge and hopefully identifying future investigations on the embryos of viviparous mammals.

Mammals

Inactive mammals have an overriding inhibitory, muscarinic, cholinergic tone on the heart imposed via the Xth cranial nerve, the vagus (1, 2). The vagus also transmits instantaneous, beat-to-beat control of f_H (1, 4). Power spectral analysis of short-term variability (STV) in the frequency domain of f_H in adult humans and other mammals reveals three frequency regions with two 'low'-frequency peaks (approx. 0.05 Hz – 3 cycles per minute and 0.1 Hz – 6 cycles per minute) and one 'high'-frequency peak (0.25 Hz – 15 cycles per minute) (5). The region at 0.05 Hz is thought to be related to compensatory changes in peripheral vasomotor tone involved with thermoregulation. The 0.1 Hz region has been related to blood pressure control via the baroreceptor reflex (5, 6). The high-frequency peak is respiration-related variability. The heart in healthy, fit mammals accelerates during inspiration and slows during exhalation (7, 8), and this relationship is termed respiratory sinus arrhythmia (RSA). It is controlled by variable efferent input supplied by the vagus nerve.

Efferent (motor) activity in the vagus nerve arises from vagal preganglionic neurons (VPN) that innervate ganglia sited on visceral organs, including the heart and lungs. VPN distributed in two major locations in the brainstem of mammals, the dorsal vagal motonucleus (DVN) and the ventro-lateral nucleus ambiguus (NA). While 70% of VPN are located within the DVN, cell bodies of cardiac VPN (CVPN) are concentrated in the NA, with about 80% of them in this location (1). The NA is anatomically very close to the location of the ventral respiratory group, including the Pre-Botzinger complex that is considered the primary area for respiratory rhythmogenesis in mammals. CVPN in the NA receives a direct, feed-forward cholinergic, inhibitory input from these neighboring inspiratory neurons causing them to fire with respiration-related and cardiac-related rhythms (1, 9). Activity in CVPN is also affected indirectly by feedback from lung stretch receptors, entering via the nucleus of the solitary tract that gate activity arising from baroreceptor afferents (10, 11). Respiratory activity accordingly silences the discrete population of CVPN in the NA during inspiration so that their inhibitory input to the heart is withdrawn, causing f_H to rise during inspiration (1, 10), generating RSA. The responses are instantaneous because they are relayed by rapidly conducting myelinated efferent axons leaving the CVPN in the NA, classified as B-fibers on the basis of their conduction velocities (3–15 m/s).

The smaller proportion of CVPN located within the DVN activated by stimulation of pulmonary C-fibers but unaffected by stimulation of arterial baroreceptors or the respiratory cycle (12). These neurons show regular activity but this is not rhythmic, and their efferent axons supplying the heart lack myelin sheaths so have slow conduction rates, classifying them as C-fibers. They have relatively minor, slowly developing effects on heart rate that may provide tonic control of routine f_H (12). So there are two functionally different populations of CVPN in the mammalian brainstem, identified by their different locations, afferent connections, efferent activity, and the conduction velocity of their efferent axons (12–14). The control they exercise over f_H and HRV arises late in embryogenesis. Accordingly, monitoring f_H can indicate healthy development of the central nervous system (CNS), a valuable diagnostic tool for obstetricians (see below).

DOI: 10.1201/9780367494018-8

The following factors contribute to RSA in mammals:

1. **CVPN in two major locations in the brainstem**, the DVN and the NA, having different afferent connections and generating very different efferent activities.
2. Central communication between CVPN in the NA and inspiratory neurons in the ventral respiratory group, generating respiration-related activity (RRA) in the CVPN by **feed-forward control**.
3. Activation of pulmonary stretch receptor stimulation during ventilation providing **feedback control**, gating the baroreceptor response.
4. **Modulation of respiratory activity** from the effects on chemoreceptors of changes in the respiratory gases, CO_2, and O_2.
5. **Rapid conduction** (3–15 m/s) of efferent activity along the myelinated axons of CVPN within the NA, (B-fibers) exerting instantaneous, beat-to-beat control of the heart.
6. **Mechanical effects** on the heart and associated blood vessels due to ventilatory movements of the thoracic cavity, which can also stimulate mechanoreceptors.

Phylogeny

Fish

Vertebrates evolved as fish, breathing water, which is much more viscous and dense than air, limiting the diffusion rates and solubility of gases. Fish sustain oxygen uptake with a counter-current flow of blood and water over the gills with rates of flow matched according to their oxygen capacity (15, 16). Both flows are pulsatile (15, 17) and cardiorespiratory coupling (CRC) has been demonstrated by power spectral analysis of cardiac intervals (18, 19). Its abolition by cardiac vagotomy reduced oxygen uptake (20). The physiological basis of respiration-related changes in f_H varies between the major groups of fishes. In bony fishes (class Teleostei), CRC is under reflex, feedback control following stimulation of chemoreceptors by mild hypoxia. This generates an increase in ventilatory effort plus a reflex bradycardia that matches f_H to ventilation rate (15, 21, 22). It is termed the primary response and is opposite in kind to the 'secondary response', a hypoxic tachycardia, shown by mammals (23), though their fetus retains the primary response (see below). In cartilaginous fishes (sharks and rays; class Chondrichthyes), the heart is not innervated by the sympathetic arm of the ANS, so operates solely under an inhibitory vagal tonus (1, 15). Efferent activity recorded from a cardiac branch of the vagus in a catshark, *Scyliorhius canicula*, showed larger units that fired with RRA plus smaller units that were less active but responded to hypoxia (24). They showed CRC in normoxia, generated by central feed-forward control from CVPN, traced to two locations (15). Activity recorded centrally from these CVPN characterized them as: (1) CVPN in the DVN, where they are mixed with respiratory motor neurons (RMN) and showed RRA, generating CRC; (2) an isolated group of CVPN located outside of the DVN that showed low levels of activity, increasing during hypoxia, to generate a bradycardia. These are opposite in both location and function to the mammalian CVPN, but in both animals one cell group interacts with neighboring RMN to generate RRA, characterized as CRC in the catshark and as RSA in the mammal. The cardiac branches of the vagus in the catshark contain myelinated fibers and have conduction velocities

similar to B-fibers in mammals, enabling this efferent, RRA to drive the heart on a beat-to-beat basis, generating CRC (2, 15). Physical stimulation of gill arches caused activity in both groups of CVPN, with a resultant marked bradycardia, identifying a role for mechanoreceptors in reflex control of f_H. This is opposite in kind to the mammalian response to stimulation of lung stretch receptors, which causes an increase in f_H, recognized as part what separates the primary and secondary responses to hypoxia.

Air-breathing fish

The aquatic environment is prone to hypoxia, particularly in tropical habitats. In response, many fish species resort to air-breathing (AB), using a wide range of different air-breathing organs (ABO) in the buccal cavity or as extensions of the gut. Surfacing is accompanied by a tachycardia (25–28) causing increased perfusion of the ABO. These changes in f_H are considered a homologue of RSA in mammals (26, 28). This increase in f_H is a response to stimulation of stretch receptors in the ABO plus central chemoreceptors leading to release of an inhibitory vagal tonus on the heart (25), as is the case for mammals (1). The true 'lungfish' (class Dipnoi) evolved along with primitive tetrapods in the Devonian era. They show regular surfacing behavior, accompanied by instantaneous increases in f_H. Power spectral analysis characterized this as RSA, supported by CVPN in multiple locations in the brainstem plus vagal efferent fibers with myelin sheaths having conduction velocities typical of mammalian B-fibers (28).

Amphibians and reptiles

Unlike mammals, the amphibians and most reptiles have an incompletely divided ventricle, with blood flow from the heart to the systemic and pulmonary circuits controlled independently (3, 29). They breathe sporadically, with the onset of each bout of breathing, particularly after a dive, accompanied by an immediate increase in f_H and pulmonary blood flow (Q_{pul}), which is primarily due to a release of vagal tone on the heart and pulmonary artery (3). Although oscillations in blood gases (PaO_2 and $PaCO_2$) and/or pH drive these breathing patterns, the immediate increases in f_H and pulmonary blood flow at the onset of each bout of breathing suggests central interactions (29, 31). Anatomical evidence indicates a close proximity of the centers responsible for respiratory rhythmogenesis and the vagal motoneurons involved in cardiovascular regulation in both amphibians (29) and reptiles (30), while physiological studies indicate the importance of central interactions (31). The immediate effect may be due to inhibition of CVPN, releasing an inhibitory vagal tonus on the heart, as described in mammalian RSA, though the resultant increase is maintained throughout the period of ventilation. The adult, amphibious bullfrog, *Lithobates catesbeianus*, has an inhibitory vagal tone on the heart of only around 10% (2). This may relate to the concentration of all its VPN into the DVN with no trace of a ventro-lateral 'NA'. This is in marked contrast to the high levels of cardiac vagal tone on the heart of the aquatic toad, *Xenopus laevis*, which varies from 80% at 5°C to 320% at 25°C (2). *Xenopus* has a clearly demarked group of VPN, including CVPN, outside of the DVN that contains about 30% of cell bodies, constituting an amphibian NA (29). It shows marked and rapidly developed changes in f_H when surfacing after periods of submersion. Turtles and tortoises (primitive anapsids) have a large proportion of VPN (40–50%) in ventro-lateral nuclei that could form an equivalent of the NA (2, 32). In the South American caiman, *Caiman latirostris* (a primitive crocodilian), the majority of VPNs are in the DVN, but there is a discrete lateral cell group outside the DVN containing about 12% of VPNs and designated as the NA (33). Both groups show marked, rapidly developed tachycardias on surfacing from a dive. In the more recently evolved squamate reptiles (lizards and snakes), a relatively sparse distribution of VPNs outside of the DVN seems to be the rule (34). In the rattlesnake, *Crotalus durissus*, 95% of VPNs are in the DVN, while ~4% of VPNs are located in scattered ventrolateral locations outside the DVN (35). Despite the lack of a discrete NA, the rattlesnake displayed a clear, high-frequency component in the power spectrum of HRV that was respiration-related, developed at low f_H and was abolished by atropine (35). Remotely monitored snakes with low settled f_H showed clear respiration-related HRV, which was supported by myelinated efferent fibers in the vagus nerve, and was accordingly designated as reptilian RSA (36). Whether this relationship is generated centrally or as a result of peripheral reflexes has not been determined. Afferent activity, associated with stimulation of lung stretch receptors, has been recorded from the vagus nerve in rattlesnakes. However, this does not rule out a role for central interactions in the generation of respiration-related HRV.

Birds

Birds evolved endothermy from their reptilian ancestors separately from mammals. Like mammals they breathe continuously and rhythmically, to supply their high metabolic rate. They lack a diaphragm and through ventilate the lungs into air sacs (37). Lung stretch receptors have been identified in lungfish, amphibians, reptiles, and mammals but not in birds, which possess intrapulmonary chemoreceptors sensitive to CO_2 (37). The respiratory rhythm in birds arises from a Central Pattern Generator (CPG) in the medulla that generates activity driving respiratory muscles, as seen in mammals. Cardiac vagal tone predominates in control of the heart (2), with bilateral vagotomy causing a tripling of heart rate in the pigeon and duck. In the duck, VPNs are located predominantly in the DVN with only 3% of cell bodies in the NA, though 30% of CVPN are in this location, suggesting that they may have a central role in generating HRV (33). Clear indications of respiration-related oscillations in heart rate, similar to mammalian RSA, were recorded in spontaneously breathing ducks. The peak accelerations in heart rate were eliminated during induced apnea (38), implying that cardio-inhibitory activity from CVPNs is modulated by respiration, as described in mammals (see above). Respiration-related HRV, recorded remotely from shearwaters, *Calonectris leucomelas*, using ECG dataloggers, revealed clear high-frequency peaks in the power spectrum at a frequency which matched the respiratory rate (39). Injection of antagonists to the ANS revealed that control of HRV was predominantly from the parasympathetic arm, as described for mammalian RSA. There is clear evidence of myelination of the vagus nerve in birds and HRV has been attributed to fast-conducting myelinated vagal nerves (2).

Ontogeny

Fish

A beating heart appears early in development in all vertebrate embryos, even in fish when diffusion over the surface of the egg from the surrounding water would still provide sufficient oxygen to maintain aerobic metabolism. There is a progressive rise in f_H throughout embryogenesis, linked to increasing levels of circulating catecholamines and the early appearance of β-adrenergic

receptors on the heart. This is followed by a decline immediately prior to hatching (40) that signals the onset of neural control of f_H from the parasympathetic arm of the ANS, which becomes effective at hatching (2, 41). These patterns are reflected in the development of embryos from all other groups of vertebrates (amphibians: 42; reptiles, 43; birds, 44; mammals, 45). The late onset of parasympathetic control of the heart is an important part of the preparation for hatching or birth so that measuring HRV is a vital part of monitoring progress of the embryo or fetus.

Amphibians

Amphibian embryos hatch as gill-bearing, water-breathing larvae then metamorphose into lung and skin-breathing adults, providing models for examining the ontogenetic changes that occur in the CNS during the transition from aquatic to aerial breathing. Larval 'tadpoles' of the bullfrog *Lithobates catesbeianus* have β-adrenergic receptors on the heart immediately after hatching with cholinergic tone appearing later then lost at metamorphosis (42). In the neotenous axolotl, *Ambystoma mexicanum*, which retains larval features, including gills for water breathing, into adult life, efferent axons in the vagus nerve, some of which innervate the heart, arise solely from VPN in the DVN. After induced metamorphosis, with loss of the gills and a switch to lung breathing, the number of labeled VPN doubled, with 15% of them relocated into a ventro-lateral amphibian NA. The levels of HRV increase, indicating induction of an amphibian 'RSA' (33).

Reptiles

Many reptiles are oviparous, with shelled eggs laid on land. Cholinergic receptor-mediated regulation is absent until the time of hatching (43). Alligator embryos lack central nervous control of f_H in response to hypoxia but do exhibit a vagally mediate hypertensive baroreflex response during the final 30% of ontogeny. The hypotensive baroreflex was absent in embryos but appeared in hatchlings (2, 46). In green iguanas, *Iguana iguana*, both β-adrenergic and muscarinic cholinoceptors are present on the heart from 10% of incubation time, though the onset of a cardiac vagal tonus was delayed until immediately before hatching (47). In an early embryo of the green iguana, VPN were restricted to a discrete DVN close to the fourth ventricle (Taylor and Sartori unpublished observation), while in juveniles VPN were located both in the DVN and in a lateral nucleus. The establishment of a cholinergic cardiac tonus at hatching may be correlated with the onset of central respiratory rhythmicity and active ventilation (2). The importance of migration of CVPN into a reptilian NA is likely to relate to the switch to the CPG for air-breathing at the time of hatching.

Birds

Although cardiac muscarinic and adrenergic receptors are found in embryonic birds during the first quarter of incubation, the inhibitory vagal control of f_H is absent until close to hatching (2). A high-frequency oscillation appearing immediately prior to the onset of air breathing was identified as RSA (48) and was associated with external 'pipping' (the process of breaking through the egg shell during hatching) (49). Spectral analysis of HRV revealed that this avian RSA was mediated by the parasympathetic system (50). The separation of VPNs to form the NA arises by ventro-lateral migration from the DVN during embryological development, as described in the cat (51).

The human fetus

The fetal heartbeat can be audibly detected from about 24 to 26 weeks onwards and from 6 weeks using ultrasound. There is a gradual fall in baseline rate from about 14 weeks gestation, thought to be due to increasing parasympathetic (vagal) tone. Animal and human studies (6, 52, 53) indicate parasympathetic dominance, producing a slower rate than the spontaneous depolarization rate of the sino-atrial (SA) cells. In later pregnancy, as the fetus matures, activity of higher brain centers also influence fetal heart rate (FHR).

Raised base heart rate and decelerations have long been linked with fetal compromise. Cardio-tocography (CTG) records FHR and uterine activity simultaneously, allowing additional parameters such as short-term variability and patterns of deceleration and acceleration to be taken into consideration. In response to hypoxia, the fetus can only decrease demand by producing a reflex bradycardia, i.e. the 'primary response', a vagally mediated mechanism (see above). On intra-partum CTG, this response is recognized as 'early' or 'V-shaped' decelerations with a normal base rate and good STV. 'Late' or 'U-shaped' decelerations are associated with chronic hypoxia and developing acidemia (54), causing direct effects upon the heart. A concomitant rise in base rate and reduced STV are consistent with a loss of vagal tone and catecholamine release with a worsening prognosis. Monitoring STV is important as it represents rapidly acting control systems responding to central and peripheral inputs. Furthermore, it carries useful physiological information but to appreciate this requires more than 'eyeballing' patterns. An ability to separate the components of STV (see above), particularly those that reflect the functional integrity of the CNS, represents an important advance. Respiratory sinus arrhythmia (RSA) meets these requirements as it is a mechanism that matches lung ventilation with perfusion so can act to maximize respiratory effectiveness at critical times. The existence of RSA in the human fetus is well recorded (55–58).

Exploration of RSA in the fetus can be facilitated by induction of fetal breathing movements (FBM), which, in the healthy fetus are accompanied by RSA. Human FBM can be detected simply by observing the maternal abdomen in the later weeks of pregnancy but can be done much earlier and more reliably using ultrasound. FBM is diaphragmatic and sporadic. Perhaps it plays a part in stimulating growth of the lungs and in developing the respiratory musculature in readiness for the sudden transformation to air breathing in the immediate neonatal period. Clearly, FBM play no part in gas exchange. Their presence reflects an intact system linking the respiratory center in the CNS, the phrenic neural efferents, and the diaphragm. Integrity of the fetal brain cortex is not essential to the generation of FBM, and they have been reported in anencephalic fetuses (59), but destruction of the forebrain in fetal sheep abolishes FBM (60). Acute fetal hypoxia diminishes FBM (61, 62), but prolonged hypoxia sees the fetus adjust with return of FBM within 3–16 hours (63).

FBM driven by the respiratory center produce little change in intra-thoracic pressure since the lungs are fluid-filled and not inflated. Vagotomy, to eliminate pulmonary stretch receptors, has little impact on FBM (64), demonstrating that lung stretch receptor activity is minimal or absent and does not modulate heart rate. Accordingly, fetal RSA is generated solely by feed-forward control from central interactions between CVPN innervating the heart and the respiratory center. Depression of the respiratory center by general anesthesia abolished RSA (65). Groome et al.

identified a high-frequency peak in the fetal HRV spectrum on occasions when no FBM could be detected, though this need not rule out the presence of central respiratory activity (58).

In gestations less than 24 weeks, FBM tend to be highly irregular in both rate and amplitude and a variety of patterns is seen (64). The episodes, their rate, and amplitude tend to become more regular as gestation progresses. Beyond 34 weeks, episodes of regular FBM activity occur. This coincides reasonably closely with the development of RSA seen in 'healthy' premature neonates (7). In later pregnancy, FBMs are linked to fetal behavioral state (66, 67). These observations reflect maturation and developing integration of the CNS.

Brown et al. demonstrated that the high-frequency heart rate oscillations (RSAs) are directly associated with FBM and occur at the same frequency (68). A commercially available continuous wave Doppler machine was used to record blood flow in the fetal descending aorta. This detected both FBM and FHR accurately enough to perform auto-regressive spectral analysis to identify RSA in the antenatal period. Purpose-built transducers would improve sampling rate and increase resolution of the apparatus. Thus, RSA is demonstrable in the healthy human fetus in the later weeks of pregnancy using a safe, noninvasive method. The presence of RSA under these circumstances indicates an intact and functioning CNS able to integrate the respiratory center with vagal cardio-motor efferents. However, its application to fetal monitoring in labor proved problematic, since contractions make it difficult to maintain accurate positioning of the transducer to obtain a stable signal. Healthy, term neonates born after showing RSA are likely to experience normal outcomes, whereas those failing to show RSA in the latter stages of fetal development may be compromised (69) and show long-term incapacities (70).

References

1. Taylor EW, et al. Physiol Rev. 1999; 79(3):855–916.
2. Taylor EW, et al. J. Exp. Biol. 2014; 217:690–703.
3. Taylor EW, et al. In: *Cardio-respiratory control in vertebrates.* Glass ML, Wood SC, eds. Heidelberg: Springer Nature; 2009. p. 285–315.
4. Bootsma M, et al. Am J Physiol. 1994; 266:H1565–H1571.
5. Akselrod S, et al. Science. 1981; 213:220–222.
6. Akselrod S, et al. Am J Physiol. 1985; 249:H867–75.
7. Thompson CR, et al. Early Hum Dev. 1993; 31(3):217–28.
8. Grossman P, et al. Biol Psychol. 2007; 74:263.
9. Jordan D, et al. In: *neurogenesis of Central respiratory rhythm.* Lancaster: MTP Press; 1985. p. 370–378.
10. Spyer KM, In : *Central regulation of autonomic functions*, New York, Oxford University Press; 1990. p. 168–188.
11. Jordan D. In: In *cardiovascular regulation.* Jordan D, Marshall JM, eds. London: Portland Press; 1995. p. 1–14.
12. Jones JF, et al. J Physiol. 1995; 489:203–214.
13. Daly MB, et al. J Physiol. 1989; 417:323–341.
14. Jones JF. Exp Physiol. 2001; 86(6):797–801.
15. Taylor EW In: *Fish physiology* Vol. 12B. New York NY: Academic Press; 1992. p. 343.
16. Milsom WK, et al. In: *Physiology of elasmobranch fishes: B internal processes.* New York NY: Academic Press; 2016.
17. Piiper J, et al. Int Rev Physiol. 1977; 14:219–253.
18. Campbell HA, et al. J Exp Biol. 2004; 207(Pt 11):1969–1976.
19. Taylor EW, et al. Physiol Biochem Zool. 2006; 79(6):1000–1009.
20. Campbell HA, et al. J Exp Biol. 2007; 210:2472–2480.
21. Taylor EW, et al. J Exp Biol. 2009; 212:906–913.
22. Leite CAC, et al. J Comp Physiol A Neuroethol Sens Neural Behav Physiol. 2009; 195(8):721–731.
23. Daly MB, et al. J Physiol. 1958; 144:148–166.
24. Taylor EW, et al. J Appl Physiol. 1982; 53:1330–1335.
25. Graham JB. *Air-breathing fishes: evolution, diversity, and adaptation.* San Diego: Academic Press; 1997.
26. McKenzie DJ, et al. J Exp Biol. 2007; 210:4224–4232.
27. McKenzie DJ, et al. J Exp Biol. 2012; 215:1323–1330.
28. Monteiro DA, et al. Sci Adv. 2018; 4(2):eaaq0800.
29. Wang T, et al. Comp Biochem Physiol A Mol Integr Physiol. 1999; 124(4):393–406.
30. Filogonio R, et al. Am J Physiol Regul Integr Comp Physiol. 2020; 319(2):R156–R170.
31. Wang T, et al. Respir Physiol Neurobiol. 2004; 140:63–76.

32. Leong SK, et al. J Autono. Nerv Syst. 1984; 11:373–382.
33. Taylor EW, et al. Exp Physiol. 2001; 86(6):771–776.
34. Duran LM, et al. Comp Biochem Physiol A Mol Integr Physiol. 2020; 240:110607.
35. Campbell HA, et al. J Exp Biol. 2006; 209:2628.
36. Sanches PVW, et al. J Exp Biol. 2019; 222(Pt 9):jeb197954.
37. Schied P, et al. In: *Handbook of physiology. The respiratory system. control of breathing.* Bethesda, MD: Am Physiol Soc. 1986; sect.3, 2(3):815–832.
38. Butler PJ, et al. Respir Physiol. 1983; 53:109–127.
39. Carravieri A, et al. Physiol. Biochem. 2016; DOI: 10.1086/686894.
40. Rombough P In: *Cardiovascular development: from molecules to organisms.* New York NY: Cambridge University Press; 1997. p. 145.
41. Miller SC, et al. J Exp Biol. 2011; 214(Pt 12):2065–72.
42. Burggren WW In: *Mechanisms of systemic regulation. Respiration and circulation.* Berlin: Springer-Verlag; 1995. p. 175–197.
43. Birchard GF, et al. J Comp Physiol B. 1996; 166(8):461–466.
44. Crossley DA, et al. Am J Physiol. 2000; 279:R1091–R1098.
45. Peleg D, et al. J Clin Endocrinol Metab. 1986; 62(5):911–914.
46. Crossley DA, et al. J Exp Biol. 2005; 208:31–39.
47. Sartori MR, et al. Comp Biochem Physiol A Mol Integr Physiol. 2015; 188:1–8.
48. Moriya K, et al. Comp Biochem Physiol A Mol Integr Physiol. 1999; 124(4):461–8.
49. Tazawa H, et al. Comp Biochem Physiol A Mol Integr Physiol. 1999; 124(4):511–21.
50. Shah R, et al. Poult Sci. 2010; 89(1):135–144.
51. Windle WF. J Comp. Neurol. 1933; 58:643–723.
52. Pomeranz B, et al. Am J Physiol. 1985; 248(1 Pt 2):H151–H153.
53. Pagani M, et al. Circ Res. 1986; 59:178–193.
54. Cahill A, et al. Am J Obstet Gynecol Suppl. 2016; 214(1):S194–S195.
55. Dawes GS, et al. Am J Obstet Gynecol. 1981; 140(5):535–44.
56. Divon MY, et al. Am J Obstet Gynecol. 1985; 151(4):425–8.
57. Cerutti S, et al. Clin Phys Physiol Meas. 1989; 10 Suppl B:27–31.
58. Groome LJ, et al. Early Hum Dev. 1994; 38(1):1–9.
59. Manning FA. Postgrad Med J 1977; 61:116.–22.
60. Robinson JS, et al. Am J Obstet Gynecol. 1980; 137:729–34.
61. Boddy K, et al. J Physiol. 1974; 243:599–618.
62. Koos BJ, et al. J Appl Physiol. 1987; 62(3):1033–9.
63. Bocking AD, et al. J Appl Physiol. 1988; 65:2420–6.
64. Boddy K, et al. Br Med Bull. 1975; 31(1):3–7.
65. Joels N, et al. J Physiol. 1956; 133(2):360–72.
66. Nijhuis JG, et al. Early Hum Dev. 1983; 9(1):1–7.
67. Kozuma S, et al. Biol Neonate. 1991; 60 Suppl 1:36–40
68. Brown JS, et al. J Biomed Eng. 1992; 14:263–7.
69. Thompson CR, et al. 2021 (in preparation).
70. Doussard-Roosevelt JA, et al. Child Dev. 1997; 68(2):173–86.

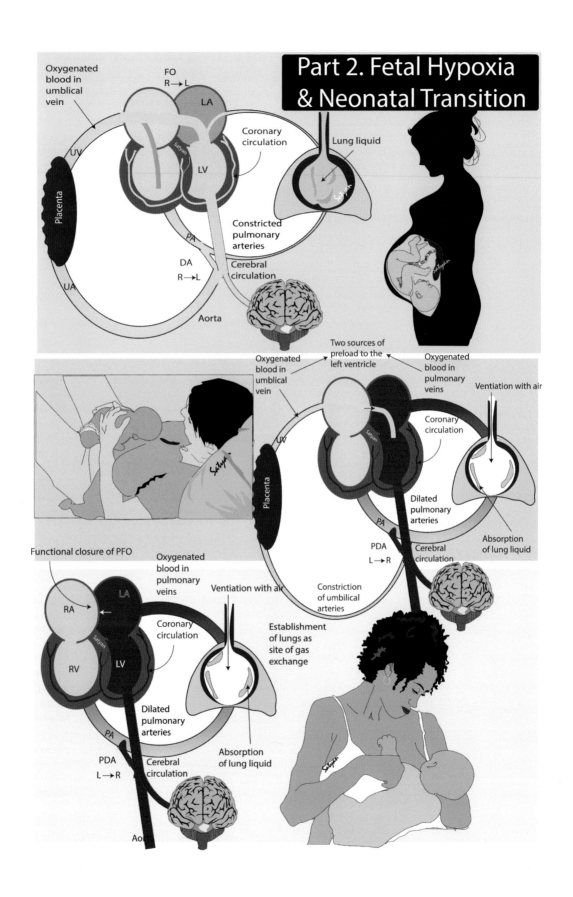

Part 2. Fetal Hypoxia & Neonatal Transition

Part 2
Fetal Hypoxia and Neonatal Transition

Edited by Satyan Lakshminrusimha

FETAL AND NEONATAL OXYGEN ENVIRONMENT

Payam Vali, Robin H. Steinhorn and
Satyan Lakshminrusimha

Contents

Introduction

The fetal environment and circulatory patterns are very different from that of extrauterine life. The fetus has evolved to thrive and grow in a relative hypoxemic environment and has adapted several mechanisms in response to changes in oxygen concentration in the blood to ensure optimal oxygen delivery to the brain and heart. The fetus's predominant oxygen carrying molecule, the hemoglobin, also differs to that of the older infant and adult for its significantly higher oxygen-carrying capacity. The presence of complex congenital heart lesions can result in alterations of fetal circulation that can have severe consequences on the developing fetal brain and heart, which can present as life threatening defects during the transition from the fetal to postnatal circulation. In this chapter, we will review the fetal circulation, the effect of oxygen on fetal pulmonary and cerebral blood flow, the role of fetal hemoglobin in oxygen delivery, and explore maternal hyperoxygenation as a therapy to improve fetal well-being in the presence of congenital heart defects (CHDs) or as a tool to risk stratify fetuses with CHD.

Fetal circulation

Remarkable observations made by Sabatier and Wolff in the late 18th century suggested that the higher oxygenated blood from the umbilical vein is preferentially directed to the ascending aorta to supply the heart and brain (1). This hypothesis was later confirmed studying the fetal circulation in lambs with the introduction of the radionuclide-labeled microsphere technique (2) and recently validated by fetal human and lamb studies using blood T2 magnetic resonance imaging (MRI) relaxometry (3).

The total venous return to the fetal heart is made up from blood coming back from the inferior vena cava (IVC), the superior vena cava (SVC), the pulmonary veins, and the myocardium (Figure 9.1). The IVC contributes to most of the venous return, representing approximately 50% of the cardiac output. Blood entering the heart from the SVC makes up approximately 30%, while the pulmonary veins add 15–20% and, finally, as little as 3% comes from the coronary sinus (4, 5).

Approximately two-thirds of the IVC flow is provided by the umbilical vein (UV) with the rest made up by blood draining from the lower body and the liver (6). Blood from the hepatic veins rejoins blood from the ductus venosus and enters the

thoracic IVC. The thoracic IVC contains two streams of blood: a stream of well oxygenated blood emerging from the left liver and ductus venosus and another stream of less oxygenated blood from the right liver and abdominal portion of the IVC (7). The richer oxygenated blood from the thoracic IVC (O_2 saturation [SO_2] ≈70%) is preferentially diverted by the crista dividens into the left atrium through the foramen ovale (where it mixes with the poorly oxygenated blood returning from the pulmonary veins), and then into the left ventricle through the mitral valve. Thus, the higher oxygenated UV blood (SO_2 80%) streams to the left atrium and is ultimately pumped out of the left ventricle guaranteeing the highest oxygen delivery to the heart and brain (preductal aorta SO_2 ≈58 – 65%). The lower oxygenated blood from the SVC and IVC entering the right ventricle (through the right atrium) pumped into the pulmonary artery (SO_2 ≈50%) is mostly diverted through the ductus arteriosus to supply the lower body and nonessential organs. The difference in SO_2 of fetal oxygen supply (UV) and return (umbilical artery) in fetal sheep is ≈30%, whereas the arterio-venous difference across the fetal cerebral circulation is ≈25% (7). Blood T2 MRI relaxometry studies have recently estimated the magnitude of streaming in the human fetal circulation by demonstrating an SO_2 gradient between the ascending aorta (68 ± 10%) and the main pulmonary artery (49 ± 9%; P < 0.001) (3). The differences in SO_2 between major vessel pairs (UV-descending aorta [≈30%] and UV-ascending aorta [≈20%]) within the human and sheep fetus were similar (3).

In utero, the fetus has limited breathing movements, decreased muscle activity and does not expend significant energy to maintain thermoregulation. The fetus can, therefore, thrive in a hypoxemic environment and several protective mechanisms maintain the fetus in such a state. When maternal ewes are exposed to 100% oxygen, the partial pressure of arterial oxygen (PaO_2) rises from a baseline of ≈100 mm Hg in room-air to > 400 mm Hg, whereas the UV PaO_2 (25–35 mm Hg) supplying the fetus only increases to 40–50 mm Hg; (7) the placenta, therefore, serving as the major barrier to hyperoxic injury to the fetus. In addition, the small rise in fetal oxygen tension results in an increase in pulmonary blood flow that leads to a greater proportion of de-oxygenated blood returning from the pulmonary veins, ultimately, into the left ventricle, thus, further limiting a substantial increase in the aortic saturation and, effectively, reducing oxygen toxicity to the vital organs (5).

DOI: 10.1201/9780367494018-9

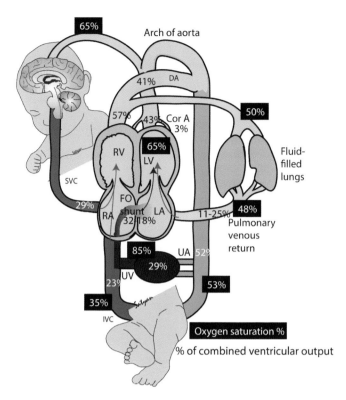

FIGURE 9.1 Fetal circulation. Circulatory pattern in a normal human fetus at late gestation. The numbers shown as percents in italics represent percentage of combined ventricular output based on data from human fetuses. The numbers in *dark boxes* represent oxygen saturation based on data from fetal lambs. *Blue shade* indicates lower oxygen saturation. Cor A, coronary arteries; DA, ductus arteriosus; FO, foramen ovale; IVC, inferior vena cava; LA, left atrium; LV, left ventricle; RA, right atrium; RV, right ventricle; SVC, superior vena cava; UA, umbilical arteries; UV, umbilical vein. (Modified from Lakshminrusimha and Steinhorn, Polin and Fox. *Fetal and Neonatal Physiology* 5th ed. Copyright Satyan Lakshminrusimha.)

Fetal pulmonary vascular resistance, cerebral circulation, and the effects of oxygen

The placenta functions as the organ of gas exchange during gestation and the mammalian fetus has evolved to divert blood away from the lungs by maintaining a high pulmonary vascular resistance (PVR). The thick muscular coat and cuboidal endothelium of the fetal pulmonary arteries contribute to the elevated PVR (8, 9). Mechanical factors (fluid-filled alveoli compressing the pulmonary arterioles), (10) and the interaction of vasodilator (e.g. prostacyclin and endothelium-derived nitric oxide) and vasoconstrictor (e.g. endothelin-1 and thromboxane) mediators on the pulmonary artery smooth muscles cells (11) account for other factors responsible in maintaining PVR high during fetal growth.

The volume of blood entering the pulmonary circulation is dynamic and changes during fetal development. During the canalicular stage of lung development (16–24 weeks gestation), the pulmonary circulation receives ≈13% of the cardiac output because the cross-sectional pulmonary vasculature is low, maintaining a higher PVR. In the saccular stage (25–36 weeks gestation), pulmonary vessels proliferate, which causes a drop in PVR and a peak pulmonary blood flow that reaches 25–30% of cardiac output. Finally, at near term gestation, fetal pulmonary vessels

develop greater sensitivity to oxygen with resultant pulmonary vasoconstriction and a reduction of fetal pulmonary blood flow to ≈16–21% of cardiac output (4, 7, 12, 13).

In sheep experiments ventilated with a fraction of inspired oxygen of 0.06, no change in PVR was demonstrated in response to fetal hypoxemia at 100 days (0.7 gestation), whereas fetal lambs at 0.9 gestation (132–138 days) saw their PVR double (14). The changes in PVR in response to an increase in fetal blood oxygen tension follow a similar pattern. Fetal lambs at 94–101 days (0.6–0.7 gestation) do not experience a meaningful difference in PVR when the maternal sheep is exposed to high oxygen concentrations, whereas a significant drop in PVR is observed in fetal lambs that are 135 days (0.9 gestation) (15, 16). Comparably, when providing 60% oxygen by face mask to pregnant woman at 20–26 weeks gestation no change in fetal pulmonary blood flow was appreciated, but pulmonary blood flow increased by a mean of almost 25% in fetuses at 31–36 weeks gestation (17).

The pulmonary circulation helps to maintain cerebral oxygen delivery within a narrow range by redirecting the pulmonary and systemic blood flows by altering the amount of blood shunting through the foramen ovale and ductus arteriosus. Following supraphysiologic oxygen concentrations in pregnant ewes, the relative small increase in oxygen saturation in the fetal ascending aorta can be explained by (1) reduction in oxygen uptake from the placenta owing to diversion of blood from the terminal villi to secondary and stem villi, (2) redistribution of blood to the left and right liver lobes owing to constriction of the ductus venosus (18), and (3) higher fetal blood oxygen content decreasing PVR and increasing pulmonary blood flow (19), thus causing more desaturated blood to return from the pulmonary veins into the left atrium, effectively buffering the oxygen saturation in the left ventricle. An increase in pulmonary venous return also leads to higher left atrial pressure and less oxygenated blood from the UV streaming into the left atrium. Furthermore, cerebral blood flow is very sensitive to oxygen. Ventilation of fetal lambs with a 100% oxygen reduced cerebral blood flow by over 30% as measured by the radionuclide-labeled microsphere technique (20). Conversely, fetal hypoxemia increases PVR, reduces pulmonary venous return, lowering left atrial pressure, and facilitating oxygen-rich blood from the UV to enter the left atrium through the foramen ovale, thereby maximizing oxygen delivery to the brain. In addition, reducing the PO_2 down to 12 mm Hg in fetal sheep by providing low oxygen gas mixtures to the pregnant ewes caused a two to threefold increase in fetal cerebral blood flow (21).

Role of fetal hemoglobin in oxygen delivery

Erythropoiesis begins in the fetal liver at approximately six weeks gestation and serves as the major site of red blood cell production until the third trimester when the bone marrow takes over. The hemoglobin (Hb) in erythrocytes functions to carry oxygen to the tissues and is determined by the amino acid configuration of the globin chains. Hemoglobin F (HbF) contains two alpha and two gamma chains ($\alpha_2\gamma_2$), which predominates in the fetal circulation. Hemoglobin A (HbA) is made up by two alpha and two beta chains ($\alpha_2\beta_2$) and becomes the predominant Hb, six months after birth. The conformation of Hb changes depending if it is in the deoxygenated state (T or tense form) or oxygenated state (R or relaxed form). Once oxygen binds to the globin chains, an alteration in its configuration facilitates further oxygen binding and as oxygen is released from Hb, a change in configuration toward the tense state enables unloading of oxygen (22). This property of Hb to change its structure promotes the loading and unloading of oxygen. In addition, the affinity of oxygen to bind Hb depends on the partial pressure of oxygen (PO_2) in the blood. At high PO_2 (eg the intervillous space of the placenta for the fetus or the lungs in postnatal life), as Hb accepts oxygen, it becomes progressively easier for the next heme group of the molecule to pick up oxygen and become fully saturated. Conversely, at the level of the tissue, unloading of oxygen shifts the Hb to the R state, which enables more oxygen release. This relationship can be better appreciated when plotting PO_2 against oxyhemoglobin saturation–revealing the characteristic sigmoidal oxyhemoglobin dissociation curve.

HbF has a higher oxygen affinity compared to HbA and is therefore represented by a leftward shift on the Hb dissociation equilibrium. HbF is saturated at 50% (P50) at a PO_2 of approximately 19 mm Hg compared to HbA, which has a P50 of 27 mm Hg (23). In the intervillous space of the placenta, because of the relatively low PO_2 at which transfer of oxygen is achieved, the higher affinity of HbF favors oxygen uptake in the fetus. Other important factors that affect Hb oxygen affinity include the effect of temperature, pH, and partial pressure of carbon dioxide (CO_2) and the concentration of organic phosphates, particularly 2,3-diphosphoglycerate (2,3-DPG). 2,3-DPG acts as an allosteric regulator and binds with the deoxy form of HbA between the two beta chains, effectively decreasing Hb oxygen affinity and shifting the dissociation curve to the right (24). 2,3-DBG has a diminished effect on HbF. The advantage of greater oxygen affinity of HbF lies in its ability to become nearly saturated at relatively low blood oxygen tensions. The possible disadvantage in oxygen delivery to fetal tissues is offset by the steep HbF dissociation, so that a small decrease in oxygen tension results in a major fall in oxyhemoglobin saturation and unloading of oxygen to the tissues. In the adult, a decrease in PO_2 from 100 mm Hg (in arterial blood), which lies on the flat portion of the dissociation curve, to 40 mm Hg (in venous blood) results in a release of oxygen amounting to approximately 5 mL/dL. For the fetus, the difference between the umbilical venous PO_2 (35 mm Hg) and the umbilical arterial PO_2 (25 mm Hg), with both values falling on the linear portion of the dissociation curve, results in a similar release of oxygen to the tissues of 4 mL/dL (7). Despite its affinity for oxygen, during periods of severe hypoxemia, HbF may better maintain oxygen delivery compared to HbA (25). Rapid postnatal decline in HbF in extremely preterm infants has been associated with morbidities such as bronchopulmonary dysplasia (BPD) (26).

Maternal hyperoxia

Maternal oxygen therapy for fetal heart disease

Maternal oxygen administration resulting in a rise in fetal blood oxygen tension has been demonstrated over six decades ago (27) and remains common practice to this day in an attempt to lessen fetal distress during labor, while existing evidence does not suggest effectiveness of this approach on perinatal outcome (28) (Figure 9.2). A plausible link between alterations in fetal oxygen delivery and aberrant brain growth in fetuses with severe CHD has led to a newfound interest, in recent years, to study maternal hyperoxygenation as a potential therapy to enhance cardiac flow and promote left ventricular development in certain types of CHD or as a tool to facilitate perinatal risk stratification for fetuses with CHD.

At the turn of the century, evidence emerged that approximately 20% of infants with complex CHD demonstrate white

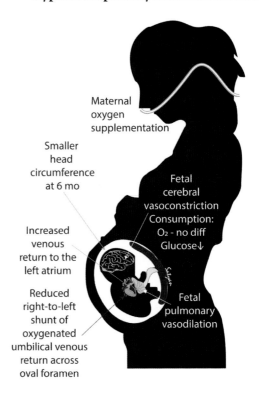

FIGURE 9.2 Summary of results from maternal oxygenation studies for fetal congenital heart disease. Oxygen supplementation in the mother can cause fetal pulmonary vasodilation and increased pulmonary venous return to the left atrium. Concerns about reduced right-to-left oval foramen shunt and cerebral vasoconstriction and its effect on brain growth require further evaluation. (Copyright Satyan Lakshminrusimha.)

matter injury before surgery (29). Soon thereafter, studies using magnetic resonance imaging (MRI) showed significant differences in white matter microstructure between infants with CHD compared to healthy newborns (30). Brain maturity of term infants with CHD has been shown to be equivalent to 35-week gestation premature brains (31), and evaluation by quantitative MRI revealed that brain volumes in fetuses with CHD diverge from expected normal during the third trimester (32). A recent study measuring cerebral oxygen consumption using phase-contrast MRI in fetuses with severe CHD and normal controls has shown an association between reduced fetal cerebral oxygen consumption with impaired brain growth, raising the possibility that cerebral development could be improved by maternal oxygen therapy (33).

Experiments in fetal lambs have shown that reducing the volume of blood entering or being ejected by the left ventricle results in a smaller sized chamber (34), and human fetuses with aortic stenosis may develop progressive left ventricular hypoplasia. Enhancing blood flow to the left ventricle and aorta could, therefore, improve cardiac development. As described in more detail in a previous section of this chapter, the fetal pulmonary vasculature's response to changes in oxygen increases with gestation with a peak blood flow to the lungs reaching 25–30% at approximately 20 weeks gestation then dropping down to <20% by near term. Greater pulmonary blood flow increases pulmonary venous return to the left atrium, but the increase in left ventricle volume may be less than expected. The pressure gradient between the right and left atrium is approximately 2–3 mm Hg and more blood returning into the left atrium from the pulmonary veins could increase left atrial pressure that would impede the umbilical vein blood streaming into the left atrium (35). Phase-contrast MRI studies have shown that there is an inverse relationship between pulmonary blood flow and foramen ovale shunt, (4) and maternal hyperoxygenation can cause a reduction of foramen ovale flow, thereby not significantly altering left ventricular output (17).

There are conflicting reports in the literature on the effects of maternal hyperoxygenation on improved development of left-sided heart structures, compounded by important variations in study protocols in respect to the duration of oxygen administration and fetal gestation when therapy was begun. In a study of 13 fetuses with left-sided cardiac hypoplasia, maternal hyperoxygenation (4-hour intervals three times/day for 1–4 weeks) at 33–38 weeks gestation resulted in increased left ventricle area size in seven subjects and increased dimension of the mitral valve in 8 subjects (36). These findings were not reproduced in a study of 9 fetuses with hypoplastic left heart exposed to maternal hyperoxygenation (8 hours/day for 4–12 weeks) at 26–34 weeks gestation compared to 9 control fetuses with hypoplastic left heart syndrome with no significant differences in cardiac dimensions observed between the groups (37).

The fetal cerebral vasculature is highly responsive to changes in oxygen and the untoward effects of increased fetal blood oxygen tension from maternal hyperoxygenation warrant careful consideration. Cerebral vasoconstriction to higher oxygen content in fetal blood is likely a protective response to maintain oxygen delivery to the brain constant and prevent oxidative stress. Experiments in fetal lambs at 133–137 days (0.85–0.9 gestation) who were ventilated at 100% demonstrated a drop in cerebral blood flow to 32% of control values, but because the concentration of blood oxygen was higher, there was no significant reduction in oxygen delivery to, or consumption by, the brain (20). Nevertheless, the significantly lower cerebral blood flow following hyperoxygenation caused a 56% fall in glucose delivery to the brain and a 27% reduction in glucose consumption. Glucose is the major source of energy for the brain, and any reduction in glucose delivery should be cause for concern. The lamb experiments were of relatively short duration, however, and it is not clear if compensatory mechanisms may alter glucose delivery and/or consumption during chronic hyperoxygenation. A recent study evaluating the effect of chronic maternal hyperoxygenation in 9 fetuses with hypoplastic left heart showed no difference in neurodevelopmental outcomes at 12 months of age compared to 9 patients with a similar cardiac defect who served as controls (38). The authors, nonetheless, reported concerning findings that the fetal skull biparietal diameter growth was significantly slower and that a smaller head circumference was observed at 6 months of age in the fetuses who were subjected to maternal hyperoxygenation. Questionable benefits on fetal cardiac development and a possible adverse effect on neurodevelopment provide strong arguments for maternal hyperoxygenation studies to be curtailed (35) and serve as a good reminder that studies evaluating maternal hyperoxygenation need to evaluate long-term neurological outcomes.

Maternal hyperoxygenation for risk stratification of fetal CHD

Fetal echocardiography has been instrumental in prenatal diagnosis of CHD, but may not reliably provide information on the physiological impact the fetal to postnatal transition in circulation could have on cardiac output. In hypoplastic left heart syndrome with an intact septum, the increase in pulmonary blood flow and resulting increased venous return that occurs at birth can rapidly cause pulmonary edema (owing to an increase in left atrial pressure from the inability of the blood to escape) and low cardiac output (39). The circulatory transition at birth may, however, be more nuanced with other types of CHD. Maternal hyperoxygenation, by simulating the fetal to neonatal transition by increasing pulmonary blood flow *in utero*, can offer more insights into the circulatory transition from fetus to neonate at birth in the presence of CHD (40). Maternal hyperoxygenation as a diagnostic tool could, therefore, enhance preparation and planning for the delivery of newborns with complex CHD (e.g. need for extracorporeal membrane oxygenation or urgent balloon atrial septostomy). The effect of maternal hyperoxygenation can be evaluated by fetal echocardiography by assessing pulmonary vasoreactivity or foramen ovale flow. Furthermore, advancement in MRI technology provide promising opportunities to study hemodynamic changes (41) as well as reliably measure fetal oxygen saturations (3), and implementation of magnetic resonance fetal imaging techniques will undoubtedly improve our understanding of fetal development.

Maternal oxygen therapy for *in utero* fetal resuscitation

Maternal oxygen administration results in a modest elevation of fetal PaO_2 (27). A Cochrane review conducted in 2012 reported that prophylactic oxygen administration to mothers led to a higher incidence of acidotic cord pH (<7.20) (28). More recently, a randomized noninferiority trial of women in labor with category II fetal heart tone tracing showed that maternal oxygen (10 liters per minute via a nonrebreather face mask) did not reduce umbilical arterial lactate levels (3.4 mM/L: 95% CI 3.0–3.8 with oxygen and 3.5 mM/L: 95% CI 3.1–4.0 with air, p = 0.69) (42). More trials are being planned to address maternal oxygen use during fetal distress (43).

References

1. The Fetal Cardiopulmonary Circulation. Acta Pædiatric. 1957; 46(s112):11–14.
2. Rudolph AM, et al. Circ Res. 1967; 21(2):163–184.
3. Saini BS, et al. J Physiol. 2020; 598(15):3259–3281.
4. Prsa M, et al. Circ Cardiovasc Imaging. 2014; 7(4):663–670.
5. Lakshminrusimha S, et al. J Perinatol. 2016; 36 Suppl 2:S3–S11.
6. Rudolph AM. Circ Res. 1985; 57(6):811–821.
7. Rudolph A In: *Congenital diseases of the heart: clinical-physiological considerations.* 3rd ed. Hoboken, NJ, USA: Wiley-Blackwell; 2009.
8. Hislop A, et al. J Anat. 1972; 113(Pt 1):35–48.
9. Levin DL, et al. Circulation. 1976; 53(1):144–151.
10. Fineman JR, et al. Annu Rev Physiol. 1995; 57:115–134.
11. Lakshminrusimha S, et al. Clin Perinatol. 1999; 26(3):601–619.
12. Rasanen J, et al. Circulation. 1996; 94(5):1068–1073.
13. Kinsella JP, et al. Am J Physiol. 1994; 267(5 Pt 2):H1955–H1961.
14. Lewis AB, et al. Circ Res. 1976; 39(4):536–541.
15. Morin FC, et al. Am J Physiol. 1988; 254(3 Pt 2):H542–H546.
16. Morin FC, et al. J Appl Physiol (1985). 1992; 73(1):213–218.
17. Rasanen J, et al. Circulation. 1998; 97(3):257–262.
18. Sorensen A, et al. Ultrasound Obstet Gynecol. 2011; 38(6):665–672.
19. Konduri GG, et al. Pediatr Res. 1993; 33(5):533–539.
20. Iwamoto HS, et al. Pediatr Res. 1991; 30(2):158–164.
21. Cohn HE, et al. Am J Obstet Gynecol. 1974; 120(6):817–824.
22. Bell SG. Neonatal Netw. 1999; 18(2):9–15.
23. Maurer HS, et al. Nature. 1970; 227(5256):388–390.
24. Arnone A. Nature. 1972; 237(5351):146–149.
25. Wimberley PD. Scand J Clin Lab Invest Suppl. 1982; 160:1–149.
26. Hellstrom W, et al. Arch Dis Child Fetal Neonatal Ed. 2021; 106(1):88–92.
27. McClure JH, et al. Am J Obstet Gynecol. 1960; 80(3):554–557.
28. Fawole B, et al. Cochrane Database Syst Rev. 2012; 12:CD000136.
29. Mahle WT, et al. Circulation. 2002; 106(12 Suppl 1):I109–I114.

30. Miller SP, et al. N Engl J Med. 2007; 357(19):1928–1938.
31. Licht DJ, et al. J Thorac Cardiovasc Surg. 2009; 137(3):529–536.
32. Limperopoulos C, et al. Circulation. 2010; 121(1):26–33.
33. Sun L, et al. Circulation. 2015; 131(15):1313–23.
34. Fishman NH, et al. Circulation. 1978; 58(2):354–364.
35. Rudolph AM. Pediatr Res. 2020; 87(4):630–633.
36. Kohl T. Pediatr Cardiol. 2010; 31(2):250–263.
37. Lara DA, et al. Ultrasound Obstet Gynecol. 2016; 48(3):365–372.
38. Edwards LA, et al. Fetal Diagn Ther. 2019; 46(1):45–57.
39. Olivieri L, et al. J Am Coll Cardiol. 2011; 57(20):e369.
40. Schidlow DN, et al. Am J Perinatol. 2018; 35(1):16–23.
41. Porayette P, et al. Prenat Diagn. 2016; 36(3):274–281.
42. Raghuraman N, et al. JAMA Pediatrics. 2018; 172(9):818–823.
43. Bullens LM, et al. Trials. 2018; 19(1):195.

FETAL OXYGENATION DURING MATERNAL HYPOXIC ILLNESS

Fabiana Postolow and Shyamala Dakshinamurti

Contents

Maternal hypoxia and fetal outcomes

During the 2009 pandemic H1N1 influenza outbreak in Canada, 1473 ICU admissions and 428 deaths were ascribed to H1N1 (1). Pregnant women comprised under 1% of the population, but 5% of H1N1-related deaths. H1N1-positive pregnant women proved four times more likely to be hospitalized compared to nonpregnant (2). In a case series of 6 pregnant women with H1N1, all were persistently hypoxic despite high PEEP, 100% oxygen ventilation, and broad-spectrum antimicrobial therapy; 2 required extracorporeal oxygenation. 5 of 6 pregnant women had hypoxic fetuses; 3 infants survived, 2 without significant hypoxic encephalopathy sequelae (3). Similar data were reported in Australia/New Zealand during the same pandemic: Compared with nonpregnant women, pregnant H1N1 influenza patients had a sevenfold increased risk of ICU admission; women above 19 weeks' gestation, 13-fold greater. Of 64 pregnant women in ICU, 44 were mechanically ventilated and 14 required ECMO; 7 died. There were 7 stillbirths or infant deaths, attributed to hypoxic-ischemic injury (4).

The influenza epidemic of 1918 and Asian flu epidemic of 1957 also reported 30% to 50% maternal mortality (5). SARS had a similar impact; pregnant women had a case fatality rate of 25%; 50% of pregnant patients required ICU admission and 33% mechanical ventilation, compared with 20% ICU admissions among nonpregnant adults. Placental findings in SARS patients included thrombosis and infarcts; a 50% spontaneous miscarriage rate was ascribed to severe maternal respiratory compromise, not transplacental infection (as viral particles were absent in products of conception) (6). While data are yet limited, SARS-CoV-2 (COVID-19) also appears to pose a greater risk during pregnancy; pregnant women are more likely than nonpregnant women to be admitted to intensive care (10.5 versus 3.9 per 1000 cases), to require mechanical ventilation (2.9 versus 1.1 per 1000), or to die (1.5 versus 1.2 per 1000) (7). Placental abnormalities including intraplacental thrombi are more common in pregnant women with COVID-19 (8). Reported fetal complications of COVID-19 include miscarriage 2%, IUGR 10%, and preterm birth 39% (9), though other studies have reported fetal risks to be similar to those of uninfected women (10). Early neonatal COVID-19 infection is reported in up to 3% of tested infants (10), despite scant evidence for transplacental vertical transmission of the virus (11).

But in the smaller subset of pregnant women with COVID-19 developing critical respiratory failure before 37 weeks, pregnancy loss or preterm birth is reported as high as 60%, ascribed mainly to maternal hypoxia (10).

Acute respiratory distress syndrome (ARDS) is characterized by acute hypoxemia and increased alveolar-capillary permeability resulting from pulmonary inflammation, complicating COVID-19, and other infections. The incidence of ARDS in pregnancy is higher than in the general population, and the reported frequency of pregnant patients requiring mechanical ventilation increased from 36 cases per 100,000 births in 2006 to 60 per 100,000 in 2012 (12). Pregnant women admitted to ICU with ARDS have a 35% fetal mortality rate, exceeding the maternal mortality (20%) (13), while a study of pregnant women admitted to ICU for all nonobstetrical causes (mainly hypotension) listed only 1% neonatal deaths and 15% fetal deaths (14). These data highlight fetal risk during severe maternal hypoxia.

Placental buffering of maternal hypoxia

The notion that the fetus is the "perfect parasite" has of course long been debunked; the placenta functions as both nutrient- and oxygen-sensor, such that maternal deprivation of nutrients results in placental modulation of resources allocated to the fetus, altering somatic growth and metabolism (15). However, the high morbidity and mortality observed in fetuses during maternal hypoxic respiratory failure trigger the question: Is there a threshold for adequate fetal oxygenation? Fetal outcomes in the context of maternal critical illness reveal the complex nature of hemodynamic and oxygenation relationships between mother, placenta, and fetus (Figure 10.1).

The placental circulation comprises high flow, low resistance spiral arteries, usually held in a maximally dilated state but capable of a brisk α-adrenergic constrictor response (16). Uterine blood flow increases to 20% of maternal cardiac output by the third trimester, derived entirely from the gravid increase in maternal cardiac output and circulating blood volume, so blood flow to other maternal organs is not curtailed during a normal pregnancy. The low resistance in the placental circuit drops maternal systemic vascular resistance by 30% (17).

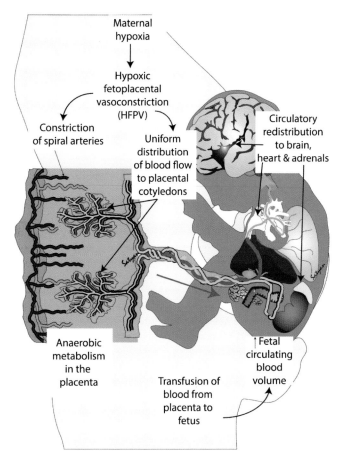

FIGURE 10.1 Compensatory mechanisms for mild to moderate maternal hypoxia. Placental hemodynamic and metabolic adaptations preserve fetal oxygen supply during moderate maternal hypoxia. (Copyright Satyan Lakshminrusimha.)

During the third trimester, the umbilical vein carrying oxygenated blood to the fetus has a PO_2 between 20 and 35 mm Hg, much lower than the PO_2 of maternal arterial blood (18). However, while the relationship between maternal and fetal PO_2 is not linear, owing to the distinct oxygen affinities and carrying capacities of adult and fetal hemoglobins, maternal and fetal arterial oxygen contents relate linearly, resulting in an umbilical venous oxygen content comparable to that of adult arterial blood (19). Hence, fetal tissues are not hypoxic; oxygen delivery is sufficient to meet demand. Returning umbilical arterial blood has a median PO_2 19 to 22 mm Hg (20), but can range from 10 to 30 mm Hg (21), dependent on fetal oxygen extraction. Infants suffering hypoxic morbidities have lower umbilical artery PO_2, although this absolute value is not predictive (22).

The placental circulation is intrinsic to hypoxia adaptation. Maternal hypoxia induces placental vasoconstriction by means of hypoxic fetoplacental vasoconstriction (HFPV), via inhibition of vascular smooth muscle potassium channels leading to membrane depolarization that activates voltage-gated calcium channels, causing calcium influx and activation of the smooth muscle contractile apparatus, akin to the mechanisms of hypoxic pulmonary vasoconstriction (23). As in the lung, HPFV appears to be a homeostatic mechanism ensuring placental recruitment for optimal oxygen delivery to the fetus. Radiolabeled perfusion studies reveal an inhomogenous blood flow pattern among placental cotyledons when breathing room air, indicating variable circuit

resistance; parts of the placenta do not receive blood flow sufficient for gas exchange. Maternal hypoxia (FiO_2 10–12%) increases uniformity of placental flow distribution, thereby increasing the efficiency of placental oxygen exchange (24). During the second half of pregnancy, fetuses return a third of their cardiac output to the placental circulation; but as they approach term, this volume drops to 20%, and even lower in growth-restricted fetuses, as umbilical blood is recirculated more extensively to fetal vital organs (25). During acute hypoxia in pregnant sheep, while maternal and fetal arterial blood pressure, heart rates, and total placental blood flow are unchanged, the placental blood volume decreases by 21% over 30 minutes of hypoxia, with a precisely reciprocal increase in fetal blood volume, suggesting placental vasoconstriction during fetal hypoxia also causes a significant placental transfusion to the lamb fetus augmenting fetal circulating volume. These hemodynamic changes persist for 30 min following resolution of hypoxia and may constitute a rapid protective mechanism against fetal deoxygenation (26).

During moderate maternal hypoxia, the placenta also adapts its metabolism to be anaerobic, sparing oxygen for fetal use so the fetus still receives oxygen adequate to its needs. In a study of late gestation mice, hypoxia at FiO_2 13% (commensurate with 3700m altitude) induces beneficial changes in placental morphology improving gas exchange surface and nutrient transport, increasing placental glucose uptake without altering other nutrient utilization (27). Unchanged protein utilization is also reported in placentas of humans gestating at moderate altitude (28). Photoacoustic imaging of placental regional circulation in pregnant rats during hypoxia shows that the placenta protects the fetus from experiencing oxygen variations during maternal hypoxia down to FiO_2 5% for 4 minutes (29). Preferential anaerobic consumption of glucose by the placenta spares oxygen, but limits the availability of glucose for the fetus. Thus, fetal IUGR in moderate maternal hypoxia is associated not with fetal hypoxia, but with fetal hypoglycemia and hypoinsulinemia (30).

The fetal impacts of preplacental hypoxia (reduced oxygen content of maternal blood due to altitude, respiratory illness, anemia, etc.), or of uteroplacental hypoxia (normally oxygenated maternal blood has restricted entry into uteroplacental circuit, as in preeclampsia), are similar (31). The effect of chronic maternal hypoxia on uterine artery flow and infant birth weight has been examined in altitude-dwelling cohorts of recent migrants versus multigenerationally altitude-adapted populations in Tibet. Umbilical artery diameter and blood flow are higher in the adapted population, protecting uteroplacental oxygen delivery and averting altitude-associated IUGR; while in the unadapted population, the impact of 3600 m altitude on uterine blood flow is comparable to the effect of preeclampsia on mothers at 3100m altitude (32). Uteroplacental perfusion is regulated by the local ratio of nitric oxide to endothelin generation, which in acute hypoxia is augmented by induction of nitric oxide synthase, but in chronically hypoxic vessels favors endothelin (33). Hypoxia also causes adrenergic activation (34), triggers HIF1α-mediated arterial remodeling (35) and fetal growth restriction (36) pathways, and decreases uterine sensitivity to nitric oxide (37), impairing uteroplacental blood flow (34) and slowing the trajectory of fetal growth at altitude (38). Positive maternal physiological adaptations protecting the fetus at altitude include increased total cardiac output, a higher rate of ventilation resulting in hypocapneic protection of alveolar oxygen (32), and induction of placental nitric oxide synthase (35). Despite these, mean birth weight in unadapted populations falls by 100 g per 1000 m altitude gain (39).

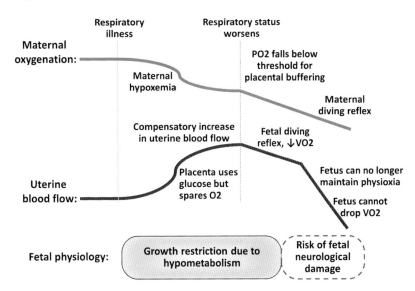

FIGURE 10.2 Schematic of the fetal environment during maternal critical illness. Uterine blood flow increases as maternal oxygenation decreases, due to compensatory redistribution of flow, while placental oxygen-sparing metabolism maintains fetal oxygen delivery. When maternal oxygenation falls below the threshold for placental buffering, the decreased uterine blood flow can initially be buffered by fetal blood flow redistribution and metabolic restriction. However, during severe cardiopulmonary illness, initiation of the maternal diving reflex markedly curtails uterine blood flow, leading to fetal compromise.

Impaired placental oxygen transport also curtails oxygen delivery, which triggers fetal metabolic adaptation (40), slowing third trimester fetal growth, and dropping fetal oxygen utilization to safely below the level of oxygen delivery (34).

However, there appears to be a threshold somewhere between 13% and 10% FiO_2, below which the placenta no longer adapts its glucose metabolism to support fetal resource allocation; and in severe hypoxia (FiO_2 10%, roughly equal to 5800 m altitude), all bets for the fetus are off. Placental and fetal vascularity is impaired, diffusion barrier thickness increased, and placental amino acid transfer to the fetus impaired (27). When homeostatic metabolic responses to oxygen restriction are exhausted, fetal hypoxia does ensue – a drop in maternal arterial oxygen saturation to 85% drops fetal umbilical vein saturation from 70% to 55% – but the fetus handles this by blood flow redistribution toward brain and heart (16). This circulatory redistribution response to hypoxia is confirmed by phase-contrast MRI studies in asymmetrically IUGR fetuses (40). The mammalian "diving reflex" response to hypoxia includes breath-holding; slow heart rate due to parasympathetic stimulation of the cardiac pacemaker; diminished blood flow to nonvital organs due to sympathetic vasoconstriction while sparing flow to brain, heart, and adrenals; and a gradual increase in mean arterial pressure (41). These adaptations, highly developed in aquatic or hibernating mammals, also form the basis of a more rudimentary "master switch" for lowering metabolic rate in humans during asphyxial stressors such as drowning and parturition (42). In instrumented sheep, maternal hypoxia to PaO_2 35 mm Hg results in a small increase in umbilical circuit vascular resistance, no change in umbilical blood flow, but a rapid 50% drop in fetal oxygen consumption, associated with a decrement in fetal heart rate (43). In rhesus monkeys, moderate maternal hypoxia (FiO_2 15%) causes fetal bradycardia without otherwise altering fetal circulation; oxygen delivery to the fetus remains directly related to the quantity of oxygen delivered to the uterus. Increased shunting of SVC flow across the foramen ovale protects fetal brain and coronary perfusion (19). Brain sparing

due to preferential flow redistribution is confirmed by MRI blood oxygen signal intensity measures in animal models of hypoxic pregnancy (44, 45).

Severe maternal hypoxia (FiO_2 10% or less) eventually decreases afferent uterine blood flow, impairing oxygen supply to the placenta, and resulting in fetal hypoxia and acidosis indicating tissue oxygen starvation (19). At this level of hypoxia, maternal hemodynamic responses preserve the mother's vital organs and not the fetus's, shifting cardiac output away from uterine circulation and toward maternal brain and heart (16). This reflex effectively reduces circulating volume on the fetal side of the placenta. A study of near-term sheep subject to a 30-minute normocapneic hypoxic challenge revealed fetoplacental blood volume decreased by 8%, while fetal arterial and venous pressures increased; fetal blood volume did not return to normal until 30 minutes after resolution of maternal hypoxia (46). Fetal tissue oxygenation can no longer be protected, as uterine blood flow is jettisoned by the maternal circulation's diving reflex during severe hypoxia, and the fetal circulation becomes compromised. Initial fetal vasoconstriction preserves cerebral blood flow, while brain electrical activity quickly flattens to decrease oxygen consumption; subsequently, hypoxia-induced fetal hypotension results in cerebral hypoperfusion and asphyxia (47). The impact of progressively worsening maternal hypoxia on placental and fetal oxygen homeostasis is summarized in Figure 10.2.

Supportive care for maternal critical illness and impacts on fetal physiology

Critical illness complicates 0.3 to 1.8% of pregnancies. Approximately 25% of maternal ICU deaths occur antepartum, 25% intrapartum, and 50% postpartum (48). Patients with primary obstetric disorders including preeclampsia, hemorrhage, and sepsis represent 50 to 80% of pregnant ICU admissions (49), but have a better prognosis. Nonobstetrical critical illnesses in pregnant women include ARDS, asthma, pneumonia, drug use, complicated urinary infections, thromboembolism, trauma, autoimmune disorders, and endocrine disorders; maternal mortality ranges 12–20%. Fetal prognosis is guarded in patients with nonobstetrical causes of ICU admission; in a study of 93 such pregnant women in ICU, 32 fetal losses were reported, with 10 neonates requiring intensive care (16).

Respiratory support
Pregnant women are disproportionally affected by respiratory illnesses, with increased infectious morbidity and high mortality rate. Respiratory adaptations associated with pregnancy place the pregnant woman at risk of respiratory compromise during critical illness. Oxygen consumption increases 20–33%. Progesterone stimulates a 30% increase in minute ventilation, achieved by an increase in tidal volume without changing respiratory rate. But increased chest wall circumference, widening of the costal angle, and elevation of the diaphragm start even before increases in uterine size, maternal body weight or intra-abdominal pressure, caused by ligamentous relaxation due to the hormone relaxin. Elevation of the diaphragm by the gravid uterus and altered chest wall shape reduce functional residual capacity, residual volume, and expiratory reserve volume (50). During mechanical ventilation, reduced chest wall compliance during pregnancy compounded by low lung compliance from ARDS may result in severe lung derecruitment when low tidal volumes are used. High PEEPs used in nonpregnant patients with severe ARDS may not be well tolerated hemodynamically during pregnancy, as elevated intrathoracic pressures restrict venous return into the thorax, negating the adaptive high cardiac output state (51).

Pregnant women maintain a near-normal pH, despite co-existing respiratory alkalosis and bicarbonate-losing metabolic acidosis (49). The maternal-fetal CO_2 gradient is normally 10–13 mm Hg. This gradient, as well as adequate blood flow at both sides of the placenta, must be preserved to facilitate diffusion of carbon dioxide from fetus to mother (51). In context of ARDS, the use of a permissive hypercapnia lung-protective ventilation strategy improves maternal morbidity and mortality. In contrast, severe maternal respiratory alkalosis should be avoided, as this can promote uterine vasoconstriction (52). Consequences of hypercapnia in the fetus are not well understood; however, acidosis is known to be deleterious to oxygen delivery. Bicarbonate diffusion across the placenta is slow, hence infusion of bicarbonate-based solutions to the mother may not correct fetal acidemia (51).

Cardiovascular support
Fetal oxygen saturation is dependent on adequate placental blood flow and transfer of O_2 across the placenta is driven by oxygen content. Apart from the hemodynamic effects of maternal hypoxia and ventilation, maternal hypotension can directly impair uterine blood flow.

To meet rising metabolic demand, maternal cardiovascular adaptations include a 50% increase in cardiac output accomplished by a rightward shift along the Starling curve, increased heart rate, and decreased systemic vascular resistance. Arterial blood pressure reaches its nadir at 28 weeks and increases to normal near term. Maternal blood volume increases by roughly 1200 ml; this increased preload augments cardiac output. Plasma volume increases disproportionally to red cell mass, leading to dilutional anemia and a decreased plasma oncotic pressure, predisposing pregnant patients to pulmonary edema. Normal cardiovascular changes of pregnancy thus mimic a distributive

preshock picture, with relative peripheral vasodilation and low blood pressure, increased heart rate, and high cardiac output (51).

Uterine perfusion is proportional to systemic arterial pressure, exhibiting autoregulation when maternal mean pressure drops below 40 mm Hg (17), a critical point below which placental resistance rises. Uterine circulatory responses vary considerably between conscious and anesthetized subjects. Anesthetized sheep challenged with endotoxin rapidly deteriorate in cardiac output, blood pressure, and uterine blood flow to lethality in 3 hours; while unanesthetized sheep tolerate 3 times that dose of endotoxin without hemodynamic decompensation (53). Similarly, maternal hypovolemia in unanesthetized sheep results in fetal bradycardia but not hypotension, while anesthetized fetal sheep cannot tolerate maternal blood loss (54). These findings suggest a large sympathetic contribution to placental autoregulation in maternal shock, which is damped by anesthesia.

Supportive measures during maternal shock include volume, inotropy, and pressors. Among these, pressors should be used with caution and after volume expansion (16), as α-adrenergic agents effects directly vasoconstrict the uteroplacental vasculature, impeding uterine blood flow and negating the beneficial effects of increased maternal blood pressure (55). Norepinephrine, epinephrine, and dopamine all restrict uterine blood flow, leaving ephedrine and phenylephrine as preferred options. However, a permissive hypotensive resuscitation strategy, restoring maternal mean arterial pressure to 60 mm Hg, may be sufficient to protect placental perfusion pressure without exacerbating maternal hypoxia from low-pressure pulmonary edema (56).

Cardiac arrest occurs in 1:20,000 to 1:50,000 pregnancies. The limited cardiac output provided by cardiopulmonary resuscitation efforts has devastating effects on the fetus (16). Management of cardiac arrest in pregnancy requires patient position modification to avoid aortocaval compression, by manual uterine displacement; and consideration of emergency cesarean section for the maternal indication of supporting venous return, if return of spontaneous circulation does not occur by 4 minutes of CPR (57).

Thermoregulation
Maternal fever impairs fetal ability to lower its VO_2 (16), increasing fetal metabolic rate and promoting fetal tachycardia which demands additional oxygen consumption (58) fever is an independent risk factor for fetal neurological compromise (59). Pyrexia triggers maternal hyperventilation, which is associated with increased uterine blood flow, but this does not improve umbilical blood flow, placental transfer of glucose, or fetal glucose uptake (60). Management of fever during maternal critical illness is thus pertinent to management of fetal hypoxia.

Extracorporeal membranous oxygenation (ECMO)
Use of ECMO has increased in the past decade, as a salvage therapy for patients with cardiopulmonary failure where oxygen saturation is refractory to mechanical ventilatory support. Although maternal ARDS remains a major indication for ECMO, ECMO is also used in pregnant patients with other pulmonary catastrophes, with improved fetal and maternal outcomes (61). In a metanalysis of ECMO in pregnant or postpartum patients (12), indications were ARDS (66%), cardiogenic shock (17%), amniotic fluid embolism (8%), and postpartum hemorrhage (5%). Maternal survival was 77%; fetal survival was 69%. Survival rates for pregnant and postpartum women on ECMO are higher than in ARDS untreated by ECMO, while major complications are low,

supporting early adoption of ECMO for cardiopulmonary failure in pregnancy (62).

Maternal exposure to wildfires and air pollution

Areas affected by wildfire smoke report elevated levels of air pollutants, including particulate matter (PM), carbon monoxide (CO) and other volatile organic compounds associated with adverse pregnancy outcomes. The smallest group of particulate matter ($PM_{2.5}$, diameter <2500 nm) enter maternal alveoli and cross the capillary network, inducing inflammation. PM with diameter <500 nm can pass the placental barrier during gestation, while those <240 nm are able to reach the fetal bloodstream, influencing fetal organ development and metabolism (63). Maternal exposure to 5 $\mu g/m^3$ increments in $PM_{2.5}$ starting early in pregnancy is associated with a 50% increased risk of pregnancy-induced hypertension, and adverse neonatal outcomes including stillbirth, congenital anomalies, fetal growth restriction and preterm birth (64).

Less is understood about the obstetrical or neonatal impact of short- to medium-term (days to months) maternal exposures, such as that caused by woodsmoke during Australia's extensive wildfires during 2019–2020. Following wildfires in California in 2003, smoke-exposed infants weighed on average 6.1g less at birth than unexposed infants, with infants exposed during second trimester having the largest weight reduction 9.7 g (65). Data from Colorado wildfires 2007–2015 indicated that each 1 $\mu g/m^3$ increase in wildfire smoke $PM_{2.5}$ exposure during first trimester of pregnancy was associated with a 14% increase in gestational diabetes and 15% increase in gestational hypertension; and during second trimester with a 13% increased risk of preterm birth (66).

$PM_{2.5}$ may not be the only smoke constituent causing adverse birth outcomes following fire exposure; the role of CO in fetal hypoxia is discussed below.

Smoking and vaping during pregnancy

Cigarette smoke liberates over 4000 compounds, including nicotine, CO, tar, benzene, and heavy metals. Nicotine has high lipid solubility, crossing the placenta to the fetal bloodstream, where it has sympathomimetic properties decreasing umbilical blood flow, increasing vascular resistance in the feto-placental compartment (67). Additionally, cigarette smoke contains 4% CO; in pregnant smokers, the blood carboxyhemoglobin level is 3%. The carboxyhemoglobin level in newborns of nonsmoking mothers approaches 2%, but increases to 6–9% if the mother smokes. Chronic exposure to CO during first and second trimesters can produce significant intrauterine growth restriction, presumably due to chronic fetal hypoxia (68).

Use of electronic cigarettes (EC) among pregnant women is increasing, as EC is perceived as less harmful and an aid for smoking cessation (69). EC aerosols provide a rapid plasma level of nicotine approaching that achieved by cigarettes. Exclusive EC users and dual-users both have an elevated greater risk of SGA and preterm birth (70). In animal models, EC exposure reduces fetal weight while markedly decreasing maternal uterine artery and fetal umbilical artery blood flow (67). Studies of early gestational EC vaping also show dysregulation in pulmonary gene expression, inhibiting postnatal lung development (71), and

altered gene expression in the developing frontal cortex (72), effects ascribed to EC aerosol constituents of other than nicotine. EC do not produce CO; other harmful compounds, such as aldehydes and nitrosamines, are produced albeit at a lower level than conventional cigarette smoking (69).

Carbon monoxide intoxication

CO comprises <0.001% of the atmosphere, but 20% of vehicle exhaust fumes, 30% in gas heating circuits; and in smoke from explosions and fires, the CO concentrations can reach 60% (73). Maternal CO inhalation due to combustion fumes or burns is a special case of maternal hypoxemia due to hemoglobin occupancy and highlights the interrelationship between maternal oxygen-carrying capacity and that of fetal hemoglobin.

CO inhalation inhibits oxygen transport and delivery. As CO has 210 times greater affinity for hemoglobin than does O_2, and greater affinity still for fetal hemoglobin (68), the protection from hypoxia usually afforded by fetal hemoglobin is upended. Acute maternal CO intoxication causes fetal hypoxia by decreasing oxygen carriage on maternal hemoglobin, and also by transplacental diffusion of CO to the fetus (74). CO binds to fetal hemoglobin 2.5–3 times more strongly than to adult hemoglobin, resulting in a 10–15% higher fetal carboxyhemoglobin concentration, left-shifting the fetal hemoglobin–oxygen dissociation curve, preventing the release of oxygen. CO tightly binds myoglobin, impairing the ability of myoglobin to act as an oxygen reservoir in hypoxic tissues, and inducing cardiac arrythmias. CO displaces oxygen from cytochrome C oxidase, damaging mitochondrial respiration (75). Respiratory uncoupling also occurs in cyanide intoxication, a common comorbidity with CO inhalation from an enclosed fire, especially in presence of plastics (75).

The impact of fetal CO injury depends on gestational age and the severity of poisoning. Studies of anoxic encephalopathy after CO inhalation reveal the vulnerability of periventricular white matter and brainstem, followed by thalamus and the cerebral cortex (76). Fetal risk is significant once the mother exhibits symptoms of altered consciousness and after prolonged duration of exposure (77). In a prospective study of CO poisonings during pregnancy, fetal outcomes correlated with severity of maternal symptoms, though not with maternal CO levels, as fetal CO may be unpredictably higher (78). Fetal toxicity outstrips maternal toxicity. While maternal mortality for CO intoxication is 19–24%, fetal mortality rates are 36–67% (79). Maternal treatment of CO poisoning begins with administration of 100% oxygen. But the half-life of CO is 4 times greater in fetus than mother. CO's high affinity for fetal hemoglobin dictates that fetal carboxyhemoglobin concentration will continue to rise after maternal levels reach a plateau, requiring >40 hours to normalize even after maternal carboxyhemoglobin normalizes (75). Fetal outcome in comatose CO-intoxicated patients remains dismal when treated with normobaric oxygen alone. Hyperbaric oxygen is strongly indicated for pregnant women with altered consciousness or a carboxyhemoglobin level >20% (80). ECMO has been reported for successful treatment of CO poisoning with multiorgan failure, but may not displace CO from hemoglobin more rapidly than normobaric hyperoxia (81).

Overall, fetal outcomes during maternal hypoxia depend on placental and fetal adaptation and the complex dynamics of fetal gas exchange, as much as on maternal supportive measures.

References

1. Helferty M, et al. CMAJ. 2010; 182(18):1981–7.
2. Cox S, et al. Obstet Gynecol. 2006; 107(6):1315–22.
3. Oluyomi-Obi T, et al. J Obstet Gynaecol Can. 2010; 32(5):443–7.
4. ANZIC Influenza Investigators and Australasian Maternity Outcomes Surveillance System. BMJ. 2010; 340:c1279.
5. Greenberg M, et al. Am J Obstet Gynecol. 1958; 76(4):897–902.
6. Wong SF, et al. Am J Obstet Gynecol. 2004; 191(1):292–7.
7. Zambrano LD, et al. MMWR Morbidity and Mortality Weekly Report. 2020; 69(44):1641–7.
8. Prabhu M, et al. BJOG. 2020; 127(12):1548–56.
9. Dashraath P, et al. Am J Obstet Gynecol. 2020; 222(6):521–31.
10. Adhikari EH, et al. JAMA network open. 2020; 3(11):e2029256.
11. Edlow AG, et al. JAMA network open. 2020; 3(12):e2030455.
12. Zhang JJY, et al. J Intensive Care Med. 2019:885066619892826.
13. Collop NA, et al. Chest. 1993; 103(5):1548–52.
14. Cartin-Ceba R, et al. Crit Care Med. 2008; 36(10):2746–51.
15. King JC. J Nutr. 2016; 146(7):1437S–44S.
16. Aoyama K, et al. Crit Care. 2014; 18(3):307.
17. Assali NS, et al. Eur J Obstet Gynecol Reprod Biol. 1978; 8(1):43–55.
18. Meschia G. Clin Chest Med. 2011; 32(1):15–9.
19. Jackson BT, et al. Am J Physiol. 1987; 252(1 Pt 2):R94–101.
20. Tang J, et al. Arch Gynecol Obstet. 2019; 299(3):719–724.
21. Monneret D, et al. Clin Biochem. 2019; 67:40–7.
22. Raghuraman N, et al. Am J Perinatol. 2018; 35(4):331–5.
23. Hampl V, et al. Physiol Res. 2009; 58 Suppl 2:S87–93.
24. Power GG, et al. J Clin Invest. 1967; 46(12):2053–63.
25. Kiserud T, et al. Ultrasound Obstet Gynecol. 2006; 28(2):126–36.
26. Jaroslov F, et al. Am J Obstet Gynecol. 1975; 122(3):316–22.
27. Higgins JS, et al. J Physiol. 2016; 594(5):1341–56.
28. Vaughan OR, et al. J Appl Physiol (1985). 2020; 128(1):127–33.
29. Arthuis CJ, et al. PLoS One. 2017; 12(1):e0169850.
30. Zamudio S, et al. PLoS One. 2010; 5(1):e8551.
31. Kingdom JC, et al. Placenta. 1997; 18(8):613–21.
32. Moore LG, et al. Am J Phys Anthropol. 2001; 114(1):42–53.
33. Julian CG, et al. Am J Physiol Regul Integr Comp Physiol. 2008; 295(3):R906–15.
34. Hutter D, et al. Int J Pediatr. 2010; 2010:401323.
35. Schaffer L, et al. Am J Physiol Regul Integr Comp Physiol. 2006; 290(3):R844–51.
36. Ream M, et al. Am J Physiol Regul Integr Comp Physiol. 2008; 295(2):R583–95.
37. Lorca RA, et al. Hypertension. 2019; 73(6):1319–26.
38. Krampl E, et al. Ultrasound Obstet Gynecol. 2000; 16(1):9–18.
39. Moore LG. High Altitude Medicine & Biology. 2003; 4(2):141–56.
40. Zhu MY, et al. Am J Obstet Gynecol. 2016; 214(3):367 e1–e17.
41. Gooden BA. Integr Physiol Behav Sci. 1994; 29(1):6–16.
42. Hagen JB. Hist Philos Life Sci. 2018; 40(1):18.
43. Parer JT. Eur J Obstet Gynecol Reprod Biol. 1980; 10(2):125–36.
44. Wedegartner U, et al. Radiology. 2006; 238(3):872–80.
45. Cahill LS, et al. J Cereb Blood Flow Metab. 2014; 34(6):1082–8.
46. Brace RA. Am J Obstet Gynecol. 1986; 155(4):889–93.
47. Gunn AJ, et al. Clin Perinatol. 2009; 36(3):579–93.
48. Wanderer JP, et al. Crit Care Med. 2013; 41(8):1844–52.
49. Zieleskiewicz L, et al. Anaesth Crit Care Pain Med. 2016; 35(Suppl 1):S51–S57.
50. Guntupalli KK, et al. Chest. 2015; 148(4):1093–104.
51. Honiden S, et al. J Intensive Care Med. 2013; 28(2):93–106.
52. Brower RG, et al. N Engl J Med. 2000; 342(18):1301–8.
53. Zugaib M, et al. Surg Gynecol Obstet. 1979; 149(3):337–42.
54. Nuwayhid B, et al. Am J Obstet Gynecol. 1978; 132(6):658–66.
55. Fishburne JI, et al. Am J Obstet Gynecol. 1980; 137(8):944–52.
56. Yu YH, et al. Resuscitation. 2009; 80(12):1424–30.
57. Vanden Hoek TL, et al. Circulation. 2010; 122(18 Suppl 3):S829–61.
58. Morishima HO, et al. Am J Obstet Gynecol. 1975; 121(4):531–8.
59. Impey LW, et al. Am J Obstet Gynecol. 2008; 198(1):49 e1–6.
60. Andrianakis P, et al. Exp Physiol. 1994; 79(1):1–13.
61. Agerstrand C, et al. Ann Thorac Surg. 2016; 102(3):774–9.
62. Naoum EE, et al. J Am Heart Assoc. 2020; 9(13):e016072.
63. Luyten LJ, et al. Environ Res. 2018; 166:310–23.
64. Melody SM, et al. Environ Pollut. 2019; 244:915–25.
65. Holstius DM, et al. Environ Health Perspect. 2012; 120(9):1340–5. Epub 2012/05/31.
66. Abdo M, et al. Int J Environ Res Public Health. 2019; 16(19):3720.
67. Orzabal MR, et al. Transl Res. 2019; 207:70–82.
68. Aubard Y, et al. BJOG. 2000; 107(7):833–8.
69. McDonnell BP, et al. BJOG. 2020; 127(6):750–6.
70. Wang X, et al. Preventive Medicine. 2020; 134:106041.
71. McGrath-Morrow SA, et al. PLoS One. 2015; 10(2):e0118344.
72. Lauterstein DE, et al. Int J Environ Res Public Health. 2016; 13(4):417.
73. Sinkovic A, et al. Inhalation Toxicol. 2006; 18(3):211–4.
74. Longo LD. Am J Obstet Gynecol. 1977; 129(1):69–103.
75. Culnan DM, et al. Ann Plast Surg. 2018; 80(3 Suppl 2):S106–12.
76. Delomenie M, et al. Case Rep Obstet Gynecol. 2015; 2015:687975.
77. Greingor JL, et al. Emerg Med J. 2001; 18(5):399–401.
78. Koren G, et al. Reprod Toxicol. 1991; 5(5):397–403.
79. Elkharrat D, et al. Intensive Care Med. 1991; 17(5):289–92.
80. Bird SB. Toxicology Open Access. 2017; 3(4):134.
81. Teerapuncharoen K, et al. Respir Care. 2015; 60(9):e155–60.

HEMODYNAMICS OF THE CIRCULATORY TRANSITION

Graeme R. Polglase, Martin Kluckow, Andrew W. Gill and Stuart B. Hooper

Contents

The normal circulatory transition at birth

The transition of a fetus to a newborn is perhaps the greatest physiological challenge that we must all overcome if we are to survive after birth. Before birth, the future airways of the lungs are liquid-filled, and the lungs play no role in gas exchange (1). Instead, gas exchange occurs across the placenta and the majority of right ventricular output by-passes the lungs and passes through the ductus arteriosus (DA) to enter the descending aorta (Figure 11.1) (2). As much of this blood is directed through the placenta, the right ventricle provides the majority of blood flow through the organ of gas exchange in the fetus, just as it does in the adult (lung) (3). Similarly, due to the presence of the ductus venosus (DV) and foramen ovale (FO), highly oxygenated umbilical venous blood passes directly into the left atrium and left ventricle (2). Thus, the left ventricle in the fetus receives highly oxygenated blood from the organ of gas exchange, just as occurs in newborns and adults (Figure 11.1), and provides the majority of preload for the left ventricle in the fetus, just like it does in the adult (3–5). As the lungs must take over the role of the gas exchange at birth, the circulation has to undergo a massive reorganisation so that the lungs can: (i) Become the sole recipient of blood exiting the right ventricle and (ii) become the sole provider of preload (venous return) for left ventricular output. It is very important not to overlook this second role as it is critical for cardiac function after birth.

Effect of the onset of respiration on the cardiovascular transition

The two key physiological adaptations that must occur at birth are 1) the neonatal lungs must take over the role of gas exchange from the placenta and 2) the fetal circulation must transition to the newborn circulation to allow transfer of oxygenated blood from the lungs throughout the body. Importantly, lung aeration is the critical aspect of a successful transition at birth, which supports the focus of stimulating breathing and early initiation of respiratory support within the first minute of life in resuscitation guidelines worldwide. At birth, lung aeration decreases pulmonary vascular resistance (PVR) which increases pulmonary blood flow (PBF) and redirects right ventricular output through the lungs (2). The precise mechanisms for the reduction in PVR by lung aeration have been debated for decades and includes (a) increased vasodilator release, particularly nitric oxide (NO) (6);

(b) increases in regional oxygenation; (c) entry of gas into the lungs (7, 8); (d) increase in lung recoil caused by the formation of an air/liquid interface and the creation of surface tension within the lung following aeration (9); and (e) recent evidence indicates that a neural reflex may mediate the lung aeration induced increase in PBF (10).

Regardless of the mechanism, the result of the decrease in PVR is that right-to-left shunting of blood through the DA decreases, and flow in the umbilical artery also decreases (11), if the cord remains unclamped. In effect, the lung and placenta compete with one another for both right and left ventricular output due to the ongoing presence of the DA (Figure 11.1) (11). If the decrease in PVR precedes umbilical cord clamping (UCC), cord clamping greatly increases PBF due to a large increase in left-to-right shunting through the DA (3–5). This results from the loss of the low-resistance placental circulation, which increases systemic vascular resistance and promotes blood flow from the systemic into the pulmonary circulation. This reversal in DA blood flow is a normal and important feature of the cardiovascular transition at birth, irrespective of the timing of cord clamping (see below), but it is transient (1–2 h) in normal healthy infants (12).

Umbilical venous return is lost following UCC and so the left ventricle becomes solely dependent upon pulmonary venous return for preload (4). While this has implications for the timing of UCC in relation to lung aeration (see below), the large contribution of left-to-right shunting through the DA to PBF immediately after birth indicates that the left ventricle contributes to its own preload (12). That is, shortly after birth, a left ventricle – DA – lung – left ventricle short circuit develops (Figure 11.1) which is a normal feature of the fetal-to-neonatal cardiovascular transition immediately after birth (12–14). The significance of this is unclear, but as the "short circuit" includes all preductal arteries (Figure 11.1), it would appear that these vessels retain a privileged position within the newborn circulation. It may also offer an opportunity for the output of both ventricles to gradually come into balance before the DA closes and the circulations separate.

In view of a large amount of left-to-right shunting in the DA, venous return to the right ventricle must decrease, which may induce left-to-right shunting through the FO. While it is widely assumed that flow through the FO is unidirectional (15), bidirectional flow has been observed both in fetal sheep following cord clamping and left-to-right shunting has been observed in premature infants (16). Indeed, the presence of bidirectional flow is

DOI: 10.1201/9780367494018-11

Fetal and Adult circulations

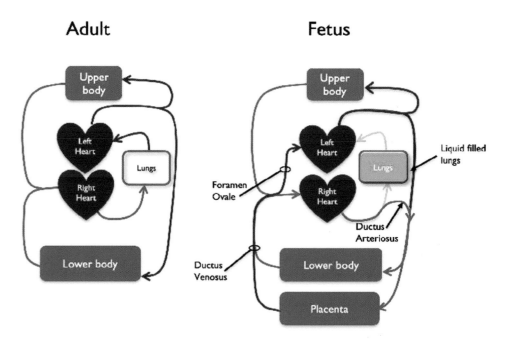

FIGURE 11.1   Schematic diagram of the circulation in the adult and fetus. While the fetal circulation is structurally more complex than the adult, the two circulations are functionally similar, differing only due to the different sites of gas exchange in the fetus and adult. Indeed, in the fetus, the right ventricle provides the majority of blood flow to the organ of gas exchange (placenta), just like it does in the adult (lung), due to the DA which shunts blood from the pulmonary artery into the descending aorta. Similarly, the left ventricle receives most of its venous return from the organ of gas exchange, just like it does in the adult, which passes from the umbilical vein through the DV and foramen ovale directly into the left atrium.

somewhat normal in the first 24–48 hours. This may also help balance preload and output from both ventricles before the two circulations eventually separate. On the other hand, left-to-right shunting through the FO can only occur if left atrial pressure exceeds right atrial pressure, which is thought to be the primary mechanism driving closure of the FO (15). As such, the contribution of the left ventricle and left-to-right shunting through the DA to PBF and pulmonary venous return may help to increase left atrial pressure above right atrial pressure and facilitate closure of the FO.

Cardiovascular effects of UCC at birth and the role of lung aeration

During fetal life, PBF is low and contributes little to the supply of preload for the left ventricle, which instead primarily comes from umbilical venous return (2, 17). Thus, after birth the supply of preload for the left ventricle must switch from umbilical venous to pulmonary venous return (3). However, before this can happen, the lungs must aerate so that PBF can increase and provide the left ventricle with preload (4, 12). As such, when UCC occurs before the lungs have aerated, the loss of umbilical venous return causes a loss of preload and a sudden reduction in cardiac output (4). Cardiac output remains low until the lungs aerate and PBF increases to restore venous return to the left ventricle (4). In addition, due to the loss of the low-resistance placental circulation, UCC rapidly increases systemic vascular resistance, causing a rapid and large increase in arterial pressure (30% increase in 4

heartbeats) (4). As a result, UCC before lung aeration not only causes a loss in ventricular preload but also causes a large increase in after load, which likely contributes to the reduction in cardiac output (4). A further consequence of UCC before lung aeration is the removal of the newborn's only source of gas exchange: The placenta. This results in a rapid fall in arterial and cerebral oxygenation (18) which can only be reversed by the lungs taking over the role of gas exchange. Perhaps the best evidence of the role of UCC before lung aeration on cardiac output is from a study detailing the heart rate changes from birth in normal healthy well oxygenated infants (19). Up to 50% of normal healthy infants were found to be bradycardic (heart rate <100) within the first minute of birth, which was difficult to explain by a hypoxia-mediated bradycardia (19). Instead, they suggested that the loss of umbilical venous return due to UCC, reduced cardiac output, which was reflected by a decrease in heart rate (19), consistent with that observed in animal studies (4). Importantly, these animal studies also demonstrated that if lung aeration and the increase in PBF occurs before UCC, the reduction in cardiac output and subsequent bradycardia is avoided. This is now referred to as physiological-based cord clamping (PBCC) and provides an additional or alternative explanation for the benefits of delayed UCC (3, 5, 20).

Physiological-based cord clamping

At birth, if the lung aerates and PBF increases before the cord is clamped, then PBF is able to immediately take over the role of providing preload for the left ventricle following cord clamping

(3, 4). This avoids the reduction in cardiac output caused by the loss of umbilical venous return with UCC (4). In addition, cord clamping after lung aeration mitigates the increase in arterial pressure caused by UCC, because the lung becomes an alternate (to the placenta) low-resistance pathway for blood flow (4, 12). As a result, left-to-right shunting through the DA increases, leading to a further increase in PBF and venous return to the left ventricle (12). Further, aeration of the lungs before UCC provides the newborn with an alternative source of oxygen so that upon UCC, a fall in systemic and cerebral oxygenation is prevented (18). On the other hand, immediate UCC after birth causes a reduction in cardiac output that is sustained until the lungs aerate and PBF increases (4). Thus, if lung aeration is delayed, cardiac output will remain reduced, which increases the risk of hypoxic/ischemic brain injury if the infant is hypoxic. Then, after lung aeration, cardiac output is rapidly restored, causing a rebound in arterial pressure and a large increase in cerebral blood flow (4). It is not surprising therefore that one of the noted benefits of delaying UCC until after breathing onset is a reduction in intraventricular hemorrhage (IVH) (21).

Influence of hypoxia on the transition at birth

The term "birth asphyxia" is commonly used to describe severely asphyxic infants that are bradycardic (detected by ECG), apneic, have little or no tone, and may lack a detectable pulse. However, asphyxia is a continuum that ranges from the mild to the very severe, and the type of assistance an infant requires likely depends on where it is along that continuum. The cardiovascular response to progressive asphyxia is well established (22). If it is severe and protracted, myocardial contractility diminishes and heart rate and arterial blood pressures decrease with decreasing cardiac output (23, 24) until eventually a complete loss of cardiac function (indicated by very low blood pressures and little to no ventricular outputs) is obtained. At this stage, chest compressions and adrenaline are required to restore oxygenation and cardiac output (25).

The underlying physiology of asphyxiated newborns is very different to that of normoxic newborns. The cardiovascular response to asphyxia (26, 27) involves both an increase and redistribution of cardiac output to increase perfusion and maintain oxygen delivery to vital organs, including the heart and brain (29). This is achieved via vasoconstriction of vascular beds in less vital organs (e.g. skeletal muscle) and dilation of vessels in vital organs including the brain (28, 29). This adaptation is aimed at fetal survival and maintaining brain oxygenation but may severely compromise the newborn at birth. Although systemic vascular resistance increases during fetal hypoxia, placental resistance remains low and cardiac output is directed away from high resistance systemic vascular beds toward the placenta, resulting in a reduction in fetal blood volume (28). In addition, as the cerebral vascular bed is maximally vasodilated, cerebral blood flow autoregulation is impaired and brain flow becomes pressure passive (30). Thus, the brain is unable to protect itself from fluctuations in blood pressure or flow. After birth, asphyxiated newborns can only survive if they rapidly aerate their lungs, which increases PBF, restores cardiac output, and increases blood oxygen content and delivery to the brain (25). However, if restoration of the circulation occurs too rapidly, the brain is exposed to significant fluctuations in pressure and flow, increasing the risk of cerebrovascular injury.

Research using experimental animal models has investigated approaches that can be used to resuscitate asphyxic infants at birth. However, many of these studies have used newborns hours to days after birth (31, 32). More recently, studies have utilised asphyxiated lambs to better understand the transitional haemodynamics during hypoxia (33–37). These studies have shown a profound and rapid rebound hypertension (with mean BP ~50 mmHg above control levels), higher cerebral blood flows and increased oxygen delivery upon return of spontaneous circulation (ROSC) (Figure 11.2). As this response is so rapid in onset, the cerebral resistance vessels, which normally protect the microvasculature from high blood pressures, may still be dilated. If so, these high pressures could be directly transmitted onto the cerebral microvasculature and tissue, potentially causing injury. Thus, it is possible that a more rapid restoration and a greater post-asphyxial rebound response are injurious to the brain (36).

Recent studies in severely asphyxic and asystolic lambs have shown that it is possible to mitigate the post-asphyxial hypertension by resuscitating lambs with the umbilical cord intact (36, 37). While the presence of an intact cord had no effect on the time taken for ROSC, the presence of the low-resistance placental circulation was found to greatly reduced the rebound hypertension (by 20–30 mmHg). The caveat to this finding was that if UCC was only delayed for a minute or two, and therefore occurred during the peak of the rebound sympathetic response, the hypertension tended to be worse (37). Nevertheless, these studies have highlighted the concept that the post-asphyxial rebound response may contribute to the brain injury (and seizures) associated with severe birth asphyxia. Furthermore, it raises the possibility that if the post-asphyxial rebound response can be avoided, its contribution to brain injury may also be avoided.

Resuscitation with an intact umbilical cord – Moving toward the clinic

The logistics of helping infants, particularly very preterm infants, aerate their lungs with an intact umbilical cord was, until recently, thought to be unfeasible. However, recent feasibility studies have demonstrated that the logistical issues are not insurmountable (38, 39). One study (baby-directed UCC study; baby-DUCC) assessed the feasibility of stabilising preterm infants (>32 weeks) with the cord intact by placing the baby on the mother's legs (40). They found that stabilising infants, as indicated by regular stable breathing, with the cord intact, prevented the bradycardia evident in normal healthy infants immediately after birth. Another study (ABC) has used a purpose-built resuscitation table (Concord Table, Concord Neonatal, the Netherlands) that allows for more extensive resuscitation and monitoring of the infant while the umbilical cord remains intact (38, 39). Recent safety and feasibility studies in very preterm infants (<30 weeks) have shown that all necessary interventions for cardiopulmonary stabilization can be performed, while the infant remains attached to the umbilical cord (38, 39). They also observed less bradycardia and hypoxia at birth, supporting the concept of a more stable haemodynamic transition. As the average cord clamping time was over 4 minutes (38, 39), this approach also allows preterm infants to maximally benefit from placental transfusion, while not delaying the onset of resuscitation. Trials are now focussing on PBCC, rather than a time-based approach, in subgroups of infants that will likely experience a long delay between birth and lung aeration. These include very preterm infants (<28 weeks), newborns

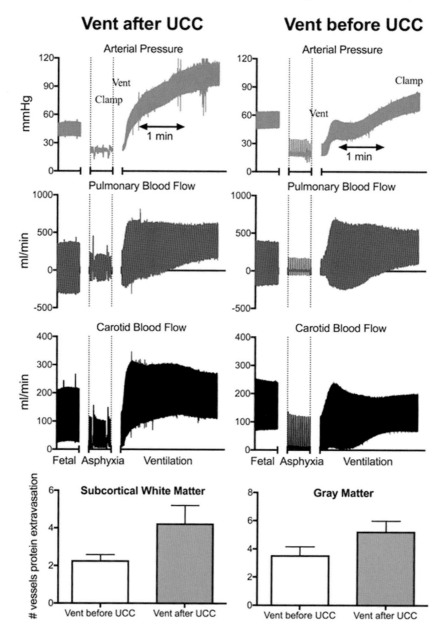

FIGURE 11.2 Effects of ventilation after or before UCC on carotid arterial pressures and flows and PBF. Recordings taken prior to asphyxia (fetal), at the end of asphyxia (asphyxia), and upon ventilation onset (ventilation). The lower panel shows increased protein extravasation into brain parenchyma (BBB breakdown) in asphyxiated lambs where lungs are aerated after clamping of the umbilical cord (vent after UCC vs. vent before UCC).

with a congenital diaphragmatic hernia (41–43), and potentially in the future, asphyxiated infants.

Conclusion

The transition to newborn life is complex, and rapid aeration of the lungs is critical to facilitate a successful transition. Experimental evidence in animals is now clearly supportive of the importance of lung aeration prior to clamping of the umbilical cord, which may underlie the majority of the benefits demonstrated in delayed cord clamping trials. Additionally, these benefits may be greater in infants requiring resuscitation at birth. This has led to preclinical and clinical studies focusing on resuscitation of newborns

with an intact cord. The outcome of these trials may lead to a paradigm shift in the way infants requiring resuscitation at birth are managed in the delivery room; however, more studies around the feasibility and safety of these interventions are required.

References

1. Harding R, et al. J Appl Physiol. 1996; 8 1(1):209–24.
2. Rudolph AM. Annu Rev Physiol 1979; 41:383.–95.
3. Hooper SB, et al. Pediatr Res. 2015; 77(5):608–14.
4. Bhatt S, et al. J Physiol. 2013; 591(8):2113–26.
5. Hooper SB, et al. Arch Dis Child Fetal Neonatal Ed. 2015; 100(4):F355–60.
6. Gao Y, et al. Physiol Rev. 2010; 90(4):1291–335.
7. Teitel DF, et al. Pediatr Res. 1990; 27(4):372–8.
8. Sobotka KS, et al. Pediatr Res. 2011; 70(1):56–60.

9. Hooper SB. Exp Physiol. 1998; 83(6):833–42.
10. Lang JA, et al. J Physiol. 2017; 595(5):1593–606.
11. Blank DA, et al. Arch Dis Child Fetal Neonatal Ed. 2018; 103(6):F539–46.
12. Crossley KJ, et al. J Physiol. 2009; 587(Pt 19):4695–704.
13. van Vonderen JJ, et al. Pediatr Res. 2014; 75(3):448–52.
14. van Vonderen JJ, et al. Neonatology. 2014; 107(2):108–12.
15. Dawes GS, et al. J Physiol. 1955; 128(2):384–95.
16. Evans N, et al. J Pediatr. 1994; 125(5):786–92.
17. Rudolph AM. Circ Res 1985; 57:811.–21.
18. Polglase GR, et al. PLoS One. 2015; 10(2):e0117504.
19. Dawson JA, et al. Arch Dis Child Fetal Neonatal Ed. 2010; 95(3):F177–81.
20. Hooper SB, et al. Matern Health Neonatol Perinatol. 2016; 2:4.
21. Niermeyer S, et al. Semin Fetal Neonatal Med. 2013; 18(6):385–92.
22. Dawes GS. *Foetal and neonatal physiology: A comparative study of the changes at birth.*
    Chicago: Year Book Medical Publishers; 1968.
23. Klingenberg C, et al. Arch Dis Child Fetal Neonatal Ed. 2013; 98(3):F222–7.
24. Sobotka KS, et al. PLoS One. 2014; 9(11):e112264.
25. Sobotka KS, et al. Pediatr Res. 2015; 78(4):395–400.
26. Dawes GS, et al. J Physiol. 1960; 152:271–98.
27. Sobotka KS, et al. PLoS One. 2016; 11(1):e0146574.
28. Polglase GR, et al. Clin Perinatol. 2016; 43(3):469–83.
29. Van Bel F, et al. Acta Paediatr Scand. 1990; 79(8-9):756–62.
30. Herrera-Marschitz M, et al. Adv Neurobiol. 2015; 10:169–98.
31. Dannevig I, et al. Neonatology. 2011; 99(2):153–62.
32. Solevag AL, et al. Arch Dis Child Fetal Neonatal Ed. 2011; 96(6):F417–21.
33. Rawat M, et al. Children (Basel). 2019; 6(4):52.
34. Vali P, et al. Pediatr Crit Care Med. 2017; 18(8):e370–e377.
35. Vali P, et al. J Vis Exp. 2018; (138):57553. doi: 10.3791/57553.
36. Polglase GR, et al. Arch Dis Child Fetal Neonatal Ed. 2018; 103(6):F530–F8.
37. Polglase GR, et al. Front Physiol. 2020; 11:902.
38. Brouwer E, et al. Arch Dis Child Fetal Neonatal Ed. 2019; 104(4):F396–F402.
39. Knol R, et al. Arch Dis Child Fetal Neonatal Ed. 2018; 103(5):F493–F7.
40. Blank DA, et al. Resuscitation. 2018; 131:1–7.
41. Kashyap AJ, et al. Arch Dis Child Fetal Neonatal Ed. 2020; 105(1):18–25.
42. Horn-Oudshoorn EJJ, et al. Arch Dis Child Fetal Neonatal Ed. 2020; 105(4):449–454
43. Lefebvre C, et al. Resuscitation. 2017; 120:20–25.

OXYGEN DURING POSTNATAL STABILIZATION

Maximo Vento and Ola D. Saugstad

Contents

Introduction

Fetal to neonatal transition in mammals is characterized by a precise sequence of circulatory and respiratory changes that contribute to the establishment of an adult-type circulation and airborne respiration. As a consequence, there is an abrupt increase in oxygen availability that fulfills the increased energy requirements of multicellular organisms (1). Despite the exquisite physiologic arrangements that regulate this sequence of events, almost 10% of all newly born infants, and especially those born prematurely, will require resuscitative interventions to achieve an adequate postnatal adaptation (2). In the newborn period, resuscitation requires lung expansion, reducing pulmonary resistance, improving lung compliance, and achieving a functional residual capacity. All these changes improve alveolar-capillary gas exchange and arterial blood oxygenation (3).

The lungs, the thoracic cage, and respiratory muscles only mature late in gestation (4). Moreover, surfactant and the antioxidant enzymatic and nonenzymatic defenses especially in males are not readily available until the last weeks of gestation (5). Hence, preterm infants, and especially very preterm infants with gestational ages below 32 weeks, frequently experience difficulties to establish effective respiration immediately after birth. Immaturity and surfactant deficiency leads to an uneven lung ventilation with hyperventilated areas coexisting with atelectasis and the inability to establish a functional residual capacity. As a consequence, the premature baby is at increased risk of developing hypoxemia, hypercapnia, and increased work of breathing characteristic of respiratory distress syndrome (RDS) with hypoxemic respiratory failure. Therefore, prenatal interventions, such as the administration of antenatal steroids, and postnatal resuscitation with positive pressure ventilation and oxygen supplementation constitute essential interventions necessary to overcome respiratory insufficiency (6).

Oxygen has been widely accepted as the most relevant drug for preterm resuscitation. However, there are still important aspects regarding its use in the immediate postnatal period that has not yet been answered. It would be necessary to address the optimal initial inspired fraction of oxygen (FiO₂), the oxygen saturation (SpO₂) target ranges in the first minutes after birth, and how to titrate oxygen according to the infant's response. Of note, oxygen in excess leads to hyperoxemia and direct tissue damage secondary to oxidative stress, activation of pro-inflammatory and pro-apoptotic pathways, and other mechanisms (5). At the other extreme, hypoxemia especially when combined with bradycardia significantly enhances the risk for intraventricular hemorrhage

(IVH) and death. Both these situations increase mortality and/or short long-term morbidities in survivors (7).

The aim of the present chapter is to critically analyze the most relevant and recent literature concerning the use of oxygen in the delivery room (DR) to help neonatologists optimize the management of preterm infants during postnatal stabilization.

Oxygen *in utero* and during fetal-to-neonatal transition

During late gestation, the arterial partial pressure of oxygen ranges between 25 and 30 mmHg in the fetus and 80–90 mmHg in the mother. Oxygen gradient between mother and fetus drives oxygen across the intervillous space of the placenta. Oxygen content in fetal blood is low during embryogenesis and progressively rises during fetogenesis reaching a saturation plateau at around 14-20 weeks postconception of 50–60%. Thereafter, oxygen saturation slowly decreases to values of 45–50% in the last trimester (8). Oxygenated blood is redirected through circulatory shunts at the *foramen ovale* and *ductus arteriosus* to the lung, brain, and cardiac circulation. The brain and heart are extremely dependent on aerobic metabolism (9). Immediately after birth, newly born infants initiate profound inspiratory movements reaching negative pressures of as low as −40 to −50 cm H₂O that contribute to lung expansion and extrusion of lung fluid from the respiratory airways and alveoli to the interstitium. In addition, increased oxygen content causes vasodilatation of the lung vasculature, drop of the vascular resistance, closure of intra-and-extra-cardiac shunting, and redirection of the ventricular output to the lungs (7). PaO₂ rises to 70–80 mmHg in the first 5–10 min after birth; and arterial oxygen saturation (SpO₂), reflecting the percentage of hemoglobin that is saturated with oxygen, oscillates between 95% and 100% once the fetal-to-neonatal transition is completed (7).

Evolving arterial oxygen saturation in the first minutes after birth

Dawson et al. merged databases from three research groups that included term and preterm newborn infants who did not need resuscitation or oxygen supplementation upon stabilization. With these data, they assembled an oxygen saturation range graph with centiles for a term and late preterm babies for the first 10 minutes after birth (10). Reference ranges for term infants have been adopted by international guidelines to establish target SpO₂ recommendations minute by minute. Thus, recommended ranges

DOI: 10.1201/9780367494018-12

for SpO_2 are at 1 min 60–65%, 2 min 65–70%, 3 min 70–75%, 4 min 75–80%, 5 min 80–85%, and 10 min 85–95% (11). However, the reference ranges for preterm infants were based on a smaller population of 136 late preterm infant (33^{+6} to 36^{+6} weeks gestation). The percentiles for preterm infants did not reflect the evolving SpO_2 in very preterm infants ≤32 weeks GA in the first minutes after birth (10). Vento et al. (12) retrieved minute by minute SpO_2s and heart rate (HR) in very preterm infants ventilated with positive pressure and air mimicking the real clinical situation in the DR. The results of this study showed that very preterm infants on mask ventilation achieved higher SpO_2s and stabilized significantly earlier than preterm infants as shown in Dawson's nomogram (12).

Delaying cord clamping has been recommended by international guidelines in the last decade and widely accepted as a routine intervention in the DR (5, 11, 13). Delaying cord clamping contributes to the hemodynamic stabilization of the newborn infant increasing the left ventricular preload and afterload, decreasing pulmonary vascular resistance and facilitating pulmonary gas exchange (14). Hence, aerating the lung and increasing pulmonary blood flow before umbilical cord clamping could avoid the reduction of cardiac preload and output as a consequence of immediate cord clamping (14). Based on these assumptions, several clinical studies have reported the feasibility of ventilating newborn infants with patent cord although no improvement in outcomes has been yet reported (15–18).

Recently, reference ranges for term infants born by vaginal delivery, delayed cord patency for more than one minute, and not needing resuscitation or oxygen at birth have been constructed (19). Minute by minute data for HR and SpO_2 were registered during the first 10 minutes after fetal expulsion. Significantly higher values for SpO_2 for the 10th, 50th and 90th centiles compared with Dawson's reference range (10) for the first 5 minutes and for HR for the first 1–2 minutes after birth were reported (19). Hence, in healthy newly born by vaginal delivery and with delayed cord clamping > 60 seconds, higher SpO_2 and HR were achieved in the first 5 minutes after birth compared with term neonates born but with immediate cord clamping (19).

Initial inspired fraction of oxygen (FiO_2) for resuscitation in the delivery room

The 2015 international guidelines (11, 13, 20) strongly recommend initiating resuscitation of preterm infants < 32 weeks gestational age with a low oxygen concentration (21–30%) acknowledging that the evidence that supports this recommendation is of moderate-quality. The recent 2019 European Consensus Guidelines on the management of RDS (5) advocates the use of FiO_2 of 0.21–0.30 as initial gas admixture for preterm infants <28 weeks' gestation and 0.30 for babies 28–31 weeks. Oei et al (21) launched an international survey that showed that the majority (77%) of neonatologists targeted SpO_2 between the 10th and 50th percentiles of Dawson's reference range for full-term infants (10) and would start with an FiO_2 0.3. Interestingly, most participants acknowledged lack of sufficient evidence and recommended further research (21). It could be hypothesized that the use of lower initial FiO_2 would reduce the oxygen load and the oxidative stress upon stabilization. Oxidative stress has been linked as a causative agent to a series of neonatal conditions including bronchopulmonary dysplasia (BPD), retinopathy of prematurity (ROP), necrotizing enterocolitis (NEC), or intraventricular hemorrhage (IVH) among others (22, 23). In two randomized controlled trials, the initiation of resuscitation with high initial FiO_2 (0.9 or 1.0) with subsequent

titration resulted in increased oxidant stress and BPD incidence compared to starting with 0.21 or 0.30 (24, 25). In contrast, when the difference between higher (≥0.60) and lower (≤0.30) initial FiO_2 was reduced, no differences in clinical outcomes or biomarkers of oxidative stress were found in two randomized controlled trial (RCT) blinded for the air/oxygen blender (26, 27). Contrarily, a nonblinded RCT performed in extremely premature infants (<28 weeks' gestation) raised concerns about the optimal strategy to supplement oxygen to extremely preterm infants. The TO2RPIDO study randomized infants <32 weeks GA to air or 100% oxygen. SpO_2 was targeted to 65% to 95% at 5 minutes and 85% to 95% at NICU admission (28). A total of 287 infants with a mean GA of 28.9 weeks were included. In a nonprespecified *post hoc* analysis, infants <28 weeks GA had increased of mortality of almost 4-fold if initially started with air, compared with 100% O_2 (RR 3.9; 95% CI 1.1–13.4) (28). It should be underpinned that this study was underpowered to address this post hoc hypothesis reliably and the trial was ceased per recommendation of the Data and Safety Monitoring Committee due to loss of equipoise for the use of 100% oxygen (28). Further, Oei et al. (29) performed a systematic review of the outcomes of infants ≤28 +6 weeks gestation randomized to resuscitation with low (≤0.3) versus high (≥0.6) FiO_2 at delivery in 8 RCT that fulfilled these requirements. They did not find differences in the overall risk of death or other common preterm morbidities including BPD, NEC, ROP, PDA, or IVH after resuscitation was initiated at delivery with lower or higher FiO_2 (29). Accumulated evidence of the last decade has been reported by two major systematic reviews and meta-analyses. Lui K et al. (30) performed a Cochrane systematic review of 10 RCTs that included 914 infants. No significant impact was assessed on death at discharge or relevant neonatal conditions such as ROP, periventricular leukomalacia (PVL), IVH, NEC, BPD, or PDA and neurodevelopmental outcome in preterm infants ≤32 weeks' gestation with lower (<0.4) or higher (≥0.4) initial FiO_2 titrated to target oxygen saturations (30). Almost simultaneously, Welsford et al. (31), in a systematic review and meta-analysis that included 10 RCT and 4 cohort studies totaling 5697 preterm infants <35 weeks gestation, compared higher (>50%) versus lower (<50%) initial FiO_2 for resuscitation in the DR. This study also failed to show differences in short-term mortality, long-term mortality, neurodevelopmental impairment, or other relevant preterm morbidities in the neonatal period (31). However, the authors pointed out that the majority of the subgroup of newborns ≤32 week's gestation required oxygen supplementation upon stabilization (31).

Higher initial FiO_2: Critical appraisal of recent evidence

Despite the results of both meta-analyses (30, 31) ongoing studies have approached the best option to stimulate respiration and achieve suitable SpO_2s in the DR in preterm infants ≤ 28 weeks' gestation. Crawshaw et al. (32). using phase contrast X-ray imaging studied the effect of mask ventilation upon the glottis and epiglottis status and showed that immediately after birth both remained predominantly closed rendering IPPV ineffective. Of note, after lung aeration, the larynx was predominantly open allowing noninvasive ventilation to efficiently ventilated the lung (32). Hence, in apneic preterm infants, noninvasive ventilation may render inefficient because of the glottis remaining close. However, tactile stimulation is a potent stimulator of spontaneous breathing and therefore should be routinely applied to avoid tracheal intubation (33). Dekker et al. (34), based on the inhibitory effect of hypoxia on spontaneous breathing, hypothesized that the use of high FiO_2

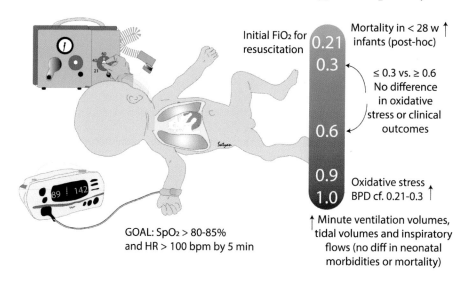

FIGURE 12.1 An infographic summarizing the results of randomized controlled trials and post hoc analysis and meta-analyses comparing low vs. high initial fraction of inspired oxygen (FiO₂) for resuscitation of preterm infants. SpO₂ – oxygen saturation by pulse oximetry, BPD – bronchopulmonary dysplasia, HR – heart rate. (Copyright Satyan Lakshminrusimha.)

would reduce the risk of hypoxia and increased the respiratory drive at birth. Preterm kittens were randomized to receive CPAP immediately after birth with either 21% or 100% oxygen. If apnea occurred, intermittent positive pressure ventilation (IPPV) was applied with 21% or 100% to the 21% group and remained at 100% for kittens who started with 100%. Kittens receiving 21% oxygen had an unstable respiratory pattern as compared with kittens on 100% oxygen. Apneas that required IPPV were significantly more frequent in kittens initially resuscitated with 21% and recovery after apneas showed also a more unstable pattern of respiration in kittens on 21%. Thus, initiating resuscitation with 100% contributed to a stable respiratory pattern and decreased the risk for apneas (34). This group translated the results of their experiments into a small randomized controlled clinical trial in which preterm infants <30 weeks' gestation were initially ventilated with FiO₂ 0.3 (n=20) vs. 1.0 (n=24) (35). The primary outcome was minute volume of spontaneous breathing. Other clinical and oxidative stress parameters were also measured. Minute volumes, tidal volumes and mean inspiratory flow rate were significantly higher in the 100% oxygen group and the duration of mask ventilation significantly shorter. Oxygenation in the first 5 minutes was significantly higher and the duration of hypoxemia significantly shorter in infants in the 100% group. No differences in the oxidative stress marker were found. However, mortality and relevant morbidities in the neonatal period such as BPD, IVH, NEC, or length of hospital stay were not different between groups (35). Despite the improvement in the immediate postnatal period, using 100% oxygen had no positive impact on clinical outcomes in the neonatal period. The beneficial effect of an initial ventilation with pure oxygen was limited to the stabilization period in the DR and did not influence longer-term clinical outcomes.

Our aim should be to reach SpO₂ of 80–85% within 5 minutes of life. It has been shown that despite the initial FiO₂ there is little difference in the SpO₂ achieved in the first 2–3 minutes after birth. Moreover, often reliable SpO₂ readings are not achieved until this time elapses. Hence, the chance to correctly adjust FiO₂ to achieve a SpO₂ of 80% at five minutes is limited to a time span of 2–3 minutes. This is one of the strong arguments for starting with 100% oxygen, to reach targeted saturations and then titrate down.

However, doing so we only improve the infant's response in the first minutes but not the longer-term outcomes. In addition, there is a risk of unexpectedly prolonging hyperoxia with inherent deleterious consequences. Very careful titration is necessary; exactly the same as when starting with lower oxygen and increasing FiO₂ rapidly if needed to avoid hypoxemia and its consequences.

To date, we still lack a SpO₂ reference range for very preterm infants; nor we have established saturation goals in the first minutes after birth. In the study by Dekker et al (35), oxygen load was apparently lower in babies receiving lower than higher initial FiO₂ in the first minutes after birth and titrating thereafter. However, there is no evidence supporting what is more detrimental either the oxygen load exposure or the peak concentration of oxygen. In this regard, the study by Dekker et al. measured 8-iso-prostaglandin F2α (8iPGF2α) at 1 and 24 hours after birth and did not find a significant increase (35). Not all isoprostanes always reflect the presence of hyperoxic oxidative stress. In this regard, isofurans are the most reliable biomarkers to assess oxidative damage to lipids caused by hyperoxia (36). Oxygen concentration differentially modulates the formation of isoprostanes and isofurans. As oxygen concentrations increase, the formation of isofurans is favored, whereas the formation of isoprostanes becomes disfavored (36). This could explain why despite using 100% oxygen, the levels of isoprostanes did not increase as expected. However, the results of previous studies clearly correlate the use of higher oxygen concentrations with oxidative stress and increased incidence of oxidative-stress associated conditions especially BPD (24, 25). Oei et al. (37) analyzed data from 768 infants <32 weeks GA enrolled in 8 RCT initially resuscitated with higher (≥0.6) or lower (≤0.3) initial FiO₂. Babies who, independent from the initial FiO₂, did not reach a SpO₂ of 80% within 5 minutes after birth had higher mortality, more severe IVH, and poorer neurodevelopmental outcome compared to those who reached this level of oxygenation (37).

These and other findings reflected in comprehensive updated reviews and meta-analyses should be taken into consideration before generalizing the use of high initial FiO₂ in extremely preterm infants (37). An infographic summarizing current evidence on initial FiO₂ for resuscitation of preterm infants is shown in Figure 12.1.

Final considerations

The key for this conundrum resides in the ability to achieve SpO$_2$s between 80% and 85% within the first five minutes after birth in very preterm infants <32 weeks' gestation independently of the initial FiO$_2$, gender or type of delivery. Reaching an adequate oxygenation and avoiding episodes of bradycardia in the first five minutes after birth seems essential to enhance postnatal stability and avoid death or serious complications such as IVH (38, 39).

With the present evidence consensus guidelines recommend to initiate resuscitation of infants 28–31 weeks with an initial FiO$_2$ of 0.21–0.30 guiding oxygen titration up and down with the use of pulse oximetry aiming to achieve SpO$_2$ of 80–85% and HR >100 bpm within 5 minutes (5, 11, 13, 20).

References

1. Lara-Cantón I, et al. Children (Basel). 2019; 6(2):29
2. Vento M, et al. Semin Fetal Neonatal Med. 2020; 25:101088.
3. Alphonse RS, et al. Antioxid. Redox Signal. 2012; 17:1013–1040.
4. Vento M, et al. Antioxid. Redox Signal. 2009; 11:2945–2955.
5. Sweet DG, et al. Neonatology. 2017; 115:432–450.
6. Torres-Cuevas I, et al. Front. Pediatr. 2016; 4:29.
7. Gao Y, et al. Physiol. Rev. 2010; 90:1291–2010.
8. Vento M, et al. Semin Fetal Neonatal Med. 2013; 18:324–329.
9. Vali P, et al. Children (Basel). 2017; 4:67.
10. Dawson JA, et al. Pediatrics. 2010; 125:e1340–e1347.
11. Wyckoff MH, et al. Circulation 2015; 132 (Suppl. 2):S543–S560.
12. Vento M, et al. Arch Dis Child Fetal Neonatal. 2013; 98:F228–F232.
13. Wyllie J, et al. Resuscitation. 2015; 95:249–263.
14. Hooper SB, et al. Semin Fetal Neonatal Med. 2019; 24:101033.
15. Katheria A, et al. J Pediatr. 2016; 176:75–80.e3.
16. Winter J, et al. Am J Perinatol. 2017; 34:111–116.
17. Pratesi, et al. Front Pediatr. 2018; 6:364.
18. Brouwer E, et al. Arch Dis Child Fetal Neonatal Ed. 2019; 104:F396–F402.
19. Padilla-Sánchez C, et al. J Pediatr. 2020; 227:149–156.e1.
20. Perlman JM, et al. Circulation. 2015; 132(16 Suppl 1):S204–S241.
21. Oei JL, et al. Acta Paediatrica. 2016; 105:1061–1066.
22. Saugstad OD, et al. Pediatr Res. 2019; 85:20–29.
23. Saugstad OD. Pediatr Res. 1988; 23(2):143–50.
24. Vento M, et al. Pediatrics. 2009; 124:e439–449.
25. Kapadia VS, et al. Pediatrics. 2013; 132:e1488–98.
26. Rook D, et al. J Pediatr. 2014; 164:1322–1326.e3.
27. Aguar M, et al. EPAS 2014; 3843:540.
28. Oei JL, et al. Pediatrics. 2017; 139:e20161452.
29. Oei JL, et al. Arch Dis Child Fetal Neonatal Ed. 2017; 102:F24–F30.
30. Lui K, et al. Cochrane Database Syst Rev 2018; 5(5):CD010239.
31. Welsford M, et al. Pediatrics. 2019; 143:e20181828.
32. Crawshaw JR, et al. Arch Dis Child Fetal Neonatal Ed. 2018; 103:F112–F119.
33. Kuypers K, et al. Arch Dis Child Fetal Neonatal Ed. 2020 Nov; 105(6):675–679.
34. Dekker, et al. Front Pediatr. 2019; 7:427.
35. Dekker J, et al. Front Pediatr. 2019; 7:504.
36. Roberts LJ, et al. Brain Pathol. 2005; 15:143–8.
37. Oei JL, et al. Arch Dis Child Fetal Neonatal Ed. 2018; 103:F446–F454.
38. Saugstad OD, et al. J Pediatr. 2020; 227:295–299.
39. Lara-Cantón, et al. Front Pediatr. 2020; 8:12.

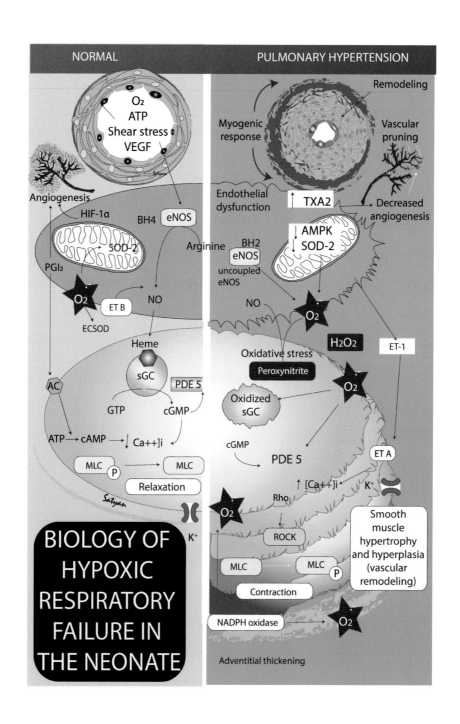

Part 3

Biology of Hypoxic Respiratory Failure in the Neonate

Edited by Steven H. Abman

HYPOXIA AND PULMONARY ARTERY STRUCTURE

Csaba Galambos and Steven H. Abman

Contents

Pulmonary arterial structure in the postnatal lung

Pulmonary arteries are conducting vessels that provide pathways to the flow of deoxygenated blood to reach the alveolar capillaries for gas exchange. As the pulmonary circulation travels from proximal to distal parts of lung, the pulmonary arterial vascular tree undergoes successive stages of branching, and structure that is characterized by gradual decrease in diameter and wall thickness, gradually leading to the distal vasculature that normally lacks a muscular coat. The various arterial segments between the pulmonary trunk and the alveolar capillaries have specialized niches with diverse neighboring cells and matrix composition, many of which are developmentally regulated that lead to unique patterns of vasoreactivity, growth responses with age, and the ability to adapt to various injuries with appropriate repair. These structural differences, linked to vessel size and function, have distinct histologic correlates.

Overall, the pulmonary arteries are generally grouped into elastic and muscular types that are composed of 3 microanatomical components: Tunica intima, tunica media, and tunica adventitia. Tunic intima, the thinnest layer lining the inner aspect of the artery, is a single layer of endothelial cells that sit on an elastic membrane. The internal elastic lamina separates tunica intima from tunica media. The tunica media is the major component of the arterial wall and composed mainly of elastic fibers in elastic type arteries and smooth muscle in muscular type arteries. The outermost layer of all types of arteries is the tunica adventitia, which harbors a vast amount of collagen-rich matrix with embedded scattered fibrocytes. Tunica adventitia is separated from tunic media by external elastic lamina.

The most proximal and largest arteries are of elastic type and have a diameter of roughly 1 mm. A characteristic feature is that the media contains multiple parallel elastic lamina embedded in a mixture of smooth muscle cells, collagen, and other types of extracellular matrix. The function of these arteries is related to their elasticity, which allows to expand and retract following large amount of blood inflow during heart contractions. In normal condition, the pulsatile stretch recoil of the elastic arteries allows smooth transition to continuous, low-velocity blood flow and low pressures in in the distal arteries and capillaries (1).

The transition from elastic to muscular-type arteries takes place at a diameter around 500 micrometer, where the elastic arteries gradually lose their elastic tissue within the media with the exception of external elastic lamina. Pulmonary arteries with an external diameter between 500 and 70 micrometer constitute the muscular type. These medium-sized arteries play crucial roles in governing arterial pressure and regulating the distribution of blood flow within the pulmonary vascular tree in response to vasoconstrictor and vasodilator stimuli. The media is composed of smooth muscle cells with a circular orientation. Between the smooth muscle cells are minimal amount of collagen and reticulin fibers. When compared to systemic arteries of similar diameter, the tunica media or wall of pulmonary arteries is much thinner and the lumen is larger, which reflects the difference in pressure between the systemic and normal pulmonary vascular circulation. In principle, the muscular arteries travel with the bronchi and larger bronchioles, and the diameter of the PA is generally smaller than that of the accompanying airway.

In addition to conventional branches, numerous small vessels branch off of pulmonary arteries that are not accompanied by neighboring airways. They are termed supernumerary arteries, whose function and structure are poorly understood. The media to diameter ratio of a conventional pulmonary artery is generally constant so when the diameter is known the thickness can be predicted. The media thickness of pulmonary artery is generally expressed as the percentage of external diameter and ranges from 2.8 to 6.8%, when the lung is fully extended before fixation (2). Some authors note that pulmonary arteries of muscular wall thickness up to 25% can be occasionally observed in healthy lungs, raising the possibility that the functional state pulmonary arteries may not be uniform (3). The percentage of wall thickness changes in accordance with its associated airway size (4). Importantly, the most notable changes take place at the site where the pulmonary artery enters the distal acinus. The intra-acinar arteries are no longer accompanied by an airway, their external diameter decreases to the level of 70 micrometer, and they lose their muscular coat. This thinning of the media is a gradual process, which evolves from containing a full smooth muscle coat to lacking smooth muscle more distally, with an intermediate vessel segment containing smooth muscle bundles that run a spiral course. Once the pulmonary arteries lose their muscle coat, they are virtually

DOI: 10.1201/9780367494018-13

indistinguishable from the intra-acinar veins on routine histologic sections. These precapillary arterial segments harbor occasional precursor smooth muscle cells, or pericytes within their wall. The intima of nonmuscular intra-acinar arteries is composed of a single endothelial layer resting on a thin basement membrane (5).

Pulmonary arterial structure in the fetus

The overall structure of pulmonary arterial circulation is markedly different in fetal lung. In addition to high vascular tone leading to the high pulmonary vascular resistance that characterizes the fetal lung, a number of distal pulmonary arteries rapidly proliferates during the later stages of lung development, including the late canalicular and saccular stages. Postmortem angiograms of fetal and neonatal lung often show minimal background filling when compared to those of older infants, children and adults, indicating markedly reduced vascular development in the fetus and newborn (6). During fetal life, there is constant growth, as reflected by increased branching and remodeling of the pulmonary arterial system. The lumen of muscular pulmonary arteries is narrow and the media is thick. Pulmonary arterial smooth muscles cells are round in shape and densely packed in a thick arterial wall with narrow lumen (7). The diameter to thickness ratio is constant and observed in the range of 15-25% (8). The total amount of muscle tissue in the lung increases with gestational age and parallels the growing number of pulmonary arteries. Mechanisms that contribute to the maintenance of high resting tone in the fetal lung are not completely understood, but include mechanical factors such as compression of fetal pulmonary arteries by the fluid filled alveolar space, the lack of rhythmic (breathing) distension, the presence of low resting alveolar and arteriolar oxygen tensions, high myogenic tone and an altered balance of vasoactive mediators that favor vasoconstriction (9).

Pulmonary arterial structure during transition to birth

At birth, marked remodeling of the fetal pulmonary arterial system takes place to accommodate the physiologic changes that are essential for survival. Rhythmic air-breathing movements begin, blood flow to the placenta is lost, the heart pumps high volume of pulsatile flow to the lung, and extrapulmonary shunt pathways close. As the result, the lung is filled with oxygenated air and pure deoxygenated blood enters the pulmonary bed for gas exchange. In support of this, the pulmonary arteries acutely expand and adapt to high flow as lung vascular resistance drops 8-10 folds to accommodate the entry of the entire cardiac output. The sudden hemodynamic change broadcasts a sudden transition of fetal to adult type arteries. During the first 24 hours, there is marked and progressive thinning and dilatation of muscular and nonmuscular pulmonary arteries. The partially muscularized arteries become nonmuscularized, completely muscularized arteries become partially muscularized, and the larger vessels of the muscular layer become thin. This program continues throughout the first weeks of life before achieving adult values within the first 3 months of age (10) along with a reduction in pulmonary vascular resistance. Gradual and slower thinning of media takes place in the first one and one and half years to reach that of adult size (8). The media becomes thinner from the hilum to the capillary bed without a reduction in the amount of vascular

smooth muscle. Rather, the smooth muscle cells re-orient and change shape rapidly after birth, as their surface to volume ratio increases as the smooth muscle cells become stretched around larger vessels (7, 9). As the endothelial cells spread out, their length increases along with the surface-to-volume ratio, leading to increased lumen diameter and decreased resistance (7). The reduction of muscular coat correlates with decreased vasoreactivity, especially in the small, precapillary arteries (7). The swollen endothelial cells of tunica intima within nonmuscularized arteries become flattened at birth. There is a rapid increase in the endothelial and smooth muscle surface-to-volume ratio as the cells spread within the vessel wall to increase lumen diameter and thus lower pulmonary resistance. This change in smooth muscle cell shape is associated with de-polymerization of cytoskeletal and contractile proteins. Reorganization of actin filament network occurs when the adult wall-thickness-to-diameter ratio is achieved (11).

Pulmonary arterial structure in PPHN

Persistent pulmonary hypertension of the newborn (PPHN) develops when the cardiopulmonary system fails to adapt to the normal oxygen-rich environment following birth. The intra- and extra-cardiac shunts remain open, the smooth muscle walls of pulmonary arteries fail to thin, the vessel diameter remains small, and high vascular tone dominates the pulmonary circulation. As a consequence, pulmonary vessel resistance remains high, deoxygenated blood does not reach the pulmonary acinus, alveolar capillaries are not recruited for gas-exchange and marked hypoxemia of the newborn ensues. Histologically, extension of the smooth muscle layer to intra-acinar arteries is a key pathologic process, in addition to the above-mentioned abnormalities (Figure 13.1). Intra-acinar arteries are virtually nonmuscularized in fetal life and at birth. Distal extension of arterial smooth muscle into these vessel takes place only postnatally, beginning normally about six months of age, and is competed in adolescent years. The pathologic vascular remodeling characteristic of PPHN represents new muscle development, as opposed to the persistence of fetal vessel musculature or fetal vessel vasoconstriction (12). In addition to small arteries, elastic arterial pathology in PPHN has been observed, including loss of distensibility (13) and increased stiffness (14). Ultrastructurally, lack of reorganization of smooth muscle cell cytoskeleton along with γ-actin isoform abundance is seen (10, 15).

Effect of hypoxemia on fetal pulmonary arterial remodeling in PPHN

Oxygen tension in the fetal pulmonary circulation is low (approximately 17 to 25 mm Hg), and vasoconstriction in response to low oxygen tension may contribute to high pulmonary vascular resistance in the fetus (16, 17). Reducing blood PO_2 to fetal values markedly increases pulmonary vascular resistance in newborn lambs (18). Hypoxic pulmonary vasoconstriction increases over the last trimester of gestation, when a cross-sectional area of the vascular bed is increasing rapidly. Decreasing oxygen tension in fetal lamb at 103 days of gestation does not increase pulmonary vascular resistance, but in the 130- to 138-day fetus it doubles the resistance (19). Conversely, increasing oxygen tension before 100 days gestation does not decrease pulmonary vascular resistance, but by 135 days gestation (with term roughly 150 days), increased oxygen tension decreases pulmonary vascular resistance and

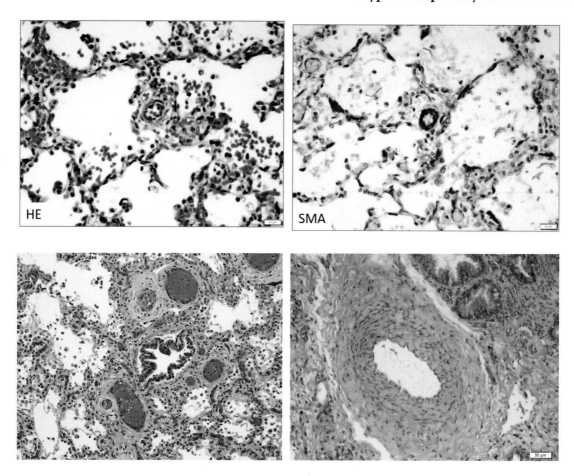

FIGURE 13.1 Histopathology of PPHN. Autopsy studies demonstrate that muscularization of distal and intra-acinar pulmonary arteries are consistently present in PPHN, in addition to variable degrees of dysmorphic vessels and reduced alveolarization. The muscularized media is highlighted by immunostaining with smooth muscle actin (SMA). In normal conditions under 6 month of age, intra-acinar arteries are thin, and devoid of smooth muscle cells. The lower panels illustrate pulmonary vascular and related alveolar hypoplasia in alveolar capillary dysplasia (left), and severe pulmonary artery remodeling in an infant with severe chronic lung disease (right).

increases pulmonary blood flow to normal newborn levels (20). Although the mechanism by which low fetal oxygen tension regulates pulmonary vascular resistance is not known, it may do so in part through regulation of nitric oxide, endothelin, and prostacyclin (21–24). Acidemia increases pulmonary vascular resistance and accentuates hypoxic vasoconstrictor responses, indicating that pH may modulate the effects of oxygen on pulmonary vascular resistance (25). What exactly causes PPHN is not entirely understood, but *in utero* stresses leading to hypoxia adversely affecting pulmonary vascular growth, remodeling, and reactivity in the fetus is a major driver (Figure 13.2). Hypoxic vasospasm of the pulmonary arteries is a key and early driver of PPHN (26).

Hypoxia-responsive genes: The role of HIF-derived signals in PPHN

Hypoxia inducible factors (HIFs) are considered to play a key role in pulmonary vascular signaling, pulmonary arterial vasoconstriction, and pathologic remodeling. HIFs are heterodimers consisting of oxygen-sensitive α-subunits (*HIF-1α, HIF-2α*) and constitutively expressed β subunits. Hypoxia stabilizes the α subunit leading to nuclear accumulation and activation of multiple target genes (27). HIFs are highly conserved transcription factors that are expressed in multiple cell types, and control the

oxygen-dependent expression of numerous genes (27). The fetus is programmed to develop under hypoxic conditions, and HIF expression is essential to normal fetal lung development. Basal HIF expression has been reported to be higher in the fetal relative to the adult lung (28), and deletion of the HIF gene is lethal during fetal life.

After birth, chronic hypoxia through HIFs induces pulmonary vascular abnormalities characteristic of PPHN (29–31). Heterozygous mice lacking one *HIF-1α* allele display attenuated hypoxia-induced pulmonary vascular remodeling and pulmonary hypertension (32), Targeted silencing of smooth muscle *HIF-1α* expression rescues the development of pulmonary vascular remodeling and pulmonary hypertension (33), consistent with a key role for *HIF-1α* in the pulmonary vascular response to hypoxia. Elevated HIF expression and activity in lungs and pulmonary arterial smooth muscle cells has been linked to abnormal gene expression seen previously in PPHN lambs. PPHN vascular cells exposed to hypoxia showed increased HIF signaling that was mediated by stretch via mitochondrial reactive oxygen species and NFκB. Together these data suggest that elevated HIF signaling may contribute to pulmonary vascular remodeling and pulmonary hypertension in PPHN. However, more recent studies suggest that augmentation of HIF activity improves lung vascular

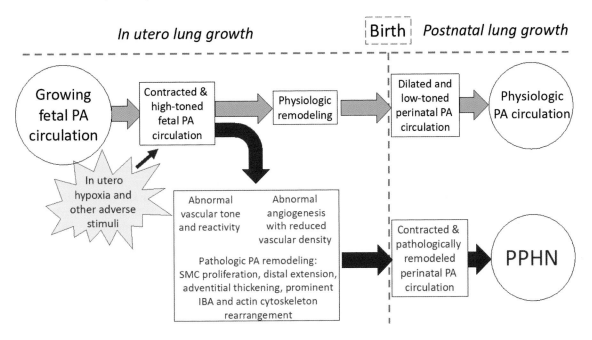

FIGURE 13.2 Schematic of pulmonary vascular disease in PPHN.

growth and prevents the development of pulmonary hypertension in antenatal and postnatal (hyperoxia) models of bronchopulmonary dysplasia, suggesting a more complex role of HIF regulation on lung vascular growth and structure (34).

Endothelial cell dysfunction, increased vascular tone, and resistance

The innermost layer of pulmonary arteries is made of endothelial cells (EC), in intimate contact with the smooth muscle layer and the blood being conducted within the pulmonary artery. Endothelial cells are capable of detecting changes in oxygenation, circulating factors, flow, and pressure in the blood and regulate smooth muscle homeostasis. In fact, oxygen-induced pulmonary vasodilation in the fetus is at least partly mediated by the release of nitric oxide (NO) (35, 36). Hypoxic remodeling of EC is minimal but may be characterized by cellular hypertrophy, subendothelial space widening, edema, and minimal collagen and elastin fiber deposition (37). During hypoxemic stimulus and in PPHN, there is limited fibrointimal proliferation early as opposed to that seen with later or more severe diseases associated with PAH (38, 39). While there are conflicting *in vivo* data regarding the extent of pulmonary artery endothelial cell proliferation according to the specific animal model and postnatal age, however, with the exception of neonatal calves, the degree of smooth muscle cell proliferation in most models of hypoxic pulmonary hypertension is low (40–42). The proliferative response of EC in hypoxic conditions is controversial, and pulmonary hypertension is not likely an effect of hypoxia alone, as in vitro studies demonstrate growth inhibition with acute (24 h) or chronic hypoxia (5 days) compared with normoxia (43, 44). Conflicting data showing human EC proliferation in serum containing media at 1% hypoxia for 72 h have been reported, but growth was inhibited at earlier time points; there were no data at later time points (45). Subendothelial thickening can be observed in response to chronic hypoxic exposure. Hypoxia induces an increase in EC permeability, the influx of vasoactive mediators, and plasma proteins and subsequent activation of vascular wall proteases, which all contribute to remodeling (46–48). Changes in EC barrier function,

induced by hypoxia, have been associated with alterations in actin stress fiber formation, increased cell stiffness, and contraction, all of which appear to be mediated by activation of MAP kinase and/ or Rho kinase (49). These hypoxia-induced alterations in cell shape and structure, resulting in increases in permeability, could result in exposure of smooth muscle cells to circulating vasoactive substances. They also contribute to the development of subendothelial edema, which is commonly observed. Hypoxia has significant effects on the regulation of synthesis and secretion of vasoactive factors and inflammatory cytokines in EC. Hypoxia causes EC to induce a vasoconstrictive environment through decreased production and/or activity of prostacyclin and nitric oxide as well as increased production of endothelin, serotonin, leukotrienes, and other mediators (50–52). Thus, whereas hypoxia induces important EC changes that can directly lead to intimal thickening and remodeling, probably equally important are the indirect signals capable of recruiting circulating cells and inducing local cellular proliferation and smooth muscle contraction, hypertrophy, and even hyperplasia.

Hypoxic vasospasm, smooth muscle cell phenotype, and actin cytoskeletal rearrangement

Hypoxic vasospasm with right to left extracardiac shunting marks the initial presentation of PPHN (26). This implies vasoactive change within small pulmonary arteries. Animal models of PPHN exposed to postnatal hypoxia pulmonary arterial smooth muscle cells retain their shape and low surface to volume ratio. Neither the normal postnatal reduction in arterial smooth muscle content nor the normal transient postnatal reduction of actin content is seen in PPHN pulmonary arteries. Both human PPHN subjects and hypoxic animal models exhibit persistently polymerized actin (10).

Dynamic reorganization of smooth muscle cells depends of the function of actin cytoskeleton in early PPHN that includes smooth muscle cell lengthening, position readjustment with increased cellular overlap locally controlled by *Rho, Rac* and *Cdc42* pathways that are hypoxia-sensitive. Pulmonary arteries exposed to hypoxia promotes actin polymerization, actin incorporation into cytoskeletal filaments, which is linked to increased thromboxane-induced vasoconstriction. Vasoconstriction induces actin polymerization in hypoxic pulmonary arteries, which is actin isoform dependent. Hypoxia induces α and γ actin isoforms in vitro and in PPHN vessels. Upon treatment with a vasoconstrictive agent, the polymerization consisted mainly of γ isoforms. Although changes in vascular reactivity may precede many structural changes, increased distal muscularization of small pulmonary arteries is generally associated with heightened vascular tone and hypoxic reactivity (15).

Restructured adventitia: Outward remodeling of pulmonary arteries

Adventitia, the outermost portion of the pulmonary arteries, consist of a 3D network of extracellular matrix, nutritional vessels (i.e. the vasa vasorum), nerves, and a variety of resident cells including fibroblasts, progenitor cells, and inflammatory cells. The ontogeny of adventitia is poorly understood, but in fetal life adventitia appears to be thick; gradual thinning and increase in density takes place until the pulmonary arteries acquire structures seen in adulthood. With prolonged hypoxia, the adventitia becomes thicker and denser and is characterized by matrix deposition, expansion of the vasa vasorum, and proliferation of resident cells including fibroblasts, progenitor cells, and macrophages (52). These changes appear to affect medial smooth muscle cell structure, organization, activity, and cause external lamina disruption (53). Moreover, under hypoxia, the fibroblasts of adventitia, through epigenetic mechanisms, acquire an "activated" phenotype (54, 55) and regulate vascular function directly or indirectly (52).

Hypoxia in newborn calves uniquely induces marked changes of the adventitia, as characterized by thickening, cellular proliferation, and extracellular deposition of altered collagen and elastin content (56). During development, fetal calf pulmonary artery fibroblasts are highly proliferative and synthetic, a phenotype that nearly disappears shortly after birth; however, this phenotype persists or reappears during high altitude-induced hypoxia and neonatal fibroblasts become both highly synthetic and highly proliferative. Although systematic studies of adventitia in human newborn with PPHN are lacking, it has been suggested that the hypoxemic adventitia significantly affects vascular remodeling and contributes to high pulmonary vascular resistance.

Bronchial circulation: Recruitment of intrapulmonary bronchopulmonary anastomoses

Both hemodynamically and metabolically, the lung provides important communications between the right and left heart. The lung includes a "double circulation" – the pulmonary and systemic (bronchial) systems, and although considered distinct, there can be key interactions between these systems, contributing to normal lung physiology as well as to disease (57). The pulmonary artery supplies the capillary bed of the alveolar wall, while the bronchial artery supplies the hilar structures as well as the capillary bed in the wall of intrapulmonary airways (bronchi and bronchioli), the pulmonary arteries, veins, lymphatics, nerve structure, and the pleura. The capillary bed from these structures, like the capillary bed of the alveoli, drains to the pulmonary veins; the blood from only the hilum returns to the azygos system. Additional components include the vascular network of microvasculature connections from transpleural-systemic to PA anastomoses, whose contribution diminishes with development

and maturation (58–61). However, in pathologic conditions, these special connecting vascular networks may contribute significantly to the remodeling of the entire pulmonary circulation. Structurally, the bronchial arteries are similar to those of systemic arteries, with a relatively thick muscular media and a well-defined internal elastic lamina. The external elastic lamina is either absent or incompletely developed, rarely visible as a thin and fragmentated membrane. The intima is thin and composed of a single layer of endothelial cells. The diameter of bronchial arteries is significantly smaller than that of the accompanying airway and pulmonary artery, sometimes they are not even visible on histologic sections. The bronchial arteries are usually situated next to bronchial veins within the peri-bronchial connective tissue and within the adventitia of pulmonary arteries and pulmonary veins. The capillary networks in the walls of bronchi and bronchioli are situated both inside and outside of the bronchial muscle coat supplying the mucosa and muscular coat, respectively (62). Vasa vasorum, the microvascular network supplying vessels, formed by micro branches of the bronchial arteries in the lung, supply the muscular type arteries through adventitia. They do not penetrate the media or intima, hence there is no communication between vasa vasorum and the lumen of pulmonary arteries (63). Bronchial arteries also give supply to the pleura and may enter the interlobular septum to give supplying branches to the walls of pulmonary veins, lymphatics and nerve structures. These vessels are inconspicuous but can be visible in histologic sections in pathological conditions.

The bronchial circulation must play a significant role by providing nutrition and oxygen to the growing lung *in utero*. Because alveolar hypoxemia, a common cause of hypoxic pulmonary hypertension in children and adults, does not exist in fetal life, pathologic effects of hypoxemia may take place via compromised blood flow and/or pressures within the bronchial circulation. These could be abnormalities within the bronchial circulation proper, or other congenital abnormalities effecting the heart and cardiopulmonary hemodynamics. More study is needed to explore the role of bronchial circulation in PPHN. In newborn calves, expanded vasa vasorum of bronchial circulation was observed in chronic hypoxic conditions, suggesting that vasa vasorum may be a conduit for inflammatory cells and/or circulating progenitors to bring about hypoxic responses in the tunica media (64, 65).

Relatively little is known about the underlying developmental biology of the bronchial circulation. Based on examination of one normal and one abnormal human embryo, early studies suggested that pulmonary and bronchial vessels develop independently on 7th and 9–12th gestational weeks, respectively (66, 67). However, extensive studies with specific antibody labeling and injection methods identified one common vascular plexus that gave rise to both the pulmonary and bronchial vasculature. These data suggest the feasibility of development of an extensive anastomosing system between the intrapulmonary bronchial system and the pulmonary vascular tree, seen in the normal lung (68).

Intrapulmonary bronchopulmonary anastomoses (IBA) are preexisting pathways that provide the anatomic structure for blood communication between the pulmonary arterial and bronchial arterial vascular system. When recruited, blood is able to flow from PA to BA, or vice versa, from PA to BA, depending on the local hemodynamic conditions and needs. When PA-BA flow takes place, much of the deoxygenated blood from PA flows to the bronchial vascular system including the bronchial microvessels, vasa vasorum, and bronchial veins, which in turn become expanded. Similarly, in the normal scenario, blood is drained by the pulmonary veins to the left atrium. However, during PA-BA shunt process, the blood bypasses the alveolar capillaries and does not get oxygenated leading to significant systemic hypoxia. These pathways are suggested to be widely open during fetal life; most are closed at birth and remain closed during normal conditions to adulthood (69, 70). It is difficult to know how frequently IBA are recruited in a diseased lung; it is agreed that their number increases in pathologic conditions (71, 72). There is tremendous size variation in their range between 15 and 500 micrometer, which would accommodate the bubbles during an agitated-saline test for right-to-left shunts which has been demonstrated in certain diseases with recruited IBAs (73). Although the exact regulation of intrapulmonary right-to-left shunt is not known, hypoxemia, extreme exercise, catecholamines, and prostacyclin have been shown to generate intrapulmonary right-to-left shunt (74–77). In fact, in babies who died of severe PPHN due to alveolar capillary dysplasia (78, 79), bronchopulmonary dysplasia (80), congenital diaphragmatic hernia (81), or meconium aspiration syndrome (82), IBA were recruited leading to intractable hypoxemia and death. Intriguingly, regulation of the IBA closure at birth appears similar to that of ductus arteriosus (DA) (79). Persistently open IBA, similar to DA, could lead to right-to-left shunt, mixture of pulmonary and bronchial blood, and hypoxic lung tissues in fetal life, possibly contributing the myriad of hypoxia-induced changes manifesting immediately after birth as PPHN. We propose that in addition to the right-to-left extrapulmonary shunt that marks the initial presentation of PPHN, open intrapulmonary shunt pathways (i.e. IBA) could also contribute to the pathobiology of PPHN.

Summary

Although low oxygen tension exists in the normal fetus, the lung and its circulation undergo tremendous growth and development. However, with additional decreases in PaO_2 from placental insufficiency or other adverse stimuli, hypoxia can alter diverse and complex transcriptional programming *in utero*, leading to altered pulmonary vascular growth and structure. Remarkable structural changes take place in the normal fetus at birth, which are partly mediated by the increase in oxygen tension, supporting the normal adaptations of lung structure during the first months of life. In the setting of PPHN, sustained elevation in pulmonary artery pressure and resistance in addition to hypoxia disrupt this transition and can cause sustained changes in remodeling of the pulmonary circulation. Sustained or progressive changes in pulmonary vascular disease further stimulate aberrant vascular structure, leading to more severe disease. A greater understanding of mechanisms underlying pulmonary vascular growth and remodeling, especially in response to hypoxia, will lead to more focused targets for therapeutic interventions and improved clinical outcomes.

References

1. Martinez-Lemus LA, et al. Physiology (Bethesda). 2009; 24:45–57.
2. Heath D, et al. J Pathol Bacteriol. 1958; 76(1):165–174.
3. Wagenvoort CA, et al. In: *Pathology of pulmonary hypertension.* Wagenvoort CA, Wagenvoort N, eds. New York, NY: John Wiley & Sons; 1977. p. 31.
4. Elliott FM, et al. Clin Radiol. 1965; 16:193–198.
5. Meyrick B, et al. Clin Chest Med. 1983; 4(2):199–217.
6. Geggel RL, et al. Clin Perinatol. 1984; 11(3):525–549.
7. Lakshminrusimha S, et al. Clin Perinatol. 1999; 26(3):601–619.
8. Wagenvoort CA, et al. Lab Invest. 1961; 10:751–762.
9. Abman SH, et al. In: *Tissue oxygen deprivation: developmental, molecular and integrative function.* Haddad G, Lister G, eds. New York NY: Marcel Dekker, 1996. p. 367–432.
10. Hall SM, et al. J Anat. 2000; 196(Pt 3):391–403.
11. Haworth SG, et al. Cardiovasc Res. 1981; 15(2):108–119.
12. Hall SM, et al. J Pathol. 1992; 166(2):183–193.
13. Tozzi CA, et al. Am J Respir Crit Care Med. 1994; 149(5):1317–1326.
14. Dodson RB, et al. Am J Physiol Lung Cell Mol Physiol. 2014; 307(11):L822–L888.
15. Fediuk J, et al. Can J Physiol Pharmacol. 2015; 93(3):185–194.
16. Fineman JR, et al. Annu Rev Physiol. 1995; 57:115–134.
17. Morin FC, 3rd, et al. Am J Respir Crit Care Med. 1995; 151(6):2010–2032.
18. Rudolph AM. Annu Rev Physiol 1979; 41:383.–395.
19. Lewis AB, et al. Circ Res. 1976; 39(4):536–541.
20. Morin FC, 3rd, et al. J Appl Physiol. 1992; 73(1):213–218.
21. McQuillan LP, et al. Am J Physiol. 1994; 267(5 Pt 2):H1921–H1927.
22. Morin FC 3rd. Pediatr Res. 1989; 25(3):245–250.
23. Shaul PW, et al. Am J Physiol. 1993; 265(2 Pt 2):H621–H628.
24. Shaul PW, et al. Am J Physiol. 1992; 262(2 Pt 2):H355–H364.
25. Rudolph AM, et al. J Clin Invest. 1966; 45(3):399–411.
26. Dakshinamurti S. Pediatr Pulmonol. 2005; 39(6):492–503.
27. Shimoda LA, et al. J Appl Physiol. 2014; 116(7):867–874.
28. Resnik ER, et al. Proc Natl Acad Sci USA. 2007; 104(47):18789–18794.
29. Allen KM, et al. J Pathol. 1986; 150(3):205–212.
30. Tulloh RM, et al. Am J Physiol. 1997; 272(5 Pt 2):H2436–H2445.
31. Ambalavanan N, et al. Pediatr Res. 2005; 57(5 Pt 1):631–636.
32. Yu AY, et al. J Clin Invest. 1999; 103(5):691–696.
33. Ball MK, et al. Am J Respir Crit Care Med. 2014; 189(3):314–324.
34. Hirsch K, et al. Am J Respir Crit Care Med. 2020; 202(8):1146–1158.
35. Abman SH, et al. Am J Physiol. 1990; 259(6 Pt 2):H1921–H1927.
36. Cornfield DN, et al. Am J Physiol. 1992; 262(5 Pt 2):H1474–H1481.
37. Stenmark KR, et al. Am J Physiol Lung Cell Mol Physiol. 2009; 297(6):L1013–L1032.
38. Guignabert C, et al. Semin Respir Crit Care Med. 2017; 38(5):571–584.
39. Heath D, et al. Histopathology. 1990; 16(6):565–571.
40. Belknap JK, et al. Am J Respir Cell Mol Biol. 1997; 16(4):366–371.
41. Meyrick B, et al. Lab Invest. 1980; 42(6):603–615.
42. Stenmark KR, et al. Annu Rev Physiol. 1997; 59:89–144.
43. Tucci M, et al. Am J Physiol. 1997; 272(5 Pt 1):C1700–C1708.
44. Yu L, et al. J Vasc Res. 2011; 48(6):465–475.
45. Porter KM, et al. PLoS One. 2014; 9(6):e98532
46. Botto L, et al. Respir Res. 2006; 7(1):7.
47. Rabinovitch M. Clin Chest Med. 2001; 22(3):433–449, viii.
48. Stenmark KR, et al. Circ Res. 2006; 99(7):675–691.
49. An SS, et al. Am J Physiol Cell Physiol. 2005; 289(3):C521–C530.
50. Aaronson PI, et al. Respir Physiol Neurobiol. 2002; 132(1):107–120.
51. Chen YF, et al. J Cardiovasc Pharmacol. 2000; 35(4 Suppl 2):S49–S53.
52. Faller DV. Clin Exp Pharmacol Physiol. 1999; 26(1):74–84.
53. Stenmark KR, et al. Annu Rev Physiol. 2013; 75:23–47.
54. Li M, et al. J Immunol. 2011; 187(5):2711–2722.
55. El Kasmi KC, et al. J Immunol. 2014; 193(2):597–609.
56. Zhang H, et al. Circulation. 2017; 136(25):2468–2485.
57. Mecham RP, et al. Science. 1987; 237(4813):423–426.
58. Jones RC, et al. In: *Current pulmonology,* Vol 8. Simmons DH, ed. Chicago IL: Year Book Medical publishers; 1987. p. 175–210.
59. Berrocal T, et al. Radiographics. 2004; 24(1):e17.
60. Castañer E, et al. Radiographics. 2006; 26(2):349–371.
61. Gao Y, et al. Physiol Rev. 2010; 90(4):1291–335.
62. Burri PH. Biol Neonate. 2006; 89(4):313–322.
63. Reid A, et al. Med Thorac. 1962; 19:215–219.
64. Wagenvoort CA, et al. In: *Pathology of pulmonary hypertension,* Wagenvoort CA, Wagenvoort N, eds. New York NY: John Wiley & Sons; 1977. Chapter 3, p. 35.
65. Duong HT, et al. Angiogenesis. 2011; 14(4):411–422
66. Davie NJ, et al. Am J Physiol Lung Cell Mol Physiol. 2004; 286(4):L668–L678.
67. Boyden EA. Am J Anat. 1970; 129(3):357–368.
68. Boyden EA. Anat Rec. 1970; 166(4):611–614.
69. DeRuiter MC, et al. Circulation. 1993; 87(4):1306–1319.
70. Verloop MC. Acta Anat (Basel). 1948; 5(1-2):171–205.
71. McMullan DM, et al. J Am Coll Cardiol. 2004; 44(7):1497–500.
72. Wagenvoort CA, et al. Lab Invest. 1967; 16(1):13–24.
73. Murillo H, et al. Semin Ultrasound CT MR. 2012; 33(6):473–484.
74. Lovering AT, et al. Injury. 2010; 41 Suppl 2(0 2):S16–S3.
75. Lovering AT, et al. J Appl Physiol. 2008; 104(5):1418–1425.
76. Eldridge MW, et al. J Appl Physiol. 2004; 97(3):797–805.
77. Laurie SS, et al. J Appl Physiol. 2012; 113(8):1213–1222.
78. Charan NB, et al. Am Rev Respir Dis. 1986; 134(1):89–92.
79. Galambos 78 C, et al. J Pediatr. 2014; 164(1):192–195.
80. 79. Galambos C, et al. Thorax. 2015; 70(1):84–85.
81. Galambos C, et al. Ann Am Thorac Soc. 2013; 10(5):474–481.
82. Acker SN, et al. J Pediatr. 2015; 166(1):178–183.
83. Ali N, et al. J Pediatr. 2015; 167(6):1445–1447.

ANIMAL MODELS OF PPHN AND VASOCONSTRICTOR SIGNALING IN HYPOXIA

Candice D. Fike and Judy L. Aschner

Contents

Neonatal pulmonary hypertension (PH) is a spectrum of disorders caused by *in utero* and postnatal insults to the developing pulmonary circulation. The clinical presentation can be sudden or insidious. Persistent pulmonary hypertension of the newborn (PPHN) manifests acutely in the immediate perinatal period, often accompanying life-threatening processes, including sepsis and hypoxic-ischemic events. In infants with chronic cardiopulmonary disorders, PH may be clinically unrecognized until the infant is dying from right-sided heart failure. The breadth of knowledge needed to understand the pathophysiology and devise therapies for the broad spectrum of neonatal PH has led to the creation of numerous experimental models in animals at different developmental stages. To create PH, investigators manipulate environmental and hemodynamic conditions known to impact pulmonary vascular tone and/or structure. To achieve meaningful translational relevance to human newborns, the ideal stimulus both elevates tone and causes pertinent structural changes in the pulmonary vasculature, mimicking the pathophysiology of human newborns with treatment-resistant PH.

The objectives of this chapter are:

- Describe various injurious stimuli, developmental stages, and animal species that are used to create neonatal models of PH (Figure 14.1)
- Discuss the contribution of endogenously produced vasoconstrictors to the development of PH in neonatal animal models

Hypoxia

Pulmonary arteries of newborns, including humans, constrict in response to low oxygen tension. Investigators have created models of PH in large animal species, such as lambs (1) and piglets (2, 3) to study acute hypoxic PPHN. In these models, catheters are placed *in vivo* at a few hours or days of postnatal age. Pulmonary arterial pressure (PAP), left atrial pressure, and cardiac output are measured and used to calculate pulmonary vascular resistance (PVR). An acute increase in PVR is elicited by ventilation with a hypoxic gas mixture and hemodynamic responses to vasodilators, vasoconstrictors, or antagonists of vasoconstrictor pathways are measured (1). Blood can be collected to measure levels of metabolites that might mediate acute hypoxia-induced pulmonary vasoconstriction (3).

Chronic hypoxic models of PH have been created to study the type of PH associated with chronic lung diseases and some forms of congenital heart disease. To reflect prolonged postnatal insults to the pulmonary circulation, hypoxic exposure is initiated when the animals are a few hours to a few days of age and continued for a few days to a few weeks of life. Both normobaric and hypobaric hypoxic conditions have been used. During the initial hours to days of hypoxic exposure, elevated PVR can be attributed to a reactive, vasoconstrictor response, which is largely reversible with vasodilators. With extended duration of hypoxia, the media of pulmonary arterial walls thickens, and contributes to a fixed elevation in PVR, with poorer responses to vasodilators (4).

Postnatal models of chronic hypoxia-induced PH have been developed in both large and small species, including calves (5), piglets (6–8), rabbits (9), mice (10), and rats (11, 12). An advantage of large animals is that they can be instrumented *in vivo* to obtain the hemodynamic measurements needed to calculate the magnitude of elevation in PVR and to assess vascular dysfunction by measuring responses to vasoconstrictors and vasodilators. The pulmonary arteries of large animals can be harvested for in vitro studies of vascular dysfunction. Enough pulmonary arteries can be collected to measure protein levels and metabolite production to evaluate signaling abnormalities underlying vascular dysfunction and remodeling. Right ventricular hypertrophy (RVH) can be evaluated post-mortem, providing another metric of PH.

It is technically challenging, if not impossible, to obtain a similar array of information in small rodent models of chronic hypoxia-induced PH. The measurements needed to accurately determine *in vivo* PVR cannot be directly obtained in these tiny newborn animals. Echocardiography has been used to provide

DOI: 10.1201/9780367494018-14

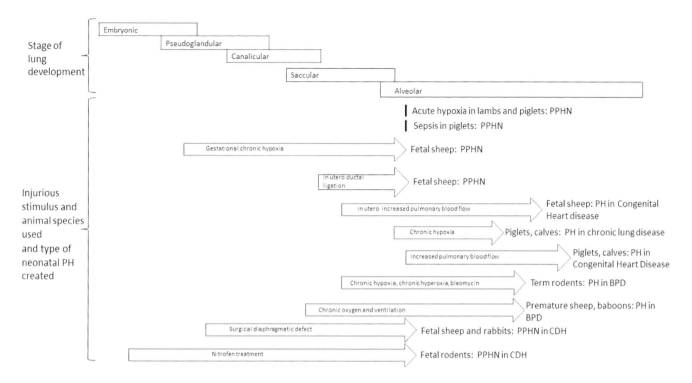

FIGURE 14.1 Neonatal models of pulmonary hypertension. Exposure to injurious stimuli used in various animal species at different developmental stages of lung development to create neonatal models of PH.

noninvasive *in vivo* estimates of PVR (11, 13). Most commonly, RVH is evaluated post-mortem to reflect PH. However, the timing and degree of elevation in PVR and RVH may not be the same and the signaling abnormalities underlying RVH may differ from those causing pulmonary vascular dysfunction and remodeling. Few investigators have been able to collect small pulmonary arteries from newborn rodents to perform in vitro studies (12). Samples of parenchymal lung tissue, not pulmonary vessels, are most often collected and used to perform assays for signaling derangements. Signaling abnormalities in parenchymal lung tissue may not accurately reflect the pulmonary circulation.

Notable advantages of small rodent models are cost and the ability to modify and selectively target protein expression at the genetic level. Rodent species born at term are at an immature saccular stage of lung development whereas the lungs of humans and large animals, including pigs and calves, born at term are at the beginning of the alveolar stage of lung development. When exposed postnatally to chronic hypoxia, lung alveolar development is impaired in rats and mice, simulating the pathologic changes found in premature human infants with bronchopulmonary dysplasia (BPD). Use of these small rodent models may therefore provide information pertinent to understanding the pathogenesis and impact of therapies on the development of PH in premature human infants with BPD.

Fetal models are needed to understand *in utero* insults to the pulmonary circulation. Although lowered oxygen tension increases PVR in fetal animals, it has been challenging to create PH using *in utero* chronic hypoxia (14). Successful models of chronic hypoxia-induced PH have been created in fetal sheep by husbandry of the pregnant ewe at high altitude (15), and may provide information relevant to PH that develops *in utero* and presents at birth as PPHN.

Lung injury from hyperoxia or bleomycin treatment

Hyperoxia is an oxidant stress that injures the lung parenchyma and pulmonary vasculature of newborns of many species, including humans. Animal models of chronic hyperoxia exposure have been used to simulate the PH that develops in human infants treated with supplemental oxygen for underlying lung disease. In rodent models, the animals are raised in chambers filled with hyperoxic gas mixtures, >60% oxygen, from birth until a few days to weeks of postnatal age (16). Paradoxically, but similar to the impact of chronic hypoxia, newborn rodents exposed to chronic hyperoxia develop RVH and pulmonary vascular remodeling and exhibit impaired alveolar development similar to that found in human premature infants who develop BPD. These rodent models have improved knowledge about the pathogenesis of BPD-associated PH in human preterm infants.

The chronic hyperoxic rodent model has been modified to include additional stressful conditions experienced by premature human infants. Postnatal growth restriction is common in premature infants with BPD and is associated with an increased risk of PH. Increasing the number of pups per litter limits milk intake and causes postnatal growth restriction in newborn rodents. Combining chronic hyperoxia with postnatal growth restriction causes particularly severe pulmonary arterial wall thickening and RVH in newborn rodents (17). Premature infants with BPD are frequently exposed to supraphysiological levels of oxygen with alternating periods of hypoxia due to severe desaturation episodes. To mimic this situation, newborn rats are exposed to hyperoxia from birth until day 14, then recovered in air with or without intermittent hypoxia for an additional 14 days. A greater degree of PH develops in the animals recovered in intermittent hypoxia than in animals recovered in room air (18). Combining chronic hyperoxia with additional relevant stresses should provide information about the mechanisms underlying the increased susceptibility for PH experienced by subgroups of infants with BPD.

Newborn rodents have been used to develop models of PH associated with inflammatory lung injury. Lungs of newborn rats (19) or mice (13) receiving daily or weekly intraperitoneal injections of bleomycin sulfate, commencing on the day of birth and continuing for 14–21 days, have greatly increased numbers of alveolar and interstitial neutrophils and macrophages (19). Histologically mimicking lung and pulmonary vascular changes found in human infants with BPD and PH, alveolar development is impaired and RVH and pulmonary vascular wall thickening develop in bleomycin-treated rodents.

Large animals have also been used to create PH associated with lung injury. In these models, premature lambs and baboons are delivered by C-section during the canalicular or saccular stage of lung development (sheep: 125–131 days gestation, 80–85% gestation; baboons: 134–147 days gestation, 65–75% gestation). The animals are intubated at delivery, given surfactant, placed on mechanical ventilators, and given supplemental oxygen for days to weeks. Similar to pathologic features found in premature human infants with BPD, pulmonary capillary growth is reduced and alveolarization is impaired in lungs of chronically ventilated premature lambs and baboons (20, 21). PVR fails to decline in the first postnatal weeks, in vivo responses to pulmonary vasodilators are altered, and pulmonary arterial walls are thickened in preterm lambs chronically ventilated for 3 weeks (22).

The premature sheep and baboon models reproduce the clinical setting of respiratory failure requiring prolonged ventilation and oxygen supplementation experienced by human premature infants. Catheters can be placed in these large animals to facilitate in vivo physiologic studies during the evolution of BPD and PH. The major limitations of these relevant preterm models are the cost and complexity of intensive care required to support the animals. This contrasts with rodents born at term with lungs at the saccular stage of development, who do not need respiratory support to survive but are too small to use for accurate in vivo hemodynamic studies. Nonetheless, both the hyperoxic term rodent and chronically ventilated premature sheep and baboon models have informed our understanding of the PH that develops in human premature infants with BPD.

Fetal ductal ligation

In utero constriction of the ductus arteriosus causes changes in the pulmonary vasculature of fetal sheep similar to those found in some human infants with PPHN, including those exposed to maternal prostaglandin synthetase inhibitors. To create ductal constriction models, the late gestation (126–135 days gestation; normal length is approx. 147 days) fetus undergoes operative surgical ligation of the ductus arteriosus, or has an inflatable occluder placed on the ductus to maintain chronic constriction (23, 24). After placing catheters needed to monitor fetal PVR, the fetus is replaced in the ewe's uterus and the pregnancy allowed to continue. Within a few days following ductal ligation or constriction, fetal PVR is increased. At operative delivery at term, pulmonary vascular walls are thickened, pulmonary vascular responses are abnormal, PVR is elevated, and RVH has developed in the ductal ligation lambs. Thus, this model can be used to inform mechanisms and therapies for PPHN with in utero onset.

Sepsis

Newborn infants who become septic in the perinatal period sometimes develop PPHN. To simulate this clinical scenario, catheters for hemodynamic measurements are placed in vivo in piglets when the animals are a few hours to days old (2, 3). Live washed Group B streptococcus or other bacterial organisms are infused, PVR is elevated within minutes, and hemodynamic responses to vasodilators or vasoconstrictors are measured. Blood can be collected for plasma levels of metabolites that might cause the bacterial-induced pulmonary vasoconstriction.

Increased pulmonary blood flow

Infants with congenital heart lesions associated with increased pulmonary blood flow often develop PH. Postnatal models have been developed to evaluate the impact of increases in blood flow on the entire lung, one lung, or to only one lobe of the lung. At postnatal ages ranging from 4–6 days (25) to 1–3 months (26, 27), increased flow to the entire lung of newborn piglets is achieved by sewing a graft to create an aortopulmonary shunt or by anastomosing the left subclavian artery to the pulmonary arterial trunk. Piglets studied 1 to 3 months after shunt placement have elevated PAP and thickened pulmonary arteries, with more severe changes found in the animals with the shunts placed at younger ages. In a model of unilateral increased pulmonary blood flow in calves (28), the left pulmonary artery (LPA) is anastomosed to the aorta within the first week of life. Ten weeks later, PAP in the unshunted right lung is normal with only mild thickening of small pulmonary arteries in that lung; in contrast, in the shunted left lung PAP is elevated and pulmonary arteries exhibit a marked degree of wall thickening or obliteration of their lumens. To evaluate the impact of delivering high flow under systemic pressure to one lung, the aorta is anastomosed to the left lower lobe pulmonary artery in newborn piglets (29). Eight weeks later, PVR is elevated and the pulmonary arteries of the shunted lobe have severe wall thickening. Differences in vasoreactivity are found in pulmonary arteries of the shunted versus unshunted lobes (30).

Models of increased flow to the entire lung have also been developed by surgically anastomosing a graft between the ascending aorta and main pulmonary artery in late gestation fetal lambs (31). The lambs are allowed to deliver spontaneously at term gestation. Although initially asymptomatic, the lambs develop clinical signs of pulmonary overcirculation and heart failure over 6–8 weeks. The gradual development of these physiologic symptoms is accompanied by an increase in PAP, altered pulmonary vascular reactivity and pulmonary arterial wall thickening.

To evaluate the impact from increased pulmonary blood flow without a concomitant increase in PAP, an LPA ligation model has been developed in fetal lambs (31). Similar to the shunt model, lambs undergo LPA ligation at late gestation, are allowed to deliver spontaneously at term, then studied 4–6 weeks later. Unlike the shunt lambs, the LPA ligation lambs have minimal elevation in PAP, no pathologic increase in pulmonary vascular wall thickness, and exhibit less altered pulmonary vascular reactivity. Findings in the different shunt models can provide knowledge about the pathophysiology of PH found in infants with different forms of congenital heart disease who experience different biomechanical stresses.

Congenital diaphragmatic hernia

Many infants with congenital diaphragmatic hernia (CDH) present acutely with PPHN at birth, and some develop a more chronic form of PH postnatally. Experimental animal models have been developed to help understand the structural and functional abnormalities of the pulmonary circulation found in infants with CDH who exhibit PPHN at birth. In surgical models, CDH is induced by creating left diaphragmatic defects in fetal sheep at 60–90 days gestation (term is 140–145 days) (32) and in fetal rabbits at day 23 of gestation (term is 31 days) (33, 34). When delivered by C-section at term, the pulmonary arterial tree is abnormally muscularized and the pulmonary vascular bed is reduced in lungs of lambs and rabbits with CDH. More severe pulmonary vascular abnormalities are found in the lung on the side of the diaphragmatic defect. CDH lambs also have hemodynamic evidence of pulmonary vascular dysfunction and PH, with PAP approaching aortic pressure (35) and elevations in PVR (36). A limitation of the surgical models is that the diaphragmatic defect is created relatively late in gestation when compared to the onset of the defect in many human fetuses. Thus, information from these surgical models may not accurately reflect the early pathogenesis of lung and pulmonary vascular abnormalities found in human infants with CDH and early herniation.

Experimental CDH has also been created by giving one oral dose of nitrofen (2,4-dichlorophenyl-p-nitrophenyl ether) to pregnant rodents on day 9 or 12 of gestation (37, 38). When delivered by C-section at term, 60–80% of the fetuses have either a right or left diaphragmatic hernia. Animals with a diaphragmatic hernia have hypoplastic lungs, pulmonary arteries with thickened walls and abnormal dilator and constrictor responses, and a decrease in the cross-sectional area of the pulmonary vascular bed affecting both ipsilateral and contralateral lungs. An advantage of this model is that the nitrofen is given before formation of the lung and diaphragm, so that the timing of the development of the CDH is similar to that in humans. A disadvantage is that the relevance to human infants of the teratogenic effect of nitrofen is unknown. Nonetheless, both the nitrofen and surgical models of CDH can be used to understand the pathophysiology and develop therapies for human infants with CDH.

Vasoconstrictors

It is generally accepted that vasoconstrictors, including those discussed below, contribute to the development of neonatal PH.

Thromboxane

The arachidonate metabolite thromboxane (TXA2) is a potent pulmonary vasoconstrictor. Levels of thromboxane B2 (TXB2), the stable metabolite of TXA2, are elevated in the plasma of some human infants with PPHN (39) and in pulmonary arterial endothelial cells isolated from the fetal ductal ligation lamb model of PPHN (40). Plasma levels of TXB2 are elevated in the septic piglet model, but not in the acute hypoxic piglet model of PPHN (2, 3). TXB2 production is elevated in lungs of chronically hyperoxic newborn rats (41) and in pulmonary arteries from piglets with chronic hypoxia-induced PH (6). Pulmonary arterial smooth muscle cells from piglets with chronic hypoxia-induced PH exhibit hypersensitivity and hyperresponsiveness to TXA2 (42). Treatment with TXA2 synthase inhibitors ameliorates chronic hypoxia-induced PH in newborn piglets (7, 43) and completely reverses sepsis-induced elevations in PVR (2). Ample evidence

supports TXA2 involvement in some forms of PPHN and in some types of postnatal PH.

Leukotrienes

Leukotrienes (LTs) are potent vasoconstrictors produced by arachidonate metabolism via the lipoxygenase pathway. Tracheal aspirates of human infants with PPHN have increased amounts of LTs (44). LT antagonists reverse elevations in PVR in the acute hypoxic lamb model of PPHN (1). LT biosynthesis inhibitors prevent PH in the newborn rat bleomycin lung injury model (45). Albeit limited, data from experimental animal models supports a role for LTs in some types of neonatal PH.

Cytochrome P450 metabolites of arachidonic acid

Cytochrome P450 (CYP450) metabolism of arachidonic acid results in the formation of the four regioisomers of epoxyeicosatrienoic acids (EETs), their corresponding dihydroxyeicosatrienoic acids (DHETs), and 19- and 20-hydroxyeicosatetraenoic acids (HETEs). EETs are generally dilators. HETEs are constrictors in most vascular beds, including the neonatal pulmonary circulation (46). The only available information about HETEs in newborn models of PH is that HETE amounts are increased, and the pulmonary arterial constrictor response to 15-HETE is augmented in lungs of chronically hypoxic newborn rabbits (47).

Isoprostanes

Isoprostanes are a complex family of compounds produced nonezymatically from arachidonic acid via a free radical-catalyzed mechanism. Lung isoprostane levels are elevated in both chronically hyperoxic (48, 49) and chronically hypoxic (11, 50) newborn rodent models of PH. Newborn rats with chronic hyperoxia-induced PH have exaggerated pulmonary constrictor responses to isoprostanes (51). Antioxidants reduce lung isoprostane levels and prevent RVH in chronically hyperoxic newborn rats (48). Evidence limited to data from newborn rodent models suggests that isoprostanes may play a role in some types of postnatal PH.

Serotonin

There is extensive evidence that serotonin (5-HT) contributes to the pathogenesis of PH in adults. Interest in 5-HT and neonatal PH arose with reports that human infants born to mothers treated during pregnancy with selective 5-HT reuptake inhibitors (SSRIs) have an increased risk of PPHN. Infusion of 5-HT and SSRIs elicits pulmonary vasoconstriction in late-gestation fetal sheep (52). 5-HT levels are elevated in pulmonary arterial endothelial cells isolated from the fetal ductal ligation lamb model of PPHN (53). 5-HT signaling is increased, and 5-HT receptor antagonists inhibit PH in bleomycin-treated mice (13). The pulmonary vasoconstrictor response to 5-HT is augmented in chronically hyperoxic newborn rats (54). Yet, pulmonary arterial vasoconstriction to 5-HT is impaired in fetal lambs who develop PH during gestation at high altitude (55). The role of 5-HT signaling in neonatal forms of PH is not yet fully characterized and may vary dependent on the form of PH.

Endothelins

Endothelins (ETs) are a family of vasoactive peptides with 3 distinct isoforms, ET-1, ET-2, and ET-3. Two distinct receptors, ETA and ETB, mediate the hemodynamic effects of the ETs. Of the ETs, ET-1 is the best characterized and its role in the development of neonatal PH the best studied. ET-1 has complex pulmonary vasoactive effects, including potent pulmonary vasoconstriction and vasodilation. Plasma levels of ET-1 are elevated in human neonates with severe PPHN (56). Lung ET-1 content and ET-1 mRNA expression are increased, ETA-mediated pulmonary vascular constriction is augmented, and ETB receptor mRNA expression and ETB-mediated pulmonary vascular dilation are reduced in the lamb ductal ligation model of PPHN (57, 58). Moreover, ETA receptor antagonist treatment inhibits the development of PPHN in the ductal ligation model (59).

Human infants with CDH have elevated plasma levels of ET-1 (60) and greater lung expression of ETA than ETB receptors (61). In the surgical lamb model of CDH, plasma ET-1 levels increase dramatically a few hours after delivery (35), and pulmonary vascular ETA receptor activity is increased while ETB receptor function is reduced (36). A selective nonpeptidic ETA receptor antagonist acutely improved hemodynamic evidence of PH in lambs with surgically induced CDH (35). Pulmonary arteries of nitrofen-treated rats with CDH have elevated expression of ET-1 and ETA receptors (38) and exaggerated responses to ET-1 (37). Whether abnormal ET-1 signaling is a marker or a mediator of PPHN in CDH is not yet clear.

Alterations in lung or plasma ET-1 levels have been found in newborn piglets with chronic hypoxia-induced PH (8), mice with chronic hypoxia-induced PH (10), and newborn rats with chronic hyperoxia-induced PH (41, 49). An orally active ETA receptor antagonist inhibited PH in chronically hypoxic newborn piglets (8). Pulmonary vascular wall thickening and RVH were inhibited in chronically hypoxic newborn mice treated with an ETA receptor antagonist (62) and in chronically hyperoxic newborn rats treated with a mixed ETA/ETB receptor antagonist (49). Treatment for three months with the dual endothelin-receptor antagonist, bosentan, prevented pulmonary vascular wall thickening and elevations in PAP in piglets with increased pulmonary blood flow due to the surgical anastomosis of the left subclavian artery to the pulmonary arterial trunk at 3 weeks of age (27). One month of treatment with an ETA receptor antagonist inhibited the elevation in PVR and pulmonary vascular wall thickening in lambs with increased pulmonary blood flow from in utero placement of an aortopulmonary shunt (63). However, the timing and length of treatment with ETA receptor antagonists merits further consideration because lambs with PH induced by fetal aortopulmonary shunts exhibit temporal alterations in ET-1 signaling (64). Pulmonary vascular ETB receptor expression is elevated at 1 month, but by 2 months the expression of ETB receptors has returned to normal and its predominant localization has shifted from endothelial cells, where it mediates dilation, to smooth muscle cells, where it mediates constriction. Thus, the optimal ET-1 receptor antagonist strategy may need to change during the progression of pulmonary vascular disease. Nonetheless, there is a substantial body of evidence that abnormal ET-1 signaling is not just a marker of disease but that it contributes to the pathogenesis of some types of neonatal PH.

Reactive oxygen species and their sources

Elevated levels of reactive oxygen species (ROS), such as superoxide and hydrogen peroxide, are found in the pulmonary arteries of lambs with PPHN induced by in utero fetal ductal ligation (65, 66), in newborn piglets (67) and newborn rats (50) with chronic hypoxia-induced PH, and in lambs with high flow-induced PH from in utero aortopulmonary shunts (68). Antioxidants or ROS scavengers improve pulmonary vascular responses in most of the aforementioned newborn animal models of PH (12, 50, 65–67). Prolonged treatment with ROS scavengers or antioxidants inhibits PH in chronically hypoxic

and chronically hyperoxic newborn rats (48, 50). Sources of the elevated ROS have been identified in some of the newborn models of PH and include NADPH oxidase enzymes (65, 67–69), uncoupled eNOS (67, 68, 70), xanthine oxidase (50), and mitochondria (12, 69, 71). Therapies that reduce ROS by targeting their sources improve aberrant pulmonary vascular responses (12, 50, 70–72). ROS production is reduced and PH is inhibited by targeting xanthine oxidase with allopurinol treatment in chronically hypoxic newborn rats (50). Mitochondrial-specific antioxidant treatment prevents RVH in chronically hyperoxic newborn mice (69). Reducing ROS by restoring uncoupled eNOS with L-citrulline treatment ameliorates chronic hypoxia-induced PH in newborn piglets (73). Thus, there is abundant evidence that ROS are involved in the pathogenesis of numerous forms of neonatal PH. However, ROS are integral to normal signaling processes in many organs and vascular beds, including the pulmonary circulation. Therapeutic strategies that reduce ROS should be limited to benign agents that target the sources of aberrant ROS and do not cause adverse effects in other vascular beds and organs.

References

1. Schreiber MD, et al. Ped Res. 1985; 19:437–41.
2. Gibson RL, et al. Ped Res. 1988; 23:553–6.
3. Hammerman C, et al. Am J Dis Child. 1988; 142:319–25.
4. Durmowicz AG, et al. NeoReviews. 1999; e99–e102.
5. Stenmark K, et al. J Appl Physiol. 1987; 62:821–30.
6. Fike CD, et al. Am J Physiol Lung Cell Mol Physiol. 2003; 284:L316–L323.
7. Fike CD, et al. J Appl Physiol. 2005; 99:670–6.
8. Perreault T, et al. Pediatr Res. 2001; 50:374–83.
9. Baker EJ, et al. Am J Physiol Heart Circ Physiol. 1995; 268:H1165–H1173.
10. Ambalavanan N, et al. Ped Res. 2007; 61:559–64.
11. Kantores C, et al. Am J Physiol Lung Cell Mol Physiol. 2006; 291:L912–L922.
12. Sheak JR, et al. Am J Physiol Heart Circ Physiol. 2020; 318:H470–H483.
13. Delaney C, et al. Am J Physiol Lung Cell Mol Physiol. 2019; 314:L871–L881.
14. Papamatheakis DG, et al. Curr Vasc Pharmacol. 2013; 11:616–40.
15. Papamatheakis DG, et al. Pulm Circ. 2013; 3:757–80.
16. O'Reilly M, et al. Am J Physiol Lung Cell Mol Physiol. 2014; 307:L948–L958.
17. Wedgwood S, et al. Ped Res. 2020; 87:472–9.
18. Mankouski A, et al. Am J Physiol Lung Cell Mol Physiol. 2017; 312:L208–L216.
19. Lee AH, et al. Am J Respir Cell Mol Biol. 2014; 50:61–73.
20. Bland RD, et al. Ped Res. 2000; 48:64–74.
21. Maniscalco WM, et al. Am J Physiol Lung Cell Mol Physiol. 2002; 282:L811–L823.
22. Bland RD, et al. Am J Physiol Lung Cell Mol Physiol. 2003; 285:L76–L85.
23. Morin FC. Ped Res. 1989; 25:245–50.
24. Abman SH, et al. J Clin Invest. 1989; 83:1849–58.
25. Fike CD, et al. Am J Physiol Lung Cell Mol Physiol. 2001; 281:L475–L482.
26. Rendas A, et al. J Thorac Cardiovasc Surg. 1979; 77:109–18.
27. Rondelet B, et al. Circulation. 2003; 107:1329–35.
28. Fasules J, et al. J Appl Physiol. 1994; 77:867–75.
29. Bousamra IIM, et al. J Thorac Cardiovasc Surg. 2000; 120:88–98.
30. Pfister SL, et al. J Thorac Cardiovasc Surg. 2011; 141:425–31.
31. Kameny RJ, et al. Am J Respir Crit Care Med. 2019; 60:503–14.
32. Adzik NS, et al. J Pediatr Surg. 1985; 20:673–80.
33. Roubliova X, et al. J Pediatr Surg. 2004; 39:1066–72.
34. Wu J, et al. Hum Reprod. 2000; 15:2483–8.
35. Kavanagh M, et al. Br J Pharmacol. 2001; 134:1679–88.
36. Thebaud B, et al. Am J Physiol Lung Cell Mol Physiol. 2000; 278:923–32.
37. Coppola CP, et al. J Surg Res. 1998; 76:74–8.
38. Okazaki T, et al. J Pediatr Surg. 1998; 33:81–4.
39. Hammerman C, et al. J Pediatr. 1987; 110:470–2.
40. Mahajan CN, et al. Ped Research. 2015; 77:455–62.
41. Jankov RP, et al. Am J Resp Crit Care Med. 2002; 166:208–14.
42. Hinton M, et al. Am J Physiol Lung Cell Mol Physiol. 2006; 290:L375–L384.
43. Hirenallur-S DK, et al. Pulm Circ. 2012; 2:193–200.
44. Stenmark KR, et al. N Engl J Med. 1983; 309:77–80.
45. Ee MT, et al. Am J Physiol Lung Cell Mol Physiol. 2016; 311:L292–L302.
46. Fuloria M, et al. Am J Physiol Lung Cell Mol Physiol. 2004; 287:L360–L365.
47. Zhu D, et al. Circ Res. 2003; 92:992–1000.
48. Jankov RP, et al. Ped Research. 2000; 48:289–98.
49. Jankov RP, et al. Ped Research. 2001; 50:172–83.
50. Jankov RP, et al. Am J Physiol Lung Cell Mol Physiol. 2008; 294:L233–L245.
51. Belik J, et al. J Appl Physiol. 2004; 96:725–30.
52. Delaney C, et al. Am J Physiol Lung Cell Mol Physiol. 2011; 301:L937–L944.
53. Delaney C, et al. Am J Physiol Lung Cell Mol Physiol. 2013; 304:L894–L901.

54. Dumas de la Roque E, et al. PLoS One. 2017; 12:e1073044.
55. Goyal R, et al. Reprod Sci. 2011; 18:948–62.
56. Rosenberg AA, et al. J Pediatr. 1993; 123:109–14.
57. Black SM, et al. Ped Res. 1998; 44:821–30.
58. Ivy DD, et al. Pediatr Res. 1996; 39(3):435–42.
59. Ivy DD, et al. J Clin Invest. 1997; 99:1179–86.
60. Keller RL, et al. Am J Respir Crit Care Med. 2010; 182:555–61.
61. de Lagausie P, et al. J Pathol. 2005; 205:112–8.
62. Ambalavanan N, et al. Ped Res. 2005; 57:631–6.
63. Fratz S, et al. Am J Physiol Lung Cell Mol Physiol. 2004; 287:L592–L597.
64. Fratz S, et al. Circulation. 2011; 123:916–23.
65. Brennan LA, et al. Circ Res. 2003; 92:683–91.
66. Wedgwood S, et al. Am J Physiol Lung Cell Mol Physiol. 2005; 289:L660–L666.
67. Fike CD, et al. Antioxid Redox Signal. 2013; 18(14):1727–38.
68. Grobe AC, et al. Am J Physiol Lung Cell Mol Physiol. 2006; 290:L1069–L1077.
69. Datta S, et al. Am J Physiol Lung Cell Mol Physiol. 2015; 309:L369–L377.
70. Konduri GG, et al. Am J Physiol Heart Circ Physiol. 2007; 292:H1812–H1820.
71. Afolayan et al. Am J Physiol Lung Cell Mol Physiol. 2012; 303:L870–L879.
72. Fike CD, et al. Am J Physiol Lung Cell Mol Physiol. 2008; 295:L881–L888.
73. FikeFike CD, et al. Am J Resp Cell Mol Biol. 2015; 53:255–64.

HYPOXIA AND ENDOTHELIAL DYSFUNCTION IN THE LUNG

Emily Callan and Girija Ganesh Konduri

Contents

Endothelial regulation of neonatal pulmonary arterial tone

The human fetal pulmonary circulation is characterized by pulmonary vasoconstriction, facilitated by a low-oxygen environment, resulting in less blood flow to the lung. The elevated pulmonary vascular resistance (PVR) allows the majority of right ventricular output to bypass the nonrespiring lungs during fetal life. After ~31 weeks of gestational age, the fetal pulmonary vasculature demonstrates an increase in reactivity, particularly to changes in oxygen tension (1, 2). At birth, PVR rapidly decreases with a subsequent rise in pulmonary blood flow as the lungs take over gas exchange function (2, 3). This pulmonary vasodilation occurs in response to mechanical distension of the lung, shear stress, and most importantly, an increase in alveolar and systemic oxygen tension. This change in vascular tone is mediated by endothelial cell (EC) signals transmitted to adjacent smooth muscle cells (SMC) through paracrine mediators, direct ligand-receptor interactions by the Notch-signaling pathway, and coordination of direct contact at connexin-gap junction or cadherin-adherens junctions. The best-studied paracrine signals are vasodilators such as prostaglandins (PGs) (4), nitric oxide (NO) (5) and vascular endothelial growth factor (VEGF) (5, 6), and vasoconstrictors endothelin-1 (ET-1), thromboxane A_2 (TxA_2), and platelet-activating factor (PAF) (7). The ability of the endothelium to orchestrate these changes facilitates autonomous regulation of tone, which is intrinsic to the pulmonary vascular bed (6).

Effects of hypoxia on endothelial cell signaling

Hypoxia acutely elicits vasoconstriction in the lung, a response that is distinct and opposite to several systemic vascular beds. While the mechanisms involved in this unique pressor response of pulmonary circulation to hypoxia at the cellular level remain unknown, changes in vasoactive mediator release and structural adaptations have been well characterized as summarized below (Figure 15.1). This review focuses on the contribution of endothelial cells (ECs) to this response, although SMC also responds directly to a decrease in the oxygen tension, as reviewed in the other chapters in this book.

Hypoxia effects on NO-cGMP signaling

Hypoxia has been shown to decrease NO levels acutely in the pulmonary arteries and ECs, a response that is distinct from systemic vascular beds where hypoxia leads to NO-dependent vasodilation in an attempt to increase systemic oxygen (O_2) delivery (8). Chronic hypoxia decreases the activity and expression of endothelial nitric oxide synthase (eNOS) and uncouples the function of eNOS in the lungs of newborn piglets (Figure 15.1) (8, 9). Exogenous L-arginine and L-citrulline, precursors for NO and tetrahydrobiopterin (BH4), the required cofactor for eNOS, improve NO levels and attenuate hypoxia-induced pulmonary hypertension in newborn piglets (10). These studies show that the pulmonary vascular bed has a unique response to hypoxia, in part, through its differential effects on NO biology. The mechanism(s) of downregulation of eNOS function and expression in hypoxia remain unclear. Although oxygen is a required substrate for NO synthesis, the activity of eNOS is generally not limited by changes in O_2 tension over the physiologic range. The specific effects of hypoxia on cGMP levels and protein kinase G (PKG) expression and function in pulmonary artery ECs (PAECs) are less clear. In the fetal lamb model of PPHN which is achieved via *in utero* ductal constriction, NO levels and the expression and function of eNOS in PAECs are significantly decreased (11, 12). Both mRNA and protein levels of eNOS are strikingly decreased in PAECs from PPHN lambs, associated with increased promoter area methylation of the eNOS gene in the estrogen response element and histone modifications that lead to epigenetic silencing of the eNOS gene (13). Similar to these changes in the lamb model of PPHN, NO metabolites and eNOS expression are decreased

DOI: 10.1201/9780367494018-15

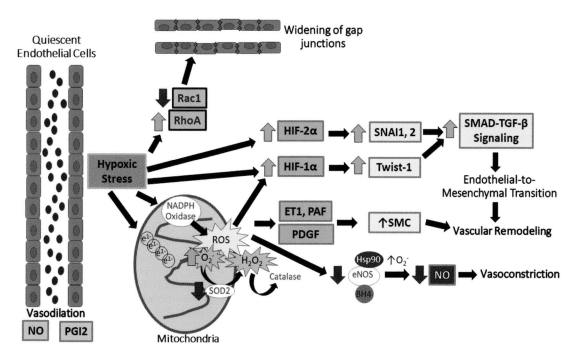

FIGURE 15.1 Role of endothelium in the response to hypoxia. Quiescent pulmonary vascular endothelium (left) maintains low pulmonary vascular tone through tonic release of NO and PGI2 in response to shear stress. In response to hypoxia, ECs contract via increased RhoA activity; this widens gap junctions and increases permeability. Sustained hypoxia leads to HIF-1/2α stabilization, which signals several transcription factors to increase Twist1-dependent or SNAI1/SNAI2-dependent endothelial-mesenchymal transition and/or SMC hyperplasia through release of pro-mitotic signals, ET-1, PAF and PDGF. Activation of ROS by hypoxia leads to mitochondrial dysfunction and eNOS uncoupling, with feed-forward ROS generation.

in neonates with PPHN (14). A decrease in cGMP-PKG signaling downstream of NO in the vascular SMCs was also previously demonstrated in fetal lambs with PPHN (15). Ductal constriction in the fetus leads to elevation in pulmonary artery (PA) pressure, without a decrease in fetal PO_2, and provides insights into the effects of pulmonary hypertension, without coexisting hypoxia. These studies together show that endothelial-derived NO plays a significant role in modulating the response of pulmonary vasculature to hypoxia and in PPHN.

Cyclooxygenase (COX) and prostaglandins (PGs)

PGs, particularly prostacyclin (PGI2) and prostaglandin E2 (PGE2), are important pulmonary vasodilators in the fetus and newborn (Figure 15.1). These PGs are primarily produced by ECs via COX-1, which is the isoform with constitutive activity (2, 16). COX-1 expression increases in late gestation with a subsequent increase in PGI2 levels from the third trimester, lasting until one month after birth (2, 8). PGE2 levels also rise late in the third trimester (2, 8). PGs mediate their vasodilator effects by the activation of adenylyl cyclase (AC) in the adjacent SMCs, which increases intracellular cyclic adenosine monophosphate (cAMP) levels (2, 16). Protein kinase A (PKA) mediates the downstream vasodilator signaling initiated by cAMP (2, 17). Hypoxia stimulates COX-1 function resulting in increased PGI2 synthesis, allowing for ECs and SMCs to adapt to hypoxia (8). While the pulmonary vasculature is more sensitive to the vasodilator effects of cGMP analogs compared to cAMP analogs in the fetal lamb model, PGs serve an important role in modulating vascular tone during periods of extreme hypoxia (18). Studies in the fetal lamb model of PPHN demonstrated a coordinated downregulation of

COX-1 and PGI2 synthase expression and increased TxA_2 synthase expression in PAECs (19). These changes lead to decreased levels of PGI2, increased levels of TxB_2, the stable metabolite of TxA_2, and impaired angiogenesis function of PAECs in PPHN (19). Exogenous PGI2 restores angiogenesis function to PPHN PAEC (19). These studies suggest that PG signaling plays an important role in pulmonary vascular development and adaptation to physiologic stresses.

Contribution of reactive oxygen species (ROS) to hypoxia signaling in endothelial cells (EC)

One of the early signaling events that occurs in lung cells in response to hypoxia is increased generation of ROS (20). Hypoxia leads to increased mitochondrial superoxide (O_2^-) generation, primarily due to electron leak from the electron transport chain (ETC) complexes I and III (21). Superoxide dismutase 2 (SOD2) in the mitochondrial matrix dismutes O_2^- to hydrogen peroxide (H_2O_2), which is then efficiently degraded by catalase to maintain normal ATP production through oxidative phosphorylation, which is necessary for normal endothelial function (22). However, prolonged hypoxia increases ROS to greater-than-physiological levels in both endothelial and smooth muscle cells, which then results in ROS-induced vasoconstriction via downstream signaling events that promote calcium influx (20, 21). SOD2 levels were found to be decreased in PPHN PAECs, thereby lowering the threshold for ROS to stimulate vasoconstriction (23). Therefore, efficient regulation of mitochondrial and cytosolic ROS levels is necessary for physiologic pulmonary vasodilation and angiogenesis to occur during normal birth-related transition (23–25).

The low-oxygen environment during fetal life normally induces basal release of mitochondrial ROS, which stimulate growth factors and increase hypoxia-inducible factor-1α (HIF-1α) levels that together upregulate angiogenesis. HIF-1α serves as a major transcription factor for growth factors, such as VEGF, to promote lung parenchymal and vascular growth in the fetus. Prolyl hydroxylases, which function as oxygen sensors in the cell, degrade HIFs in normoxic conditions, but due to their inhibited activity in hypoxic conditions, HIFs become stabilized (26). Postnatally, when the neonate is challenged by hypoxia, mitochondrial ROS generation rises along with HIF-1α levels, which leads to vascular remodeling and disrupted angiogenesis (24, 25, 27). However, it is important to recognize that basal expression of HIF-1α is needed for proper SMC response to hypoxia since targeted deletion of HIF-1α gene from SMC results in an accentuated response in PH secondary to hypoxia (28, 29). Consistent with the critical role of HIF-1α and HIF-2α in lung development, HIF augmentation by PHD inhibitors preserves lung alveolar and vascular growth in a rat model of bronchopulmonary dysplasia (BPD) induced by intraamniotic endotoxin (30).

In the setting of hypoxia and PPHN, ROS levels also increase via membrane-bound NADPH oxidases, resulting in the formation of O_2^-, H_2O_2, and peroxynitrite from O_2^- reacting with NO. The increased levels of ROS eventually lead to uncoupling of eNOS function. Under normal conditions, eNOS generates NO in the presence of its cofactor, BH4, and eNOS activity is enhanced through modulation by a chaperone protein, Heat Shock Protein 90 (Hsp90) (31). When eNOS is uncoupled as a consequence of ROS oxidizing BH4 and decreased interactions with Hsp90, O_2^- is generated instead of NO, leading to decreased cGMP mediated vasodilation, which was shown to occur in the lamb model of PPHN (Figure 15.1) (11, 32). Uncoupled eNOS then increases ROS further in a feed-forward process, leading to vasoconstriction in PPHN lambs (25, 32). In the lamb model of PPHN, the use of intratracheal recombinant human SOD (rhSOD) improves oxygenation and restores eNOS function, suggesting that an increase in ROS contributes to impaired adaptation of PVR at birth in PPHN (24). In summary, diminished expression of SOD2 and eNOS and uncoupled function of eNOS in PPHN together amplify the effects of hypoxia on endothelial ROS levels, leading to impaired vasodilation, disrupted angiogenesis, and failed adaptation at birth (11, 23, 25, 33).

Structural changes in endothelial cells

Both acute and chronic hypoxia are common causes of PPHN as low oxygen tension can lead to endothelial dysfunction through structural and molecular signaling events (34). The PVR in neonates remains relatively higher in the first few days of postnatal life which renders them vulnerable to pulmonary hypertension in response to hypoxia. The presence of fetal shunts also makes them susceptible to acute hypoxemia as a result of pulmonary hypertension, compared to adults (35–37). During normal postnatal transition, the pulmonary arteries dilate in part from the ECs increasing their surface area, spreading rapidly, losing junction-associated VE-cadherin microfilaments, and shear-stress induced release of endogenous vasodilators, all of which serve to facilitate relaxation of the blood vessel wall.

In animal models, exposure to chronic hypoxia results in failure of this postnatal adaptation with subsequent preservation of the fetal phenotype (34). Specifically, the newborn piglet models of PPHN show PAEC shape distortion, low surface area-to-volume ratio, and interdigitated cell-cell contacts with associated microfilaments after exposure to hypoxia (Figure 15.1) (34). PAEC dysfunction following hypoxia compounds the lack of normal structural adjustments with the increased release of vasoconstrictors ET-1 and PAF and decreased release of vasodilators NO and PGI2 (38, 39). Hypoxia also leads to increased endothelial permeability and inflammatory mediator expression, and these cumulative effects create an increase in vascular tone with subsequent elevation of PVR (39).

Rho kinase (ROK) pathway

Rho GTPases, crucial regulators of the actin cytoskeleton which include Rac1 and RhoA, control EC phenotype and permeability in the pulmonary vasculature. These Rho GTPases are activated by hypoxia (34, 39) and may contribute to the pathogenesis of chronic hypoxia-induced pulmonary hypertension (34). While this pathway is active in both ECs and SMCs, this section will focus on their effects in ECs. Rac1 and RhoA exert antagonizing effects on the barrier function of endothelium (39), where Rac1 supports adhesion by initiating the assembly and development of endothelial junctions while RhoA destabilizes endothelial junctions by increasing actomyosin contractility (Figure 15.1) (34, 39). Acute hypoxia inhibits Rac1 and activates RhoA in normal adult PAECs, leading to diminished endothelial barrier function (40). Comparable studies in a neonatal porcine model of PPHN show that PAECs even in normoxia have baseline alterations in structure, with increased amounts of stress fibers, increased permeability, and altered Rho GTPase activity (34). When these PPHN PAECs are then exposed to acute hypoxia, they develop stress fibers with increased permeability; lose junctional VE-cadherin; and show profoundly decreased Rac1 and increased RhoA levels (34). With PPHN PAECs having an altered cytoskeleton at baseline, they have limited ability to adapt to hypoxia, resulting in a worsening phenotype as demonstrated by their inability to produce a vasodilatory state.

Role of VEGF and HIF-1

In ECs, increased HIF-1α in pulmonary hypertension has been shown to mediate the metabolic switch to glycolysis, remodeling of the pulmonary arteries and impairment of angiogenesis function (41). These studies were done in the adult animal models of pulmonary hypertension and in the neonatal model of PPHN induced by prenatal ductus arteriosus constriction or hypoxia exposure. HIF-1α expression in these models is stimulated to excessive levels by mitochondrial H_2O_2 production in addition to hypoxia, resulting in a shift from oxidative phosphorylation to glycolysis with the induction of Hexokinase-2, pyruvate dehydrogenase kinase and other glycolytic genes in PPHN (27). Reducing aberrant HIF-1α signaling in PPHN improves angiogenesis function and increases VEGF levels (27). In contrast, the basal expression of HIF-1α promotes lung growth and protects against hypoxia-induced pulmonary hypertension (42). These studies together suggest that HIF-1α has dual roles: physiological levels promote angiogenesis during normal lung development; whereas aberrant expression leads to remodeling and impaired angiogenesis.

The role of HIF-1 and HIF-2α signaling is also context dependent. Recent studies, as pointed out above, demonstrated that augmenting HIF signaling through preventing its degradation or by increasing cGMP levels, promotes lung alveolar and vascular growth (30, 43). In this context of decreased lung growth due to perinatal LPS or hyperoxia, preserving HIF-1α levels maintains the levels of VEGF, activated Akt and eNOS, all of which are important growth signals in the lung. Therefore, future therapies targeting HIF signaling will need to consider the specific context and whether the lung disease represents altered lung development or abnormal vascular adaptation to pre- and postnatal stress.

Vascular remodeling in hypoxia and PPHN

Autopsy studies on neonates who die of PPHN reveal a marked increase in the thickness of media and adventitia of the small pulmonary arteries, extension of the muscle layer into non-muscular arteries, and microthrombi occlusions within the small pulmonary arteries (44). These structural changes support the concept that these alterations in the pulmonary circulation occur *in utero*, and these adjustments are associated with increased expression of genes that promote vasoconstriction over vasodilation, such as ET-1 (45).

The vascular remodeling that occurs in the pulmonary arteries in PPHN consists of ECs undergoing increased apoptosis while SMCs show increased proliferation (46). The subsequent rise in PVR precipitates hypoxemia due to extrapulmonary shunting of deoxygenated blood (44). The role of endothelium in the vascular remodeling in hypoxia and PPHN involves loss of vasodilator and gain of vasoconstrictor signals. Under physiologic conditions when the vasculature is quiescent, SMC show more contractile and less synthetic phenotype. This phenotype with decreased proliferation is maintained by the constant relay of signals from EC. Both NO and PGI2 released by EC inhibit SMC proliferation and maintain SMC in a differentiated state (47, 48). In response to hypoxia or injury, EC release vasoconstrictors that also have a strong pro-mitotic effect on the SMC. These include ET-1, PAF, and platelet-derived growth factor (PDGF) and inhibition of this signaling attenuates remodeling in hypoxia-induced pulmonary hypertension (7, 47, 49).

Hypoxia and endothelial-mesenchymal transition (endo-MT) in the pulmonary circulation

In addition to inciting SMC hyperplasia through the release of vasoactive mediators, EC can undergo mesenchymal transition in response to hypoxia or injury (Figure 15.1). Endo-MT has been mostly studied in animal models and patient derived samples in adult pulmonary hypertension. Several transcription factors and microRNA (miRNA) have been identified as initiators of this process in the EC, leading to their transition to acquire a smooth muscle or fibroblast morphology. ECs have inherent plasticity, thereby allowing them to induce changes in their own phenotype (36). The endo-MT entails ECs losing their morphology and cell-specific markers, such as PECAM (CD31), in order to acquire a mesenchymal-like phenotype, characterized by markers including α-smooth muscle actin (α-SMA) (50), S100a4 (fibroblast-specific protein, FSP1), and transgelin (TAGLN) (36, 51). Exposure of adult rats and pulmonary microvascular ECs (PMVECs) to hypoxia led to the increased expression of mesenchymal cell proteins, α-SMA, collagen type I alpha 1 chain (Col1A1), and collagen type III alpha 1 chain (Col3A1), along with decreased expression of CD31 (52). These changes were dependent on increased HIF-1α levels, which also increased the expression of transcription factor, Twist-1. Conversely, knockdown of HIF-1α and Twist-1 in PMVECs decreased the expression of mesenchymal markers (52).

Similarly, endothelial Twist-1 levels increased in cultured ECs and in adult mice exposed to hypoxia (53). Twist-1, in turn, mediates the endo-MT transition and pulmonary artery remodeling in hypoxia-exposed mice via activation of transforming growth factor-β2 (TGF-β2) (53). Overexpression of Twist-1 is associated with decreased VE-cadherin levels, further demonstrating the changing phenotype (54). In patients with idiopathic pulmonary arterial hypertension (IPAH), lung microvascular ECs show increased expression of HIF-1α and HIF-2α, decreased CD31 and VE-cadherin levels, and increased α-SMA and TAGLN levels. The IPAH cells also show increased expression of Zinc-finger transcription factors, SNAI1 and SNAI2 (55). Interestingly, deletion of HIF-2α, but not HIF-1α, attenuated the levels of SNAI1 and SNAI2 and decreased the endo-MT in these cells as well as in hypoxia-exposed mice (55). These data together suggest that hypoxia exposure can initiate vascular remodeling by endo-MT through related, but distinct, roles of HIF transcription factors, HIF-1α and HIF-2α in adult pulmonary hypertension. Endo-MT contributes to the extension of SMCs into the peripheral arteries and pulmonary arterial wall muscularization in pulmonary hypertension (36). Although pulmonary vascular remodeling has been well studied in PPHN, the role of endo-MT and the specific mechanisms that regulate this process in PPHN remain unclear since these studies were performed in adult mouse and rat models.

Micro-RNA-mediated endo-MT

MiRNA are highly conserved noncoding RNA molecules that serve to regulate gene expression negatively at the post-transcriptional level (36). MiRNA dysregulation occurs during pulmonary arterial hypertension via their control of endo-MT as well as effects on VEGF signaling (36, 56, 57). A specific miRNA, miR-126a-5p, has been implicated in the endo-MT that occurs in pulmonary hypertension (36). Inhibition of this particular miRNA leads to increased expression of CD31, and conversely, overexpression of miR-126a-5p leads to increase in S100a4 in neonatal rat pulmonary microvascular ECs (RPMECs) (36). These findings demonstrate that a single miRNA can regulate vascular integrity and angiogenesis, providing a new target for modulating vascular remodeling and function.

In summary, ECs play a prominent role in the vascular remodeling in response to hypoxia or other stresses that lead to persistent pulmonary hypertension, both through proliferative signaling to SMC and by undergoing transformation to mesenchymal morphology.

Role of endothelial cells in angiogenesis in PPHN

Previous studies in the fetal lamb model of PPHN demonstrated a decrease in the angiogenesis function of PAECs *in vitro* (25, 58, 59) and decreased capillary number and vessel density *in vivo* (33, 60). These changes can potentially lead to persistently high PVR in severe PPHN (59, 61). These findings are in contrast to the models of adult pulmonary arterial hypertension (PAH) where an increase in angiogenesis has been reported in response to chronic hypoxia (62) or injection of monocrotaline which induces extensive remodeling with plexiform lesions. These studies suggest that pulmonary hypertension in the fetus and neonate induces unique disruptions that impair vascular and, interestingly, alveolar development in the maturing lung (33, 60). We will briefly review the angiogenesis function of ECs which initiate this process and present evidence of their altered phenotype in PPHN based on extensive studies performed in the fetal lamb model.

Regulation of physiologic angiogenesis

Previous mechanistic studies of angiogenesis have been largely done in the developing retina and not in maturing lung vasculature. There is evidence that the majority of new blood vessels form by an angiogenesis process during the saccular and alveolar phases of lung development in the late-gestation fetus. Angiogenesis is a carefully orchestrated process that requires the vasculature to sense physiologic signals in the environment for activation, express specific ligand-receptor pairs of angiogenesis mediators, and commit ECs to specific roles through the changes in EC phenotype (Figure 15.2).

Hypoxic cells that are at a distance from the vessels release VEGF, which then guides the endothelial branching morphogenesis (2). Sprout formation is initiated when the ECs in existing vessels sense the VEGF gradient across the hypoxic tissue. The subpopulation of ECs with a higher expression of the functional VEGF receptor, VEGFR2 (Kdr), respond to the signal by acquiring filopodia, thereby adopting the migratory phenotype (Figure 15.2). These migratory cells then initiate contact with neighboring migratory cells from another sprout to induce branch formation. This cascade is executed when the migratory cells express higher levels of a specific Notch ligand, delta-like 4 (Dll4), in response to VEGF. Dll4 activates the Notch1 receptor in cells immediately adjacent to them via paracrine signals, preventing them from acquiring the migratory phenotype and instead promoting their commitment to a proliferative morphology required for sprout elongation (Figure 15.2). Since the migratory cells are positioned at the tip of the sprout, these are labeled as tip cells while the adjacent proliferative cells are referred to as stalk cells (Figure 15.2). The extent to which this process is reproduced in the lung vasculature is unclear; however, these ligands are expressed in PAECs in the late-gestation, saccular lung (33). The tip and stalk cells also differ in their expression of angiopoietins, Ang-1 and Ang-2, with the tip cells showing higher expression of Ang2 and stalk cells displaying elevated expression of Ang1 and its functional receptor, Tie2.

The expression of particular ligands and phenotype commitment are also linked to EC metabolic activity. Proliferation requires both ATP and metabolic intermediates generated through oxidative phosphorylation for basic biosynthetic reactions to occur efficiently. The migratory tip cells have a higher metabolic demand and show increased levels of glycolytic enzyme, 6-phosphofructo-2-kinase/fructose-2,6-biphosphatase 3 (PFKFB3). In contrast, the stalk cells generate ATP primarily through mitochondrial oxidative phosphorylation. It is unclear whether a change in metabolism leads to alterations in ligand-receptor expression or vice versa but remains an important paradigm to delineate the mechanisms of vascular disease. Here we briefly describe the alterations in angiogenic signals and EC metabolism in PPHN models, followed by a discussion of the potential connections based on *in vitro* mechanistic studies to restore metabolism to PPHN PAECs.

Alterations in angiogenic signal expression in PPHN

Previous studies in the fetal lamb model revealed that PPHN PAECs have reduced expression of eNOS and VEGF, associated with excess ROS signaling (58, 63). PAECs from PPHN lambs also exhibit decreased proliferation and migration and an increase in apoptosis *in vitro* (63). Restoring NO levels or scavenging ROS can independently improve these *in vitro* angiogenesis measures (25, 58). Restoring eNOS function through either supplementation of its cofactor, BH4, or stimulation of its upstream kinase, 5'AMP-activated protein kinase (AMPK), also improves angiogenesis function (63, 64). These data suggest that both depletion of NO and an increase in ROS play mechanistic roles in the impaired angiogenesis function in PPHN. The downstream signaling events that lead to decreased angiogenesis, however, remain unknown. Recent studies in retinal vasculature and ischemic systemic vascular beds revealed that endothelial metabolism is mechanistically linked to the expression of specific angiogenic signals and the phenotype of ECs. These studies suggested that investigation of endothelial metabolism and its influence on angiogenic signal expression may reveal new insights into decreased angiogenesis in PPHN.

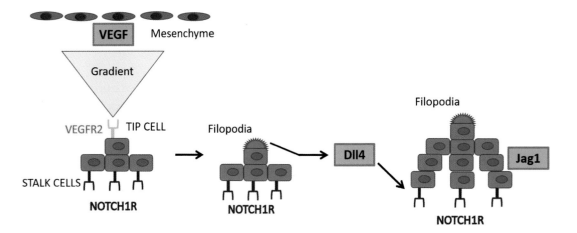

FIGURE 15.2   Role of notch signaling in angiogenesis. During normal angiogenesis, ECs in the existing vessels sense the VEGF gradient from hypoxic mesenchymal cells. The subpopulation of EC with a higher expression of VEGF functional receptor VEGFR2 are activated and become migratory, extending filopodia, and express the notch ligand, Dll4. Activation of Notch1 receptor in adjacent EC by Dll4 induces the transformation of those cells to a proliferative phenotype and induces expression of the notch ligand, Jagged1 (Jag1). Proliferation of these stalk cells elongates the sprout, positioning tip cells to make contact with tip cells from an adjacent sprout, to initiate branch formation.

Regulation of mitochondrial biogenesis and angiogenesis

Impaired mitochondrial function was shown to be a component of decreased vasodilation in PPHN (22). Studies in fetal lamb PPHN model have shown increased mitochondrial oxidative stress in PPHN PAECs (65) associated with significantly decreased ATP levels, indicating diminished utilization of oxidative phosphorylation (22, 23). PPHN PAECs also show a decrease in mitochondrial number and ETC complex protein expression, necessitating the shift away from oxidative phosphorylation to glycolysis (23, 33).

AMPK is a key metabolic sensor that regulates cellular bioenergetics, including mitochondrial function (Figure 15.3) (66). In the presence of energy depletion, AMPK is sensitized to phosphorylation by upstream kinases, liver kinase B1 (LKB1) and calmodulin-dependent protein kinase kinase 2 (CaMKK2/beta) (66). PAECs in PPHN demonstrate a coordinated downregulation of LKB1 and CaMKK2 levels and decreased phosphorylation of AMPK (33, 64). Decreased AMPK activity leads to reduced function of its downstream targets, eNOS and mitochondrial transcription factor, peroxisome proliferator-activated receptor gamma coactivator-1α (PGC-1α) (Figure 15.3) (25, 33). These changes lead to decreased mitochondrial biogenesis with subsequent reduction in the mitochondrial ETC complex proteins and mitochondrial number (33). AMPK agonist metformin, and allosteric AMPK activator A769662, increase PGC-1α levels, mitochondrial ETC complex proteins, and mitochondrial number (33). These data collectively show that PPHN is associated with decreased AMPK signaling and decreased mitochondrial function. The mechanistic link between these metabolic alterations in PPHN and decreased angiogenesis remains an area of active investigation.

A potential link between these metabolic alterations and decreased angiogenesis was suggested by Notch ligand alterations in PPHN as well as the response to pharmacologic activation of AMPK *in vitro* in PPHN PAECs and in intact fetal lambs. Expression of Dll4, a tip cell marker, is robustly upregulated in PPHN, while the stalk cell and proliferation marker, Jagged1, is downregulated (33). These changes were associated with impaired *in vitro* capillary tube formation and EC migration in PPHN PAECs. Both metformin and A769662 restored the Notch ligand balance in PAECs by increasing Jagged1 and decreasing Dll4 expression to control levels and restored the angiogenesis function of PAEC (33). These studies overall suggest that altered metabolic activity of PAECs due to AMPK dysfunction programs the dysmorphic angiogenesis in PPHN.

Additional metabolic alterations in pulmonary hypertension include downregulation of peroxisome proliferator-activated receptor gamma (PPARγ), a member of a nuclear receptor family (67), which is highly expressed in blood vessels throughout fetal lung development (59, 68). In the experimental models of pulmonary hypertension and chronic lung disease (CLD), PPARγ activation protects the lungs from injury and pulmonary hypertension in the setting of hypoxia (59, 69). PPARγ regulates eNOS protein expression and activity as shown by studies in PPARγ-knockout mice that generate less NO compared to controls (59). PPARγ agonists increase endogenous NO production and eNOS protein levels in PPHN PAECs, which is associated with restored capillary tube formation (59). Whether restoring metabolic function of PAEC would increase angiogenesis to normal levels in the developing lungs in pulmonary hypertension, requires further investigation.

Conclusion

ECs play a central role in the regulation of vascular tone in response to hypoxia. Endothelial dysfunction leads to both acute and chronic changes in pulmonary vasculature, resulting

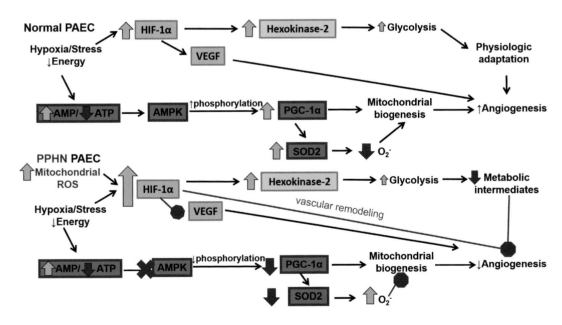

FIGURE 15.3 The role of HIF-1α and AMP-activated protein kinase (AMPK) in normal and abnormal adaptation responses of pulmonary artery endothelial cells (PAEC) to stressors. During transient hypoxia or other stresses that decrease energy availability, PAEC respond by HIF-1α-mediated upregulation of glycolysis, while AMPK activation increases mitochondrial biogenesis by the increased expression of transcription cofactor, PGC-1α. This leads to tissue angiogenesis, to maintain the balance of oxygen and nutrient supply with metabolic demand. In the abnormal adaptation of PPHN, excess HIF-1α and decreased AMPK function lead to predominance of glycolysis and loss of mitochondrial oxidative phosphorylation. This causes vascular remodeling and decreased angiogenesis.

in increased pulmonary artery pressure and PVR through complex signaling pathways. These changes include altered release of vasoactive mediators, vascular remodeling, and dysmorphic angiogenesis. Endothelial cell-targeted therapies to restore the EC function and reprogram the vasculature to quiescent state are currently unavailable and remain an active area of investigations. Additionally, the role of endothelium is critical in restoring lung vascular and parenchymal growth in a variety of neonatal lung diseases that present with hypoxia, including PPHN and bronchopulmonary dysplasia with/without pulmonary hypertension. Strategies to restore endothelial cell metabolism and angiogenesis offer potential targets for new therapeutic advances in this area.

Acknowledgments

Supported by RO1HL 136597-01A1 from NHLBI and multi-year innovative research grant and Muma Endowed Chair in Neonatology from Children's Research Institute of Children's Wisconsin (GGK).

References

1. Rasanen J, et al. Circulation. 1998; 97(3):257–262.
2. Gao Y, et al. Physiol Rev. 2010; 90:1291–1335.
3. Rasanen J, et al. Circulation. 1996; 94(5):1068–1073.
4. Shaul PW, et al. J Cardiovasc Pharmacol. 1993; 22(6):819–827.
5. Brenner BM, et al. J Clin Invest. 1989; 84(5):1373–1378.
6. Abman SH, et al. Am J Physiol. 1990; 259(6 Pt 2):H1921–H1927.
7. Ibe 7 BO, et al. Am J Physiol Lung Cell Mol Physiol. 2005; 288(5):L879–L886.
8. Shaul PW, et al. Am J Respir Cell Mol Biol. 1994; 11(4):432–438.
9. Fike CD, et al. Am J Physiol. 1998; 274(4):L517–L526.
10. Dikalova A, et al. Am J Physiol Lung Cell Mol Physiol. 2020; 318(4):L762–L772.
11. Konduri GG, et al. Am J Physiol Heart Circ Physiol. 2003; 285(1):H204–H211.
12. Villamor E, et al. Am J Physiol. 1997; 272(5 Pt 1):L1013–L1020.
13. Ke X, et al. Physiol Genomics. 2018; 50(10):828–836.
14. Villanueva ME, et al. Pediatr Res. 1998; 44(3):338–343.
15 Chester M, et al. Am J Physiol Lung Cell Mol Physiol. 2011; 301(5):L755–L764.
16. Nair J, et al. Semin Perinatol. 2014; 38(2):78–91
17. Acarregui MJ, et al. Biochim Biophys Acta. 1998; 1402(3):303–312.
18. Gao Y, et al. Am J Physiol Lung Cell Mol Physiol. 2005; 288(2):L213–L226.
19. Mahajan CN, et al. Pediatr Res. 2015; 77:455–462.
20. Desireddi JR, et al. Antioxid Redox Signal. 2010; 12(5):595–602.
21. Smith KA, et al. J Physiol. 2019; 597(4):1033–1043.
22. Afolayan AJ, et al. Am J Physiol Lung Cell Mol Physiol. 2016; 310(1):L40–L49.
23. Afolayan AJ, et al. Am J Physiol Lung Cell Mol Physiol. 2014; 306(4):L351–L360.
24. Farrow KN, et al. Antioxid Redox Signal. 2012; 17(3):460–470.
25. Teng RJ, et al. Am J Physiol Lung Cell Mol Physiol. 2009; 297(1):L184–L195.
26. Shimoda LA et al. Am J Respir Crit Care Med. 2011; 183(2):152–156.
27. Makker K, et al. Physiol Rep. 2019; 7(3):e13986.
28. Barnes EA, et al. FASEB J. 2017; 31(2):650–662.
29. Ball MK, et al. Am J Respir Crit Care Med. 2014; 189:314–324.
30. Hirsch K, et al. Am J Respir Crit Care Med. 2020; 202(8):1146–1158.
31. Pritchard KA Jr, et al. J Biol Chem. 2001; 276(21):17621–17624.
32. Konduri GG, et al. Am J Physiol Heart Circ Physiol. 2007; 292(4):H1812–H1820.
33. Rana U, et al. Am J Respir Cell Mol Biol. 2020; 62(6):719–731.
34. Wojciak-Stothard B, et al. Am J Physiol Lung Cell Mol Physiol. 2006; 290(6): L1173–L1182.
35. Stenmark KR, et al. Circ Res. 2006; 99(7):675–691.
36. Xu Y, et al. Hypertens Res. 2017; 40(6):552–561.
37. Yang Q, et al. Vasc Pharmacol. 2015; 73:20–31.
38 Haworth SG. Heart. 2002; 88(6):658–664.
38. Wojciak-Stothard B. Postgrad Med J. 2008; 84(993):348–353.
39. Wojciak-Stothard B, et al. Am J Physiol Lung Cell Mol Physiol. 2005; 288(4):L749–L760.
40. Fijalkowska I, et al. Am J Pathol. 2010; 176(3):1130–1138.
41. Barnes EA, et al. FASEB J. 2017; 31(2):650–662
42. Park HS, et al. Am J Respir Cell Mol Biol. 2013; 48(1):105–113.
43. Murphy JD, et al. J Pediatr. 1981; 98(6):962–967.
44. Wedgwood S, et al. Antioxid Redox Signal. 2003; 5(6):759–769.
45. Schultz A, et al. Hypertension. 2019; 74(4):957–966.
46. Kadowaki M, et al. Respir Res. 2007; 8(1):77.
47. Wedgwood S, et al. Nitric Oxide. 2003; 9(4):201–210.
48. Zucker MM, et al. Biochim Biophys Acta Mol Basis Dis. 2019; 1865(6):1604–1616.
49. Lin F, et al. IUBMB Life. 2012; 64(9):717–723.
50. Cooley BC, et al. Sci Transl Med. 2014; 6(227):227ra34.
51. Zhang B, et al. Int J Mol Med. 2018; 42(1):270–278.
52. Mammoto T, et al. Am J Resp Cell Mol Biol. 2018; 58(2):194–207.
53. Ranchoux B, et al. Circulation. 2015; 131(11):1006–1018.
54. Tang H, et al. Am J Physiol Lung Cell Mol Physiol. 2018; 314(2):L256–L275.
55. Caruso P, et al. Arterioscler Thromb Vasc Biol; 2010; 30(4):716–723.
56. Grant JS, et al. Cell Mol Life Sci. 2013; 70(23):4479–4494.
57. Gien J, et al. Am J Respir Crit Care Med. 2007; 176(11):1146–1153.
58. Wolf D, et al. Am J Physiol Lung Cell Mol Physiol. 2014; 306(4): L361–L371.
59. Grover TR, et al. Am J Physiol Lung Cell Mol Physiol. 2005; 288(4):L648–L654.
60. Hopkins N, et al. J Anat. 2002; 201(4):335–348.
61. Howell K, et al. J Physiol. 2003; 547(Pt1):133–145.
62. Teng RJ, et al. Am J Physiol Lung Cell Mol Physiol. 2011; 301(3):L334–L345.
63. Teng RJ, et al. Am J Physiol Lung Cell Mol Physiol. 2013; 304(1):L29–L42.
64. Afolayan AJ, et al. Am J Physiol Lung Cell Mol Physiol. 2012; 303(10):L870–L879.
65. Hardie DG, et al. Nat Rev Mol Cell Biol. 2012; 13(4):251–262.
66. Ameshima S, et al. Circ Res. 2003; 92:1162–1169.
67. Abbott BD, et al. PPAR Res. 2010; 2010:690907.
68. Crossno JT, et al. Am J Physiol Lung Cell Mol Physiol. 2007; 292(4):L885–L897.

EFFECTS OF HYPOXIA ON PULMONARY VASCULAR SMOOTH MUSCLE CONTRACTION AND RELAXATION

Shyamala Dakshinamurti, Anjali Y. Bhagirath and Robert P. Jankov

Contents

Introduction

The normal postnatal pulmonary vasculature is characterized by extremely low resistance and high compliance, which is essential to the accommodation of the entire cardiac output while keeping the pressure gradient low. The contractile state of pulmonary vascular smooth muscle is therefore critical to cardiorespiratory homeostasis. While acute hypoxic pulmonary vasoconstriction (discussed in detail elsewhere in this volume) is an adaptive physiological response to decreased regional alveolar O_2, a transition from physiologically beneficial to pathologically persistent vasoconstriction occurs when hypoxia is severe, sustained, and/or generalized, e.g., secondary to placental dysfunction, high altitude or severe pulmonary diseases, or in persistent pulmonary hypertension of the newborn (PPHN). It has been long understood that chronic hypoxia leads to altered pulmonary vascular physiology and structure, via increased local production and activity of various smooth muscle constrictors/mitogens that act through stimulation of G-protein-coupled receptors (GPCRs), including endothelin-1, thromboxane A_2, serotonin, and angiotensin-II. In parallel, hypoxia leads to decreased content and/or activity of smooth muscle dilators/anti-mitogens, including nitric oxide (NO) and prostacyclin (PGI_2). In this chapter, we will discuss known pathways modulating pulmonary vascular smooth muscle contraction and relaxation and their perturbations by hypoxia (Figure 16.1). Finally, we will highlight current and future prospects for pharmacological manipulation of these pathways for therapeutic benefit (Table 16.1).

Hypoxia and electromechanical coupling

In pulmonary artery myocytes, the membrane potential (E_m) rests between −40 to −60 mV, generated by the ATP-dependent electrochemical gradient of sodium and potassium ions across the plasma membrane (1). E_m is primarily maintained by outward-flowing current through the K_V voltage-sensitive potassium channel family. An inward-rectifying K_{IR} current of K+ ions prevents the membrane E_m from getting hyperpolarized (2). Membrane depolarization of vascular smooth muscle can be triggered by sympathetic nerve activity, by ligands activating membrane calcium channels, by mechanical stretch, or by inhibition of the outward K+ current (3), as the open-potential of pulmonary arterial K_V channels is reduced by hypoxia (2).

Pulmonary arteries exist in a partially contracted state due to the myogenic response, which opposes the outward stretch of blood pressure to maintain resting arterial tone. While shear stress of endothelium promotes vasodilation, the smooth muscle responds to stretch by constriction; this is true in the fetal pulmonary artery (4), and more so in PPHN pulmonary artery (5). Oscillations in systolic pulmonary pressure stretch the myocyte longitudinally, resulting in depolarization via the opening of mechanosensitive stretch-activated channels transducing an inward K+ current (6). Focal adhesions linking the extracellular matrix to the actin cytoskeleton may also act as mechanosensors, eliciting membrane depolarization (7).

Smooth muscle cells do not have voltage-gated sodium channels; their action potential is the result of calcium influx. Early depolarization opens smaller T-type calcium channels (threshold of activation −60 to −70 mV) (8), while these are quickly inactivated, this triggers the opening of large L-type voltage-dependent calcium channels (VDCC; threshold −30 to −40 mV), amplifying the influx of extracellular calcium and spiking an action potential (9). Intracellular calcium concentration ($[Ca^{2+}]_i$) in myocytes rests at 100nM (1), but rises up to 1 μM after VDCC open (10). During contraction, only a third of the increase in $[Ca^{2+}]_i$ occurs on the upstroke of the action potential; the remainder is accrued during the plateau. However, the kinetics of force development is slower than that of calcium, indicating that calcium flux is not rate-limiting (11).

Membrane depolarization is opposed by calcium-activated BK_{Ca} and calcium-independent K_{ATP} delayed-rectifier channels, which repolarize the myocyte to its resting state. Half of the decline in $[Ca^{2+}]_i$ occurs immediately after E_m repolarization (11). The ATP-dependent Na+/Ca2+ exchanger removes any calcium not taken up by intracellular stores from the cytoplasm. Acute hypoxia directly inhibits K_V and K_{Ca} outward current; chronic hypoxia downregulates K_V expression, causing membrane depolarization, opening VDCC, and thus increasing calcium influx (12).

DOI: 10.1201/9780367494018-16

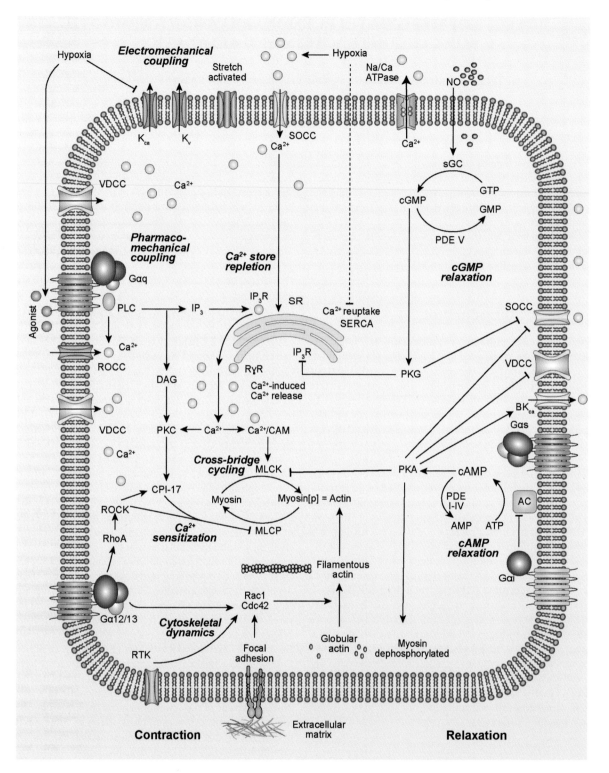

FIGURE 16.1 Contraction and relaxation pathways in the pulmonary arterial smooth muscle cell. AC, adenylyl cyclase; AMP, adenosine monophosphate; ATP, adenosine triphosphate; BK_{Ca}, large-conductance voltage-, and calcium-activated potassium channel; CAM, calmodulin; cAMP, cyclic adenosine monophosphate; cGMP, cyclic guanosine monophosphate; CPI-17, protein kinase C-activated inhibitor 17 kD protein; DAG, diacylglycerol; Em, membrane electrical potential; GMP, guanosine monophosphate; GTP, guanosine triphosphate; IP3, inositol 1,4,5-trisphosphate; IP3R, inositol 1,4,5-trisphosphate receptor; kKca, calcium-dependent potassium channel; Kv, voltage-dependent potassium channel; MLCK, myosin light chain kinase; MLCP, myosin light chain phosphatase; myosin(p), phosphorylated myosin; Na/Ca ATPase, plasmalemmal sodium calcium exchanger ATPase; NO, nitric oxide; PDE, phosphodiesterase; PLC, phospholipase C; PKA, cAMP-dependent protein kinase; PKC, calcium-dependent protein kinase; PKG, cGMP-dependent protein kinase; ROCC, receptor-operated calcium channels; ROCK, rho-associated protein kinase; RTK, receptor tyrosine kinase; RyR, ryanodine receptor; SERCA, sarcoplasmic reticulum calcium ATPase; sGC, soluble guanylate cyclase; SOCC, store-operated calcium channels; SR, sarcoplasmic reticulum; VDCC, voltage-dependent calcium channels.

TABLE 16.1 Pharmacomechanical Coupling

Drug	Mechanism of Action	Route of Administration	Indications/Uses	Clinical Status
Ambrisentan	ETA selective antagonist	Enteral	Pulmonary hypertension.	Approved in North America. No data in human neonates.
Benazepril	Angiotensin converting enzyme inhibitor	Enteral	Cardiovascular and renal diseases.	Approved in North America. No data in human neonates.
Bosentan	Dual ET receptor antagonist	Enteral	Pulmonary hypertension.	Approved in North America.
Captopril	Angiotensin converting enzyme inhibitor	Enteral	Cardiovascular and renal diseases.	Approved in North America. No data in human neonates.
Enalapril	Angiotensin converting enzyme inhibitor	Enteral	Cardiovascular and renal diseases.	Approved in North America. No data in human neonates.
Fosinopril	Angiotensin converting enzyme inhibitor	Enteral	Cardiovascular and renal diseases.	Approved in North America. No data in human neonates.
Losartan	Angiotensin II receptor antagonist	Enteral	Cardiovascular diseases.	Approved in North America. No data in human neonates.
Macitentan	Dual ET receptor antagonist	Enteral	Pulmonary hypertension.	Approved in North America. No neonatal data.
Olmesartan	Angiotensin II receptor antagonist	Enteral	Cardiovascular diseases.	Approved in North America. No data in human neonates.
Ramipril	Angiotensin converting enzyme inhibitor	Enteral	Cardiovascular and renal diseases.	Approved in North America. No data in human neonates.

Calcium Store Repletion

Drug	Mechanism of Action	Route of Administration	Indications/Uses	Clinical Status
Amlodipine	VDCC blocker	Enteral	Cardiovascular and cerebrovascular diseases.	Approved in North America. No human neonatal data.
Felodipine	VDCC blocker	Enteral	Cardiovascular and cerebrovascular diseases.	Approved in North America. No human neonatal data.
Nifedipine	VDCC blocker	Enteral	Cardiovascular and cerebrovascular diseases.	Approved in North America.
Verapamil	VDCC blocker	Enteral, systemic	Cardiovascular and cerebrovascular diseases.	Approved in North America. No human neonatal data.

Calcium Sensitization

Drug	Mechanism of Action	Route of Administration	Indications/Uses	Clinical Status
Atorvastatin	Statin (Rho inhibitor)	Enteral	Hypercholesterolemia, cardiovascular diseases.	Approved in North America. No studies in neonates.
CCG-1423	Rho inhibitor	Systemic	Antifibrotic, cerebrovascular, and cardiovascular diseases.	Experimental use only. No human data.
Fasudil	ROCK inhibitor	Systemic/inhaled	Cerebral vasospasm, stable angina, pulmonary hypertension.	Approved in China and Japan. No data in human neonates.
Fluvastatin	Statin (Rho inhibitor)	Enteral	Hypercholesterolemia, cardiovascular diseases.	Approved in North America. No studies in neonates.
Lovastatin	Statin (Rho inhibitor)	Enteral	Hypercholesterolemia, cardiovascular diseases.	Approved in North America. No studies in neonates.
NSC23766	Rho inhibitor	Systemic	Anti-fibrotic, cerebrovascular and cardiovascular diseases.	Experimental use only. No human data.
Pravastatin	Statin (Rho inhibitor)	Enteral	Hypercholesterolemia, cardiovascular diseases.	Approved in North America. No studies in neonates.
Rosuvastatin	Statin (Rho inhibitor)	Enteral	Hypercholesterolemia, cardiovascular diseases.	Approved in North America. No studies in neonates.
SAR-407899	ROCK 2-selective inhibitor	Systemic/enteral	Cardiovascular diseases.	Investigative use only (Phase 2). No neonatal data.
Simvastatin	Statin (Rho inhibitor)	Enteral	Hypercholesterolemia, cardiovascular diseases.	Approved in North America. No studies in human neonates.
Y-27632	ROCK inhibitor	Systemic/enteral	Systemic and pulmonary hypertension.	Experimental use only. No human data.

(Continued)

TABLE 16.1 Pharmacomechanical Coupling (*Continued*)

Drug	Mechanism of Action	Route of Administration	Indications/Uses	Clinical Status
NO-cGMP Signaling				
BAY 60-2770	sGC activator	Enteral	Pulmonary hypertension, cardiovascular diseases.	Investigational use only. No data in neonatal humans.
Cinaciguat	sGC activator	Enteral	Pulmonary hypertension, cardiovascular diseases.	Investigational use only. No data in neonatal humans.
Ethyl nitrite	NO donor	Inhaled	Pulmonary hypertension.	Experimental use only. No human data.
L-Arginine	NOS stimulator	Systemic/enteral	Systemic and pulmonary hypertension, erectile dysfunction, prevention of necrotizing enterocolitis, peripheral arterial disease, fetal growth restriction, preeclampsia.	Investigational use only in neonates.
L-Citrulline	NOS stimulator	Systemic/enteral	Systemic and pulmonary hypertension, erectile dysfunction.	Investigational use only. No data in human neonates.
Nitric oxide	sGC stimulator	Inhaled	Pulmonary hypertension.	Approved for use in neonates.
Riociguat	sGC stimulator	Enteral	Pulmonary hypertension, systemic sclerosis.	Approved in North America. No data in human neonates.
Sapopterin	Cofactor of eNOS, phenyl-alanine hydroxylase	Enteral	Phenylketonuria, pulmonary hypertension.	Approved for phenylketonuria. Investigational use only for pulmonary hypertension (no data in human neonates).
Sildenafil	PDE5 inhibitor	Systemic/enteral	Pulmonary hypertension, erectile dysfunction.	Approved in North America. Off-label use in neonates.
Sodium nitrite	NO donor	Systemic/inhaled	Cyanide toxicity, pulmonary hypertension.	Approved in North America for cyanide toxicity (systemic). Investigational use for pulmonary hypertension (Phase 2). No data in human neonates.
Tadalafil	PDE5 inhibitor	Enteral	Pulmonary hypertension, erectile dysfunction.	Approved in North America. No studies in human neonates.
Vardenafil	PDE5 inhibitor	Enteral	Pulmonary hypertension, erectile dysfunction.	Approved in North America. No studies in neonates.
cAMP Signaling				
Alprostadil	Prostaglandin E1 analogue	IV infusion, topical	Maintenance of ductal patency, pulmonary hypertension with right ventricular dysfunction, erectile dysfunction.	Approved in North America.
Epoprostenol	Synthetic prostacyclin	IV infusion	Pulmonary hypertension	Approved in North America. Investigational use in human neonates only.
Iloprost	Prostacyclin analogue	Systemic infusion (IV or s.c.)	Pulmonary hypertension	Approved in North America. Investigational use in human neonates only.
Milrinone	PDE3 inhibitor	Systemic infusion	Cardiac failure, pulmonary hypertension.	Approved in North America. Off-label use in neonates.
Selexipag	Prostacyclin receptor agonist	Enteral	Pulmonary hypertension	Approved in North America. No data in neonates.

TABLE 16.1 Pharmacomechanical Coupling (*Continued*)

Drug	Mechanism of Action	Route of Administration	Indications/Uses	Clinical Status
Trepostinil	Prostacyclin analog	Systemic, enteral, inhaled	Pulmonary hypertension	Approved in North America. Investigational use in human neonates only.
Multiple pathways				
Superoxide dismutase	Antioxidant, anti-inflammatory	Intratracheal	Acute and chronic lung injury.	Investigational use only.
Rosiglitazone	PPAR γ agonist	Enteral	Type 2 diabetes mellitus, cardiovascular diseases.	Approved in North America. No data in human neonates.

Hypoxia and pharmacomechanical coupling

Pharmacomechanical coupling involves activation of G-protein coupled receptors (GPCRs) by endogenous or exogenous ligands to raise intracellular calcium, without change in membrane potential (13). GPCRs signal through heterotrimeric G-proteins, consisting of Gα, Gβ, and Gγ subunits. GDP-bound Gα rests bound to Gβγ. When a circulating agonist activates a GPCR, the Gα subunit docks with the GPCR's cytoplasmic loops and exchanges GDP for GTP. This releases Gβγ to interact with effectors including phospholipase C, small GTPases or ion channels, to trigger signal transduction (14). Agonists for vasoconstrictor GPCRs abound in hypoxic PPHN; thromboxane, endothelin, and serotonin are increased in hypoxic animal models and pulmonary hypertension patients, while expression and cell surface localization of their receptors also increases (15).

To prevent uncontrolled signal amplification, termination of GPCR-G-protein signaling requires: (i) GPCR internalization and (ii) GTP hydrolysis, reverting Gα to its inactive state (16). Gα subunits have slow intrinsic GTPase activity; RGS (Regulator of G-protein Signaling) proteins increase the GTPase activity of Gα several-fold (16). GPCR internalization is triggered by its phosphorylation by second messenger-activated kinases or by G-protein receptor kinase, followed by endocytosis. Internalized GPCRs, after agonist removal and dephosphorylation, may be degraded or trafficked back to the membrane. Hypoxia inhibits GPCR desensitization by decreasing regulatory kinase activity (17), increasing receptor sensitivity to vasoconstrictors, and preventing internalization.

The 16 human Gα subunits are classified into 4 subfamilies: $Gα_s$, $Gα_{i/o}$, $Gα_{q/11}$, and $Gα_{12/13}$. $Gα_s$ activates adenylyl cyclase, while $Gα_{i/o}$ inhibits adenylyl cyclase; these are discussed under cAMP-mediated relaxation pathways. Many vascular GPCRs couple with more than one Gα family. Contractile GPCRs signal via $Gα_{q/11}$, which activates phospholipase C (PLC), increasing intracellular calcium; these GPCRs often also couple with $Gα_{12/13}$, activating small GTPase proteins Rac and Rho. Smooth muscle GPCRs implicated in PPHN vasoconstriction include endothelin receptor ET-A, coupled to $Gα_{q/11}$, $Gα_{12/13}$, and $Gα_{i/o}$; thromboxane receptor (TP), coupled to $Gα_{q/11}$, $Gα_{12/13}$, and $Gα_s$, plus FP and EP prostanoid receptors similarly coupled; serotonin receptors 5-HT$_{1B}$ ($Gα_{i/o}$-coupled) and 5-HT$_{2A/B}$ ($Gα_{q11}$-coupled); angiotensin receptor AT$_1$R ($Gα_{i/o}$ or $Gα_{q11}$-coupled); α1-adrenoceptor ($Gα_{q/11}$ and $Gα_{12/13}$-coupled); and P2Y purinoceptor ($Gα_{q11}$-coupled) (18). Hypoxia influences GPCR coupling through protein modifications increasing $Gα_q$-receptor association (19), heightening calcium responses to vasoconstrictors. Antagonists of these vasoconstrictor GPCRs used in treating PPHN are detailed in Table 16.1.

$Gα_{q/11}$ activation prompts PLC enzyme activity, producing diacylglycerol (DAG) and IP$_3$. DAG and its downstream effector protein kinase C activate receptor-operated cation channels including transient receptor potential canonical (TRPC) channels, causing calcium influx (20). Other receptor-operated calcium channels include P2X purinoceptors, activated by ATP from sympathetic nerves to evoke calcium transients (21). IP$_3$ diffuses toward IP$_3$ receptors on the endoplasmic reticulum, which release ER-stored calcium into the cytosol. Adjacent on the ER, the ryanodine receptor opens as the cytosolic calcium rises, in a mechanism termed calcium-induced calcium release, creating localized calcium sparks; these are exaggerated during pulmonary arterial hypoxia (22). The amplitude and frequency of these calcium oscillations determine actomyosin interaction.

Hypoxia and calcium store repletion

During chronic hypoxia, persistently high intracellular Ca^{2+} and sustained contraction are maintained in part by entry of Ca^{2+} from the extracellular space via L-type voltage-dependent calcium channels (VDCC), or voltage-independent TRCP channels, comprising receptor-operated (ROCC) and store-operated Ca^{2+} channels (SOCC) (23). VDCC are highly expressed and have the largest immediate influence on global intracellular calcium during contraction.

The major intracellular repository of calcium in myocytes is the sarcoplasmic reticulum (SR), a network of membranes and tubules which amplifies the intracellular calcium signal. Prompted by VDCC calcium influx or pharmacomechanical signaling, waves of calcium are released from the SR into the cytosol. This depletes SR calcium stores, requiring replenishment through store-operated calcium entry. When SR calcium decreases, calcium-sensitive proteins embedded in the SR membrane called stromal interaction molecules oligomerize and migrate to the cell membrane, where they activate SOCC (24). Capacitative calcium entry increases, while receptor-operated calcium entry is inhibited by calcium depletion of the SR; SOCC opening can sustain agonist-induced calcium oscillations in the absence of other calcium influx (25). TRPC expression increases in hypoxia; acute hypoxia also enhances capacitative calcium entry through SOCCs in pulmonary arteries, increasing resting calcium. This triggers depolarization and secondary activation of VDCCs, augmenting contraction (26).

Higher intracellular Ca^{2+} concentrations during prolonged hypoxia are maintained by the upregulation of Ca^{2+} channels, especially TRPC (12), the inhibited activity of sarcoplasmic reticulum calcium ATPase (SERCA), which transports Ca^{2+} from the cytosol back into the SR, and the inhibited activity of plasma membrane Na^+-Ca^{2+} exchanger, which exports Ca^{2+} from the cytosol to the extracellular space. SERCA gene transfer rescues both hypoxic and monocrotaline-induced pulmonary hypertension and regresses arterial remodeling (27). This indicates that impaired calcium reuptake following contraction increases $(Ca^{2+})_i$ and leads to calcium-dependent activation of smooth muscle proliferation in hypoxic conditions.

Hypoxia and actomyosin crossbridge cycling

The central contractile mechanism of vascular smooth muscle is the sliding interaction of phosphorylated myosin with actin thin filaments, resulting in shortening of the cell. Smooth muscle thick filaments consist of intertwined myosin proteins, comprising two heavy chains with ATPase activity making the myosin head; and four light chains at the neck, including two regulatory 20kD light chains activated by phosphorylation.

Myosin heavy chain (MHC) phenotype is developmentally regulated and influences force of contraction; in vessels, fetal MHC SM-1 isoforms generally generate less force than neonatal SM-2 (28). Vascular smooth muscle is tonic (slow contraction kinetics, maintenance of sustained tone), as opposed to the phasic smooth muscle in bladder, gut, or uterus (spontaneous contractile activity, fast force development) (29). The MHC amino-terminal SMB isoform characteristic of phasic muscle also appears in fetal and neonatal vasculature, especially in small muscular arteries, but disappears from the adult (30). These isoform variations may contribute to faster contractile responses in neonatal compared to adult arteries. Following prolonged hypoxia-induced remodeling of pulmonary artery, muscle MHC isoforms give way to less reactive non-muscle MHC, as part of the switch to a fibrotic phenotype (31); this is when vascular reactivity is lost.

When calcium enters a myocyte, it activates the Ca^{2+} sensor protein calmodulin; this complex activates myosin light chain kinase (MLCK), which phosphorylates serine 19 of the myosin light chain 20 kDa subunit (MLC_{20}) and initiates contraction. MLC phosphorylation enables the interaction of the myosin head with actin, and determines the velocity of contraction. When bound to ADP, myosin binds actin in a weak rigor configuration; the arrival of ATP dissolves this old crossbridge and causes a conformational change in MHC, raising the head of the myosin molecule, and forming a strong crossbridge in its new location. With the hydrolysis of ATP and release of phosphate, the myosin head 'nods' to propel the actin filament. This power stroke moves the thin filament by 100 Å, where myosin remains weakly bound to actin while awaiting its next ATP (32). Slower, tonic smooth muscles have stronger ADP binding than phasic muscle resulting in energy-efficient maintenance of tone, sometime termed latch-bridges (33). Sustained tone in pulmonary artery is calcium/

calmodulin-independent; while in agonist-induced contraction, the crossbridge cycling rate is dependent on MLCK activity. In hypertensive pulmonary vessels, the velocity of shortening increases independent of load (34), suggesting a shift toward phasic muscle behavior.

MLC dephosphorylation by myosin light chain phosphatase (MLCP) interrupts actomyosin interaction and desensitizes muscle to calcium. In a fetal PPHN model, MLCK activity is unchanged but MLCP inhibited, resulting in pulmonary hypertension (35). The balance between MLCK and MLCP activities determines contractile force, so any therapy that tips this balance toward dephosphorylation would ameliorate pulmonary arterial contraction. Two potential targets for which small molecule inhibitors have been developed are MLCK (36) and Ca^{2+}-Calmodulin kinase II (37). To date, these agents have not been tested for treatment of cardiovascular disorders.

Hypoxia and calcium sensitization

Increased sensitivity to Ca^{2+}-mediated contraction is achieved via inhibited activity of MLCP, thus increasing MLC_{20} phosphorylation (and thereby contractile activity) at a given concentration of intracellular Ca^{2+}. The predominant driver of Ca^{2+}-sensitization is increased activity of the RhoA/Rho-kinase (ROCK or ROK) pathway (38). RhoA is a small GTPase belonging to the Ras superfamily (comprising three families: RhoA, Rac, and Cdc42), which function as GTP hydrolases, active when bound to GTP and inactive when bound to GDP. This switch is turned on by guanine nucleotide exchange factors that facilitate the dissociation of GDP from RhoA, allowing GTP to bind, and is counterbalanced by GTPase-activating proteins, which increase the efficiency of GTP hydrolysis. Inactive RhoA-GDP is located in the cytoplasm while active RhoA-GTP is tethered to the plasma membrane by geranylgeranylation (prenylation) of its C-terminus. Guanine dissociation inhibitors are a third inhibitory mechanism of RhoA activity, preventing its translocation from the cytosol to the membrane.

Hypoxia stimulates RhoA activity via activation of GPCRs, through membrane depolarization, or by oxidative or mechanical stress. The downstream effector of RhoA is ROCK, a serine/threonine kinase with two isoforms (ROCK I and II), both highly expressed in vascular SMCs. Several ROCK polymorphisms have been linked to risk for RDS in preterm neonates (39), suggesting a role in cardiorespiratory homeostasis. ROCK phosphorylates the myosin-binding subunit of MLCP (MYPT1) at threonine 853 and 696, leading to suppression of MLCP activity. ROCK may also contribute to Ca^{2+} sensitization via phosphorylation of CPI-17 (at threonine 38), a small inhibitor of PP1cδ, which is the catalytic subunit of MLCP. Other effects of RhoA/ROCK activity contributing to sustained vasoconstriction include reversion to increased "fetal" levels of myogenic activity, inhibition of endothelial nitric oxide synthase (NOS) expression and activity, and suppressed activity of the actin filament severing protein, cofilin. RhoA/ROCK activity is also essential for *de novo* formation of actin filaments, and formation of the focal adhesions that are required for myosin-dependent force development and transmission.

Several small molecule kinase inhibitors possessing high specificity toward ROCK have been studied as therapeutic vasodilators (40). Among these, fasudil hydrochloride (HA-1077) has shown efficacy in pulmonary hypertensive neonatal animals (41) and human children (42). A slow-release oral formulation of fasudil (AT-877ER) improved pulmonary hemodynamics in adult pulmonary hypertensives over 3 months (43). Sustained treatment with ROCK inhibitors reversed hypoxic pulmonary vascular remodeling in neonatal rats, via antimitotic and proapoptotic effects on vascular myocytes (44). The high risk of systemic hypotension with ROCK inhibitors may be overcome by direct pulmonary delivery (45). Another translatable approach to limiting RhoA/ROCK activity is the use of HMG-CoA reductase inhibitors (statins). In addition to lipid-lowering effects, statins inhibit prenylation of Rho-GTP and thus its ability to translocate to the membrane and activate ROCK. Statins have shown efficacy in prevention and treatment of hypoxic pulmonary hypertension in neonatal animals (46). Several small molecule compounds capable of limiting Rho-GTP binding are also under development.

Hypoxia and cytoskeletal dynamics

The contractile apparatus is composed of thick (myosin) and thin (actin) filaments. Actin filaments polymerize during smooth muscle contraction and depolymerize during relaxation. Generation of mechanical tension in response to an agonist requires an increased proportion of filamentous (F) to globular (G)-actin (47). Unlike skeletal or cardiac, vascular smooth muscle contains a substantial pool of monomeric G-actin. After α-adrenergic stimulation, F-actin increases over 90%, as G-actin incorporates into the actin network (48). Cytoskeletal remodeling alters the transduction of force from cross-bridges, along the actin filaments to membrane focal adhesions. Small increments in actin polymerization create large increases in contraction.

The F:G-actin ratio is determined by GPCRs coupling to $G\alpha_{12/13}$, or tyrosine kinase receptors which activate Rho-family GTPases; these regulate actin binding, capping and sequestering proteins, controlling thin filament assembly. During pulmonary arterial hypoxia, $G\alpha_{12/13}$ signaling via RhoA, Rac or Cdc42 activates LIM kinase which inhibits cofilin, increasing actin polymerization (49).

Fetal pulmonary arterial myocytes are densely packed into a thick arterial wall with a narrow lumen. Postnatally, hypoxic arterial smooth muscle cells also have increased cell volume, more numerous focal adhesions, and loss of polarity (50). Length adaptation also reorganizes myosin filaments; a series-to-parallel change in myosin filaments doubles contraction velocity, without change in myosin phosphorylation (51). This contractile plasticity permits vascular constriction to a much smaller diameter; while cytoskeletal plasticity limits dilation upon vascular relaxation (52).

Cytoskeletal architecture is acutely sensitive to mechanical strain; at low pressure, filamentous actin is restricted to the cell periphery, but increasing pressure rapidly polymerizes actin fibers along the myocyte's long axis (53). Disassembly and remodeling of cytoskeletal filaments to permit myocyte elongation is a critical element of circulatory transition, which is not observed in PPHN (54) due to increased transmural pressure.

Smooth muscle actin includes α, β and γ isoforms; α-actin is the major component of thin filaments, which connect to cortical actin networks comprising muscular γ-actin. Cytoplasmic β- and γ-actin isoforms support internal cell structure and motility (55). α-Actin predominates in tonically contractile vascular smooth muscle; γ-actin expression increases in phasically-contractile muscle, and tissues subject to dilational stretch, including blood vessels (55). Agonists induce actin polymerization into a cortical filament scaffold comprised primarily of γ-actin. Contractile filaments exert force upon this scaffold, to shorten the cell. Gamma-actin increases in PPHN pulmonary arteries (56), possibly as a component of a tonic-to-phasic muscle switch, amplifying the velocity of shortening. Hypoxia increases polymerized actin, increasing pulmonary vasoreactivity (57). By upregulating integrins and focal adhesions connecting cytoskeleton to extracellular matrix, hypoxia also augments the transduction of external stresses to the smooth muscle cytoskeleton (58).

Hypoxia and cGMP signaling

NO is a gaseous free radical, first identified as the endothelium-derived vascular relaxing factor in 1987, essential to the maintenance of low vascular tone during postnatal life. NO is the product of the enzymatic conversion of L-arginine to L-citrulline, catalyzed by any of three isoforms of NOS: NOS1 (neuronal NOS), NOS2 (inducible NOS), and NOS3 (endothelial NOS).

NO signals either via direct interaction with smooth muscle soluble guanylyl cyclase (sGC) that catalyzes the conversion of GTP to cyclic guanosine monophosphate (cGMP) (59) or via a reaction with protein thiol groups to form S-nitrosothiols (60). sGC is composed of α and β subunits, and a single heme moiety coordinated with the β-subunit of the heterodimer via a histidine residue. NO binding to heme forms a Fe^{2+}-NO complex, stimulating cyclase activity. sGC is under redox control, active when in a reduced state. Hypoxia downregulates sGC and limits its ability to be activated by NO (61), likely via oxidation/nitration of its heme and thiol groups. cGMP activates cGMP-dependent protein kinase (PKG), which in turn mediates relaxation via phosphorylation of various targets, many of which are shared by PKA, the protein kinase activated by cyclic adenosine monophosphate (cAMP).

cGMP is hydrolyzed by phosphodiesterases (PDEs), a superfamily comprising 11 isoforms. Smooth muscle expresses predominantly PDE 1, 3, and 5, with the latter primarily hydrolyzing cGMP (62). Hypoxia upregulates PDE5 in the pulmonary vasculature (61). cGMP-PKG activity stimulates smooth muscle relaxation by (i) inhibition of Ca^{2+} influx through VDCCs and SOCCs and increased Ca^{2+} efflux via SERCA and the plasma membrane Na^+/Ca^{2+} exchanger; (ii) decreased Ca^{2+} mobilization via inhibition of IP_3 synthesis and IP_3R activity; (iii) Ca^{2+} desensitization via phosphorylation of MYPT1 serine 695 and 852, which prevents the adjacent threonine residues (696 and 853) from becoming phosphorylated by ROCK; and (iv) phosphorylation of RhoA at serine 188, increasing its binding to GDI and thus preventing membrane attachment. PKG activity also phosphorylates MYPT1 (at serine 668), which directly stimulates MLCP activity; this phosphorylation target is downregulated by chronic hypoxia.

Inhaled NO was adopted in the early 1990s as a selective and short-acting pulmonary vasodilator for newborns with hypoxemic respiratory failure. Chronic exposure to hypoxia diminishes NO-mediated pulmonary vascular relaxation in neonatal animals (41). Other NO-based therapies include inhaled ethyl nitrite (63) or sodium nitrite (64), which act as NO donors; these therapies remain investigational. Endogenous NO production may be enhanced with L-arginine or L-citrulline (65), or by supplementation with tetrahydrobiopterin (Saproterin), a cofactor necessary for NOS function. Inhibitors of arginases, which are upregulated by hypoxia and starve NOS of L-arginine substrate, have also shown promise in experimental neonatal pulmonary hypertension (66). The prototypical PDE5 inhibitor, Sildenafil, remains a mainstay of therapy for pulmonary hypertension in all age groups. Newer PDE5 inhibitors with longer activity and greater potency (e.g. Tadalafil, Vardenafil) have yet to see use in newborns. sGC stimulators (e.g. Riociguat) and activators (e.g. Cinaciguat) are highly potent vasodilators, yet to be studied in human newborns.

Hypoxia and cAMP signaling

Relaxation of pulmonary arterial myocytes can also involve vasodilator binding to $G\alpha_s$-coupled GPCRs, leading to adenylyl cyclase (AC) activation. AC interacts with activated $G\alpha_s$, converting ATP to cAMP. In opposition, $G\alpha_{i/o}$-coupled receptors inhibit AC interaction with $G\alpha_s$. In the pulmonary circuit, GPCRs coupling to $G\alpha_s$ include prostacyclin receptor (IP), prostaglandin receptor EP2 and adenosine receptor A2A (15).

While it has been assumed that one GPCR signals through one $G\alpha$ at a time, heterodimerized TP/IP receptors couple simultaneously to $G\alpha_{q/11}$ and $G\alpha_s$, biasing their signaling so that TP receptor agonists activate $G\alpha_s$ and thus AC and relaxation (67). However these receptor partnerships can be influenced by environmental factors including hypoxia (68), abruptly reverting GPCR signals toward vasoconstriction, even in the presence of a vasodilator agonist.

The nine transmembrane isoforms of AC are activated by $G\alpha_s$, most are inhibited by $G\alpha_{i/o}$, and several are activated by protein kinase C (PKC), some inhibited by PKA, some by calcium (69). Pulmonary artery myocytes primarily express AC isoform 6, with lower levels of AC2, AC3, and AC7 (70). AC6 localizes to caveolar lipid rafts associated with IP and adrenergic receptors, influences resting membrane potential, and serves as the principle vasodilator in vascular myocytes. Like guanylate cyclase (71), AC6 activity is inhibited by NO (72), which nitrosylates and inactivates the enzyme.

The concentration of cAMP is determined by AC generation of cAMP and by PDE 1-4 which hydrolyze cAMP. High intrinsic PDE activity can tightly regulate cAMP even in the presence of AC-activating or -inhibiting stimuli (73). Cyclic AMP-elevating agents can cause bronchodilation, reduce inflammation, limit apoptosis, inhibit smooth muscle proliferation promoting an antifibrotic phenotype, and vasodilate pulmonary as well as systemic arteries. In the pulmonary circuit, cAMP activates PKA, which phosphorylates signaling targets, including BK_{Ca} and voltage-dependent and -independent calcium channels (74), attenuating Ca^{2+} release. PKA also inhibits MLCK and indirectly activates MLCP, thereby dephosphorylating myosin. Hypoxia inhibits these actions of PKA (75).

Hypoxia increases the thromboxane to prostacyclin ratio, promoting pulmonary vasoconstriction. Loss of IP signaling via $G\alpha_s$ precipitates hypertension and hypoxic cardiac dysfunction (76). Several prostacyclin analogs are available for intravenous or inhaled treatment of hypoxic PPHN, limited by their relatively short half-life, and by rapid agonist-induced desensitization and internalization of IP receptors, resulting in tachyphylaxis and loss of response (77). Hypoxia also accelerates cAMP degradation. The PDE3 inhibitor milrinone prevents degradation of cAMP, promoting pulmonary vasorelaxation and cardiac

contractility. It also restores inhibitory phosphorylation of the thromboxane receptor (78). Milrinone has been effective in treating NO-refractory PPHN (79).

In this review, we have not touched upon the effects of hypoxia on smooth muscle phenotype, matrix deposition, or proliferative activation; these topics are covered in full in other chapters. The effects of hypoxia on the complex contractile machinery of pulmonary arterial smooth muscle create a multiplicity of therapeutic targets, many of which can be harnessed for the amelioration of hypoxic pulmonary hypertension during its vasoconstrictive phase.

References

1. Makino A, et al. Compr Physiol. 2011; 1(3):1555–1602.
2. Archer SL, et al. J Clin Invest. 1998; 101(11):2319–2330.
3. Nelson MT, et al. Am J Physiol. 1990; 259(1 Pt 1):C3–C18.
4. Storme L, et al. Pediatr Res. 1999; 45(3):425–431.
5. Belik J. Pediatr Res. 1995; 37(2):196–201.
6. Davis MJ, et al. Physiol Rev. 1999; 79(2):387–423.
7. Walsh MP, et al. J Cereb Blood Flow Metab. 2013; 33(1):1–12.
8. Pluteanu F, et al. Am J Physiol Cell Physiol. 2011; 300(3):C517–C525.
9. Tykocki NR, et al. Compr Physiol. 2017; 7(2):485–581.
10. Orallo F. Pharmacol Ther. 1996; 69(3):153–171.
11. Burdyga T, et al. Pflugers Arch. 1997; 435(1):182–184.
12. Mauban JR, et al. J Appl Physiol. 2005; 98(1):415–420.
13. Somlyo AP, et al. Acta Physiol Scand. 1998; 164(4):437–448.
14. Oldham WM, et al. Nat Struct Mol Biol. 2006; 13(9):772–777
15. Strassheim D, et al. Vessel Plus. 2018; 2:29.
16. Hendriks-Balk MC, et al. Eur J Pharmacol. 2008; 585(2-3):278–291.
17. Santhosh KT, et al. Br J Pharmacol. 2014; 171(3):676–687.
18. Iyinikkel J, et al. Br J Pharmacol. 2018; 175(15):3063–3079.
19. Sikarwar AS, et al. Am J Respir Cell Mol Biol. 2014; 50(1):135–143.
20. Hofmann T, et al. Nature. 1999; 397(6716):259–263.
21. Burnstock G, et al. Circ Res. 1986; 58(3):319–330.
22. Zheng YM, et al. J Gen Physiol. 2005; 125(4):427–440.
23. McFadzean I, et al. Br J Pharmacol. 2002; 135(1):1–13.
24. Reddish FN, et al. Int J Mol Sci. 2017; 18(5):1024.
25. Croisier H, et al. PLOS ONE. 2013; 8(7):e69598.
26. Wang J, et al. Am J Physiol Lung Cell Mol Physiol. 2005; 288(6):L1059–L1069.
27. Prieto-Lloret J, et al. Cardiovasc Res. 2014; 103(2):189–191.
28. Chern J, et al. Pediatr Res. 1995; 38(5):697–703.
29. Horiuti K, et al. J Gen Physiol. 1989; 94(4):769–781.
30. White SL, et al. Am J Physiol. 1998; 275(2 Pt 1):C581–C589.
31. Packer CS, et al. Am J Physiol. 1998; 274(5 Pt 1):L775–L785.
32. Vale RD, et al. Science. 2000; 288(5463):88–95.
33. Fuglsang A, et al. J Muscle Res Cell Motil. 1993; 14(6):666–677.
34. Packer CS, et al. Can J Physiol Pharmacol. 1985; 63(6):669–674.
35. Belik J, et al. Pediatr Res. 1998; 43(1):57–61.
36. Xiong Y, et al. Front Pharmacol. 2017; 8:292.
37. Pellicena P, et al. Front Pharmacol. 2014; 5:21.
38. Somlyo AP, et al. J Physiol. 2000; 522 Pt 2:177–185.
39. Kaya G, et al. Pediatr Neonatol. 2017; 58(1):36–42.
40. Uehata M, et al. Nature. 1997; 389(6654):990–994.
41. McNamara PJ, et al. Am J Physiol Lung Cell Mol Physiol. 2008; 294(2):L205–L213.
42. Li F, et al. Pediatr Cardiol. 2009; 30(3):363–366.
43. Fukumoto Y, et al. Circ J. 2013; 77(10):2619–2625.
44. Ziino AJ, et al. Pediatr Res. 2010; 67(2):177–182.
45. Gosal K, et al. Am J Respir Cell Mol Biol. 2015; 52(6):717–727.
46. Wong MJ, et al. Am J Physiol Lung Cell Mol Physiol. 2016; 311(5):L985–L999.
47. Gunst SJ, et al. Am J Physiol Cell Physiol. 2008; 295(3):C576–C587.
48. Cipolla MJ, et al. FASEB J. 2002; 16(1):72–76.
49. Veith C, et al. Proteomics. 2013; 13(1):75–88.
50. Vogler M, et al. PLOS ONE. 2013; 8(7):e69128.
51. Seow CY, et al. J Appl Physiol (1985). 2000; 89(3):869–876.
52. Tuna BG, et al. Basic Clin Pharmacol Toxicol. 2012; 110(1):35–41.
53. Flavahan NA, et al. Am J Physiol Heart Circ Physiol. 2005; 288(2):H660–H669.
54. Haworth SG. Exp Physiol. 1995; 80(5):843–853.
55. Vandekerckhove J, et al. J Mol Biol. 1978; 126(4):783–802.
56. Hall SM, et al. J Anat. 2000; 196(Pt 3):391–403.
57. Weise-Cross L, et al. Am J Physiol Heart Circ Physiol. 2018; 314(5):H1011–H1021.
58. Blaschke F, et al. Biochem Biophys Res Commun. 2002; 296(4):890–896.
59. Lucas KA, et al. Pharmacol Rev. 2000; 52(3):375–414.
60. Lima B, et al. Circ Res. 2010; 106(4):633–646.
61. Jernigan NL, et al. Am J Physiol Lung Cell Mol Physiol. 2002; 282(6):L1366–L1375.
62. Rybalkin SD, et al. Circ Res. 2003; 93(4):280–291.
63. Moya MP, et al. Lancet. 2002; 360(9327):141–143.
64. Jankov RP, et al. Am J Physiol Lung Cell Mol Physiol. 2018; 315(5):L742–L751.
65. Fike CD, et al. Am J Respir Cell Mol Biol. 2015; 53(2):255–264.

66. Grasemann H, et al. Am J Physiol Lung Cell Mol Physiol. 2015; 308(6):L503–L510.
67. Ibrahim S, et al. Arterioscler Thromb Vasc Biol. 2013; 33(1):60–66.
68. Porzionato A, et al. Front Physiol. 2018; 9:697.
69. Hanoune J, et al. Annu Rev Pharmacol Toxicol. 2001; 41:145–174.
70. Jourdan KB, et al. Am J Physiol Lung Cell Mol Physiol. 2001; 280(6):L1359–L1369.
71. Gladwin MT. J Clin Invest. 2006; 116(9):2330–2332.
72. McVey M, et al. J Biol Chem. 1999; 274(27):18887–18892.

73. Creighton JR, et al. Am J Physiol Lung Cell Mol Physiol. 2003; 284(1):L100–L107.
74. Cuinas A, et al. Life Sci. 2016; 155:102–109.
75. Barman SA, et al. Lung. 2005; 183(5):353–361.
76. Rohlicek CV, et al. Cardiovasc Res. 2005; 65(4):861–868.
77. Schermuly RT, et al. Respir Res. 2007; 8:4.
78. Santhosh K, et al. Br J Pharmacol. 2011; 163(6):1223–1236.
79. McNamara PJ, et al. Pediatr Crit Care Med. 2013; 14(1):74–84.

CELLULAR OXYGEN SENSING, MITOCHONDRIAL OXYGEN SENSING AND REACTIVE OXYGEN SPECIES

Jason Boehme and Emin Maltepe

Contents

Introduction

Molecular O_2, as the terminal electron acceptor of the mitochondrial electron transport chain (ETC), is essential to sustain the high rate of cellular energy production required for the normal function of mammalian cells and tissues. It allows the catabolism of carbohydrates, lipids, and other nutritive substrates to be efficiently paired to the production of ATP via the Krebs cycle and the maintenance of a proton motive force across the inner mitochondrial membrane. Conversely, excessive O_2 is potentially injurious to cells, and tissue hypoxia can be both protective and adaptive in various developmental and physiologic states. O_2 delivery must therefore be tightly coordinated, and highly responsive, to the metabolic demands of the tissue.

Specifically adapted cell types that sense and coordinate the physiologic responses to alterations in local oxygen tension are found in the carotid body, adrenal medulla, neuroepithelial bodies, and the vascular cells of the pulmonary arteries, ductus arteriosus, and fetoplacental arteries (1). However, the primary focus of this chapter will be oxygen sensing and the role of reactive oxygen species (ROS), specifically in regard to the pulmonary vasculature and pulmonary arterial (PA) myocytes.

Hypoxic pulmonary vasoconstriction (HPV) describes the acute vasoconstriction of the pulmonary arteries in response to hypoxia, which is distinctive from the corresponding reaction of mild vasodilation that is observed in the systemic arteries (2). This hypoxic response is somewhat variable throughout the pulmonary arterial tree, but is most consistent and pronounced in the small resistance pulmonary arteries (3). The primary stimulus to HPV is alveolar hypoxia, though there is some effect exerted by hypoxemia of the pulmonary arterial (mixed venous) blood, as well as a detectable, but seemingly small, influence by the bronchiolar arterial supply (3, 4). It is important to note that HPV within the context of the whole organism is a complex and multifactorial process. There are distinct temporal phases, including an acute phase 1 reaction that develops over the first 0–30 minutes of hypoxic exposure (generally peaking within the first 5 minutes), and a delayed phase 2 reaction of greater intensity that develops more gradually over the next 6–8 hours (plateauing at about 2 hours in human adults) (3, 5–7). Different experimental preparations have shown the vascular endothelium to be noncontributory or only partially contributory to the phase 1 response, while phase 2 is heavily dependent on the endothelium and other modulating factors such as acid-base status, presence of erythrocytes, inflammatory mediators, hormones, gasotransmitters, and neurohumoral activation (3, 5).

Canonical receptors and ion channels involved in hypoxic pulmonary vasoconstriction

Consensus holds that at least the initial hypoxic vasoconstrictive response is intrinsic to the pulmonary vascular smooth muscle, and great attention has been focused on the mechanisms by which these myocytes sense and respond to local O_2 tension. A central model has emerged that converges on the downstream modulation of K$^+$ and Ca^{++} channels in response to hypoxia, ultimately resulting in increased cytoplasmic Ca^{++} and arterial smooth muscle cell contraction.

K$^+$ channels

Early experimental work demonstrated that inhibition of K$^+$ channels mimicked the effects of hypoxia on PA rings and myocytes. Hypoxia was shown to inhibit outwardly directed K$^+$ currents at the cell membrane, causing membrane depolarization and myocyte contraction in pulmonary, but not systemic arteries (8, 9). Studies with various selective pharmacologic inhibitors identified the family of voltage-gated (K$_V$) K$^+$ channels as being O_2 sensitive, with receptor-specific antibodies identifying K$_V$ 1.5 and 2.1 as the major contributors to the outward K$^+$ current inhibited by hypoxia (10). The importance of K$_V$ 1.5 in this role was further demonstrated using gene knockout approaches (11).

There has also been interested in the family of twin pore (K$_{2P}$) K$^+$ channels, particularly the TASK channels, which are believed to be open and contributory to the outward K$^+$ current under relevant physiologic conditions. Some evidence suggested that TASK-1 is indeed responsive to hypoxia (12), while more recent studies in knockout mice demonstrated no role in acute HPV, but

DOI: 10.1201/9780367494018-17

some participation in sustained phase 2 HPV in the pre-acinar arteries (13).

Multiple studies suggest that the inhibition of O_2 sensitive K^+ channels is mediated via their interactions with ROS and redox pairs, likely through modulation of thiol-containing residues of the pore-forming units (3, 14). However, other mechanisms have been described, including inhibition of Kv currents mediated by an isoform of protein kinase C (PKC-ς), in response to both ceramide production (15) and through agonism of thromboxane endoperoxide receptors (16).

Ca^{++} channels

The classic model holds that inhibition of outward K^+ current and membrane depolarization results in activation and opening of voltage-dependent Ca^{++} channels (VDCCs) leading to an influx of cytoplasmic Ca^{++} and smooth muscle contraction (9). Inhibition of Ca^{++} channels or removal of Ca^{++} from extracellular media in perfusion studies is shown to abrogate or diminish HPV (3, 17). However, voltage-gated Ca^{++} channels are not sufficient on their own to mediate HPV and appear to contribute only partially to the phase 1 response (18). Ca^{++} release from stores within the sarcoplasmic reticulum (SR) through both the ryanodine receptor (RyR), and inositol triphosphate receptor (IP_3R) Ca^{++} channels, appears to be important for both the initial and sustained release of Ca^{++} in response to hypoxia (19). Both RyRs and IP_3Rs are potentially activated by cellular ROS through distinct mechanisms. ROS inhibit FK506 Binding Protein 12.6 from interacting with and stabilizing RyRs in the closed conformation on the SR membrane, resulting in activation (20), while H_2O_2 activates Ca^{++} release in a Phospholipase-C (PLC)-dependent manner, presumably through PLC-mediated production of IP3 and activation of IP_3R channels (21).

Depletion of Ca^{++} from the SR triggers store operated Ca^{++} entry (SOCE) when the SR Ca^{++} sensor, stromal interacting molecule-1 (Stim1), redistributes and activates plasma membrane pore-forming multimers of Orai and/or transient receptor potential canonical (TRPC) channel proteins, allowing continued Ca^{++} influx from the extracellular space. Components of this process are also implicated in the cascade of HPV, which is suppressed by the pharmacologic blockade of SOCE. TRPC 6 null mice do not exhibit phase 1 of HPV, while Stim1 knockdown suppresses phase 2. Attenuation of HPV observed in transient receptor potential vanilloid (TRPV 4) knockout mice may also be due to participation of this channel in SOCE (22).

Of note, the TRP pores respond to other signals and participate in receptor operated Ca^{++} entry (ROC), in addition to SOCE. Experimental work has shown that TRPC6 in particular contributes to HPV through a mechanism involving activation by diacylglycerol (DAG), another metabolite arising from activity of the aforementioned PLC (22, 23).

Redox theories of hypoxic pulmonary vasoconstriction: Effects of hypoxia on the mitochondrial electron transport chain, ROS generation and cellular energy production

As noted in the discussion of canonical ion channels, the production of ROS is widely implicated as the upstream controlling mechanism that provokes the downstream effectors of HPV. The mitochondrial ETC is widely believed to be the primary sensor of cellular O_2 tension and source of these regulatory ROS-mediated signals. However, there is ongoing controversy as to the precise nature of the mitochondrial response to hypoxia. During electron flux through the ETC, uncoupled electrons can escape predominantly from complexes I and III, and interact with molecular O_2 to form superoxide ($O_2^{\cdot-}$) anions. These $O_2^{\cdot-}$ anions are transformed rapidly into hydrogen peroxide (H_2O_2) which widely mediates downstream signaling.

The Redox theory holds that electron escape from the ETC and the resulting production of $O_2^{\cdot-}$ is directly proportional to electron flow through the chain, and that hypoxic slowing of overall flow through the ETC results in diminished mitochondrial ROS (24). This hypoxic decrease in ROS production was initially demonstrated by Archer and colleagues in studies using the redox sensitive probes luminol and lucigenin in perfused lungs (24, 25). Additional studies demonstrated relaxation of PAs in response to exogenous H_2O_2 and other oxidants, as well as constriction in response to the antioxidants CoQ_{10} and duroquinone (26, 27). Most recently, work using transfection of more sophisticated targeted redox probes has demonstrated decreased ROS generation by complex I in response to hypoxia (28).

However, work by Chandel et al. challenged this model, demonstrating a hypoxic increase in the production of mitochondrial ROS arising primarily from complex III (29, 30). Subsequent work by several groups, utilizing varied methodologies such as FRET-based redox sensors and compartment-specific targeted protein sensors, have provided additional data demonstrating increased mitochondrial ROS in response to hypoxia (31, 32). Supportive additional data have shown that exogenous ROS scavengers and adenoviral expression of the H_2O_2 scavenger periredoxin-5 in the mitochondrial intermembrane space inhibit HPV and hypoxic cytosolic Ca^{++} influx (33, 34). This model of increased hypoxic ROS signaling is consistent with the previously discussed evidence for parallel ROS-mediated activation of SR Ca^{++} release from RyR and IP_3R channels (20, 21), while the redox theory invokes the centrality of K_V inhibition, membrane depolarization, and activation of membrane VDCCs (1).

Perhaps unsurprisingly, these differing theories of mitochondrial ROS production have led to divergent models of acute mitochondrial O_2 sensing.

Complex I

One model implicates the mitochondrial complex I subunit Ndufs2 (NADH dehydrogenase ubiquinone iron-sulfur protein 2) as the site of ETC O_2 sensing. This model arose from initial observations that pharmacologic inhibitors of complex I in the ETC mimic features of hypoxia in both pulmonary and systemic vasculature, as well as other O_2-responsive tissues. Work by Dunham-Snary et al., proponents of the redox theory of mitochondrial ROS, shows that pulmonary artery smooth muscle cells (PASMCs), but not renal arterial SMCs, decrease mitochondrial H_2O_2 production and increase cytosolic Ca^{++} in response to acute hypoxia. siRNA knockdown of Ndufs2 in rat PASMCs eliminated this hypoxic rise in Ca^{++}, while knockdown of Ndufs1, the Rieske Fe-S protein (RISP) in Complex III, and COX4i2 did not. Nebulization of the same Ndufs2 siRNA into the lungs of intact rodents was subsequently shown to eliminate HPV in these animals (28).

Complex III and IV

Following the initial description of increased mitochondrial ROS arising from complex III in response to hypoxia (30), it was shown that conditional deletion of the complex III RISP from PASMCs inhibited the hypoxic rise in mitochondrial ROS and abolished the hypoxic increase in cytosolic Ca^{++} in these cells

(31). More recent work by Sommer et al. provides additional mechanistic explanation for the increase in mitochondrial ROS in response to hypoxia and implicates complex IV as the primary site of O_2 sensing. Using rodent knockouts of the complex IV subunit 4 isoform 2 (Cox4i2), a subunit preferentially expressed in the PA myocytes and often under the control of hypoxic responsive promoters, they showed that these animals lacked acute HPV, and that SMCs from the precapillary arteries did not exhibit typical hypoxia induced increases in superoxide production and cytosolic Ca^{++}, or cellular membrane depolarization. They further demonstrated that the Cox4i2 subunit mediates hyperpolarization of the mitochondrial membrane potential ($\Delta\Psi_m$) in response to hypoxia, and that this hyperpolarization of $\Delta\Psi_m$ triggers the observed increase in ROS production at complex III, as has been described previously (35, 36). In a complimentary approach, they introduced expression of an alternative oxidase (AOX) from *Ciona intestinal*is into lung tissue. This enzyme accepts electrons from reduced ubiquinol (generated by complexes I and II) and directly reduces O_2 to H_2O, creating a branch in the ETC and allowing bypass of electrons through the downstream complexes III and IV. This branch pathway prevented hypoxic mitochondrial membrane hyperpolarization, ROS production, and HPV. Interestingly, this data showed somewhat higher (though still reduced) O_2 consumption in these cells and overall more oxidized NAD^+/$NADH$ under hypoxia, suggesting ongoing engagement of complex I (and AOX) when not limited downstream by complex III/IV (37).

ATP and energetic intermediates

The work by Sommer et al. suggests a mechanism in which hypoxic inhibition of the distal ETC stalls respiration and results in proximal electron accumulation, provoking $\Delta\Psi_m$ hyperpolarization and increased ROS production. It is possible that other, indirect, energetic shifts may also contribute to the observed hyperpolarization of $\Delta\Psi_m$ as they note. There have also been several studies suggesting baseline differences in ATP production via oxidative metabolism between pulmonary compared to systemic arterial myocytes (28, 38). Previous groups have described that during acute hypoxia, both PA and systemic myocytes exhibit an overall decrease in mitochondrial O_2 consumption, which coincides with the onset of HPV in the PAs (38). This is associated with reduction of cytochromes within the ETC complexes (38) and accumulation of reduced forms of the cofactors NADPH and NADH relative to their oxidized counterparts (39). Interestingly, even in the face of prolonged and relatively severe hypoxia, PA myocytes maintain steady ATP levels. ATP is often buffered through the energetic intermediate metabolite phosphocreatinine (PCr), which exhibits transient, but inconsistent, decreases in the face of hypoxia in the PA myocytes. However, the PA smooth muscle is notably better at maintaining hypoxic PCr levels than systemic arterial smooth muscle (40). It is uncertain precisely how the PA myocytes adapt in this regard, though work on urinary tract smooth muscle suggests a relatively high baseline contribution of glycolysis to total ATP production (~30%), that can be significantly increased in the setting of hypoxia (41). This maintenance of persistent high levels of ATP as well as an intact Pi/ATP ratio has largely argued against a role for ATP-mediated activation of AMP-activated protein kinase (AMPK). However, there is some evidence to suggest that AMPK may augment the HPV response through separate means of activation such as ROS and Ca^{++}-dependent phosphorylation (42, 43).

Other sources of ROS and antioxidant mechanisms in PA myocytes

"Reactive oxygen species" describes a group of both free radical, and non-radical, oxygen-containing species that have one or more unpaired electrons in their outer orbital layer, making them highly reactive with other biomolecules. Given this reactivity, they can be injurious to cells at high concentrations, but at low concentrations serve important cellular signaling functions. The primary ROS involved in these signaling activities are superoxide ($O_2^{\cdot-}$) and hydrogen peroxide (H_2O_2). $O_2^{\cdot-}$ is limited to intracellular signaling by a short diffusion distance and an inability to traverse lipid membranes freely. It can alter enzyme activity through interactions with iron–sulfur centers or various (often heme-containing) co-factors. $O_2^{\cdot-}$ is dismutated spontaneously or enzymatically to the more stable H_2O_2, which can diffuse farther and easily pass through lipid membranes. Furthermore, H_2O_2 has broader capacity to alter enzymatic function through oxidation of cysteine thiol groups, rendering the oxidized sulfur-containing groups more reactive and prone to formation of disulfide bridges (43–46).

The **NAD(P)H Oxidases (NOXs)** are a family of membrane-bound, multimeric oxidases that generate $O_2^{\cdot-}$ through reduction of molecular O_2 using NADH or NADPH as a co-factor. NOX2 is the prototypical form initially described in phagocytes and associated with oxidative destruction of pathogens, but additional isoforms are present in various tissue distributions, including within the pulmonary vasculature and PASMCs. ROS arising from differing NOX isoforms have been implicated in both HPV and the response to more sustained hypoxia. In chronic hypoxic conditions, NOX2 has been shown to contribute to increased ROS generation, endothelial dysfunction, and development of hypoxic pulmonary hypertension (47, 48). However NOX2 does not seem to be necessary for HPV in a mouse knockout model (49). NOX4 is one of the predominant isoforms expressed in the pulmonary vasculature, and its expression is inducible in response to various stressors, particularly hypoxia. It has been shown to contribute to increased production of ROS in response to hypoxia, and to promote increased PASMC proliferation. Early studies also suggested that pharmacologic blockade of NOX4 activity attenuated HPV (43, 50). However, recent work using mouse knockout models of NOX4 suggested no effect on the response to either acute HPV or sustained hypoxia (50).

There are three members of the **superoxide dismutase** (SOD) family which are characterized by distinct cellular localizations and catalytic metal ions. Two of the family members utilize Cu/Zn, and are localized to the cytosol (SOD1) or exported to the extracellular space (SOD3), respectively. SOD2 uses a Mn ion and is localized to the mitochondrial space. These enzymes convert 2 $O_2^{\cdot-}$ radicals into H_2O_2 and molecular O_2, and all three are expressed in lung tissue. The expression and activity of this family of enzymes are often altered in hypoxic and other models of pulmonary vascular disease, and experimental manipulation has revealed them to play important roles in attenuating oxidative vascular stress and vascular remodeling in various pathologic conditions (44, 51).

Glutathione peroxidases (Gpxs) are selenium-containing proteins that catalyze the conversion of H_2O_2 to water, using reduced glutathione (GSH) as a cofactor. There are 8 distinct isoforms, of which Gpx1 plays an important role in decomposing H_2O_2 generated by the mitochondria and Gpx4 has a unique role in reducing lipid hydroperoxides and preventing toxic accumulation of lipid ROS. **Catalase** is an Fe-containing enzyme that similarly decomposes H_2O_2 to water and unlike Gpx, does not require a reducing cofactor or system for regeneration, but is largely confined to the peroxisomes (44, 51).

Peroxiredoxins (Prxs) are a family of highly abundant thiol peroxidases that scavenge cellular peroxides via a cysteine active site that is oxidized by the catalytic activity of the enzyme. There are 6 family members in humans that are characterized by differing subcellular locations in the cytosol (Prx 1,2,5,6), mitochondria (Prx 3,5), and ER (Prx 4). In order to regenerate their catalytic activity, oxidized Prxs are dependent on other dithiols and reductases, particularly the thioredoxin/thioredoxin reductase/NADPH system, and GSH (52). Notably, Prxs are shown to participate in highly regulated signaling relays of H_2O_2 to redox-sensitive proteins. Given their high reactivity with H_2O_2, they are easily oxidized at low concentrations, and then interact with, and pass on this oxidative state to specific target proteins via formation of disulfide bonds. At least some of these protein targets may be simultaneously resistant to nonspecific oxidation, even at relatively high concentrations of H_2O_2 (51, 53). These relays provide fascinating insight into how low concentrations of regionally restricted ROS can enact redox modifications of selective targets without more generalized and widespread protein oxidation (46).

Chronic hypoxia and the effects of sustained mitochondrial hypoxic signaling

Hypoxia that is sustained will eventually lead to vascular adaptations that are not acutely reversible, and ultimately, pathologic pulmonary vascular remodeling. This has long been recognized in humans and other animals ascending to high altitudes, who develop elevated pulmonary artery pressure (PAP) that, after as little as 36 hours, cannot be completely normalized by O_2 administration or other inhibitors of HPV (3). Similarly, prolonged exposure to altitude results in the occurrence of high altitude pulmonary hypertension (PH) and associated vascular remodeling amongst resident populations (54). Animal models routinely employ chronic hypoxia or states of pseudo-hypoxia as methods of provoking PH. Although the transition from acute HPV to chronic vascular adaptation remains incompletely understood, it is well established that the response to chronic hypoxia is heavily mediated by oxygen responsive transcription factors, of which, the hypoxia inducible factors (HIFs) are the archetypal and most important examples.

The HIFs are hetero-dimeric transcription factors composed of a stable beta subunit (ARNT/HIF-β), and a constitutively transcribed and translated alpha subunit (HIF-α) that is rapidly targeted and degraded at normal O_2 tensions. This canonical regulation via coordinated destruction is mediated by hydroxylation of proline residues in the HIF-α subunit, which allows binding of the von Hippel-Lindau (VHL) protein and recruitment of the E3 ubiquitin ligase complex that ubiquinates the HIF-α subunits, targeting them for proteasomal degradation. The initial hydroxylation reaction is mediated by the prolyl-hydroxylases (PHDs), a family of α-ketoglutarate dependent dioxygenases with an Fe-containing catalytic site. In hypoxic conditions, the hydroxylation activity of the PHDs is inhibited, allowing hypoxic accumulation of HIF-α subunits, which are able to then dimerize with HIF-β to broadly regulate transcription. It is important to note that beyond this canonical mechanism, additional factors including ascorbate, Fe, and the metabolites α-ketoglutarate and succinate are also shown to regulate HIF activity, as do other post-translational modifications (55, 56).

Given that molecular O_2 is a required substrate for PHD-mediated hydroxylation, early models theorized that hypoxic substrate limitation directly slowed the enzymatic reaction allowing HIF-α accumulation. However, evidence soon revealed that cells lacking functional mitochondria did not exhibit hypoxic HIF stabilization (57). Careful work performed with pharmacologic inhibitors and genetic knockout strategies targeting the ETC have subsequently confirmed an essential role of mitochondrial ROS in the regulation of PHD and HIF activity. This regulation is not completely understood, though a recently proposed mechanism suggests that oxidative stress results in homo-dimerization of PHD2 via disulfide bridge formation, inhibiting hydroxylase activity (58). As with the literature relating to HPV, controversy persists as to whether mitochondrial ROS are increased or decreased in response to hypoxia (56, 59). However, elegant work by Martinez-Reyes et al. in this field creates a fascinating parallel to the work of Sommer et al. discussed in the previous section. Through depletion of mitochondrial DNA, they eliminated ETC function and aerobic respiration, but were able to restore a mitochondrial membrane potential ($\Delta\Psi_m$) through genetic knockout of the F0F1-ATPase inhibitor ATPIF1. This allows the F1 component of the ATPase to pump H^+ in a retrograde fashion across the inner mitochondrial membrane, consuming glycolytic ATP in the process. In this manner, the cells are able to establish a $\Delta\Psi_m$, despite the lack of a functional ETC or tricarboxylic acid (TCA) cycle. They then demonstrated that the presence of $\Delta\Psi_m$, even in the apparent absence of mitochondrial respiration, was able to restore mitochondrial ROS production and hypoxic HIF stabilization (60).

The importance of HIF signaling in the development of hypoxic PH is illustrated by the rare disorder Chuvash syndrome (or Chuvash polycythemia) that is characterized by enhanced HPV, polycythemia, and the development of PH. This syndrome arises from homozygous mutations in the VHL gene, impairing its ability to interact with the hydroxylated HIF-1α and HIF-2α subunits. Despite a normoxic environment, these patients develop an analog of hypoxic PH due to inappropriate HIF signaling (59). This phenotype can be replicated through forced HIF expression in animal models, while animals with heterozygous HIF-1α or HIF-2α deletion exhibit limited pulmonary vascular remodeling and attenuated development of PH when exposed to chronic hypoxia. Additional insight has emerged using molecular techniques that allow for the genetic manipulation of HIF levels in specific cell lines. HIF-1α is shown to be of particular importance in the myocytes, where it promotes distal migration and expansion of PASMCs, increased muscularization of the arterial wall, and elevations in right ventricular pressure in response to chronic hypoxia (54). Notable alterations in myocyte biology that have been implicated in the HIF-mediated development of hypoxic PH include increased cytosolic Ca^{++} via regulation of TRPC cation channels, increased expression of the Na^+/H^+ exchanger (NHE) ion channel, leading to elevated cytosolic pH, and alterations of cellular metabolism promoting increased glycolytic activity and repressed mitochondrial respiration (54, 59, 61). HIF-2α, which is predominantly expressed in the endothelium, promotes chronic hypoxic PH through various mechanisms including increased expression of Endothelin-1 (ET1), a potent vasoconstrictor and PASMC mitogen, along with other factors that exert growth effects on the PASMCs such as CXCL12. HIF-2α is further implicated in the regulation of Nitric Oxide production via its transcriptional targeting of Arginase-1, and the regulation of endothelial to mesenchymal transition (54, 61). It must be emphasized that HIF-1α and HIF-2α are exceptionally broad transcriptional regulators with wide-reaching effects on cellular behavior, growth, and metabolism. They are heavily implicated in varied etiologies of PH, and the pathways highlighted above represent an extremely truncated overview of their many important targets and interactions, the full extent of which are beyond the limited scope of this chapter.

References

1. Dunham-Snary KJ, et al. Pflugers Arch. 2016; 468(1):43–58
2. Leach RM, et al. Am J Physiol Lung Cell Mol Physiol. 1994; 266(3 Pt 1):L223–L231.
3. Sylvester JT, et al. Physiol Rev. 2012; 92(1):367–520.
4. Holzgraefe B, et al. Acta Anaesthesiol Scand. 2020; 64(7):992–1001.
5. Swenson ER. High Alt Med Biol. 2013; 14(2):101–110.
6. Dorrington KL, et al. Am J Physiol Heart Circ Physiol. 1997; 273(3 Pt 2):H1126–H1134.
7. Talbot NP, et al. J Appl Physiol. 2005; 98(3):1125–1139.
8. Post JM, et al. Am J Physiol 1992; 262(4 Pt 1):C882–C890
9. Yuan XJ, et al. Am J Physiol Lung Cell Mol Physiol. 1993; 264(2 Pt 1):L116–L123.
10. Archer SL, et al. Circ Res. 2004; 95(3):308–318.
11. Archer SL, et al. FASEB J. 2001; 15(10):1801–1803.
12. Olschewski A, et al. Circ Res. 2006; 98(8):1072–1080.
13. Murtaza G, et al. PLoS One. 2017; 12(3):e0174071.
14. Mittal M, et al. Free Radic Biol Med. 2012; 52(6):1033–1042.
15. Cogolludo A, et al. Int J Mol Sci. 2019; 20(2):411.
16. Cogolludo A, et al. Ann N Y Acad Sci. 2006; 1091:41–51.
17. McMurtry IF, et al. Circ Res. 1976; 38(2):99–104.
18. Robertson TP, et al. J Physiol. 2000; 525(3):669–680.
19. Wang J, et al. Am J Physiol Lung Cell Mol Physiol. 2012; 303(2):L161–L168.
20. Liao B, et al. Antioxidants Redox Signal. 2011; 14(1):37–47.
21. González-Pacheco FR, et al. Nephrol Dial Transplant. 2002; 17(3):392–398.
22. Reyes RV, et al. Front Physiol. 2018; 9:486.
23. Fuchs B, et al. Respir Res. 2011; 12(1):20.
24. Archer SL, et al. J Appl Physiol. 1989; 67(5):1903–1911.
25. Archer SL, et al. Circ Res. 1993; 73(6):1100–1112.
26. Burke TM, et al. Am J Physiol Heart Circ Physiol. 1987; 252(4 Pt 2):H721–H732
27. Reeve HL, et al. Exp Physiol. 1995; 80(5):825–834
28. Dunham-Snary KJ, et al. Circ Res. 2019; 124(12):1727–1746.
29. Chandel NS, et al. Proc Natl Acad Sci USA. 1998; 95(20):11715–11720
30. Chandel NS, et al. J Biol Chem. 2000; 275(33):25130–25138.
31. Waypa GB, et al. Am J Respir Crit Care Med. 2013; 187(4):424–432.
32. Smith KA, et al. J Physiol. 2019; 597(4):1033–1043.
33. Waypa GB, et al. Circ Res. 2006; 99(9):970–978.
34. Sabharwal S, et al. Biochem J. 2013; 456(3):337–346.
35. Bleier L, et al. Biochim Biophys Acta. 2013; 1827(11-12):1320–1331.
36. Sommer N, et al. Circ Res. 2017; 121(4):424–438.
37. Sommer N, et al. Sci Adv. 2020; 6(16):eaba0694.
38. Sommer N, et al. Eur Respir J. 2010; 36(5):1056–1066.
39. Leach RM, et al. J Physiol. 2001; 536(1):211–224.
40. Leach RM, et al. Am J Physiol Lung Cell Mol Physiol. 2000; 278(2):L294–L304.
41. Wendt IR. Am J Physiol Cell Physiol. 1989; 256(4 Pt 1):C719–C727.
42. Moral-Sanz J, et al. Sci Signal. 2018; 11(550):eaau0296.
43. Siques P, et al. Front Physiol. 2018; 9:865.
44. Aggarwal S, et al. Compr Physiol. 2013; 3(3):1011–1034.
45. Liemburg-Apers DC, et al. Arch Toxicol. 2015; 89(8):1209–1226.
46. Smith KA, et al. Redox Biol. 2017; 13:228–234.
47. Aggarwal S, et al. Trends Cardiovasc Med. 2010; 20(7):238–246.
48. Fresquet F, et al. Br J Pharmacol. 2006; 148(5):714–723.
49. Archer SL, et al. Proc Natl Acad Sci USA. 1999; 96(14):7944–7949.
50. Veith C, et al. Pulm Circ. 2016; 6(3):397–400.
51. Hopkins BL, et al. Redox Biol. 2019; 21:101104.
52. Cox AG, et al. Biochem J. 2010; 425(2):313–325.
53. Elko EA, et al. Antioxidants Redox Signal. 2019; 31(14):1070–1091.
54. Young JM, et al. Front Med (Lausanne). 2019; 6:93.
55. Samanta D, et al. Redox Biol. 2017; 13:331–335.
56. McElroy GS, et al. Exp Cell Res. 2017; 356(2):217–222.
57. Pan Y, et al. Mol Cell Biol. 2007; 27(3):912–925.
58. Lee G, et al. Sci Rep. 2016; 6:18928.
59. Dasgupta A, et al. Compr Physiol. 2020; 10(2):713–765
60. Martínez-Reyes I, et al. Mol Cell. 2016; 61(2):199–209.
61. Urrutia AA, et al. Biomedicines. 2018; 6(2):68.

REACTIVE OXYGEN SPECIES SIGNALING IN ANIMAL MODELS OF PULMONARY HYPERTENSION

Stephen Wedgwood, Satyan Lakshminrusimha and Robin H. Steinhorn

Contents

Introduction

Pulmonary hypertension (PH) is often due to an increase in pulmonary vascular resistance (PVR) typically associated with muscularization and fibrosis of the pulmonary arterioles, decreased pulmonary blood flow and right ventricular hypertrophy (RVH). Abnormal signaling pathways triggered by elevated reactive oxygen species (ROS) during the perinatal and postnatal periods play a substantive role in the development of PH in several animal models. ROS levels become elevated when ROS-generating enzyme systems are activated and/or when ROS scavengers are inactivated. General antioxidant therapy has been largely unsuccessful, perhaps because low-level ROS signaling is essential for normal cell function. Identifying specific components of pathways triggered by ROS to induce a specific disease may reveal more attractive targets for therapy. This chapter will discuss the mechanisms by which ROS are elevated, the subsequent target molecules, and the consequences of abnormal signaling in several models of pulmonary hypertension.

Persistent pulmonary hypertension of the newborn

Neonatal pulmonary vascular disease

At birth, complex biochemical processes regulate a dramatic decrease in PVR resulting in an 8–10-fold increase in pulmonary blood flow (1). Figure 18.1A illustrates the signaling pathways leading to pulmonary vasodilation. When the pulmonary circulation fails to adapt to postnatal life, the result is persistent pulmonary hypertension of the newborn (PPHN). PPHN is characterized by right-to-left or bidirectional extrapulmonary shunting of deoxygenated blood that produces a variable degree of hypoxemia (2). Animal models of PPHN have proved invaluable in identifying the underlying biochemical pathways that mediate the fetal-to-newborn transition and are discussed in Chapter 13. In fetal lambs, ligation, mechanical compression, or pharmacological constriction of the ductus arteriosus produces fetal and neonatal PH (3–6). Similar to pathological findings observed in newborns that die of PPHN, these lambs exhibit hypoxemia, right ventricular failure, and pulmonary vascular remodeling.

ROS and PPHN

The most severe cases of PPHN appear to have their origins in fetal stressors that induce pulmonary vascular remodeling (Figure 18.1B). Increased levels of the ROS superoxide have been found in the endothelium and vascular smooth muscle of pulmonary arteries from fetal lambs within days after antenatal ligation of the ductus arteriosus (PPHN lambs) (7, 8), and there is in vitro and *in vivo* evidence that these ROS cause significant vasoconstriction under hypoxic conditions (9). Superoxide reacts rapidly with the pulmonary vasodilator NO to form peroxynitrite ($ONOO^-$), a potent vasoconstrictor of the neonatal pulmonary vasculature (10). Multiple enzyme systems are potentially involved in ROS generation in PPHN including NADPH oxidases (Nox), membrane proteins that produce superoxide by transferring electrons from NADPH to molecular oxygen. Nox subunits p22^{phox} and p67^{phox} are elevated in pulmonary arteries isolated from fetal PPHN lambs (8, 11). Peroxynitrite inhibits NOS activity via mechanisms that include decreased association with the chaperone protein HSP90, and in turn, uncoupled eNOS further reduces NO and elevates superoxide levels in PPHN lambs (12). Superoxide levels are additionally regulated by the activities of superoxide scavengers including the superoxide dismutases (SODs). SOD activity is decreased in PPHN pulmonary arteries (8), potentially via decreased extracellular SOD (13) and mitochondrial MnSOD (14) activities.

The potent, longer-acting ROS hydrogen peroxide (H_2O_2) is elevated in PPHN pulmonary arteries (15). This may be due to

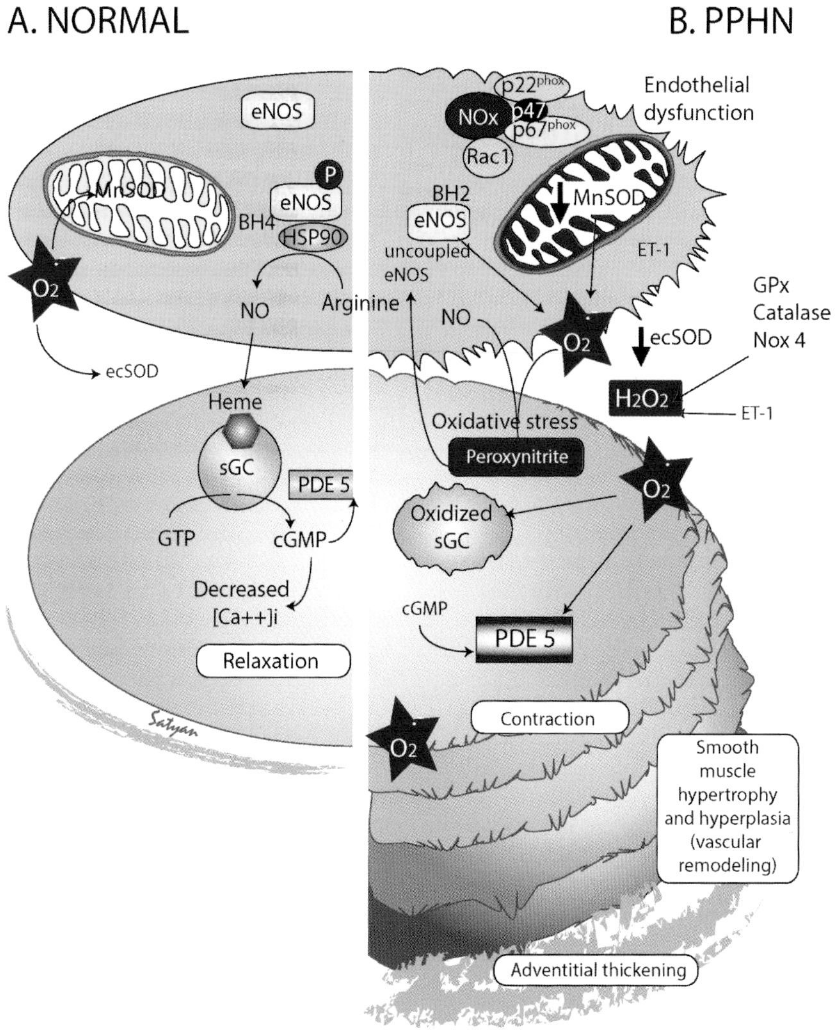

A. NORMAL

B. PPHN

FIGURE 18.1 Biochemical pathways involved in pulmonary vasodilation in normal patients and the dysfunctional pathways in patients with PPHN. Please refer to the text for the definitions of abbreviations.

increased activity of Nox4 (11), a Nox isoform that generates H_2O_2 instead of superoxide. High levels of endothelin-1 (ET-1) can stimulate H_2O_2 production (16). Furthermore, catalase and glutathione peroxidase activities are unchanged in PPHN pulmonary arteries (15) suggesting that increased H_2O_2 production and not scavenging is involved.

ROS and NO signaling in PPHN

Treating PPHN lambs postnatally with antioxidants has revealed that ROS impair multiple molecules in the NO-mediated pulmonary vasorelaxation pathway illustrated in Figure 18.1. First, the rapid reaction between NO and superoxide decreases bioavailable NO. PPHN lambs develop life-threatening hypoxemia after birth, even with ventilation with oxygen. Administration of a single dose of recombinant human SOD (rhSOD) to PPHN lambs followed by ventilation with 100% oxygen for 24 h improves oxygenation (17), decreases ROS (superoxide, H_2O_2, and peroxynitrite), and improves eNOS function by restoring levels of tetrahdrobiopterin (BH_4), a critical cofactor for eNOS that also prevents uncoupling (18). Other studies indicate that PDE5 activity is elevated in fetal and ventilated PPHN lambs, and rhSOD restores normal

levels of PDE5 activity and cGMP after birth and ventilation (19). Similarly, a single dose of intratracheal PEG-catalase improves oxygenation and increases ecSOD activity in ventilated PPHN lambs (13) and normalizes PDE5 activity and cGMP levels in their pulmonary arteries (19). PPHN lambs given a single intratracheal dose of the Nox inhibitor apocynin have improved oxygenation, decreased ROS, and decreased expression of several Nox subunits (20). Taken together, these studies highlight the roles of ROS in the pathogenesis of PPHN and suggest that general and specific antioxidant therapy may be beneficial to treat the hypoxemia and vascular dysfunction in newborn infants with PPHN.

Studies with clinically relevant steroids have also given promising results in ventilated PPHN lambs. Antenatal betamethasone improves the relaxation of pulmonary arteries to NO donors, decreases ROS, increases cGMP levels and MnSOD protein, and improves eNOS function in PPHN lambs (7). Postnatal hydrocortisone treatment improves oxygenation, decreases ROS, decreases PDE5 activity, increases cGMP levels, and increases SOD activity. Figure 18.1 illustrates the molecular pathways involved in vasorelaxation in healthy patients and the dysfunction characteristic of PPHN.

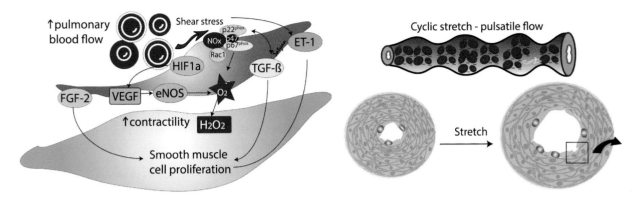

FIGURE 18.2 Molecules impacted by increased pulmonary blood flow leading to smooth muscle contraction and proliferation. Please refer to the text for the definitions of abbreviations.

In vitro studies

The animal studies discussed above have been complemented by in vitro studies to investigate further the underlying mechanisms of PPHN. Relaxation of pulmonary artery rings isolated from PPHN lambs is improved by pretreatment with rhSOD (8) and catalase (15) prior to exposure to NO donors. Smooth muscle cells exposed to cyclic stretch to mimic the sustained elevation in pulmonary pressure in PPHN display elevated ROS (21). Furthermore, Nox4 is a major source of this stretch-induced ROS (21), highlighting the importance of this enzyme in the development of PPHN. Stretch also increases the expression and activity of hypoxia inducible factor-1α (HIF-1α) via ROS generated from mitochondrial complex III thereby mimicking the increased HIF-1α detected in PPHN lungs (22). Similarly, the cell cycle regulatory cyclinD1 is elevated in PPHN lungs (11), and stretch increases cyclin D1 expression in PASMC in a Nox4- and mitochondrial complex III-dependent fashion (21). Multiple studies have shown that ROS stimulate smooth muscle proliferation suggesting a role for this pathway in the pulmonary vascular remodeling manifest in PPHN. The potent pulmonary vasoconstrictor ET-1 is elevated in PPHN lambs, and ET-1 stimulates ROS production and the proliferation of PASMC isolated from fetal lambs (23). Several antioxidants attenuate growth factor-induced PASMC proliferation (24). Furthermore, studies on pulmonary artery endothelial cells (PAEC) isolated from PPHN lambs reveal a decrease in MnSOD activity, which contributes to elevated ROS (14). ET-1 impairs angiogenesis of PPHN PAEC via activation of Rho-kinase (25) while other studies indicate a role for HIF-1α (26). The role of ROS in impaired angiogenesis of PPHN PAEC is currently unknown, but the interactions between ET-1, ROS, and HIF-1α in PASMC suggest that a central role is likely.

Increased pulmonary blood flow

Pulmonary hypertension secondary to congenital heart disease

PH is a common complication of congenital heart disease with increased pulmonary blood flow. An accurate and reliable model of a large aortopulmonary shunt was established in the late gestation fetal lamb by placing a graft between the ascending aorta and the main pulmonary artery (27). After spontaneous delivery, these lambs go on to develop morphological and physiological features that mimic the human disease. By one month of age, the shunt lambs have increased pulmonary blood flow, elevated pulmonary

artery pressure, and impaired endothelium-dependent vasodilation of intact and isolated pulmonary arteries (27).

ROS and increased pulmonary blood flow

At 4 and 8 weeks of life, shunt lambs exhibit increased superoxide, but not H_2O_2, in the pulmonary arteries (28). This is associated with multiple disruptions in superoxide generation, including increased lung expression of the Nox subunits Rac1 and p47[phox], eNOS uncoupling including a low BH_4/BH_2 ratio (28) and reduced levels of the eNOS substrate L-arginine (29), and increased xanthine oxidase (30). In addition, activity of the mitochondrial superoxide scavenger MnSOD was higher in shunt lungs relative to control lambs (31). H_2O_2 levels are increased in shunt lambs at two weeks of age correlating with reduced catalase expression, but catalase and H_2O_2 levels return to normal control levels at 4 weeks (31). These data indicate that different etiologies of PH have common (e.g. increased superoxide levels, uncoupled eNOS) and distinct (e.g. H_2O_2 levels, specific Nox subunits, endogenous antioxidant activities) underlying mechanisms.

ROS signaling with increased pulmonary blood flow

PASMC isolated from shunt lambs are hyperproliferative and exhibit elevated Nox activity (32). TGF-β levels are elevated in shunt lambs and treating fetal ovine PAEC with TGF-β increases in expression of the Nox subunits p47[phox], p67[phox], and Rac1 (33). These increases may be involved in impaired eNOS function and disrupted mitochondrial bioenergetics characteristic of cells from shunt lambs. L-arginine increases NO production and decreases ROS levels in shunt lambs, highlighting the central role of uncoupled eNOS in PH in this model (29).

Underlying pathways have been elucidated in vitro by exposing isolated pulmonary vascular cells to the biomechanical forces that pulmonary arteries are exposed to as a result of increased pulmonary blood flow. Vessels are exposed to cyclic stretch due to increased pulsatile pulmonary blood flow, and the stretch-induced increase in ROS and HIF-1α outlined in section 1D may also contribute to vascular remodeling in shunt lambs (Figure 18.2). Cyclic stretch increases ROS in lamb PASMC via Nox and TGF-β (34), while TGF-β-induced proliferation of human PASMC is dependent on Nox4-derived ROS (35). The PASMC mitogen fibroblast growth factor-2 (FGF-2) is elevated in shunt lungs (36), and stretch increases FGF-2 expression in lamb PASMC via a pathway involving Nox and HIF-1α (37). Stretch also increases FGF-2 (36) and ET-1 (38) expression in PAEC. Endothelial cells in shunt pulmonary arteries are exposed to shear stress as a result of increased pulmonary blood flow. PAEC exposed to shear stress display elevated ROS and ET-1 expression (38) and increased FGF-2 expression (36). Together these data suggest that biomechanical forces including stretch and shear contribute to pulmonary vascular remodeling in shunt lambs via positive feedback mechanisms that increase ROS levels and growth factor expression. Figure 18.2 depicts the molecules impacted by biomechanical forces resulting from increased blood flow.

Hyperoxia

PH and prematurity

Normally, the fetus thrives *in utero* under hypoxic conditions that favor lung growth. However, because the preterm lung is meant to grow in a low-oxygen intrauterine environment, it is also ill-equipped to handle oxygen administration. Preterm birth exposes the lung to relative hyperoxia at a critical developmental juncture, an event that can disrupt normal parenchymal and vascular lung development (39). The incidence of PH among extremely premature infants is as high as 18% and increases to 25–40% among premature infants with bronchopulmonary dysplasia (BPD), the chronic lung disease of prematurity that is characterized by arrested development resulting in alveolar simplification (40, 41). Although BPD is triggered by multiple factors, elevated ROS is one of the major contributors. Elevated ROS can occur prenatally due to placental insufficiency or postnatally due to oxygen exposure and pulmonary and systemic inflammatory responses (42).

Hyperoxia-induced PH in rodents

Mice and rats are born in a saccular stage of lung development equivalent to a very preterm infant and do not begin alveolarization until postnatal day 5. Neonatal rodents exposed to hyperoxia (75–95% O_2) for 14 days develop PH, RVH, pulmonary vascular remodeling, and alveolar simplification characteristic of preterm infants with BPD (43). Hypoxia-inducible factors (HIFs) are transcription factors that regulate the expression of key proteins involved in normal fetal lung vascular and parenchymal development, and exposure to oxygen triggers a pathway leading to HIF protein degradation. Targets of HIFs include vascular endothelial growth factor (VEGF) and VEGF receptor type-2 (VEGFR2), and decreases in these proteins have been reported in various animal models of BPD induced by hyperoxia (44–46), as well as in the lungs of premature infants who die with BPD (47, 48). Rodent models of PH have the added advantage of genetic manipulation to interrogate the underlying mechanisms. Hyperoxia exposure results in elevated ROS and lung injury, which are reduced in adult mice lacking the NADPH oxidase subunit Nox1, but not in mice lacking Nox2 (49). Similarly, mice lacking the Nox isoform Duox2 have reduced lung injury following oxygen exposure (50). ROS levels are also determined by antioxidant capacity. Neonatal mice treated with the mitochondrial-specific antioxidant, mito-TEMPO, are protected against impaired alveolarization and RVH (51), suggesting that mitochondrial ROS are involved in BPD pathogenesis. However, neonatal mice heterozygous for the mitochondrial antioxidant, MnSOD, do not exhibit worsened hallmarks of PH and BPD in response to hyperoxia (52), highlighting the complexity of the antioxidant systems. Lung 3-nitrotyrosine (3-NT) levels, which reflect the interaction of NO and superoxide to form peroxynitrite, are elevated in rats exposed to 75% O_2 (53). A peroxynitrite decomposition catalyst improves alveolarization, attenuates vascular remodeling, and elevates lung VEGF and VEGFR2 proteins in rats exposed to 60% O_2 (54). Metabolomics analyses of lungs and plasma from rats exposed to hyperoxia provide evidence of altered xanthine oxidase activity (55) suggesting that superoxide generators in addition to Nox are also involved in hyperoxia-induced PH and lung injury. It appears that oxygen-mediated HIF protein degradation outcompetes ROS-mediated HIF protein stabilization in this model.

In vitro studies

Studies exposing isolated pulmonary artery smooth muscle cells (PASMCs) to hyperoxia have identified potential mechanisms of oxygen-induced PH and BPD. Brief exposure to 95% O_2 increases ROS in the mitochondrial matrix, while sustained exposure increases ROS in the cytosol and elevates PDE5 activity (55). These increases are attenuated when the H_2O_2 scavenger catalase is expressed in the mitochondrial matrix, suggesting that hyperoxia initially stimulates mitochondrial superoxide production. Superoxide is converted by MnSOD to hydrogen peroxide, which can cross the mitochondrial membranes and influence the activities of proteins including PDE5. This may explain why loss of a copy of MnSOD does not attenuate hyperoxia-induced PH and BPD while superoxide scavenging does (above).

Hypoxia-induced PH in rodents

Chronic hypoxia induces pulmonary vascular remodeling in several immature animal models. This section will focus on hypoxia-induced PH to highlight similarities with other models described above. Superoxide levels are higher in pulmonary arteries from adult mice exposed to chronic hypoxia in a hypobaric chamber for 3 weeks (56). Potential sources include Nox, xanthine oxidase, and mitochondria. Mice lacking Nox2 have blunted PH and pulmonary vascular remodeling following hypoxic exposure (57). Elevated ROS can contribute to hypoxia-induced PH and remodeling by mechanisms outlined in Section "Introduction." In neonatal rats, xanthine oxidase inhibition attenuates hypoxia-induced vascular remodeling and improves endothelium-dependent pulmonary artery relaxation (58), suggesting that superoxide derived from xanthine oxidase contributes to PH in this model. SODs also regulate superoxide levels, and mice lacking ecSOD expression in smooth muscle have worsened hypoxia-induced PH and vascular remodeling (59). The role of mitochondria in oxygen sensing and signaling is controversial and is discussed in Chapter 16. Studies indicate that ROS derived from mitochondrial complex III stabilize HIF-1α and HIF-1α in response to hypoxia (60). Mice lacking smooth muscle expression of HIF-1α have attenuated PH and vascular remodeling, but still have RVH following exposure to hypoxia (61). The authors hypothesized that expression of HIF-1α in the right ventricle contributes to hypoxia-induced RVH independent of PA pressure (61). PH and vascular remodeling increase in severity when hypoxia is combined with the VEGF receptor antagonist SU5416 in rodents (62). This suggests that the decreases in VEGFR2 in neonatal rats exposed to hyperoxia or to postnatal malnutrition contributes to PH.

Summary

This review has discussed the similarities in several diverse animal models of PH. There is a central role for ROS, with Nox being a common source. ROS are ubiquitous signaling molecules, which may explain why overall, antioxidant therapy has been unsuccessful in treating PH. A common target of ROS signaling are the HIFs, and it appears that elevated HIF signaling (increased growth factor expression and pulmonary vascular remodeling) as well as decreased HIF signaling (impaired alveolar and pulmonary vascular development during hyperoxia) contribute to PH.

References

1. Dawes GS, et al. J Physiol. 1953; 121:141–162.
2. Steinhorn RH. Pediatr Crit Care Med. 2010; 11(2 Suppl):S79–S84.
3. Abman SH, et al. J Clin Invest. 1989; 83(6):1849–1858.
4. Black SM, et al. Pediatr Res. 1998; 44:821–830.
5. Morin FC. Pediatr Res. 1989; 25(3):245–250.
6. Wild LM, et al. Pediatr Res. 1989; 25(3):251–257.
7. Chandrasekar I, et al. Pediatr Res. 2008; 63(1):67–72.
8. Konduri G, et al. Pediatr Res. 2009; 66:289-294
9. Fike CD, et al. Pediatr Res. 2011; 70(2):136–141.
10. Belik J, et al. Free Radic Biol Med. 2004; 37:1384–1392.
11. Wedgwood S, et al. Antioxid Redox Signal. 2013; 18:1765–1776.
12. Konduri G, et al. Am J Physiol Heart Circ Physiol. 2007; 292:H1812–H1820.
13. Wedgwood S, et al. Antioxid Redox Signal. 2011; 15:1497–1506.
14. Afolayan AJ, et al. Am J Physiol Lung Cell Mol Physiol. 2012; 303(10):L870–L879.
15. Wedgwood S, et al. Am J Physiol Lung Cell Mol Physiol. 2005; 289(4):L660–L666.
16. Wedgwood S, et al. Am J Physiol Lung Cell Mol Physiol. 2005; 288(3):L480–L487.
17. Lakshminrusimha S, et al. Am J Respir Crit Care Med. 2006; 174:1370–1377.
18. Farrow KN, et al. Am J Physiol Lung Cell Mol Physiol. 2008; 295(6):L979–L987.
19. Farrow KN, et al. Am J Physiol Lung Cell Mol Physiol. 2010; 299:L109–L116.
20. Wedgwood S, et al. Am J Physiol Lung Cell Mol Physiol. 2012; 302:L616–L626.
21. Wedgwood S, et al. Am J Physiol Lung Cell Mol Physiol. 2015; 309(2):L196–L203.
22. Wedgwood S, et al. Front Pharmacol. 2015; 6:47.
23. Wedgwood S, et al. Am J Physiol Lung Cell Mol Physiol. 2001; 281(5):L1058–L1067.
24. Wedgwood S, et al. Antioxid Redox Signal. 2014; 21(13):1926–1942.
25. Gien J, et al. Pediatr Res. 2013 Mar; 73(3):252–262.
26. Makker K, et al. Physiol Rep. 2019 Feb; 7(3):e13986.
27. Reddy VM, et al. Circulation. 1995; 92(3):606–613.
28. Grobe A, et al. Am J Physiol Lung Cell Mol Physiol. 2006; 290:L1069–L1077.
29. Sun X, et al. Am J Respir Cell Mol Biol. 2011; 45(1):163–171.
30. Sharma S, et al. Vascul Pharmacol. 2010; 53(1-2):38–52.
31. Sharma S, et al. Am J Physiol Lung Cell Mol Physiol. 2007; 293(4):L960–L971.
32. Boehme J, et al. Am J Physiol Heart Circ Physiol. 2016; 311(4):H944–H957.
33. Sun X, et al. Redox Biol. 2020; 36:101593.
34. Mata-Greenwood E, et al. Am J Physiol Lung Cell Mol Physiol. 2005; 289:L288–L289.
35. Sturrock A, et al. Am J Physiol Lung Cell Mol Physiol. 2006; 290(4):L661–L673.
36. Wedgwood S, et al. Pediatr Res. 2007; 61:32–36.
37. Black S, et al. Am J Physiol Cell Physiol. 2008; 294:C345–C354.
38. Zhu T, et al. Pulm Circ. 2020; 10(2):2045894020922118.
39. Thebaud B, et al. Am J Respir Crit Care Med. 2007; 175(10):978–985.
40. Berkelhamer SK, et al. Semin Perinatol. 2013; 37(2):124–131.
41. Check J, et al. J Perinatol. 2013; 33(7):553–557.
42. Wang J, et al. Gene. 2018; 678:177–183.
43. Koppel R, et al. Pediatr Res. 1994; 36(6):763–770.
44. Maniscalco WM, et al. Am J Respir Cell Mol Biol. 1997; 16(5):557–567.
45. Hosford GE, et al. Am J Physiol Lung Cell Mol Physiol. 2003; 285(1):L161–L168.
46. Thebaud B, et al. Circulation. 2005; 112(16):2477–2486.
47. Bhatt AJ, et al. Am J Respir Crit Care Med. 2001; 164(10 Pt 1):1971–1980.
48. Abman SH. Adv Exp Med Biol2010; 661:323–335.
49. Carnesecchi S, et al. Am J Respir Crit Care Med. 2009; 180(10):972–981.
50. Kim MJ, et al. Antioxid Redox Signal. 2014; 21(13):1803–1818.
51. Datta A, et al. Am J Physiol Lung Cell Mol Physiol. 2015; 309(4):L369–L377.
52. Gupta A, et al. Int J Mol Sci. 2015; 16(3):6373–6390.
53. La Frano MR, et al. Metabolomics. 2017; 13:32.
54. Masood A, et al. Free Radic Biol Med. 2010 Oct; 49(7):1182–1191.
55. Farrow KN, et al. Antioxid Redox Signal. 2012; 17:460–470.
56. Fresquet F, et al. Br J Pharmacol. 2006; 148(5):714–723.
57. Liu J, et al. Am J Physiol Lung Cell Mol Physiol. 2006; 290:L2–L10.
58. Jankov R, et al. Am J Physiol Lung Cell Mol Physiol. 2008; 294:L233–L245.
59. Nozik-Grayck E, et al. Am J Physiol Lung Cell Mol Physiol. 2014; 307(11):L868–L876.
60. Guzy R, et al. Cell Metab. 2005; 1:401–408.
61. Ball MK, et al. Am J Respir Crit Care Med. 2014; 189(3):314–324.
62. Jernigan NL, et al. Adv Exp Med Biol. 2017; 967:83–103.

HYPOXIA, MYOCARDIAL METABOLIC ADAPTATION, AND RIGHT VENTRICULAR PERFORMANCE

Mark K. Friedberg

Contents

Mechanisms of hypoxia in the pulmonary hypertensive right ventricle

The high work and metabolic demand of the myocardium make it highly reliant on oxygen for energy. Even moderate hypoxia leads to a deficiency of oxygen in the myocardium. Hypoxia not only affects the right ventricle (RV) myocardium directly but also promotes pathological conditions that severely stress the RV, such as type 3 pulmonary arterial hypertension (PAH). Moreover, hypoxia and the molecular pathways it regulates affect both the pulmonary vasculature and RV myocardium through several mechanisms that impact myocardial function, inflammation, and fibrosis. Oxygen is the terminal recipient of the electron transport system, and a lack of oxygen paralyzes the cytochrome C – respiratory enzyme chain complex, creating an energy crisis (1). Reductions in oxygen delivery to the tissue can occur via low oxygen content in the blood, low oxygen-carrying capacity (e.g. anemia), or low cardiac output. At the myocardial level, RV hypoxia occurs predominantly via 2 mechanisms: (1) Reduced capillary density, often termed capillary rarefaction and (2) reduced right coronary artery perfusion pressure, for example, due to elevated RA pressures and/or decreased aortic pressures (2). These lead to RV myocardial ischemia, which is one feature of RV maladaptive physiology. Although capillary rarefaction has been found in rat models of PH, but not in pressure loading (pulmonary artery banding) (3), we recently found that capillary rarefaction occurs in both circumstances (4). This suggests that when RV pressure stress is sufficiently severe, even when secondary to mechanical pressure loading, it leads to ischemia, hypoxia, and maladaptive physiology (4).

In the pulmonary hypertensive RV, not only are there fewer coronary vessels but also coronary vascular function is impaired. Coronary endothelial dysfunction in the existing vessels further compounds myocardial ischemia, in part through endothelial adenosine monophosphate-activated protein kinase (AMPK). AMPK plays a role in the pulmonary vasculature in type 3 PAH through decreased expression of p53 and endothelial nitric oxide synthase (eNOS). In animal models of PAH secondary to metabolic left heart disease, AMPK, which is downregulated by hyperglycemia, is upregulated in the RV (5). Consequently, treatment with Metformin, in conjunction with the pulmonary vasodilator treprostinil, upregulates AMPK and ameliorates hypoxia-induced PAH, as well as improving RV contractile function (5).

RV myocardial hypoxia signaling pathways

One of the central molecular responses to hypoxia is an activation of the transcription hypoxia-inducible factor (HIF)-1α by stress-activated mitogen-activated protein kinases (MAPK). MAPK is also an important molecule in fibrosis signaling, which will be discussed below (6). HIF-1α stabilizes in hypoxic tissue, increasing its accumulation and its activity in the nucleus, thereby allowing its binding to hypoxia response elements (HRE). In the short-term, HIF-1 protects the heart from acute ischemia by increasing capillary density and by modulating glucose metabolism and calcium handling (7). However, many of the HIF-1α HRE target genes may be detrimental to RV function in the long term (8, 9). Cardiac HIF-1α stabilization is increased in patients with end-stage cardiomyopathy and in cardiac-specific HIF-1α transgenic mouse models, left ventricular (LV) pressure loading, and ageing lead to cardiac decompensation (7). The role of HIF-1α in hypoxia-induced fibrosis and inflammation, and in myocyte energy utilization in PAH, will be expanded below.

Another pathway that appears to be important to both the pulmonary vascular response and the RV myocardial response to hypoxia is the Ras homolog family member A (Rho-A) – Rho-kinase pathway. RhoA is a small guanosine triphosphate (GTP)ase that is activated by G-protein-coupled receptor ligands, leading to activated Rho kinase (ROCK) downstream. ROCK can contribute to LV heart failure and has been implicated in RV hypertrophy and dysfunction in experimental models (10). Consequently, independent of the degree of RV afterload, chronic hypoxia in neonatal rats leads to the development of RV dysfunction in association with upregulation of ROCK activity (11). Interestingly, in these experimental studies, chronic hypoxia increased RV, but not LV, RhoA, and ROCK activity (11). The role of ROCK in the hypoxic RV, independent of pulmonary vascular resistance, was partly elucidated by experiments in which inhaled ROCK inhibitors normalized pulmonary vascular resistance, with regression of RV hypertrophy, but without improvement in RV systolic dysfunction. Additionally, systemic, but not inhaled, ROCK inhibition normalized ROCK and phosphodiesterase 5 activity in the RV. These observations suggest that RhoA/ROCK activity is in part regulated by phosphodiesterase 5 activity and that pressure unloading alone does not adequately improve RV function if ROCK activity remains increased (11). Consequently, treatment

DOI: 10.1201/9780367494018-19

with the phosphodiesterase 5 inhibitor sildenafil improved RV function in these studies. These effects on the RV are particularly pertinent in hypoxia, as activation of RhoA/ROCK is also a key pathway underlying vasoconstriction and vascular remodeling in neonatal pulmonary hypertension (12). ROCK mediates smooth muscle contraction by causing calcium sensitization, and therefore may play a role during hypoxia in both the pulmonary vasculature and the myocardial coronary vasculature (13). Hence, ROCK inhibitors such as fasudil may have a vasodilator effect as well as additional direct beneficial effects on RV function (12). ROCK also regulates expression of factors that increase proliferation and inhibit apoptosis of pulmonary vascular smooth muscle cells such as platelet-derived growth factor (PDGF) and endothelin-1 (ET-1) (14, 15). These factors play a central role in regulating pulmonary vascular tone, and as will be discussed further below, are also important in RV remodelling and fibrosis that occurs in response to increased pressure-load (16, 17). However, despite the data above, while ROCK inhibitors have been shown to be effective in LV failure, their therapeutic role in RV failure needs further study (18).

Effect of hypoxia on myocardial fibrosis and inflammation

Both pulmonary hypertension, and other forms of ventricular pressure loading, can cause regional hypoxia that triggers an immune response and fibrosis. Likewise, tissue hypoxia is common in areas of inflammation (19, 20). HIF-1α promotes recruitment and migration of inflammatory cells and fibroblasts, and transverse aortic constriction in mice is associated with myocardial hypoxia and aggregation of macrophages through HIF-1α signaling (21). The HREs in HIF-1α target genes also encode several factors that are important in collagen deposition, extracellular matrix remodeling, and consequently fibrosis; these include vascular endothelial growth factor (VEGF), integrins, fibronectin, transforming growth factor (TGF)-β1, connective tissue growth factor (CTGF), PDGF, ET-1, and fibroblast growth factor (FGF)-2 (22). In monocrotaline-induced PAH in rats, caffeic acid phenethyl ester (CAPE) suppresses HIF-1α expression and PDGF production via downregulation of AKT and extracellular signal-regulated kinase (ERK) signaling (23). These effects are associated with decreased pulmonary artery smooth muscle cell proliferation and improved RV systolic performance (23). However, it is unknown whether improved RV function with CAPE treatment can occur independently of improved pulmonary vascular disease. Myocardial hypoxia also enhances fructose metabolism in human and mouse models of cardiac hypertrophy through HIF-1α activation of mutually exclusive alternative splicing of the fructose-metabolizing enzyme ketohexokinase (KHK) isoforms (24).

Thus, HIF-1 has been shown to have important roles in various hypertrophy and heart failure signaling pathways. While these pathways have been better studied in LV pressure loading, we have consistently found robust RV fibrosis in response to both mechanical pressure loading by PAB and in pulmonary hypertension models including upregulated protein expression of TGF-β1, cardiac fibroblast activation, ERK 1/2 signaling, and phosphorylation of SMAD2/3 (25). This suggests that HIF-1α immune-mediated pathways are likely at play and need further investigation. Indeed, in neonatal hypoxic PAH, plasma HIF-1α, and ET-1 levels are increased in relation to increased RV systolic pressure and RV dysfunction. However, it is unknown to

what degree the circulating HIF-1α and endothelin-1 are from the RV versus pulmonary vasculature. Thus, the relative role of ischemia and hypoxia versus the mechanical effects of pressure and increased wall stress need further elucidation and are interdependent. In a rabbit model of pulmonary arterial band induced pressure loading, we found that changed RV geometry increases regional wall stress, particularly at the RV septal hinge points with decreased myocardial function and increased fibrosis (26). In rat pulmonary artery banding models, this mechanical stress induces β-1 integrins to upregulate TGF-β1 signaling, myofibroblast activation, and RV fibrosis, independent of pulmonary vascular disease (25). However, in this normoxia model, we did not investigate HIF-1α signaling and whether it is required to promote the hyperfibrotic response. RV pressure loading by pulmonary artery banding, when sufficiently severe, can induce RV capillary rarefication, fibrosis, and dysfunction to similar degrees as monocrotaline and Sugen-hypoxia induced PAH (4). In pulmonary artery banding models, we have also found strong upregulation of ET-1, which is a powerful pulmonary vasoconstrictor and a PAH therapeutic target, to be an important driver of RV fibrosis and apoptosis, independent of increased pulmonary vascular resistance (16, 17).

Some of the metabolic pathways induced by hypoxia and/or pulmonary hypertension/pressure stress may be common to the fibroblast and the myocyte. RV fibroblasts and profibrotic signatures in PAH rodent models, as well as from patients with PAH, have been found to undergo epigenetic modulation of mitochondrial metabolism via pyruvate dehydrogenase kinase (PDK) (27), a mechanism that also underlies maladaptive RV myocyte metabolic responses that are detailed below.

Although chronic hypoxia often promotes inflammation and fibrosis, macrophage hypoxia can suppress cardiac fibrosis via oncostatin-m (OSM) secretion (28). During fibrogenesis, several subsets of monocytes/macrophages are recruited to the heart, including both proinflammatory (Ly6Chi) and anti-inflammatory (Ly6Clo) monocytes. During cardiac remodeling, Ly6Chi monocytes/macrophages accumulate in hypoxic areas in a HIF-1α dependent manner to suppress cardiac fibroblast activation. Oncostatin-m, an interleukin-6 family member, is a HIF-1α target gene and inhibits TGF-β1-mediated activation of cardiac fibroblasts via ERK 1/2-dependent phosphorylation of Small Mothers Against Decapentaplegic (SMAD). In the pulmonary arteries of Sugen 5461 plus hypoxia PAH rats and the LV of mice with transverse aortic constriction, the transmembrane glycoprotein Basigin that activates matrix metalloproteinases plays a role in hypertrophy as well as inflammation through the ERK pathway. Basigin is activated by CyPA, mechanical stretch, and angiotensin II (29), all active in RV hypertrophy and dysfunction in PAH and RV pressure-loading models (25, 30) and may therefore also play a role in RV hypertrophy (29, 31).

Origins of the Warburg phenotype and cardiomyocyte mitochondrial dysfunction in pulmonary hypertension

Aberrant energy utilization in RV cardiomyocytes plays a key role in RV dysfunction in response to stress, including in PAH and hypoxia. As energy is produced predominantly in the mitochondria, aberrant mitochondrial metabolism, and dynamics play an important role in the abnormal cardiomyocyte energy utilization in PAH, RV hypertrophy, and also in cancer, where many of these aberrant metabolic phenomena were initially described. Mitochondria generate energy in the form of ATP and also regulate cell proliferation and apoptosis. Mitochondrial dynamics encompass a number of mitochondrial activities including division (fission), union (fusion), movement (translocation), biogenesis, and quality control (mitophagy). Abnormal mitochondrial dynamics and metabolism are observed in the pulmonary vasculature, and in the RV myocardium in patients with type-1 PAH, including increased mitochondrial fission and impaired mitochondrial fusion, which results in mitochondrial fragmentation, as well as metabolic derangements of glucose metabolism (32–35). The generation of energy (ATP) from glucose normally involves close coupling between glycolysis and mitochondrial glucose oxidation, which is dependent on pyruvate generated by glycolysis. Pyruvate dehydrogenase (PDH) is the enzyme that generates pyruvate and is inhibited by its phosphorylation by the enzyme PDK. Consequently, upregulation and activation of PDK disrupt glycolysis-mitochondrial oxidation coupling. This phenomenon, termed the Warburg effect, ultimately depletes cellular energy reserve and is observed in rapidly replicating cancer cells (36, 37). Similarly, in the pulmonary hypertensive hypertrophied RV, RV cardiomyocyte PDH becomes inhibited by upregulation of PDK (38). Consequently, mitochondrial glucose metabolism is inefficient, as conversion of glucose to pyruvate via glycolysis becomes futile and the mitochondrial Krebs cycle is paralyzed, reducing generation of ATP. An increase in lactic acidosis, as unutilized pyruvate is shunted to lactate, further compounds the energy crisis and directly impairs RV and LV myocardial function. Together, this energy deficiency impairs RV cardiomyocyte contractility and overall RV function (34, 36, 39). Modulation of PDK and consequently restoration of aberrant mitochondrial energy metabolism, may therefore restore energetics in the energy starved hypertrophied and stressed RV myocardium, potentially improving RV contractility and function.

Mitochondria also regulate HIF-1α (36). Superoxide dismutase 2 (SOD2) converts toxic reactive oxygen species (ROS) produced by the mitochondrial electron transport chain into diffusible H_2O_2, that regulates HIF-1α (36). Consequently, mitochondrial ROS can be regulated by the partial pressure of oxygen and by SOD2 expression, although there is controversy as to whether hypoxia ultimately increases or decreases mitochondrial ROS production (40–42). In the Fawn-hooded rat model of PAH, a deficiency in H_2O_2 production during normoxia, via downregulation of SOD2, creates a "pseudo-hypoxic" milieu, in which normoxic activation of HIF-1α promotes PAH (43). HIF-1α further triggers PDK transcription, which as described above, ultimately shifts energy generation from oxidative glucose utilization to glycolytic metabolism. Dichloroacetate is a compound that inhibits PDK and leads to regression of chronic hypoxia-induced PAH and improves RV function in both chronic hypoxia PAH models and the Fawn-hooded PAH rat (34, 35, 37, 43–45). The mechanisms underlying this improvement include improved glucose oxidation, increased glucose oxidation, and mitochondrial nicotinamide adenine dinucleotide (NADH) mitochondrial electron flux with restoration of physiologic ROS production (44).

There is also a pathogenic role for aberrant glutamine metabolism in PAH in both the pulmonary vascular smooth muscle cells and in the RV cardiomyocyte (46–48). In MCT-induced PAH in rats, RV cardiomyocyte hypertrophy was dependent on glutaminolysis, which was reversed by the glutamine antagonist 6-diazo-5-oxo-l-norleucine (DON) (48).

Structure-function relationships in right ventricular cardiomyocytes and their role in the myocardial dysfunction in pulmonary hypertension

Although these mitochondrial metabolic and functional alterations affect both the pulmonary vascular smooth muscle cells and RV cardiomyocytes, the triggers, mechanisms, structural and functional consequences may differ. In the pulmonary vasculature, enhanced mitotic fission is initiated by elevation of cytosolic calcium, and by kinases that regulate the activation of the fission mediator, dynamin related protein 1 (Drp1), and mitosis by cyclin B-CDK1 (33, 35). Thus, in the pulmonary vasculature, the mitochondrial metabolic phenotype is driven by accelerated cell proliferation, migration, and decreased apoptosis (32). Consequently, preventing mitotic fission, by inhibiting Drp1 or enhancing mitofusin-2, causes cell cycle arrest and can improve hemodynamics in experimental models of PAH (34).

In contrast to the pulmonary vasculature, in the RV myocardium, impaired mitochondrial metabolism and dynamics are likely related, at least in part, to RV ischemia, resulting in myocardial hibernation, RV hypokinesis, and impaired RV function (34). RV ischemia, related to capillary rarefaction and impaired coronary perfusion, promotes Drp1 activation and mitochondrial fission. However, cardiac myocytes do not undergo mitosis; and mitochondrial fission in these cells increases ROS production (34). Consequently, inhibiting Drp1, mitochondrial division inhibitor-1 (Mdivi-1) or P110 (which inhibits the interaction between Drp1 and its binding partner, fission protein 1 [Fis1]) improves RV function in RV ischemia-reperfusion injury (49).

Thus, mitochondrial metabolism, morphology, and cardiac function appear to be closely related. In canine models of ischemic CHF, the number of mitochondria in LV and RV cardiomyocytes was increased, but their average size was smaller, consistent with increased fission (50). In LV dysfunction models, inhibiting mitochondrial fission preserves function, prevents cardiomyocyte apoptosis and promotes angiogenesis (51, 52). Therefore, targeting these processes may be relevant to RV failure but requires further study.

Dichloroacetate, described above as a PDK inhibitor, also modifies voltage-gated potassium channels such as Kv1.5 in the pulmonary vasculature in PAH; a pathway that also appears to be important in the RV cardiomyocyte (44). Expression of these voltage-gated potassium channels (Kv) is further downregulated by various transcription factors that are upregulated in RV hypertrophy, including HIF-1α and forkhead box protein O1 (FOXO1). In the Fawn-hooded rat model of spontaneous PAH and secondary RV hypertrophy, dichloroacetate decreased PDK4 and FOXO1expression, with activation of PDH and restoration of glucose oxidation. Dysregulation of mitochondrial HIF-1α and Kv channels not only promotes adverse pulmonary vascular remodeling but also RV dysfunction and repolarization abnormalities (38). Hypoxia decreases production of mitochondrial ROS and activates HIF-1α, which suppresses Kv channel expression in cardiac myocytes. This induces uncoupled glycolysis and glutaminolysis, which promote cardiomyocyte hypertrophy and impair cardiomyocyte contractility; the mechanism, as detailed above, appears to underlie the PAH and RVH that develop in the fawn-hooded rat model (53).

While the effects of hypoxemia have been largely negative in terms of RV function in PAH, there are potential therapeutic implications for cardiomyocyte regeneration. In mice, gradual and progressive exposure to 7% hypoxemia for 2 weeks inhibits oxidative metabolism and decreases ROS production with subsequent reduction of oxidative damage to DNA, allowing reentry of cardiomyocyte into mitosis. In the LV, this regenerative response was associated with improved recovery after myocardial infarction including decreased myocardial fibrosis and improved systolic function (54). The increased cardiac mass and regenerated myocardium were shown to originate from proliferation of preexisting cardiomyocytes rather than myocyte hypertrophy (54). In that study, chronic hypoxia significantly affected mitochondria with decreased cardiac mitochondrial cristae density, mitochondrial DNA copy number, and reduced mitochondrial Krebs cycle and fatty acid β-oxidation (54).

Chronic hypoxia affects other aspects of mitochondrial function. In rats exposed to chronic hypoxia in the setting of high altitude, cardiac mitochondrial complex I-III and mitochondrial nitic oxide synthase (NOS) activity is upregulated (55). This phenomenon can be reversed by inhibiting phosphodiesterase 5 with sildenafil (55). Indeed, phosphodiesterase 5 may be specifically upregulated in the hypertrophied RV and negatively impacts RV contractility as sildenafil was found to increase RV contractility in PAH (56). However, whether this phenomenon is truly RV specific, rather than secondary to changes in the pulmonary vasculature, is still in question as sildenafil reversed RV hypertrophy and fibrosis in the MCT PAH model, but not in rats with pulmonary artery banding (57).

In the Sugen 5461 plus hypoxia model of PAH, there are ultrastructural RV abnormalities associated with development of RV fibrosis in our and other studies (4). At the cardiomyocyte cell level, destruction of myofilaments, T-tubules, and sarcoplasmic reticulum have been demonstrated by electron microscopy (58). Interestingly, there is likely an important influence of species, as RV mitochondrial damage and fission were found in Fischer but not Sprague–Dawley rats. These cellular and histological changes were associated with RV hypertrophy and dilatation and clinical signs of RV failure including pleural effusion and hepatomegaly, with over 90% of animals dying within 6-weeks (58). RV cardiomyocyte hypertrophy in the setting of hypoxia models is mediated in part by the cell growth, proliferation, and survival regulator, mechanistic target of rapamycin (mTOR) (59). mTOR promotes pulmonary vascular smooth muscle cell proliferation and PAH. There are 2 mTOR complexes: mTOR-1 supports cell growth and mTOR-2 promotes cell survival. Dual mTOR-1/mTOR-2 inhibition reverses pulmonary vascular remodeling via increased apoptosis (59). In the RV, mTOR complex-1 is dominant, and its inhibition can ameliorate PAH-induced RV cardiomyocyte hypertrophy, RV remodeling, RV dysfunction, and fibrosis, lending a potential therapeutic target (59).

Developmental changes in myocardial metabolism in the transition of the fetal to postnatal myocardium

The dramatic changes that occur in cardiac physiology and metabolism from fetal to post-natal life lead to many adaptations including changes in the extracellular matrix and the myocyte contractile apparatus. However, these aspects are largely beyond the scope of this chapter and will not be reviewed here. Nonetheless, some of the metabolic changes that are related to the pathways discussed above are worthwhile discussing in brief.

Fetal cardiomyocytes operate in the milieu of *in utero* hypoxia, whereas adult cardiomyocytes are very sensitive to hypoxia. This transition is of interest as a basis for therapeutic intervention. The transition between these states is still incompletely understood, but occurs through several developmental adaptations. Indeed, cardiomyocytes become incapable of adapting to hypoxia shortly after birth. In mice, cardiac cellular and metabolic changes occur rapidly after birth with metabolic switches in energy utilization happening within the first post-natal week (60). In the fetus, cardiomyocytes generate energy predominantly through glycolysis and glucose oxidation (61) processes also important in the pulmonary hypertensive RV myocardium, as discussed previously. Postnatally, the rapid increase in cardiac output and energy requirements is achieved by switching from glycolysis to β-oxidation of lipids and by an increase in the number of mitochondria (62). The proliferation of mitochondria occurs, in part, through increased Pgc1α/β expression (63). Beyond the number of mitochondria, their morphology is important (as is the case for the maladapted pulmonary hypertensive RV). Fetal mitochondria are "fragmented" in appearance, whereas postnatal mitochondria appear elongated, consistent with the post-natal metabolic switch (61). Fusion of mitochondria occurs through mitofusin proteins and is associated with increased post-natal lipid β-oxidation (64, 65). This adaptation allows for more ATP to be generated per unit of glucose (66). In part, this adaptation occurs via HIF-1α, as hypoxia-induced HIF-1α inhibits mitochondrial biogenesis (67–69). The transcription factor heart- and neural crest derivatives-expressed protein 1 (Hand1) is under direct control by HIF-1α and thus hypoxia (70). The downstream effects of Hand1 are wide, including mitochondrial function, metabolism, and susceptibility to ischaemia in cardiomyocytes (70). Indeed, Hand1 is one of several genes normally expressed in the fetus and upregulated again in the adult cardiomyocyte during heart failure. Hand1 determines oxygen consumption by inhibition of lipid metabolism in the fetal and adult cardiomyocyte, leading to downregulation of mitochondrial energy generation (70). Thus, as in RV failure, preferential selection of energetic substrate is determined by ambient oxygen levels, and regulation of cellular lipid oxidation is a key mechanism to determine oxygen consumption. Experimental inhibition of lipid metabolism by etomoxir, a carnitine palmitoyl transferase (CPT)-1 antagonist that prevents mitochondrial long-chain fatty acid import, shifts energy metabolism to glycolysis, leading to lower myocardial oxygen consumption, and protects against myocardial ischemia (71). Neonatal rats exposed to hypoxia develop decreased lipid content and altered acyl-carnitine metabolism, similar to the effects of persistent Hand1 expression on lipid metabolism (72).

The role of hypoxia through HIF-1α in determining the metabolic and functional maturation of cardiomyocytes is also observed in human pluripotent stem cell-derived cardiomyocytes (hPSC-CMs). hPSC-CMs, cultured in the presence of glucose, use primarily aerobic glycolysis and aberrantly upregulate HIF-1α and downstream lactate dehydrogenase A (73). Conversely, glucose deprivation promotes oxidative phosphorylation and represses HIF-1α. Inhibition of HIF-1α or lactate dehydrogenase A results in a switch from aerobic glycolysis to oxidative phosphorylation, together with an increase in mitochondrial content and cellular ATP levels, and improves functional gene expression, sarcomere length, and contractility (73). Thus, the HIF-1α-lactate dehydrogenase A axis seems to inhibit maturation, at least of hPSC-CM, while inhibition of HIF-1α allows their metabolic and functional maturation (73).

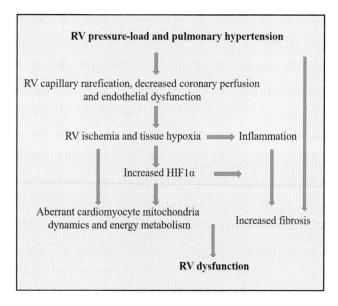

FIGURE 19.1 Right ventricular (RV) pressure-loading and pulmonary hypertension lead to RV ischemia and hypoxia through a decrease in capillary number and function and coronary perfusion pressure. Hypoxia stabilizes and activates hypoxia inducible factor (HIF)-1α to negatively impact mitochondrial function and dynamics creating an energy deficiency in the stressed RV cardiomyocyte. In parallel, HIF-1α exacerbates inflammation and fibrosis which are triggered by pressure loading through transforming growth factor-β. Together, these contribute to RV dysfunction.

Other transcription factors also play a role in the perinatal shift to lipid-based metabolism. One of these may be myeloid ecotropic viral integration site 1 (MEIS1), a transcription factor that induces glycolysis in hematopoietic stem cells. MEIS1 may play a role in the transition of cardiomyocyte metabolism from the hypoxic fetal environment to the oxygen-rich post-natal environment and concomitant switch to oxidative metabolism. In fetal, neonatal, and adult sheep, cardiomyocyte respiratory capacity increases with advancing age, in parallel to decreasing MEIS1 expression (74). Experimentally, suppression of MEIS1 leads to increased oxygen consumption in fetal, but not in postnatal cells. Similarly, MEIS1 suppression increases mitochondrial activity. Interestingly, MEIS has recently been found to also regulate the proliferation of pulmonary artery smooth muscle cells in hypoxia-induced pulmonary hypertension (75).

Summary

In summary, hypoxia profoundly impacts RV function. Many signaling pathways regulated by hypoxia, including HIF-1α, affect the pulmonary vasculature and the RV cardiomyocyte. Hypoxia signaling pathways intersect to affect inflammation, extracellular matrix remodeling, mitochondrial function, and energy generation; all of which contribute to RV dysfunction in PAH and other conditions (Figure 19.1). Some pathways that are active in the physiological hypoxia of the fetus are reactivated in the pathological hypoxia of PAH and the failing RV. Some of these signaling pathways may constitute therapeutic targets to improve RV function, especially in the setting of PAH.

References

1. Hirota K. Biomedicines. 2020; 8(2):32.
2. Sutendra G, et al. J Mol Med (Berl). 2013; 91(11):1315–1327.
3. Bogaard HJ, et al. Circulation. 2009; 120(20):1951–1960.
4. Akazawa Y, et al. J Appl Physiol (1985). 2020; 129(2):238–246.
5. Wang L, et al. Arterioscler Thromb Vasc Biol. 2020; 40(6):1543–1558.
6. Darby IA, et al. Cell Tissue Res. 2016; 365(3):553–562.
7. Holscher M, et al. Cardiovasc Res. 2012; 94(1):77–86.
8. Wang GL, et al. Proc Natl Acad Sci USA. 1993; 90(9):4304–4308.
9. Wang GL, et al. Proc Nat'l Acad Sci USA. 1995; 92(12):5510–5514.
10. Ikeda S, et al. Arterioscler Thromb Vasc Biol. 2014; 34(6):1260–1271.
11. Gosal K, et al. Am J Respir Cell Mol Biol. 2015; 52(6):717–727.
12. Xu EZ, et al. Am J Physiol Heart Circ Physiol. 2010; 299(6):H1854–H1864.
13. Somlyo AP, et al. Physiol Rev. 2003; 83(4):1325–1358.
14. Ziino AJ, et al. Pediatr Res. 2010; 67(2):177–182.
15. Jankov RP, et al. Free Radic Biol Med. 2010; 49(9):1453–1467.
16. Nielsen EA, et al. PLoS One. 2016; 11(1):e0146767.
17. Ramos SR, et al. J Appl Physiol (1985). 2018; 124(5):1349–1362.
18. Hamid SA, et al. Am J Physiol Heart Circ Physiol. 2007; 292(6):H2598–H2606.
19. Eltzschig HK, et al. N Engl J Med. 2011; 364(7):656–665.
20. Murdoch C, et al. Blood. 2004; 104(8):2224–2234.
21. Novo E, et al. J Pathol. 2012; 226(4):588–597.
22. Lokmic Z, et al. Int Rev Cell Mol Biol. 2012; 296:139–185.
23. Cheng CC, et al. Int J Mol Sci. 2019; 20(6):1468.
24. Mirtschink P, et al. Nature. 2015; 522(7557):444–449.
25. Sun M, et al. J Am Heart Assoc. 2018; 7(7):e007928.
26. Gold J, et al. Am J Physiol Heart Circ Physiol. 2020; 318(2):H366–H377.
27. Tian L, et al. Circ Res. 2020; 126(12):1723–1745.
28. Abe H, et al. Nat Commun. 2019; 10(1):2824.
29. Satoh K, et al. Circ Res. 2014; 115(8):738–750.
30. Friedberg MK, et al. Am J Respir Cell Mol Biol. 2013; 49(6):1019–1028.
31. Suzuki K, et al. Arterioscler Thromb Vasc Biol. 2016; 36(4):636–646.
32. Archer SL. N Engl J Med. 2013; 369(23):2236–2251.
33. Marsboom G, et al. Circ Res. 2012; 110(11):1484–1497.
34. Piao L, et al. J Mol Med (Berl). 2010; 88(10):1011–1020.
35. Hong Z, et al. Am J Respir Crit Care Med. 2017; 195(4):515–529.
36. Archer SL, et al. Am J Physiol Heart Circ Physiol. 2008; 294(2):H570–H578.
37. Sutendra G, et al. Cell Metab. 2014; 19(4):558–573.
38. Ryan JJ, et al. Circ Res. 2014; 115(1):176–188.
39. Stanley WC, et al. Cardiovasc Res. 1997; 33(2):243–257.
40. Semenza GL. Nat Rev Cancer. 2003; 3(10):721–732.
41. Chandel NS, et al. J Biol Chem. 2000; 275(33):25130–25138.
42. Murphy MP. Biochem J. 2009; 417(1):1–13.
43. Bonnet S, et al. Circulation. 2006; 113(22):2630–2641.
44. Michelakis ED, et al. Circulation. 2002; 105(2):244–250.
45. McMurtry MS, et al. Circ Res. 2004; 95(8):830–840.
46. Xu W, et al. Proc Natl Acad Sci USA. 2007; 104(4):1342–1347.
47. Culley MK, et al. J Clin Invest. 2018; 128(9):3704–3715.
48. Piao L, et al. J Mol Med (Berl). 2013; 91(10):1185–1197.
49. Tian L, et al. J Mol Med (Berl). 2017; 95(4):381–393.
50. Sabbah HN, et al. J Mol Cell Cardiol. 1992; 24(11):1333–1347.
51. Givvimani S, et al. PLoS One. 2012; 7(3):e32388.
52. Ong SB, et al. Circulation. 2010; 121(18):2012–2022.
53. Piao L, et al. J Mol Med (Berl). 2013; 91(3):333–346.
54. Nakada Y, et al. Nature. 2017; 541(7636):222–227.
55. Zaobornyj T, et al. Am J Physiol Heart Circ Physiol. 2009; 296(6):H1741–H1747.
56. Nagendran J, et al. Circulation. 2007; 116(3):238–248.
57. Schafer S, et al. Cardiovasc Res. 2009; 82(1):30–39.
58. Shults NV, et al. J Am Heart Assoc. 2019; 8(5):e011227.
59. Pena A, et al. Am J Respir Cell Mol Biol. 2017; 57(5):615–625.
60. Makinde AO, et al. Mol Cell Biochem. 1998; 188(1-2):49–56.
61. Lopaschuk GD, et al. Am J Physiol. 1991; 261(6 Pt 2):H1698–H1705.
62. Agata Y, et al. J Pediatr. 1991; 119(3):441–445.
63. Neary MT, et al. J Mol Cell Cardiol. 2014; 74:340–352.
64. McBride H, et al. Biochim Biophys Acta. 2013; 1833(1):148–149.
65. Papanicolaou KN, et al. Circ Res. 2012; 111(8):1012–1026.
66. Lai L, et al. Genes Dev. 2008; 22(14):1948–1961.
67. Nau PN, et al. Pediatr Res. 2002; 52(2):269–278.
68. Narravula S, et al. J Immunol. 2001; 166(12):7543–7548.
69. Zhang H, et al. J Biol Chem. 2008; 283(16):10892–10903.
70. Breckenridge RA, et al. PLoS Biol. 2013; 11(9):e1001666.
71. Lopaschuk GD, et al. Circ Res. 1988; 63(6):1036–1043.
72. Bruder ED, et al. Lipids Health Dis. 2010; 9:3.
73. Hu D, et al. Circulation. 2018; 123(9):1066–1079.
74. Lindgren IM, et al. FASEB J. 2019; 33(6):7417–7426.
75. Yao MZ, et al. Life Sci. 2020; 255:117822.

HYPOXIC REMODELING OF NEONATAL PULMONARY ARTERY AND MYOCARDIUM

Hui Zhang, R. Dale Brown, Jason Williams, Cassidy Delaney and Kurt R. Stenmark

Contents

Introduction

Infants who die with pulmonary hypertension (PH) exhibit significant remodeling along the entire longitudinal axis of the pulmonary artery (PA). These changes include thickening of the media and distal extension of smooth muscle cells (SMCs) into previously nonmuscularized vessels. There is also marked adventitial thickening with an accumulation of fibroblasts, extracellular matrix (ECM), and inflammatory cells, particularly macrophages (1, 2). While similar changes are also observed in adult forms of hypoxic PH, some aspects of the cellular responses of the neonatal pulmonary circulation are distinct. Observations in animal models suggest that the proliferative and matrix-producing potential of the neonatal pulmonary circulation in response to injury exceeds that of the adult (3, 4), which is due, in part, to the fact that PH in children is intrinsically linked to issues of lung growth and development. The timing of the pulmonary vascular injury is a critical determinant of the subsequent response of the developing lung to adverse stimuli, including hypoxia. Further, the effect of vascular disease on the right ventricle (RV) in early life is likely different than in the adult with PH. In this brief chapter, we will review mechanisms underlying hypoxia-induced changes in growth, inflammation, and matrix synthesis of neonatal vascular cells. We discuss the importance of cell type-specific responses to hypoxia, focusing particularly on SMCs and adventitial fibroblasts, as the endothelial cell is covered in other chapters within this book. We also briefly examine the response of the neonatal RV to pressure overload-induced by hypoxic PH.

Effect of hypoxia on pulmonary artery cell proliferation in the neonatal period of life

Sustained hypoxia stimulates the proliferation of pulmonary vascular cells *in vivo* (5, 6). The growth is a direct response to hypoxia and the increased pressure/mechanical stress that occurs with persistent hypoxic pulmonary vasoconstriction. Each cell type in the pulmonary arterial wall – endothelial cells, SMCs, and adventitial fibroblasts – displays unique growth responses to hypoxia. The magnitude of these responses is dependent on the duration of the stimulus, the timing of the exposure (i.e. the period of life in which the exposure occurs), and genetic predisposition. Histologic changes in the pulmonary arterial wall in response to chronic hypoxia have been extensively described (6). DNA synthesis in endothelial cells is detectable in the first 24 hours of hypoxic exposure (5, 7, 8), which occurs concomitantly with diffuse, subendothelial edema leading to subendothelial thickening.

No evidence of endothelial cell occlusion of the vessels has been reported in hypoxic forms of PH in neonates or adults. The proliferation of SMCs and medial thickening follow changes observed in the endothelium (7–9). Extension of muscle into distal arteries also occurs quickly in response to hypoxia, which is likely due to activation, migration, and proliferation of distinct SMC progenitor cells that reside in the distal vasculature (10). However, perhaps the earliest and most dramatic hypoxic growth, especially in neonates, occurs in the adventitial compartment where the fibroblast resides (5, 11). This proliferative response to hypoxia is particularly striking in resistance vessels (7). These findings support that hypoxia affects the growth of all resident cell types found *in vivo*, with each having its own unique time course.

Several studies have demonstrated that exaggerated changes in SMC proliferation observed in the neonate in response to hypoxia are probably the result of distinct properties of the neonatal SMCs compared to that of the adult (12), which has been described as a "reversion" to a fetal-like phenotype, although this phenotype is somewhat distinct from fetal cells themselves. Pulmonary artery SMCs (PASMCs) from neonatal calves, exposed to hypoxia beginning on day 1 of life, retain and or re-express enhanced fetal-like growth properties (12). As observed with normal fetal cells, PASMCs from hypoxia exposed neonatal calves exhibit increased responsiveness to maximal serum stimulation *in vitro* (Figure 20.1A, B). In addition, SMCs from the hypoxic neonatal PA have more persistent growth after serum withdrawal compared with neonatal control and adult SMCs (Figure 20.1C). Another interesting aspect of the enhanced growth properties of the neonatal SMCs is that the enhanced responsiveness to growth factors appears to be mitogen specific, including PDGF-BB and IGF-1. PASMCs from hypoxia-exposed calves have enhanced growth properties compared with neonatal control and adult cells that are at least partially dependent on activated protein kinase C (PKC) (13). The calcium-dependent isozymes of PKC and PKCα, in particular, appear to be especially important in these responses (14). Thus, retained, reexpressed, and newly acquired growth properties likely contribute to the striking hyperplasia of neonatal PASMCs *in vivo* after exposure to hypoxia.

As previously noted, of the three resident cell types in the vessel wall, the adventitial fibroblast undergoes the earliest, most dramatic, and most prolonged increase in proliferation in response to chronic hypoxia (Figure 20.2A, B) (15). Fibroblasts, likely only specific subpopulations, proliferate with greater propensity within the adventitial compartment than SMCs in response to injury or stress, including that induced by hypoxia (16, 17). Fibroblasts can also differentiate into SMC-like cells, i.e.

DOI: 10.1201/9780367494018-20

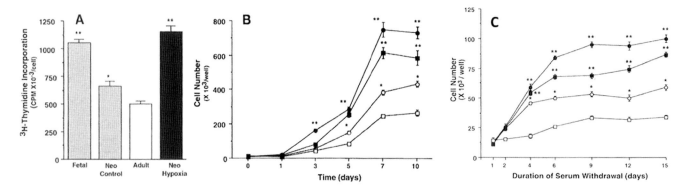

FIGURE 20.1 Neonatal PASMCs have greater proliferative response to maximal serum stimulation and more persistent growth after serum withdrawal. PASMCs from hypoxic calves and bovine fetuses have increased DNA synthesis (A) and proliferate faster (B) to maximal serum (10%) stimulation compared with neonatal (neo) control and adult cells. PASMCs from hypoxic calves and bovine fetuses have more persistent growth than neonatal control and adult cells after serum withdrawal (C). ● Neo hypoxia; ■ fetal; ○ Neo control; □ adult.

myofibroblasts, which can accumulate in the adventitia and/or migrate to the media and intimal layers of the vessel wall (Figure 20.2C) (15, 18). Fibroblasts increase or alter their profile of ECM deposition, and altered ECM can reciprocally perpetuate phenotypic change in the fibroblast and its interactions with recruited cells, such as monocytes and leukocytes (6, 15). Fibroblasts also synthesize and release molecules with potent paracrine effects on neighboring cells, such as IL-6, IL-1β, CSF-2, and TNC which have a substantial impact on macrophage phenotype (6, 19, 20).

It has been established that there is heterogeneity in fibroblast populations across tissues. Studies of fibroblasts derived from the PA's adventitia support the idea of tremendous heterogeneity in their functional characteristics. Fibroblast clones generated from the PA adventitia exhibit markedly different proliferative capabilities (16). Regarding neonatal hypoxic pulmonary hypertension, clones that consistently proliferated in response to hypoxia, and those that did not were identified. Selective contribution of one of these subsets to hypoxia-induced pulmonary vascular remodeling was suggested to be the result of the selective expansion of the "hypoxia proliferative" clones generated from the remodeled adventitia of the chronically hypoxic animals (16, 21). Populations of fibroblasts capable of proliferating in response to hypoxia do it through activation of Gαi-Gq family members, perhaps even in a ligand-independent fashion, and subsequent stimulation of PKC and mitogen-activated protein (MAP) kinase family members (16, 22). Changes in growth factor signaling likely contribute to hypoxia-induced changes in the adventitial compartment. For instance, there are reports of increased platelet-derived growth factor β receptor (PDGFβ-R) in the PA adventitial layer in PH patients (23–25). In neonatal hypoxia-induced PH, Das et al. found that hypoxia stimulates an increase in the levels and activation of PDGFβ-R in PA adventitial fibroblasts, termed PH-Fibs (Figure 20.2D, E). PDGFβ-induced proliferation was higher in PH-derived cells than controls. There was a unique dependence on transient JNK-1 phosphorylation in these cells, indicating that PDGFβ-R-JNK1 axis is integral to hypoxia-induced proliferation at this stage of development (26). Thus, it seems that a complex network of signaling pathways initiated by both G-protein-mediated signaling and a myriad of growth factors is responsible for the stimulation and proliferation of PA adventitial fibroblast in response to hypoxia, a response that is distinct among vascular wall cells.

Downstream of the aforementioned signaling pathways are transcription factors (TFs), which are involved in the proliferative response. For instance, activation of HIF1α appears to be an important regulator of replication of human PA adventitial fibroblasts under hypoxic conditions (27, 28). Hypoxia-induced activation of HIF-2α also appears critical in vascular remodeling and inflammation (29–31). Hypoxia also induces significant increases in the expression and activity of the early growth response 1 (Egr-1) gene in fibroblasts. Egr-1 contributes to the proliferative phenotype, at least partly by regulating the expression of cyclin-D and epidermal growth factor receptors (32). Numerous other TFs and transcriptional coregulators are also involved in the control of the activated PH cell phenotype. These include the pro-proliferative and proinflammatory TFs AP-1, FoxM1, NF-κb, and the antiproliferative TFs FOXO1, PPAR-γ, p53, and KLF4 (33).

It is also now evident that there are hypoxia-induced changes in fibroblast subpopulations with regard to mechanisms controlling their response to hypoxia. In some populations, the proliferative response to hypoxia is mitigated by the activation of protein kinase c-ζ. However, in populations of adventitial fibroblasts from the chronically hypoxic pulmonary vascular wall, protein kinase c-ζ is downregulated, thus abrogating an important counterbalancing pathway to control proliferation (34). It is currently unclear what controls this change in signaling, though epigenetic changes discussed below are likely involved.

Effect of hypoxia on pulmonary vascular extracellular matrix in the neonatal period of life

The phenotypic characteristics of vascular wall cells under homeostatic and pathologic conditions are regulated in part by the microenvironment and, thus, the ECM, in which they reside. This ECM provides informational cues that affect various cellular processes, including proliferation, migration, differentiation, and the synthesis of further types of matrix molecules. Thus, a balance between external signals from the matrix and local environments and the vascular cells particular intrinsic responsiveness, as was described above for neonatal vs. adult cells in response to soluble stimuli, determines the ultimate response of the cells to pathophysiologic stimuli (35–37). The expression

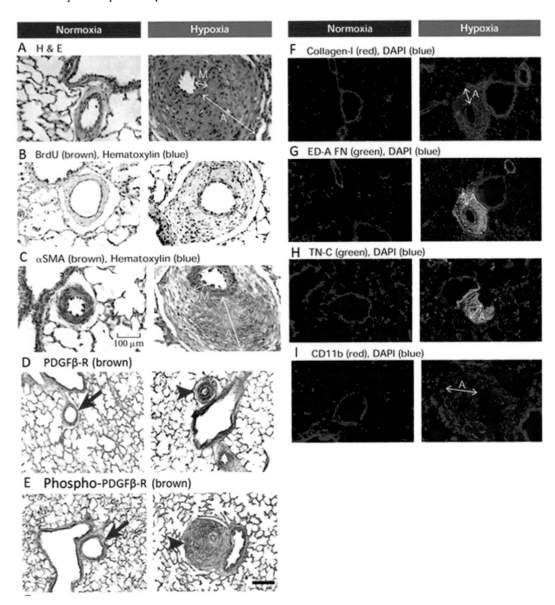

FIGURE 20.2 Pulmonary artery remodeling in hypoxia-induced pulmonary hypertension neonatal calf. Compared with control calf (normoxia), pulmonary arteries of chronically (2 wk) hypoxic neonatal calf (hypoxia) demonstrate marked adventitial thickening (A), augmented cell proliferation (BrdU; B), and myofibroblast accumulation/differentiation (α-SM-actin expression; C), elevated levels growth factors (both total and phosphorylated PDGFβ-R expression; D, E), excessive deposition of extracellular matrix proteins [type I collagen (F), cellular (ED-A) fibronectin (G), and tenascin-C (TN-C; H)] and increased recruitment of circulating leukocytes and fibrocytes (CD11b; I). H&E, hematoxylin and eosin; A, adventitia; M, media. Arrows define adventitial.

and production of many ECM proteins were observed in hypoxic neonatal calves (Figure 20.2F, G, H) and is developmentally regulated. For instance, during normal development, tropoelastin mRNA expression and elastin synthesis in lung and vascular tissues are limited to a brief period during late gestation and early postnatal life (38–40). There is significant alternative splicing of tropoelastin mRNA, which is also developmentally regulated. The frequency of alternative splicing has been shown to decrease by 10-fold in the lung over time following birth (41). These developmental differences in elastin-rich matrix are important and were demonstrated in experiments where neither fetal nor adult fibroblasts showed changes in elastin synthesis fibroblasts when grown on adult cell-derived elastin-rich matrix. However, when grown on fetal-derived cell-matrix, both fetal and adult

fibroblasts exhibited significant increases in elastin production (42). Other important constituents of the vasculature including fibronectin and collagen can also be developmentally regulated through alternative splicing changes. Also interesting and relevant to the neonatal circulation's response to hypoxia is the fact that little type-1 collagen, the collagen that imparts the greatest structural rigidity, is observed in small vessels at the time of birth. However, significant increases in type-1 collagen occur over time following birth.

Hypoxic stimuli can alter the normal developmental pattern of matrix synthesis. For instance, in newborn calves made hypoxic at birth, a dramatic increase in $\alpha 1$(I) procollagen mRNA expression is detected in resistance size pulmonary arteries within 24 hours (38). Experiments also demonstrated interruption of normal developmental expression patterns of fibronectin and tropoelastin in the pulmonary vessel wall by hypoxic exposure (38). The development-dependent differences in both type and amount of matrix proteins made in response to hypoxia support the idea that vascular changes observed in response to injurious stimuli, including hypoxia, are dependent on the point in development at which they occur. It is thus extremely important to know the precise composition of the vasculature at different developmental periods and to evaluate how that might ultimately affect responses of cells and the overall function of the vessel wall to stimuli. Thus, there is now intense interest in identifying key proteins in the PH disease processes as they may provide targets for new therapies. Unfortunately, the vast majority of work in this area has focused on mRNA changes occurring during development using whole lung tissue mRNA analysis. Studies have suggested that these approaches have a <30% chance of identifying accurately at the protein level the changes that occur.

Thus, we recently performed a detailed analysis of the pulmonary vascular proteome at different sites along its longitudinal axis under normal and pulmonary hypertensive conditions at two developmental periods. In collaboration with Dr. Hansen's laboratory at the University of Colorado, we extracted and characterized ECM and matricellular proteins, which include nearly all of the ECM proteins (>99%) within the soluble and insoluble fractions of whole tissue (PA) extracts (43–45). Over 1300 proteins were examined in decellularized proximal and distal PAs using these approaches from control and hypoxic hypertensive calves in the neonatal period and steers residing at high altitude with normal PA pressure vs. severe PH at 15 months of life. We found striking differences in the matrix composition between normal neonatal calves and 15-month-old steers without PH. These differences were observed in core ECM proteins (collagens, glycoproteins) and in matrix-associated molecules (Figure 20.3). There were also differences in the ECM proteins observed in response to either the 2-week or 15-month hypoxic exposure in these animals and the dramatic changes in the proteome of hypoxic vessels in the neonatal period (*Manuscript In Review*). Interestingly, in the neonate, pathway analysis of ECM-associated proteins revealed that among the most upregulated signaling pathways in the early stages of disease in both the proximal and distal PA are related to activation of complement and coagulation cascades (46). In addition, we found marked differences in the ECM composition of different size vessels at different times during disease progression. These observations reflect the marked heterogeneity that is now being reported in lesions observed in PH in response to injury (47). Overall, the data would support the idea that in both the proximal and distal vasculature, there is an early wound response in the newborn that is distinct from the adult, which may account for the striking changes in vascular structure that can occur in the neonatal period. We further speculate that this may further account for the greater reversibility of neonatal vascular remodeling in comparison with the adult.

Effects of hypoxia on pulmonary vascular inflammation in the neonatal period of life

In addition to changes in cellular proliferation and ECM composition and structure, numerous studies have demonstrated that PH-associated vascular remodeling is characterized by the early and persistent accumulation of mononuclear cells in the perivascular adventitia in animal models of PH, including chronically hypoxic calves (newborn) (Figure 20.2), rats, and mice, which are similar to the perivascular inflammatory infiltrates observed in human PAH in infants, children, and adults (6, 11, 48–50). It has been shown that infants and children display greater adventitial changes than adults with many forms of PH (17). Mounting evidence suggests a strong link between immune cell recruitment and inflammatory signaling in the hypoxic pulmonary circulation. In addition, evidence indicates that this inflammation is not merely a bystander but an active participant in the progression of vascular abnormalities in PH (6, 50, 51). Perinatal inflammation and immune modulation significantly impact pulmonary vascular development and appear to play a role in the progress of PH in preterm infants with bronchopulmonary dysplasia (BPD) (52, 53).

We have reported that adventitial fibroblasts that are isolated from neonatal calves with hypoxia-induced PH (termed PH-Fibs) exhibit a constitutive and persistent pro-inflammatory phenotype, which is defined by elevated expression of cytokines/chemokines and adhesion molecules, including IL-1β, IL-6, CCL2(MCP-1), CXCL12(SDF-1), CCL5(RANTES), CCR7, CXCR4, GM-CSF, CD40, CD40L, and VCAM-1 (49). In addition, PH-Fibs play a critical role in recruiting and retaining macrophages to the vessels and inducing a distinct proinflammatory phenotype of macrophages capable of contributing to chronic inflammation and fibrotic remodeling in PH (19, 49). Multiple critical pathways mediate these responses and can act in cooperative and/or combinatorial ways.

Metabolic and mitochondrial reprogramming has been increasingly recognized as hallmarks of PH, serving as central drivers of pulmonary vascular cell proinflammatory, proliferative, and fibrotic phenotypes (20, 54–57). The complex metabolic reprogramming characterized by mitochondrial abnormalities and an increase in glucose uptake and glycolysis, accompanied by increased free NADH (nicotinamide adenine dinucleotide [reduced form]) and NADH/NAD+ ratios, has been described to occur in the proinflammatory and proliferative adventitial fibroblasts isolated from neonatal calves with hypoxia-induced PH (PH-Fibs) (55–58). Furthermore, our group demonstrated that this metabolic reprogramming of PH-Fibs is regulated through a microRNA-124/PTBP1 (Polypyrimidine Tract Binding Protein 1)/PKM (Pyruvate Kinase Muscle) axis (57). Increased histone deacetylase (HDAC) activity in PH-Fibs decreases miR-124, which normally acts to maintain low levels of PTBP1. PTBP1 is an RNA splicing factor that controls PKM splicing, and when increased, the ratio of PKM2 to PKM1 is also increased. In PH-Fibs, the elevated PKM2/PKM1 ratio plays a critical role in generating aerobic glycolysis, which subsequently increases the ratio of free NADH to NAD+. The NADH-sensitive transcriptional corepressor C-terminal binding protein 1 (CtBP1) is increased in PH-Fibs and directly represses the transcriptional expression of the potent anti-inflammatory gene HMOX1 and promotes the pro-inflammatory phenotype of PH-Fibs (55). This PH phenotype can be rescued with interventions at various levels of the metabolic cascade, such as manipulation of key metabolic regulators (gene overexpression or silencing) and metabolic modulators, such as MTOB (CtBP1 inhibitor), TEPP-46 and Shikonin (PKM2 glycolytic function inhibitors) (55, 57). These findings suggest a more integrated view of PA fibroblast metabolism, which may open novel therapeutic prospects in targeting the dynamic metabolic interactions and between inflammatory mesenchymal cells in PH.

To investigate the mechanisms driving macrophage polarization within the adventitial microenvironment during PH progression, conditioned media from PA adventitial fibroblasts

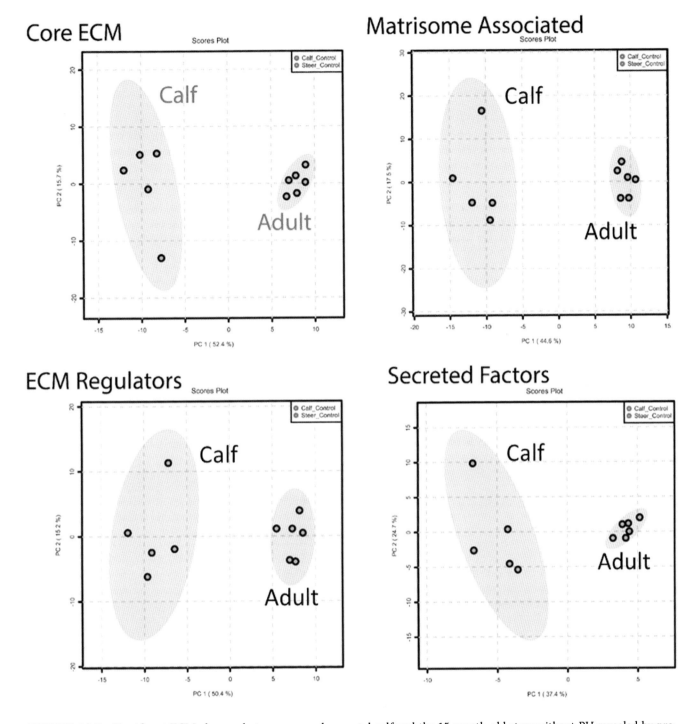

FIGURE 20.3 Significant ECM changes between normal neonatal calf and the 15-month-old steer without PH revealed by proteomic analysis. Principle component analysis (PCA) reveals clear separation between calf and steer larger proximal arteries, between the core ECM, matrix-associated molecules, ECM regulators, and secreted factors.

isolated from hypoxic pulmonary hypertensive (PH-CM), or age-matched control (CO-CM) neonatal calves were used to activate bone marrow-derived macrophages (BMDMs). RNA-Seq and mass spectrometry analyses were performed to evaluate the transcriptomic and metabolomic profiles in BMDMs. Preliminary results showed that PH-CM significantly increased the expression of genes involved in cell survival/viability, cell movement, cell recruitment, immune cell trafficking, cell–cell signaling/interaction, inflammatory responses, and carbohydrate and ROS

metabolism in BMDMs (59). These findings indicated that transcriptional and metabolic reprogramming plays a critical role in regulating macrophage polarization and further raises the possibility that targeting adventitial fibroblasts can modulate the recruitment and subsequent polarization of perivascular inflammatory monocytes/macrophages in PH (55).

Moreover, it is increasingly recognized that central components of intermediary metabolism are co-factors or substrates of chromatin-modifying enzymes (60). Thus, the concentrations of metabolic intermediates constitute a potential regulatory interface between the metabolic and chromatin states in cells, which are currently an area of intense interest. We briefly summarize the epigenetic alterations in the context of neonatal PH-Fibs. Indeed, the distinct metabolic and proinflammatory phenotypes of PH-Fibs are associated with epigenetic alterations as demonstrated by increased expression of HDAC1, HDAC2, and HDAC3 at the protein level and elevated class I HDAC catalytic activity (49, 61). HDAC inhibitors markedly reversed metabolic reprogramming and cytokine/chemokine expression in PH-Fibs and reduced their ability to induce monocyte migration and proinflammatory activation (49, 57).

We have proposed the concept that the high expression of proliferative, pro-inflammatory, and fibrotic genes in PH vascular cells is maintained by an open chromatin structure and multiple TFs via the recruitment of high levels of epigenetic regulators including the histone acetylases P300/CBP and histone acetylation readers, bromodomains (BRDs) (62). Further evaluation regarding how these aberrantly expressed genes are controlled by chromatin structure, TFs, and epigenetic regulators in pulmonary vascular cells in PH may provide new PH therapeutic strategies that target PA remodeling in addition to currently approved vasodilator therapies. Other reports in SMCs from the pulmonary hypertensive vessel wall have suggested that epigenetic regulator BRD4 (a member of the bromodomain and extra-terminal domain, BET protein family) is increased in PH cells (63). BRD4 and other BET proteins recognize acetylated-lysine residues in nucleosomal histones and other proteins such as TFs. The BRD protein then recruits other transcriptional co-factors to activate gene transcription. BRD4 inhibitors have been shown to attenuate PH in monocrotaline and sugen/hypoxia-induced rat models but have not been studied in the neonatal period of life (63, 64).

Cardiac remodeling in neonatal hypoxic PH

The pathological pulmonary vasoconstriction and remodeling of the pulmonary vasculature of PH impose a hemodynamic load that leads to remodeling and hypertrophy of the cardiac RV, and ultimately, progression to RV failure and death (65, 66). The initial responses of the RV to PH are likely compensatory and include rapid and transient increases in volume, increased contractility, and RV hypertrophy. With PH progression, declining RV function no longer meets physiological demand resulting in symptomatic heart failure, characterized by RV dilation and increased filling pressures (end-diastolic pressure and right atrial pressure). Cardiac remodeling during the progression of PH involves coordination of multiple processes, including myocyte contractility and hypertrophy, metabolism, angiogenesis, inflammation, and fibrosis, occurring among the major cell types of the myocardium, including cardiac myocytes, fibroblasts, macrophages, and vascular cells.

Despite increasing research efforts and sophistication of hemodynamic and imaging metrics, understanding of the responses of the RV to chronic PH remains incomplete. These questions are further complicated in the newborn, where the right and left ventricles undergo dramatic alterations in their respective hemodynamic loads and contractile performance owing to the perinatal transition of the cardiopulmonary circulation, combined with dramatic post-natal cell proliferation and growth of the heart. The RV differs substantially from the left ventricle (LV) in its embryonic origin and development, contractile function, and biochemical responses. Compared to the LV, the healthy thin-walled

RV is protected from hypoxia and ischemic injury by its lower O_2 demand, perfusion throughout the cardiac cycle, larger reserves of recruitable capillary flow, and O_2 extraction, and ability to further economize metabolic demand through myocyte hibernation (67). RV hypertrophy due to chronic PH pressure overload reduces RV perfusion and increases the vulnerability of the RV to the effects of hypoxia and ischemia. Capillary rarefaction has been reported as an additional cause of RV ischemia in PH (68). However, stereologic analysis has shown that the apparent diminished RV capillary density in hypoxic mouse PH, Sugen/HX rat PH, and human PAH in fact results mainly from RV hypertrophy that is incompletely compensated by increased endothelial cell proliferation, with no evidence of endothelial cell apoptosis (69). In this context, extensive studies have demonstrated that hypoxia and mechanical forces, including stretch, shear stress, and flow, act on growth factors including VEGF, basic FGF, angiopoietin and, others, to promote angiogenesis. These responses may contribute to compensatory remodeling in pressure-overload, intermittent hypoxic exposure, or exercise training and are prominent in the proliferative context of embryonic and post-natal development (70).

As discussed previously, neonatal calves exposed to environmental hypoxia have been established as a large animal model of PH that recapitulates important features of human disease (4, 71, 72). Calves respond to 2-week hypoxic exposure with RV hypertrophy measured as increased RV weight or increased wall thickness on echocardiography, accompanied by RV chamber expansion, septal flattening, systolic dysfunction, and decreased TAPSE (73, 74). Echocardiographic strain analysis further reveals decreased peak global (RV+S) longitudinal strain and peak RV free wall longitudinal strain suggesting worsened RV function (74) although these are load-dependent parameters and in part reflect developed PH (75). Moderate expansion of RV chamber, right atrium, and RV outflow tract, accompanied by septal flattening and RV systolic dysfunction, are visualized within 4 days of the initiation of hypoxic exposure and worsen progressively over the hypoxic exposure interval (*Manuscript in Review*).

These alterations in RV performance are reflected by molecular and cellular correlates of RV hypertrophic remodeling. 2-week hypoxic exposure leads to increased re-expression of skeletal muscle α-actin mRNA, characteristic of pathologic cardiac hypertrophy, and accompanied by localized disruptions of myocyte cytoskeletal organization (71, 73, 76). Despite this evidence of cardiac pathophysiology, recovery of hypertensive calves for 30 days in a normoxic atmosphere resulted in reversal of PH and disappearance of skeletal muscle α-actin mRNA (71). More recent studies from our laboratories demonstrate that cardiac myocytes from the hypertensive RV show altered patterns of contractile protein phosphorylation and abundance, yet develop similar total force and adjusted force per cross-sectional area, and mitochondrial function and integrity are also preserved in the hypertensive calf RV (77, 78). Complementing these results, cardiac fibroblasts from the PH calf RV express a transcriptomic signature enriched in gene expression related to ECM remodeling, hypoxia signaling, and production and secretion of cytokines and growth factors. Mediators released from the PH calf cardiac fibroblasts were shown to promote survival of cardiac myocytes in a de-differentiated state in vitro (79). Mechanisms of myocyte de-differentiation or hibernation initially may be protective and a pre-requisite for myocyte recovery upon release of pressure overload. A contrasting picture of gene expression appears in severe PH leading to RV failure. A recent report using transcriptomic analysis of Su5416/

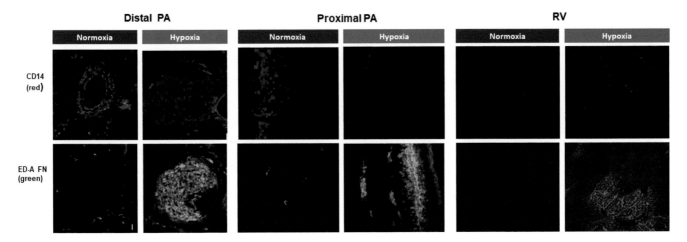

FIGURE 20.4 The hypoxic remodeling of neonatal PA and myocardium exhibits coordinate changes. Inflammatory fibrotic remodeling in distal (resistance) and proximal (conductance) PA, as well as in RV was strikingly similar as determined by CD14 and ED-A FN immunohistochemistry staining.

hypoxia or monocrotaline rat models combined with end-stage human PAH have proposed excessive cardiac fibrosis, mitochondrial dysfunction, and a failure of cell proliferation leading to capillary rarefaction as hallmarks of the failure phenotype (80). However, it remains challenging to determine mechanistically whether these processes represent a distinct maladaptive phenotype in susceptible individuals versus a failed attempt of ongoing remodeling processes to protect myocardial function from chronic PH.

Hypoxia-induced PH in experimental animals and Group 3 PH in humans are reversible in most individuals upon restoration of normoxia or reduction of pressure overload that is the driver for RV pathologic remodeling. However, a subset of susceptible individuals responds to hypoxia with severe "out-of-proportion" and irreversible PH. Developing novel biomarkers and noninvasive imaging methods to identify these at-risk individuals represents an important goal for continued research. Further, the RV shows a remarkable ability to adapt to long-term increases in pressure as occurs in congenital conditions such as Eisenmenger Syndrome or Hypoplastic Left Heart Syndromes and to recover upon surgical correction of these defects (81). Together these data demonstrate that in the face of pathologic pressure overload imposed by PH, the RV engages multiple processes to maintain physiological function while protecting the long-term survival of the cardiac myocyte. This perspective offers the hope that increased basic knowledge of RV adaptation and recovery will provide new avenues for development of cardioprotective therapies in pediatric PH.

In summary, hypoxic remodeling of neonatal PA and myocardium is distinct from the adult and is characterized by coordinate inflammatory and fibrotic remodeling throughout the cardiopulmonary system (Figure 20.4). This brief review argues for a more integrated view of hypoxia responses in the neonatal pulmonary circulation, which may ultimately lead to the development of therapeutic approaches explicitly directed at infants and children with PH.

Abbreviations

CSF-2	Colony-stimulating factor
HIF	Hypoxia-inducible factor
IGF	Insulin-like growth factor
IL-1β	Interleukin-1 beta
IL-6	Interleukin-6
PDGF	Platelet-derived growth factor
TF	Transcription factor
TNC	Tenascin C

References

1. Abman SH, et al. Prog Pediatr Cardiol. 2009; 27(1-2):3–6.
2. Abman SH, et al. Circulation. 2015; 132(21):2037–2099.
3. Rabinovitch M, et al. Am J Physiol. 1981; 240(1):H62–H72.
4. Stenmark KR, et al. J Appl Physiol (1985). 1987; 62(2):821–830.
5. Meyrick B, et al. Am J Pathol. 1979; 96(1):51–70.
6. Pugliese SC, et al. Am J Physiol Lung Cell Mol Physiol. 2015; 308(3):L229–L252.
7. Belknap JK, et al. Am J Respir Cell Mol Biol. 1997; 16(4):366–371.
8. Stiebellehner L, et al. Am J Physiol. 1998; 275(3):L593–600.
9. Dempsey EC, et al. J Perinatol. 1996; 16(2 Pt 2 Su):S2–S11.
10. Sheikh AQ, et al. Cell Rep. 2014; 6(5):809–817.
11. Stenmark KR, et al. Am J Physiol Lung Cell Mol Physiol. 2009; 297(6):L1013–L1032.
12. Xu Y, et al. Am J Physiol. 1997; 273(1 Pt 1):L234–L245.
13. Dempsey EC, et al. J Cell Physiol. 1994; 160(3):469–481.
14. Das M, et al. Am J Physiol. 1995; 269(5 Pt 1):L660–L667.
15. Stenmark KR, et al. Physiology (Bethesda). 2006; 21:134–145.
16. Das M, et al. Am J Physiol Lung Cell Mol Physiol. 2002; 282(5):L976–L986.
17. Stenmark KR, et al. Circ Res. 2006; 99(7):675–691.
18. Short M, et al. Am J Physiol Cell Physiol. 2004; 286(2):C416–C425.
19. El Kasmi KC, et al. J Immunol. 2014; 193(2):597–609.
20. Stenmark KR, et al. J Appl Physiol (1985). 2015; 119(10):1164–1172.
21. Stenmark KR, et al. Chest. 2002; 122(6 Suppl):326S–334S.
22. Das M, et al. J Biol Chem. 2001; 276(19):15631–15640.
23. Jones R, et al. Ultrastruct Pathol. 2006; 30(4):267–281.
24. Frid MG, et al. Arterioscler Thromb Vasc Biol. 1999; 19(12):2884–2893.
25. Overbeek MJ, et al. Arthritis Res Ther. 2011; 13(2):R61.
26. Panzhinskiy E, et al. Cardiovasc Res. 2012; 95(3):356–365.
27. Krick S, et al. FASEB J. 2005; 19(7):857–859.
28. Luo Y, et al. Nat Commun. 2019; 10(1):3551.
29. Smith KA, et al. Am J Respir Cell Mol Biol. 2020; 63(5):652–664.
30. Hu CJ, et al. Eur Respir J. 2019; 54(6):1900378.
31. Dai Z, et al. Am J Respir Crit Care Med. 2018; 198(11):1423–1434.
32. Banks MF, et al. J Appl Physiol (1985). 2005; 98(2):732–738.
33. Humbert M, et al. Eur Respir J. 2019; 53(1):1801887.
34. Das M, et al. Cardiovasc Res. 2008; 78(3):440–448.
35. Carey DJ. Annu Rev Physiol.1991; 53:161177.
36. Hamati HF, et al. J Cell Biol. 1989; 108(6):2495–2505.
37. Scott-Burden T, et al. J Cell Physiol. 1989; 141(2):267–274.
38. Durmowicz AG, et al. Am J Pathol. 1994; 145(6):1411–1420.
39. Stenmark KR, et al. J Clin Invest. 1994; 93(3):1234–1242.
40. Prosser IW, et al. Am J Pathol. 1989; 135(5):1073–1088.
41. Stenmark KR, et al. Annu Rev Physiol. 1997; 59:89–144.
42. Parks WC, et al. Dev Biol. 1988; 129(2):555–564.
43. Barrett AS, et al. J Proteome Res. 2017; 16(11):4177–4184.
44. Calle EA, et al. Acta Biomater. 2016; 46:91–100.
45. Goddard ET, et al. Int J Biochem Cell Biol. 2016; 81(Pt A):223–232.

46. Frid MG, et al. Glob Cardiol Sci Pract. 2020; 2020(1):e202001.
47. Tuder RM, et al. Am J Physiol Lung Cell Mol Physiol. 2020; 318(6):L1131–L1137.
48. Hansmann G. J Am Coll Cardiol. 2017; 69(20):2551–2569.
49. Li M, et al. J Immunol. 2011; 187(5):2711–2722.
50. Tuder RM, et al. J Am Coll Cardiol. 2013; 62(25 Suppl):D4–D12.
51. Rabinovitch M, et al. Circ Res. 2014; 115(1):165–175.
52. Baker CD, et al. Pediatr Allergy Immunol Pulmonol. 2014; 27(1):8–16.
53. Steinhorn RH. Pediatr Crit Care Med. 2010; 11(2 Suppl):S79–S84.
54. D'Alessandro A, et al. Antioxid Redox Signal. 2018; 28(3):230–250.
55. Li M, et al. Circulation. 2016; 134(15):1105–1121.
56. Plecita-Hlavata L, et al. Am J Respir Cell Mol Biol. 2016; 55(1):47–57.
57. Zhang H, et al. Circulation. 2017; 136(25):2468–2485.
58. Zhao L, et al. Circulation. 2013; 128(11):1214–1224.
59. Li M, et al. Front Immunol. 2021; 12:640718.
60. Gut P, et al. Nature. 2013; 502(7472):489–498.
61. Zhao L, et al. Circulation. 2012; 126(4):455–467.
62. Hu CJ, et al. J Physiol. 2019; 597(4):1103–1119.
63. Meloche J, et al. Circ Res. 2015; 117(6):525–535.
64. Meloche J, et al. Arterioscler Thromb Vasc Biol. 2017; 37(8):1513–1523.
65. Vonk Noordegraaf A, et al. Eur Respir J. 2019; 53(1):1801900.
66. Ryan JJ, et al. Circ Res. 2014; 115(1):176–188.
67. Crystal GJ, et al. Anesthesiology. 2018; 128(1):202–218.
68. Bogaard HJ, et al. Circulation. 2009; 120(20):1951–1960.
69. Graham BB, et al. Am J Respir Cell Mol Biol. 2018; 59(4):479–489.
70. Tomanek RJ, et al. Mol Cell Biochem. 2004; 264(1-2):3–11.
71. Bakerman PR, et al. Am J Physiol. 1990; 258(4 Pt 1):L173–L178.
72. Durmowicz AG, et al. Am J Physiol. 1993; 265(6 Pt 2):H2175–H2183.
73. Lemler MS, et al. Am J Physiol Heart Circ Physiol. 2000; 279(3):H1365–H1376.
74. Bartels K, et al. Anesth Analg. 2016; 122(5):1280–1286.
75. Dandel M, et al. Curr Cardiol Rev. 2009; 5(2):133–148.
76. Dirkx E, et al. Biochim Biophys Acta. 2013; 1832(12):2414–2424.
77. Walker LA, et al. Am J Physiol Heart Circ Physiol. 2011; 301(3):H832–H840.
78. Bruns DR, et al. Am J Physiol Lung Cell Mol Physiol. 2015; 308(2):L158–L167.
79. Bruns DR, et al. PLoS One. 2019; 14(8):e0220573.
80. Potus F, et al. Int J Mol Sci. 2018; 19(9).
81. van der Feen DE, et al. Eur Heart J. 2017; 38(26):2034–2041.

HYPOXIA-INDUCED EPIGENETIC MECHANISMS OF PULMONARY HYPERTENSION

Kurt H. Albertine

Contents

Introduction

Epigenetics is at the intersection of genetics and the environment, and their interaction contributes to the developmental origins of adult disease (1). For this chapter, the focus is on the epigenetic component of pulmonary artery hypertension (PAH). PAH is a vascular remodeling disease that is characterized by increased pulmonary vascular resistance and elevated pulmonary artery pressure ≥25 mmHg at rest or 30 mmHg with exercise (2). Over time, remodeling of pulmonary arteries happens through changes in pulmonary artery endothelial cells and pulmonary artery smooth muscle cells. Pulmonary artery endothelial cells become dysfunctional and pulmonary artery smooth muscle cells proliferate and migrate, changes that lead to medial hypertrophy, inflammation, and thrombosis (3). The long-term consequences are right ventricular remodeling that may lead to heart failure and death.

This chapter's focus is on epigenetics because epigenetic mechanisms regulate the magnitude and timing of gene expression in a cell-specific way, and therefore the resulting transcriptomes. Epigenetics is defined as heritable changes in the genome that redirect gene expression without affecting DNA sequence (4, 5). Epigenetic regulation directs interactions among specific DNA regions, transcription factors, and transcriptional complexes (5, 6). Epigenetic changes affect chromatin packaging and accessibility. When the epigenome in cells is altered at or during a developmentally sensitive window, a new transcriptome becomes the basis of subsequent development and responses to disease progression. For this chapter, the disease progression is PAH and its long-term consequences.

Epigenetic mechanisms in the pathogenesis of PAH

Epigenetic mechanisms include DNA methylation, histone post-translational modifications, and non-coding RNAs. Each of these mechanisms participates in the pathogenesis of PAH (7). The fidelity and diversity of these mechanisms are enormous (5). Mediators of DNA and histone epigenetic modifications are parceled into three broad groups: Writers, erasers, and readers (8–11). Writers are enzymes that directly add marks to DNA or histones (e.g. DNA methyltransferases; histone acetyltransferases; histone methyltransferases). Erasers are enzymes that directly remove marks from DNA or histones (e.g. DNA demethylases, histone deacetylases, histone demethylases). Readers are proteins that have a specialized domain that recognizes specific epigenetic marks (e.g. bromodomain, chromodomain, polycomb-group proteins). These roles will be revisited throughout this chapter.

DNA methylation

DNA methylation occurs when a methyl group is added to the 5′-carbon position of a cytosine ring for which cytosines are located next to and bound to guanines through a phosphate bond called CpG dinucleotides. CpG islands are DNA regions dense in CpG dinucleotides, which are usually confined to the promoter region of genes and typically are not methylated. In contrast, other DNA regions do not have CpG islands. Instead, such regions have sparse CpG dinucleotides that frequently are methylated. CpG islands located in coding regions tend to be associated more with exons than introns. The role of CpG islands located in coding regions tends to be in alternative exon usage.

DNA methylation involves the addition of methyl group(s) by DNA methyltransferases (DNMTs). This enzyme family, highly conserved among mammals, has five members: DNMT1, DNMT2, DNMT3A, DNMT3B, and DNMT3L. DNMT1 maintains stable methylation of daughter strands of DNA along with generations. DNMT1 plays this role by interacting with hemimethylated DNA, leading to methylation of the daughter DNA strand to restore fully methylated CpG dinucleotides.

DNA methylation at CpG islands represses gene transcription in promoter regions, thereby silencing gene expression (12). Repression of gene transcription by methylated CpG sites occurs through a number of mechanisms. One mechanism is recruitment and interaction of methylated-CpG-binding proteins (MeCPs), two of which are MeCP1 and MeCP2, which silence gene expression through their transcriptional repression domains. Another mechanism is through the formation of complexes between MeCP1 or MeCP2 and other molecular players. Complex formation condenses chromatin (13). A third mechanism is through physical obstruction of binding such that transcriptional factors/complexes cannot access promoter regions of genes (14).

DNA methylation plays a role in PAH. For example, DNA methylation epigenetically diminishes mitochondrial superoxide dismutase 2 (SOD2). SOD2 expression is significantly diminished in pulmonary artery smooth muscle cells isolated from PAH patients as well as Fawn-hooded rats, the latter of which spontaneously develop PAH (15). The mechanism by which DNA methylation downregulates SOD2 involves activation of hypoxia-inducible factor 1 alpha (HIF-1α). Activation of HIF-1α increases expression of oxygen-sensitive, voltage-gated potassium channels (Kv1.5). Consequently, oxygen sensing is impaired and

DOI: 10.1201/9780367494018-21

cytoplasmic and mitochondrial redox states are diminished (16). Supporting evidence for a causal role between DNA methylation and diminished SOD2 expression followed by downstream activation of HIF-1α and expression of Kv1.5 are provided by a series of studies that tested gain versus the loss of function along this molecular pathway (15). One supporting experiment used Sprague-Dawley rats that were treated with siRNA to inhibit SOD2 expression. The treated rats developed characteristics of PAH. The same study also overexpressed SOD2 in normal pulmonary artery smooth muscle cells. Overexpression inhibited HIF-1α expression and restored normal Kv1.5 expression. Genomic bisulfite sequencing identified selective hypermethylation of CpG islands in the promoter region and an enhancer region of intron 2 of the SOD2 gene. The increase in DNA methylation level correlated with greater expression of DNMT1 and DNMT3B in Fawn-hooded rat lungs and isolated pulmonary artery smooth muscle cells. This study also used 5-aza-2′-deoxycytidine to inhibit DNA methylation, the result of which was restored expression of SOD2 and reduced proliferation, and increased apoptosis, of pulmonary artery smooth muscle cells isolated from Fawn-hooded rats. Thus, this study provides compelling evidence for a role of DNA methylation in the pathogenesis of PAH.

Epigenetic methylation status also appears to participate in heritable PAH. Participation is suggested from genomic bisulfite sequencing of peripheral blood monocytes isolated from patients with heritable PAH (17). Specifically, methylation status in the promoter region of bone morphogenetic protein receptor type 2 (BMPR2) in the isolated monocytes was hypermethylated, resulting in downregulated expression of this receptor. The potential importance of this result is that expression of BMPR2 in lung and endothelial cells increases cell proliferation and promotes the development of PAH. However, uncertainty with this study is that methylation status of BMPR2 was not assessed in lung tissue from the patient group. Uncertainty is also made by inconsistent results from other studies. For example, patients with idiopathic PAH did not have a significant difference in the methylation status of the BMPR2 gene in peripheral white blood cells compared to healthy control study subjects (18). In another study, genomic methylation status of the BMPR2 promoter region was not different between patients with PAH and control study subjects, again using peripheral white blood cells (19). Although the results of these studies are inconsistent, perhaps related to differences in patient and disease characteristics as well as analytical approaches, they suggest that the methylation status of the BMPR2 gene may be a player in the pathogenesis of PAH.

DNA demethylation occurs via DNA demethylation enzymes. For example, the enzyme ten-eleven translocation methylcytosine dioxygenase 1 (TET1) catalyzes the conversion of 5-methylcytosine (5-mC) to 5-hydroxymethylcytosine (5-hmC), initiating steps that remove methyl groups from DNA (20). DNA demethylation of a gene promoter activates transcriptional machinery, thereby enhancing gene expression, especially gene transcription of tumor suppressor genes (21). Thus, TET1 plays a homeostatic role in regulation of cell proliferation, apoptosis, and migration in cancer biology (22). Whether TET1 participates in the pathogenesis of PAH remains to be determined.

Histone post-translational modifications

Another highly conserved epigenetic mechanism for regulating gene expression is modifying histones. A core of four pairs of histone proteins (H3, H4, H2A, and H2B) is surrounded by two-plus wraps of 147 base pairs of DNA, forming the functional unit called the nucleosome. Neighboring nucleosomes are connected by short pieces of linker DNA. The nucleosome core is the globular portion of the histone proteins and from which histone proteins extend outward as N-terminal "tails." Histone tails are a site for post-translational, covalent modifications (23). The modifications made to histone protein tails are numerous, with acetylation and mono-, di-, and tri-methylation (24) being the most studied and, therefore, the focus of the following discussion. Histone acetylation and methylation occur on lysine (K) and/or arginine (R), as do deacetylation and demethylation. Nonetheless, other histone tail marks are phosphorylation, ubiquitination, glycosylation, biotinylation, ADP-ribosylation, and SUMOylation (25).

Histone acetylation is mediated by histone acetyltransferases (HATs) (8). Histone acetylation is generally associated with gene transcription by loosening chromatin (euchromatin) to increase accessibility to transcription factors and transcription complexes. Eighteen histone acetyltransferases identified in mice and humans are placed into two general classes (type A and type B), although not all HATs fit this dual classification approach (26). Type A HATs are located in the nucleus and participate in the regulation of gene expression through acetylation of histones in nucleosomes. Type A HATS contain an acetyllysine-binding domain called bromodomain. Bromodomain assists with recognition and binding (acts as a cofactor) to acetylated lysine residues on histone tails, and therefore bromodomain is referred to as an epigenetic reader. BRD4 bromodomain is upregulated in the lung and isolated pulmonary arteries and pulmonary artery smooth muscle cells of patients with PAH compared to healthy donors (27). Relevant to the topic of this chapter, inhibition of BRD4 bromodomain in rats reversed increased muscularization of intrapulmonary arteries otherwise caused by Sugen/hypoxia. Examples of type A HATs are Gcn5, p300/CBP, and TAF$_{II}$250. In contrast, type B HATs are located in the cytoplasm of cells and acetylate histones that are newly synthesized before the histones are incorporated into nucleosomes. Unlike type A HATs, type B HATs do not have bromodomains because the targets of type B HATS in the cytoplasm are not acetylated. Once acetylated, the histones are transported into the nucleus where histone deacetylases remove the acetyl groups before the histones are assembled into nucleosomes. An example of a type B HAT is Hat1 (28).

Histone deacetylation, mediated by histone deacetylases (HDACs), typically represses gene transcription by condensing chromatin (heterochromatin) to block accessibility (11). HDACs are classified into four groups: (1) Class I HDACs (HDAC 1, 2, 3, 8) are expressed in the nucleus, (2) class II HDACs (HDACs 4, 5, 6, 7, 9, 10) are expressed in the nucleus and cytoplasm, (3) class III HDACs (Sirtuins 1-7) are expressed in the nucleus, and (4) class IV (HDAC 11) is expressed both in the nucleus and cytoplasm.

HDACs play a role in PAH as well as right and left ventricular hypertrophy. HDAC 1, 4, and 5 protein abundances are significantly greater in human lung tissue that is isolated from patients with idiopathic PAH (29). Experimental animal models of PAH that used valproic acid, an HDAC inhibitor, showed that retaining histone acetylation reduced right ventricular hypertrophy (30). The latter results are supported by another study that tested efficacy of MC1568, a class IIa HDAC inhibitor, in pulmonary artery endothelial cells *in vitro* and in experimental animal models of PAH *in vivo* (31). Likewise, HDACs regulate left ventricular hypertrophy in response to a variety of stresses (32). HDAC6 also participates in pathogenesis of PAH based on increased protein abundance in the lung and distal pulmonary arteries from patients with PAH and experimental animal models that tested blockers of HDAC6 (Tubastatin A, ACY-775, or siRNA against HDAC6) (33). Another approach used to demonstrate this regulatory role is administration of trichostatin A. This HDAC inhibitor prevented cardiac hypertrophy and fibrosis, and improved ventricular function (32). Efficacy of these HDAC inhibitors is not equal; however, leading to tests of more selective HDAC inhibitors in models of PAH (34). Examples of more selective HDAC inhibitors are suberoylanilide hydroxamic acid and Vorinostat (35). Potential advantage of using selective HDAC inhibitors is minimizing potential cardiovascular side effects (31) associated with non-selective HDAC inhibitors (36).

Histone methylation is mediated by histone methyltransferases and is associated with gene repression or activation, depending on the location of amino acids that are methylated and how many methyl groups are added per amino acid, as described above and below (8). Recognition of histone methylation on lysines, arginines, and histidines is by a protein structural domain called chromodomain (chromatin organization modifier) (37). In this regard, chromodomain is a reader of histone methylation marks (9), the functional consequences of which depend on the site of interaction (docking site) (38).

Histone demethylation is mediated by histone demethylases (39). Demethylation is by amine oxidase homolog lysine demethylase 1 (KDM1) (40) and Jumonji C (JmjC)-domain-containing histone demethylases (40). A recent study showed that Jumonji AT-rich interactive domain 1B (JARID1B) expression was upregulated in pulmonary artery smooth muscle cells isolated from a rat model of PAH (41). The downstream consequence was increased proliferation and migration of the pulmonary artery smooth muscle cells.

The preceding discussion identifies the fidelity by which histone epigenetic marks are modified. What patterns of marks are associated with upregulation or downregulation of gene expression? Insights are gained by genome-wide mapping of global patterns of histone modifications through the use of chromatin immunoprecipitation combined with DNA sequencing (so-called ChIP seq) (23). Promoters tend to be enriched with histone 3, lysine 4 trimethylation (H3K4me^3). Enhancer regions also tend to be enriched with H3K4me alone or with H3K27acetylation (H3K27ac) or H3K27me^3 (42). The body of genes tends to be enriched with H3K36me^2 (or me^3), marks that are associated with transcriptional activation. Regulation of stability of the nucleosome during RNA polymerase II transit appears to be associated with H3K4me^2 (or me^3) and H3K36me^2 (or me^3) (23). Another enrichment of the promoter and body of genes is H4K20me that may function in transcriptional initiation, promoter clearance, and nucleosome stability in the body of the gene (43). H3K4 methylation, limited to the promoter and enhancer region of genes, is associated with transcriptional activity (44). H3K9 methylation, by comparison, is associated with heterochromatin and therefore repression of gene expression (10). Other repressive marks are H3K9me^2 (or me^3) and H3K27me (45). Methyl groups can be removed from H3K9, K4, and K27 by specific lysine demethylases (KDMs). Further insight about patterns of marks is gained from analyzes of the polycomb group of proteins, which maintain transcriptional repression through their role as epigenetic readers in the pathogenesis of PAH (46). The catalytic subunit (Enhancer of zeste homolog 2, EZH2) of the polycomb repressive complex 2, for example, promotes transcriptional gene silencing by trimethylation of H3K27 (H3K27me^3). Overexpression of EZH2 in a mouse model of PAH increased proliferation and migration, and

decreased apoptosis, of human pulmonary artery smooth muscle cells (47). A causal role played by EZH2 in the pathogenesis of PAH was provided by evidence that pharmacological inhibition of EZH2 prevented production of reactive oxygen species in the lung of a mouse model of PAH (48). At the epigenetic level, H3K27me^3 was decreased in the promoter region of superoxide dismutase 1 (SOD1), which repressed SOD1 transcription and therefore its expression. Other studies support a role played by H3K27me^3 in PAH, especially with respect to proliferation, apoptosis, and inflammatory response of pulmonary vascular endothelial cells (49).

Non-coding RNAs (ncRNAs)

Non-coding RNA is functional, although not translated into a protein product. NcRNAs include micro RNA (miRNA), long noncoding RNA (lncRNA), small interfering RNA (siRNA), and Piwi-interacting RNA (piRNA). This review considers only miRNA and lncRNA in the context of the pathogenesis of PAH, because of the growing body of evidence of their participation in the disease's pathogenesis.

MiRNAs are short (21–25 nucleotides) non-coding RNAs that are processed by Drosha and Dicer to produce miRNAs that in turn are loaded onto the RNA-induced silencing complex (RISC) (50). MiRNAs within the RISC complex regulate cellular processes, such as proliferation, differentiation, or apoptosis, processes that are common to the pathogenesis of PAH (51). MiRNAs bind sequence-specifically to the 3' untranslated region (3'-UTR) of target mRNAs. Binding prevents mRNA translation by either degrading mRNA or blocking ribosomal passage (52).

Transcription of miRNAs is epigenetically controlled, including by DNA methylation and histone modifications (53). Transcription of miRNAs is triggered by cellular stress, leading to activation of stress responses (54). Among the stress responses are cellular proliferation, differentiation, migration, or apoptosis. In this regard, miRNAs regulate proliferation and migration of both pulmonary artery smooth muscle cells and pulmonary artery endothelial cells. Pathways through which these miRNA regulatory roles act include hypoxia, BMPR2, peroxisome proliferator-activated receptor gamma (PPARγ), and proproliferative signaling pathways.

Hypoxia is an important stress in the pathogenesis of PAH and acts through HIF-1α. Hypoxia stimulates the expression of numerous miRNAs, including *miR-1, -9, -cluster 17/92, -21, -27a, -27b, -138, -190, -199-5p, -210, -322, -361-5p*, and *-23a* (55–57). Their upregulated expression is associated with enhanced stabilization or increased expression of HIF-1α. For example, hypoxia leads to upregulated expression of *miR-17/92* that in turn stabilizes HIF-1α, leading to proliferation of pulmonary artery smooth muscle cells (58). *MiRNA-17/92* has pleiotropic effects in that its upregulated expression also targets signaling molecules, such as BMPR2 (described earlier in this review), that enhance survival of pulmonary artery smooth muscle cells (59). Furthermore, *miR-17/92* expression is enhanced by inflammation, which activates nuclear factor kappa B (NF-kB) and its downstream signaling pathway (60).

Hypoxia also downregulates many miRNAs that normally inhibit cell proliferation and survival of pulmonary artery smooth muscle cells and fibroblasts. An example of such a downregulated miRNA is *miR-124*, which inhibits the nuclear factor of activated T cells (NFAT) and Notch-Forkhead box O3 (Notch-FoxO3) signaling pathways (61). In addition, *miR-124* is pleotropic in that it also inhibits proliferation and migration of fibroblasts (62). Another miRNA that is downregulated by hypoxia is *MiR-204*, which inhibits NFAT and proto-oncogene tyrosine-protein kinase Src (Src) pathways (63) as well as downregulates runt-related transcription factor 2 (RUNX2) and inhibits HIF-1α (64). Hypoxia also downregulates miRNAs that target the BMP/Smad (the human homolog of *Drosophila* Mad and *C. elegans* Sma) signaling pathway, including BMPR2, through *miR-17/29, –21, –20a, –135a, and –23a* (57). *MiR-322* targets other members of the pathway, such as BMPR1 and Smad5, which promote proliferation of pulmonary artery smooth muscle cells (65). *Mir-223* has pleotropic actions because when it is downregulated by hypoxia, *Mir-223*'s downstream target, poly(ADP-ribose) synthase 1 (PARP-1), is upregulated (27). Upregulation of PARP1 promotes proliferation, and reduces apoptosis, of pulmonary artery smooth muscle cells and thus contributes to the pathogenesis of PAH.

Other miRNAs target signaling pathways downstream of tyrosine kinase receptors. Examples are *miR-140-5p*, *miR-193*-3p, and *miRNA-328*, which downregulate insulin-like growth factor 1 receptor (IGF-1R) (66), *miR-424/503* and *miR-339*, which target fibroblast growth factor 2 (FGF2) and its receptors and thereby FGF signaling (67), and *miR-34a*, which targets platelet-derived growth factor receptor alpha (PDGFRA) expression (68).

Contractility of pulmonary artery smooth muscle cells is altered in PAH (69). MiRNAs that regulate contractility are *miR-143/145* and *miR-361-5p*,(56), *miR-1*, *miR-190*, and *miR-138* (55), *miR-223* (70), and *miR-429* and *miR-424-5p* (71). These miRNAs regulate smooth muscle contractility through different molecular pathways, such as Rho/*Rho*-associated protein kinase (ROCK) pathway (72), ATP-binding cassette transporter A1 (56), voltage-dependent potassium channels (55), and calcium levels (71).

Nitric oxide (NO) production also is impacted by miRNAs. NO production in pulmonary artery smooth muscle cells and pulmonary artery endothelial cells is inhibited by several miRNAs. Among these miRNAs are *miR-138*, which targets S100A1 to downregulate endothelial nitric oxide synthase (eNOS) activation (73), *miR-199a*-5p which targets SMAD3 signaling (74), and *miR-27b*, which targets PPARγ that stabilizes the eNOS/heat shock protein 90 (HSP90) complex (75).

Peroxisome proliferator-activated receptor gamma (PPARγ) downregulates several miRNAs that, when unchecked, pathologically contribute to PAH. For example, PPARγ downregulates *miR-21* and thereby prevents this miRNA from downregulating BMPR2 and other molecular players that normally inhibit proliferation, migration, and contraction of pulmonary artery smooth muscle cells and pulmonary artery endothelial cells (76). Other miRNAs that are downregulated by PPARγ are *miR-27a* and *miR-130/301* (77).

Long ncRNAs (lncRNAs) are RNA molecules that are longer than 200 nucleotides. LncRNAs do not encode functional proteins. They are classified as sense lncRNAs, antisense lncRNAs, bidirectional lncRNAs, intronic lncRNAs, and intergenic lncRNAs (78). LncRNAs have diverse functions that include signaling, sequestering regulatory proteins or miRNAs (decoys), guiding transcription activators or repressors to specific locations (guides), and scaffolding that regulates the landscape of chromatin. LncRNAs that are circular function as transcriptional regulators (79).

Hypoxia upregulates or downregulates the expression of lncRNAs. Hypoxia upregulates the expression of lncRNAs in the lungs of patients with PAH. An upregulated lncRNA is *MALAT1*,

the consequence of which is the proliferation of pulmonary artery smooth muscle cells (80). Another upregulated lncRNA is *H19*. This lncRNA enhances the expression of angiotensin II type I receptor (AT1R) that leads to the proliferation of pulmonary artery smooth muscle cells (81). A similar outcome follows hypoxic upregulation of lncRNA *UCA1* (urothelial carcinoma-associated-1) (82), the HoxA gene cluster-lncRNA *Hoxaas3* (83), and lncRNA *PAXIP1-AS1* (84). Hypoxia also downregulates lncRNAs in the lung of patients with PAH. LncRNAs that are downregulated in this regard include *MEG3* (85), *lncRNA-p21* (86), *TCONS_00034812* (87), and *CASC2* (88). Downregulation leads to increased proliferation and cell cycle progression, and decreased apoptosis of pulmonary artery smooth muscle cells.

Summary

Epigenetic modifications participate in the pathogenesis of PAH. Epigenetic modifications act at transcriptional and post-transcriptional levels, thereby regulating gene expression. Evidence presented in this article shows that DNA methylation, histone post-translational modifications, and ncRNAs are important players in the pathogenesis of PAH or the prevention of PAH. However, no effective treatment for PAH exists. In this regard, exciting epigenetic-based therapies are being developed for cancers (89). Because PAH shares common pathological processes of increased cell proliferation and cell cycling, enhanced cell migration, and decreased cell apoptosis with cancer biology, innovative treatment opportunities may become possible to intervene in patients who would otherwise develop persistent PAH and its long-term consequence of right ventricle hypertrophy and ultimately dysfunction and failure. However, important gaps in the field remain. One gap for potential efficacy is the dearth of long-term physiological outcomes in large-animal models to correlate early-life events leading to PAH and its treatment with functional and structural outcomes later in life. Another gap is sex as a biological variable in the pathogenesis and treatment of PAH, especially its long-term outcomes. A caveat is that the field is advancing quickly, so new processes and molecular players are coming into focus, which are not included in this chapter. Although these and other important gaps in knowledge exist, the field has the exciting prospect of innovative studies to come that will test efficacy, in the context of PAH, of new therapeutics that are currently in clinical trials for cancer.

References

1. Barker DJ, et al. Lancet. 1986; 1(8489):1077–1081.
2. Barst RJ, et al. J Am Coll Cardiol. 2004; 43(12 Suppl S):40S–47S.
3. Stenmark KR, et al. Cardiovasc Res. 2018; 114(4):551–564.
4. Handy DE, et al. Circulation. 2011; 123(19):2145–2156.
5. Joss-Moore LA, et al. Biochem Cell Biol. 2014; 93(2):119–127.
6. Voss TC, et al. Nat Rev Genet. 2014; 15(2):69–81.
7. Bisserier M, et al. Vasc Biol. 2020; 2(1):R17–R34.
8. Marmorstein R, et al. Cold Spring Harb Perspect Biol. 2014; 6(7):a018762.
9. Hyun K, et al. Exp Mol Med. 2017; 49(4):e324.
10. Zhang T, et al. EMBO Rep. 2015; 16(11):1467–1481.
11. Seto E, et al. Cold Spring Harb Perspect Biol. 2014; 6(4):a018713.
12. Miranda TB, et al. J Cell Physiol. 2007; 213(2):384–390.
13. Clouaire T, et al. Cell Mol Life Sci. 2008; 65(10):1509–1522.
14. Medvedeva YA, et al. BMC Genomics. 2014; 15:119.
15. Archer SL, et al. Circulation. 2010; 121(24):2661–2671.
16. Bonnet S, et al. Circulation. 2006; 113(22):2630–2641.
17. Liu D, et al. Am J Respir Crit Care Med. 2017; 196(7):925–928.
18. Viales RR, et al. PLoS One. 2015; 10(7):e0133042.
19. Pousada G, et al. Arch Bronconeumol. 2016; 52(6):293–298.
20. Rasmussen KD, et al. Genes Dev. 2016; 30(7):733–750.
21. Tsai YP, et al. Genome Biol. 2014; 15(12):513.

22. Good CR, et al. Cancer Res. 2018; 78(15):4126–4137.
23. Zentner GE, et al. Nat Struct Mol Biol. 2013; 20(3):259–266.
24. Yun M, et al. Cell Res. 2011; 21(4):564–578.
25. Bannister AJ, et al. Cell Res. 2011; 21(3):381–395.
26. Wapenaar H, et al. Clin Epigenetics. 2016; 8:59.
27. Meloche J, et al. Am J Physiol Cell Physiol. 2015; 309(6):C363–C372.
28. Roth SY, et al. Annu Rev Biochem. 2001; 70:81–120.
29. Zhao L, et al. Circulation. 2012; 126(4):455–467.
30. Cho YK, et al. Circ J. 2010; 74(4):760–770.
31. Kim J, et al. Circulation. 2015; 131(2):190–199.
32. Xie M, et al. Trends Cardiovasc Med. 2013; 23(6):229–235.
33. Boucherat O, et al. Sci Rep. 2017; 7(1):4546.
34. Cavasin MA, et al. Circ Res. 2012; 110(5):739–748.
35. Zhao L, et al. Circulation. 2013; 127(14):e540.
36. Whittaker SJ, et al. J Clin Oncol. 2010; 28(29):4485–4491.
37. Messmer S, et al. Genes Dev. 1992; 6(7):1241–1254.
38. Lee Y, et al. Nucleic Acids Res. 2017; 45(12):7180–7190.
39. Greer EL, et al. Nat Rev Genet. 2012; 13(5):343–357.
40. D'Oto A, et al. J Med Oncol Ther. 2016; 1(2):34–40.
41. Li Y, et al. Cardiovasc Pathol. 2018; 37:8–14.
42. Zentner GE, et al. Genome Res. 2011; 21(8):1273–1283.
43. Smolle M, et al. Biochim Biophys Acta. 2013; 1829(1):84–97.
44. Cheng J, et al. Mol Cell. 2014; 53(6):979–992.
45. Aranda S, et al. Sci Adv. 2015; 1(11):e1500737.
46. Grossniklaus U, et al. Cold Spring Harb Perspect Biol. 2014; 6(11):a019331.
47. Aljubran SA, et al. PLoS One. 2012; 7(5):e37712.
48. Shi ZL, et al. Can Respir J. 2018; 2018:9174926.
49. Yu L, et al. Sci Rep. 2017; 7(1):191.
50. Filipowicz W, et al. Nat Rev Genet. 2008; 9(2):102–114.
51. Babashah S, et al. Eur J Cancer. 2011; 47(8):1127–1137.
52. Dogini DB, et al. Genet Mol Biol. 2014; 37(1 Suppl):285–293.
53. Dakhlallah D, et al. Am J Respir Crit Care Med. 2013; 187(4):397–405.
54. Emde A, et al. EMBO J. 2014; 33(13):1428–1437.
55. Mondejar-Parreno G, et al. J Physiol. 2019; 597(4):1185–1197.
56. Zhang X, et al. Exp Cell Res. 2018; 363(2):255–261.
57. Zhang Y, et al. Biomed Pharmacother. 2018; 103:1279–1286.
58. Chen T, et al. J Am Heart Assoc. 2016; 5(12):e004510.
59. Lu Z, et al. Med Sci Monit. 2016; 22:3301–3308.
60. Yang D, et al. Int J Mol Med. 2018; 41(1):43–50.
61. Wang D, et al. Circ Res. 2014; 114(1):67–78.
62. Zhang H, et al. Circulation. 2017; 136(25):2468–2485.
63. Courboulin A, et al. J Exp Med. 2011; 208(3):535–548.
64. Ruffenach G, et al. Am J Respir Crit Care Med. 2016; 194(10):1273–1285.
65. Zeng Y, et al. Sci Rep. 2015; 5:12098.
66. Sharma S, et al. Circulation. 2014; 130(9):776–785.
67. Chen J, et al. Physiol Rep. 2017; 5(18):e13441.
68. Wang P, et al. Cell Prolif. 2016; 49(4):484–493.
69. Archer SL, et al. Circulation. 2010; 121(18):2045–2066.
70. Liu A, et al. Cell Prolif. 2019; 52(2):e12550.
71. Li C, et al. Am J Physiol Cell Physiol. 2019; 316(1):C111–C120.
72. Brozovich FV, et al. Pharmacol Rev. 2016; 68(2):476–532.
73. Sen A, et al. FEBS Lett. 2014; 588(6):906–914.
74. Liu Y, et al. Biochem Biophys Res Commun. 2016; 473(4):859–866.
75. Bi R, et al. Biochem Biophys Res Commun. 2015; 460(2):469–475.
76. Green DE, et al. PLoS One. 2015; 10(7):e0133391.
77. Bertero T, et al. J Biol Chem. 2015; 290(4):2069–2085.
78. Thum T, et al. Circ Res. 2015; 116(4):751–762.
79. Bar C, et al. Circulation. 2016; 134(19):1484–1499.
80. Fredenburgh LE, et al. Circulation. 2008; 117(16):2114–2122.
81. Su H, et al. Respir Res. 2018; 19(1):254.
82. Zhu TT, et al. Pflugers Arch. 2019; 471(2):347–355.
83. Zhang H, et al. Cardiovasc Res. 2019; 115(3):647–657.
84. Jandl K, et al. J Pathol. 2019; 247(3):357–370.
85. Zhu B, et al. Biochem Biophys Res Commun. 2018; 495(3):2125–2132.
86. Wu G, et al. Circulation. 2014; 130(17):1452–1465.
87. Liu Y, et al. J Cell Physiol. 2018; 233(6):4801–4814.
88. Gong J, et al. Respir Res. 2019; 20(1):53.
89. Ahuja N, et al. Annu Rev Med. 2016; 67:73–89.

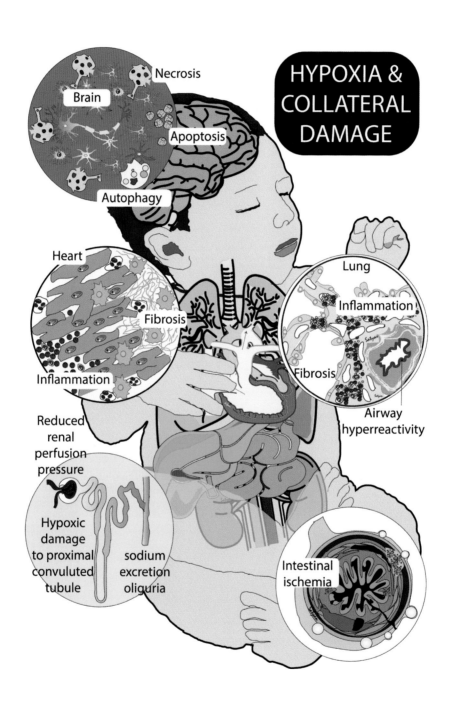

Part 4
Hypoxia and Collateral Damage

Edited by Po-Yin Cheung

THE EFFECTS OF HYPOXIA ISCHEMIA ON THE TERM BRAIN, AND A STRATEGIC APPROACH

Aravanan Anbu Chakkarapani and Nicola J. Robertson

Contents

Introduction

Intrapartum-related hypoxia-ischemia (HI) leading to neonatal encephalopathy (NE) is the second commonest preventable cause of childhood neurodisability worldwide (1) with profound psychosocial and economic consequences for families and society. The incidence of NE varies across the world, affecting 1–3.5/1000 live births in high-resource settings and ~26/1000 in low-resource settings (2). NE is a global health priority as 0.7 million affected newborns die, and 1.15 million develop NE each year (2).

Therapeutic hypothermia (HT) with intracorporeal temperature monitoring is standard care in the National Health Service, United Kingdom, and developed countries worldwide (3). Long-term follow-up has now assessed neurodevelopmental outcomes, health-related quality of life, and economic costs, confirming a persistent beneficial effect (4). With the current practice of HT, mortality due to NE has reduced from 25% in the clinical trials

DOI: 10.1201/9780367494018-22

to 9% and disability from 20% to around 16% with a reduction in the rate of cerebral palsy. However, not all children benefit from treatment, and some level of intellectual impairment may remain even in the absence of cerebral palsy (5).

Effect of hypoxia and oxidative stress in the developing brain

An enhanced understanding of neuropathology and the pathophysiology of acute brain injury in the term infant following intrapartum HI has resulted in earlier diagnosis and better localization of brain injury by using new imaging modalities and implementation of targeted neuroprotective strategies (6). The pathophysiological mechanism of HI brain injury in the term brain is an evolving process over weeks to years as shown in Figure 22.1 and neuroprotective treatments shown in Figure 22.2.

At the cellular level, three main factors combine leading to deleterious biochemical events in the primary and secondary phase of HI brain injury in term infants: (i) Regional circulatory factors (reduction in cerebral blood flow and immature cerebral autoregulation), (ii) metabolic factors (accumulation of lactate, rapid

depletion of high-energy phosphate reserves including adenosine triphosphate [ATP]), and (iii) increased regional distribution of excitatory (glutamate) synapses. Brain injury after HI evolves over hours, weeks, months, and even years; there are three main phases of injury.

Acute and latent phase

The acute or latent, or primary phase occurs within minutes of HI; the depletion of oxygen precludes oxidative phosphorylation and switches to anaerobic metabolism. Transcellular ion pump failure results in the intracellular accumulation of Na^+, Ca^{2+}, and water (cytotoxic edema) (6).

The release of excitatory neurotransmitters including glutamate, from axon terminals, occurs due to membrane depolarization. Glutamate then activates specific cell surface receptors, resulting in an influx of Na^+ and Ca^{2+} into postsynaptic neurons. The compounding effects of cellular energy failure, acidosis, glutamate release, intracellular Ca^{2+} accumulation, lipid peroxidation, and nitric oxide neurotoxicity serve to disrupt some cell's essential components with their ultimate death (primary cell death).

After resuscitation and reperfusion, the initial cytotoxic edema and accumulation of excitatory amino acids partially

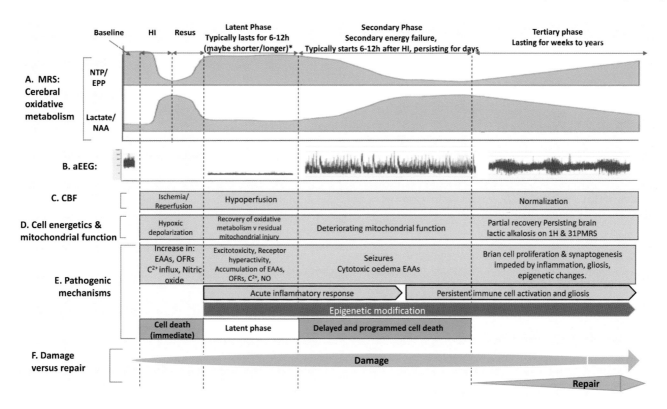

FIGURE 22.1 The evolution of injury after cerebral HI. The primary phase (acute HI), latent phase, secondary energy failure phase and tertiary brain injury phase are shown. (A) Magnetic resonance spectra showing the biphasic pattern of NTP/EPP decline and lactate/NAA increase during primary and secondary phases following the HI insult, and persisting lactic alkalosis in tertiary phase. (B) Amplitude-integrated EEG is normal at baseline; flat trace following HI, burst-suppression pattern in latent phase, emergence of seizures in secondary phase, and normalization with sleep–wake cycling in tertiary phase. (C) Latent phase includes a period of hypoperfusion associated with hypometabolism, followed by relative hypoperfusion in secondary phase. (D) Cellular energetics and mitochondrial function indicate a period of recovery in latent phase, deterioration in secondary phase, and partial recovery in tertiary phase. (E) Key pathogenic changes in each phase, including generation of toxic free radical species, accumulation of EAAs, cytotoxic edema, seizures, and inflammation. Cell lysis occurs immediately following HI, and programmed cell death occurs during the secondary phase; the latent phase is thought to represent the therapeutic window for cooling. Persisting inflammation and epigenetic changes impede long-term repair. (F) Damage is maximal in the secondary phase but persists into the tertiary phase as dysregulated inflammation and gliosis evolve. (Modified with permission from Hassell KJ, et al. Arch Dis Child Fetal Neonatal Ed. 2015;100(6):F541-52.)

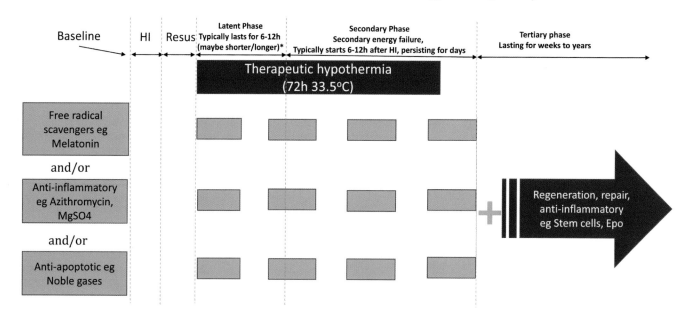

FIGURE 22.2 Future neuroprotective treatments are likely to involve a "cocktail" of therapies targeting different phases of injury. Acute therapies targeting OFR, inflammation and apoptosis should be administered as early as possible in the latent phase and through the secondary phase to target and offset evolving damage. In the tertiary phase, therapies that target regeneration, repair and inflammation are likely to be most effective. HI, hypoxia-ischemia; EAAs, excitatory amino acids; EPP, exchangeable phosphate pool; NAA, N-acetylaspartate; NO, nitric oxide; NTP, nucleoside triphosphate (this is mainly ATP); OFRs, oxygen-free radicals.

resolve, with apparent recovery of cerebral oxidative metabolism. It is believed that the endogenous inhibition of oxidative metabolism and increased tissue oxygenation happens mainly during the latent phase (7). The "therapeutic window" for HT is thought to span this period. An in-depth understanding of cerebral metabolism following HI has evolved through serial magnetic resonance spectroscopy (MRS) studies. Pre-clinical studies have shown that the latent phase duration is inversely related to insulting severity (8).

Secondary phase

The secondary phase starts with a decrease in high-energy phosphates (secondary energy failure), and evolves in parallel with on-going cellular injury. During this phase, despite adequate oxygenation and circulation in a baby undergoing intensive care, phosphocreatine (PCr) and nucleotide triphosphates fall, and inorganic phosphate (Pi) increases. Low NTP/total mobile phosphates, cerebral PCr/Pi, increased brain lactate, and an intracellular alkaline pH (pH$_i$) (9) occur during this phase; the magnitude of these changes are closely associated with subsequent neurodevelopmental outcomes (10). The onset of seizures, secondary cytotoxic edema, cytokine accumulation, and mitochondrial failure mark the secondary phase. Mitochondrial failure is a crucial step leading to delayed cell death. The degree of energy failure influences the type of neuronal death during the early and delayed stages (6).

Tertiary phase

Following on from the secondary phase, persisting dysregulation of the brain includes sensitization to inflammation or injury, increased seizure susceptibility, persistent inflammation and gliosis, impaired oligodendrocyte maturation and myelination, altered proliferation and synaptogenesis, and epigenetic alterations. This dysregulation occurs over weeks, months, and years after a hypoxic-ischemic insult

(11). Indeed, a persisting cerebral lactic alkalosis has been observed using MRS over the first year after birth in those infants with adverse neurodevelopmental outcomes (9).

Mechanisms of cell death

Cell death in the newborn brain following HI has been described as a "continuum" of necrosis, apoptosis, and autophagy. The severity of the initial insult determines the mode of cell death. If the injury is severe, it results in necrosis, while the damage is milder, resulting in apoptosis.

Necrosis

Necrosis is a passive process of lytic destruction of a single or group of cells. It starts with a cell swelling, disrupted cytoplasmic organelles, loss of membrane integrity, and eventual lysis of neuronal cells and an inflammatory process activation. The method of necrosis involves damage to the structural and functional integrity of the cell's plasma membrane and associated enzymes (e.g. Na$^+$, K$^+$ adenosine triphosphatase [ATPase]), abrupt influx and overload of ions (e.g. Na$^+$ and Ca^{2+}) and H$_2$O, and rapid mitochondrial damage and energetic collapse (12).

Apoptosis

Apoptosis is an orderly and compartmentalized dismantling of single cells or groups of cells into consumable components for nearby intact cells. It is an example of programmed cell death (PCD), termed Type I PCD. It is an ATP-driven and sometimes a gene transcription-requiring and caspase-dependent process. In contrast to necrosis, apoptosis is an active process distinguished from necrosis by the presence of cell shrinkage, nuclear pyknosis, chromatin condensation, and genomic fragmentation, events that occur in the absence of an inflammatory response. With the technical advancement of cellular and molecular biology and experimental animal studies, knowledge has been gained of the various forms of cell death in NE including apoptosis and autophagy mediated by PCD mechanisms (13).

Autophagy

Autophagy (derived from Greek *"eating of self"*) allows a cell to degrade and recycle its cytoplasm and organelles (14). Autophagy is classified as Type II PCD. A hallmark of autophagic cell death is the accumulation of autophagic vacuoles derived from lysosomes. Induced autophagy may supply energy through gluconeogenesis by protein degradation and production of an amino acid pool to maintain cellular homeostasis. However, when excess autophagy is executed, the caspase-dependent or -independent pathway of neuron death is initiated. Autophagy has a role in neurodegeneration after neonatal HI that is insult severity, time, and region-specific (15) and the development of chemical tools that prevent autophagic neuron death by specifically blocking each step of autophagy could be important.

Strategies to protect the brain

In the present era, HT is the only evidence-based treatment available for moderate to severe NE. Below, we summarize the recent network meta-analysis of HT RCTs comparing effectiveness of HT on mortality, neurodevelopmental outcome at 18 months and adverse events (16).

Therapeutic hypothermia (HT)

Currently, HT is standard care for moderate to severe NE. The optimal protocol is cooling to 33.5 ± 0.5 °C for 72 h, followed by slow rewarming 0.5 °C/h to normothermia (17). A recent network meta-analysis (where more than three treatments are compared using direct comparisons of interventions within RCTs) showed the following outcome data (16):

- *Reduction in mortality*: Whole-body cooling (Odds ratio: 0.62) (95% credible interval: 0.46–0.83); 8 trials, high certainty of evidence) was the most effective treatment, followed by selective head cooling (0.73; 0.48–1.11; 2 trials, moderate certainty of the evidence) and use of magnesium sulfate (0.79; 0.20–3.06; 2 trials, low certainty of the evidence).
- *Reduction in mortality and neurodevelopmental delay at 18 months*: Whole-body HT (0.48; 0.33–0.71; 5 trials), selective head HT (0.54; 0.32–0.89; 2 trials), and erythropoietin (Epo) (0.36; 0.19–0.66; 2 trials).
- *Reduction in cerebral palsy*: Whole-body HT (0.61; 0.45–0.83; 7 trials) and use of Epo (0.36; 0.18–0.74, 2 trials).
- *Reduction in seizures*: Whole-body HT (0.64; 0.46–0.87, 7 trials) and use of Epo (0.35; 0.13–0.94; 1 trial).

Protective mechanisms of HT

HT improves outcome through multiple pathways, with the final common pathway suppressing apoptosis and preserving neurons from further injury (18) (Figure 22.3). Recent pre-clinical and clinical trials in HT are described in Figure 22.4.

Clinical evidence

The 2013 Cochrane meta-analysis from the 11 randomized controlled trials ($N = 1505$ term and late preterm infants) showed that HT is beneficial in moderate-to-severe NE. This review concluded that HT reduces mortality without increasing significant disability in survivors. Eight of the eleven studies (1344 infants) demonstrated that HT decreased the combined outcome of death or significant neurodevelopmental disability at 18 months (46%, 312/678, vs. 61%, 409/666, in controls) (typical relative risk) (RR) 0.75, 95% confidence interval)(CI) 0.68–0.83; typical risk difference (RD) −0.15, 95% CI −0.20 to −0.10). The number needed to treat to benefit one newborn was 7 (95% CI 5–10). Eleven studies (1468 infants) supported decreased mortality with HT (25%, 186/736, vs. 34%, 250/732, in controls, RR 0.75, 95% CI 0.64–0.88) number needed to treat of 11. Eight studies (917 infants) demonstrated that HT decreases neurodevelopmental disability in surviving infants (26%, 130/495, vs. 39%, 166/422, in controls, RR 0.77, 95% CI 0.63–0.94), with a number needed to treat of 8 (19).

Long-term outcome

Long-term outcome data are currently available from 379 of the 1505 infants (25.2%) included in the Cochrane meta-analysis (19). One hundred and nine of 208 (91.3%) participants in the US National Institute of Child Health and Human Development study were assessed at 6–7 years (20). Based on this study, HT increases survival without increasing the rates of significant disability, an IQ score below 70, or cerebral palsy in surviving children. One hundred and twenty-seven of 325 infants (39%) enrolled in the European Total Body Hypothermia for NE (TOBY) trial were assessed at 6–7 years of age (21). At 6–7 years, children who had received HT (75 of 145, 52%) had a significantly higher survival with an IQ of 85 or higher than children not treated with HT (52 of 132, 39%, RR 1.31, $P = 0.04$). Follow-up of children from the Cool Cap trial reported outcomes on 62 (32 cooled, 30 controls) of 135 (46%) surviving 7–8-year-old children enrolled in the Cool Cap trial (22). Unfortunately, this follow-up study had insufficient power to determine whether treatment with HT affected long-term outcomes.

Adverse effects

Reported adverse effects of HT include sinus bradycardia, thrombocytopenia, fat necrosis, disseminated intravascular coagulopathy, and rarely pulmonary hypertension. HT has not been associated with a significant increase in the rates of major cardiac arrhythmia and hypotension or need for inotropic agents (23).

Adjunct therapies

While the effects of HT are significant, there is still an unacceptably high number of treated babies with adverse outcomes, in particular cognitive problems. Studies have shown that the current cooling protocols are optimal, and further adjustments to HT protocols (deeper and longer cooling) do not improve outcome (24, 25).

Adjunct therapies with complementary or additive effects to HT are urgently needed to improve outcomes in moderate to severe NE. In the following sections, we give an update on the current status of pre-clinical and clinical studies in a selection of promising adjunct therapies. We focus on therapies given after birth (not to the mother with fetal distress). We suggest specific therapies might be most effective when targeted at particular phases of the neurotoxic cascade (26, 27).

HT should be started as early as possible within the latent phase to optimize protection (28). Commencing HT within 6 h of birth and continuing for 72 h, spanning as much of the latent

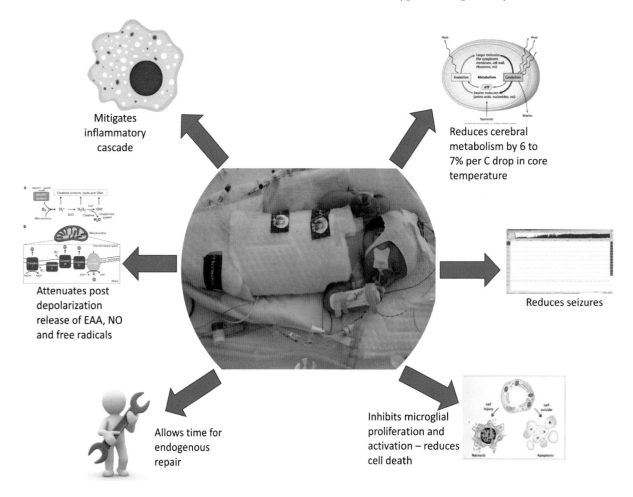

FIGURE 22.3 Multiple pathways of cooling protection.

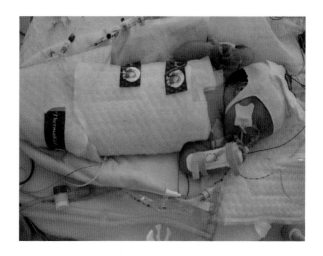

Pre-clinical studies

Cooling by 8°C for 24h leads to no protection compared to normothermia; cooling by 3.5-5.0°C is protective
(Alonso-Alconada et al., Stroke 2015)

HT >72 in the fetal sheep is deleterious on neuronal survival and microglial suppression: related to over-suppression of neuronal activity and delayed restoration of CNS microenvironment (Davidson et al., JCBFM 2015; 35:751-758; Davidson et al., Sci Rep, 2016:6:25178)

Rate of rewarming has less effect on protection than duration of HT.
Davidson et al., JCBFM: 2018; 38:1047-1059.

Clinical Trials

Cooling for 72h to 33.5°C is optimal Longer and deeper cooling deleterious
(Shankaran et al., JAMA 2017 4;318(1):57-67)

Cooling >6 and < 24h recommended, but some uncertainty in its effectiveness
(Laptook et al., JAMA 2017;318(16):1550-1560
Controversy exists (Walloe et al., Acta Pediatrica 2019 108 (7); 1190-1191

Therapeutic hypothermia induced by phase changing material (PCM) (THIN study. Aker K et al., Arch Dis Child Fetal Neonatal Ed. 2020 Jul;105(4):405-411) (Thayyil S., Arch Dis Child Fetal Neonatal Ed. 2013 May;98(3):F280-1)

FIGURE 22.4 Summary of pre-clinical studies and clinical trials. (Photograph courtesy of Mary Dinan.)

and secondary phase as possible is important, so the phase of seizures and cytotoxicity is covered. Clinical studies have shown that longer and deeper cooling is detrimental (25, 29). Pre-clinical studies have shown a U shape response to cooling; cooling by 8 °C led to no protection compared to normothermia and cooling by 3.5–5 °C provided significant protection compared to normothermia (30). HT for 48 h in the fetal sheep was less effective than 72 h cooling in the same model (31, 32), suggesting the importance of cooling duration and that clinicians should continue HT for the full 72 h, if possible. The rate of rewarming was not seen to affect protection in these fetal sheep studies (31) (Figure 22.4).

As for HT, the optimal response to some adjunct therapies is likely when they are started early in the latent phase. In the sections below, we combine the latent and secondary phases as, during these phases, adjunct therapies are likely to be co-administered with HT (Figure 22.2).

i. Acute phase and latent phase within the first 6 h after birth (latent phase typically lasts for 6–12 h, may be shorter or longer) (9):

Therapeutic hypothermia (HT), Melatonin (MEL), Magnesium Sulfate, Azithromycin (AZI), Noble gases (Xenon and Argon)

ii. Secondary phase (typically starts 6–12 h after HI and persists for days):

Continuing HT, MEL, Magnesium Sulfate, AZI, Noble gases (Xenon and Argon)

iii. Tertiary phase—lasting weeks to months:

Epo, Stem cells

Latent and secondary phase therapies

Melatonin (MEL)
Mechanisms of melatonin neuroprotection (33)

- Prevention of free radical-induced oxidative damage to the electron transport chain and mitochondrial DNA and protection against excitotoxic damage
- Down regulation of the proinflammatory transcription factor, NFκB thereby reducing neuroinflammation
- Preservation of mitochondrial integrity through stabilization and protection from nitro-oxidative damage to membrane lipids and inhibiting pro-apoptotic proteins
- Stimulation of neuronal differentiation and cell proliferation

Pre-clinical evidence
Many pre-clinical studies have shown neuroprotective benefits of MEL combined with HT. In a piglet model, compared to HT alone, intravenously administered MEL at 30 mg/kg, 10 min after HI and repeated at 24 h plus HT significantly improved cerebral energy metabolism (proton MRS), reduced cell death in deep brain and white matter, and decreased microglial activation in the cortex 48h after injury (34). *In vitro* and piglet studies suggest the therapeutic level of MEL is ~15–30 mg/L (34–36) and that MEL neuroprotection is dependent on: (i) Time taken to achieve therapeutic levels after HI and (ii) duration of exposure to therapeutic MEL levels.

Clinical evidence
Aly et al. (37) administered enteral MEL as an adjunct to HT in term NE with a total 50 mg/kg dose over 5 days, commenced within 6 h. Infants treated with MEL had reduced plasma levels

of NO and plasma superoxide dismutase after 5 days; there was also reduced white matter injury on MR, reduced seizure activity on EEG at 2 weeks and increased survival free of disability at 6 months compared with infants treated with HT. This study used the enteral route for MEL, dissolved in water. Aly et al. demonstrated a modest doubling of plasma MEL levels from baseline to day 5 with 10mg/kg/day enteral MEL (21 ± 2.4 to 42.7 ± 5.1 pg/mL ($p < 0.001$), suggesting that the intravenous route of administration is more effective in elevating plasma concentrations. Interestingly, the HT group (without enteral MEL) also showed an increase in plasma MEL from baseline to day 5 (20.6 ± 2.5 to 32.1 ± 3.5 pg/mL, $p < 0.001$), confirming an endogenous MEL response previously seen in brain injury. Larger-powered clinical studies of HT with MEL reaching therapeutic MEL levels are urgently needed.

Magnesium sulfate (MgSO$_4$)
There has been significant interest in MgSO$_4$ for perinatal neuroprotection; in many western countries, MgSO$_4$ is now standard treatment in pregnancies threatened by preterm labor at <30 weeks' gestation. Whether MgSO$_4$ is a safe and effective adjunct therapy postnatally with HT for term babies with moderate to severe NE is still unclear.

Mechanisms of magnesium sulfate neuroprotection

- Competitively antagonizes calcium ion entry within the NMDA channel
- Reduction in secondary inflammation and associated injury
- Stabilization of cell membranes
- Inhibition of free radical production
- Improved cardiovascular stability

Pre-clinical evidence
A recent systematic review of pre-clinical and clinical studies over the last 10 years (38), suggested that further pre-clinical testing is needed to determine possible differential effects of MgSO$_4$ in males and females, whether there is a specific effect of MgSO$_4$ on oligodendrocytes, and long-term effects on functional outcomes to ensure safety and to identify the optimal regimens for neuroprotection.

A recent pre-clinical piglet study comparing HT to a MgSO$_4$ bolus and constant infusion with HT was well tolerated (no hypotension) and doubled serum magnesium (0.72 vs. 1.52 mmol/L) with a modest (16%) rise in CSF magnesium. In the Mg + HT group compared to HT alone, there was overall reduced cell death and increased oligodendrocyte survival but no improvement on aEEG recovery or MRS (39). The small incremental benefit of Mg + HT compared to HT on aEEG, MRS, and regional cell death are unlikely to translate into a substantive improvement in clinical trials. Hypotension, is a common side effect of MgSO$_4$ and has previously been observed following repeated boluses of MgSO$_4$ in normothermic piglets. Given the physiological effects of HT and cardiovascular depression associated with HI, severe hypotension is a significant concern with combination therapy.

Clinical evidence
The Mag Cool study reported a favorable safety profile of MgSO$_4$ boluses with HT; however, hypotension was only broadly classified as either moderate (volume therapy and/or one inotrope) or severe (multiple inotropes) and did not report cardiovascular parameters immediately following drug administration (40). A (41) systematic review and metanalysis from 5 RCTs ($n = 182$ babies) reported no difference in the composite outcome

of moderate to severe neurodevelopmental disability at 18 months or death (RR 0.81, 95% CI 0.36 to 1.84), seizures (RR 0.84, 95% CI 0.59 to 1.19), mortality (RR 1.39, 95% CI 0.85 to 2.27), or hypotension (RR 1.28, 95% CI 0.69 to 2.38). There was a reduction noted in the unfavorable short-term composite outcome (RR 0.48, 95% CI 0.30 to 0.77) between the $MgSO_4$ and the control groups, however, the trend toward an increase in mortality in the $MgSO_4$ group was a major clinical concern.

Azithromycin
AZI (9-deoxy-9a-aza-9a-methyl-9a homoerythromycin) is a macrolide antibiotic.

Mechanisms of azithromycin neuroprotection
- Promotes anti-inflammatory phenotype expression in macrophages (termed M2 phenotype). Neuroprotective properties are thought to be mediated by promotion of microglial and/or monocyte anti-inflammatory and healing phenotype. Amantea et al. demonstrated that pharmacological inhibition of peripheral arginase (a change associated with shift of macrophages to M2 phenotype) prevented protection from AZI (42).

Pre-clinical evidence
AZI has become the macrolide of choice with a better safety profile than erythromycin. Administration is *IV in humans and large animal models; intraperitoneal injection in P7 rats* (43). Protection is dose-dependent (1.5–150 mg/kg) with a therapeutic window of up to 4.5 h. In a P7 rat Rice Vannucci model, multiple treatment protocols were evaluated (doses ranging from 15 to 45 mg/kg; treatment onset 15 min to 4 h after HI, and comparison of 1 vs. 3 injections) (43). All AZI doses improved function and reduced brain damage; efficacy was dose-dependent and declined with increasing treatment delay. Three AZI injections, administered over 48 h, improved performance on both functional measures and reduced brain damage more than a single dose (43). There is currently no data on AZI combined with HT and this needs to be assessed in pre-clinical models.

Clinical evidence
AZI has an established safety profile and a clinical trial of AZI to prevent BPD (the AZTEC trial https://aztec-trial.uk (HTA Project: 16/111/106) (ISRCTN11650227) is underway. Promising preclinical studies could quickly lead to clinical trials evaluating AZI as an adjunct to HT (26).

Noble gases (xenon and argon)
Xenon is a rare noble gas (44) and inhalation anesthetic agent. In neonatal rat and piglet studies, the combination of Xenon with cooling provided neuroprotection while neither intervention alone was as effective. Argon has shown promise as an adjunct to HT in a piglet model of NE with its neuroprotective qualities (45). Argon is more abundant than xenon. It is economical and more practical to use clinically. As yet, there are no clinical trials using argon in NE.

Mechanisms of xenon and argon neuroprotection
- Triggering gamma-aminobutyric acid (GABA) neurotransmission
- Anti-apoptotic signaling (both Argon and Xenon)
- Argon does not appear to influence NMDA receptors or potassium channels (46), which are two important mechanisms of Xenon and hypothermic protection

Clinical evidence
A recent Cochrane review (47) reported one study – the TOBY-Xe study (48), $n = 92$ infants, between 36 and 43 weeks of gestational age, 46 of whom were randomly assigned to HT only and 46 to 24 h 30% inhaled xenon plus HT. There was no evidence of short-term benefit based on the surrogate outcome measure 1H MRS Lac/NAA peak area ratio acquired from the basal ganglia and thalamus (48), confirmed subsequently at 2 years (49). This was a difficult study with the mean age of starting xenon 10 h after birth (a timing likely to be beyond the therapeutic window for xenon's action on the NMDA receptor release of glutamate). The Cochrane analysis concluded that data is inadequate to show that cooling plus xenon is safe or effective in the near term and term infants with NE. Xenon's major disadvantage is that it is difficult to use in clinical practice due to its scarcity (0.0087 ppm in the air) and high costs, along with the need for closed-circuit delivery (including cuffed tubes) and recycling systems.

Tertiary phase therapies

Erythropoietin (EPO)
EPO is a hemopoietic growth factor and pleiotropic cytokine (50). EPO can be administered intravenously or subcutaneously. It requires small volumes, so it does not impose a fluid burden.

Mechanisms of EPO neuroprotection (33)
- Prevents the secondary delayed rise in IL-1β and attenuates infiltration of leukocytes
- Activates Jak2 kinase leading to NFkB and Stat5 mobilization into the nucleus and gene expression of the antiapoptotic factors, bcl and bcl-xl (51). Reduces the expression of Fas/FasL which are part of the extrinsic apoptotic pathway (52)
- Increases glutathione peroxidase enzyme activity and decreases lipid peroxidation levels
- Inhibits the transcription of iNOS mRNA responsible for NO production and oxidative stress

Pre-clinical evidence
Recombinant human erythropoietin (rEPO) is neuroprotective in immature animals. In a recent near-term fetal sheep study, HT and rEPO independently improved neuronal survival, with greater improvement with HT. There was no improvement in any outcome after combined rEPO and HT compared with HT alone. It was concerning that the combination was associated with increased numbers of cortical caspase-3-positive cells compared with HT. These data suggest that the mechanisms of neuroprotection with HT and rEPO overlap and, thus, high-dose rEPO infusion does not appear to be an effective adjunct therapy for HT (53).

Clinical evidence
A recent systematic review and metanalysis by Razak et al. (54). from six RCTs (EPO = 5 and darbepoetin α = 1) ($n = 454$ neonates) concluded that EPO administration in neonates with NE reduces the risk of brain injury, cerebral palsy, and cognitive impairment. The results of the meta-analysis are:

i. EPO with or without HT: Five RCTs, 368 participants, RR 0.74, 95% CI 0.47–1.19, Level of evidence: Low
ii. EPO without HT: Four RCTs, 318 participants, RR 0.89, 95% CI 0.49–1.32, Level of evidence: Low
iii. Cerebral palsy risk reduced with EPO treatment without HT compared to placebo (two RCTs, 230 participants, RR 0.47, 95% CI 0.27–0.80), Level of evidence: Moderate

iv. Moderate to severe cognitive impairment risk reduced with EPO treatment without HT compared to placebo (two RCTs, 226 participants, RR 0.49, 95% CI 0.28−0.85), Level of evidence: Moderate

v. Brain injury risk reduced in EPO-treated infants (EPO with or without HT, two RCTs, 148 participants, RR 0.70, 95% CI 0.53−0.92), Level of evidence: Moderate

Wu and colleagues demonstrated that EPO treatment was associated with less MRI brain injury only in patients whose placentas exhibited no chronic histologic changes (55). The High Dose Erythropoietin for Asphyxia and Encephalopathy (HEAL) Trial (NCT02811263) will evaluate whether high-dose EPO reduces the combined outcome of death or neurodevelopmental disability when given in conjunction with HT to newborns with moderate/severe HIE (56). The HEAL trial is currently recruiting participants ($n = 501$) and estimated study completion in September 2022. Preventing Adverse Outcomes of Neonatal Hypoxic Ischaemic Encephalopathy With Erythropoietin (PAEAN trial) (NCT03079167) is also recruiting participants ($n = 300$); estimated study completion is December 2021.

Stem cell therapies
Stem cell therapy is emerging as a safe and promising therapy for neonatal diseases and clinical trials are completed or underway for NE (autologous umbilical cord cells intravenously, NCT00593242), perinatal arterial ischemic stroke (50 million allogenic bone marrow derived MSC intranasally; NCT03356821) and bronchopulmonary dysplasia (30 million huMSC/kg intratracheally; NCT03558334) (57).

Mesenchymal stromal cells (MSC) are attractive because of their low immunogenicity, self-renewing capacity, multi-lineage differentiation and secretome; human umbilical MSC (huMSC) have superior anti-inflammatory effects compared to adult MSC (58) and, as the neonatal brain is still in a developmentally active and plastic phase, MSC appear more efficient. It is understood that MSCs exert their action mainly by cell-to-cell communication through paracrine secretion of extra-cellular vesicles (EVs) that trigger reparative, anti-inflammatory, angiogenic and anti-apoptotic processes. Their multi-pathway action is a potential powerful paradigm shift for the treatment of NE.

Pre-clinical rodent studies of birth asphyxia have shown significant protection with MSCs given intracranially. As this route is not clinically translatable and the intravenous route may dilute cell delivery to the brain, the intranasal route is an attractive option for cell delivery. Intranasally administered stem cells cross the olfactory epithelium, enter a space adjacent to the periosteum of the turbinate bones, and then enter the subarachnoid space via extensions crossing the cribriform plate (59). Intranasal MSC treatment at 10 days after HI in d9 neonatal mice led to significant lesion volume reduction and improved behavioral and motor outcomes. Using fluorescence microscopy with PKH26-labelled MSC and MRI to study the kinetics of the cells, MSCs were observed to reach the lesion site within 2 h after intranasal administration and "home" to the area of injury, peaking by 12 h. EVs have been identified recently as the key mediators of stem cell signaling; EVs are naturally occurring membrane-surrounded vesicles and are released into the extracellular environment (60). The most prominent EV types are exosomes, derivatives of the late endosomal compartment (70−150 nm), and microvesicles, released from plasma membrane (100−1000 nm). Both contain specific cargo combinations of lipids, RNA, cell-adhesion molecules, cytokines, and other proteins. They mediate intercellular communication processes and transmit tailored information to specific target cells (61).

Mesenchymal stromal cells (MSC) with HT
Augmentation of HT with transplanted intraventricular MSC has been observed in P7 rats following HI, with cooling and cell transplantation started at 6 h after HI. Augmented protection was based on reduced infarct volume, TUNEL positive cells, CSF cytokine levels and improved behaviural tests. The same group showed that even if MSC transplantation was delayed to 2 days after HI, robust synergy between cooling and MSC persists (62). However, a study in P9 mice with 4 h HT after HI and MSC administered intranasally at P12 showed exacerbation of brain injury with higher pro-inflammatory cytokine levels (63).

In a piglet study of perinatal HI, compared to HT alone, IN administration of 30 million huMSC (15 million/nostril) at 24 and 48 h after HI with HT led to (i) Improved recovery of aEEG over 48 h; (ii) improved brain energy metabolism on MRS; (iii) reduced white matter injury (TUNEL positive cells). There was no effect of intravenous administration of the same number of cells. huMSC were seen to be present at 12 h after IN administration using fluorescent labeling (64).

Clinical evidence
A recent Cochrane review (65) concluded that there is currently no evidence from randomized trials of benefit or harm of stem cell-based interventions to prevent morbidity and mortality in NE.

Combination therapies targeting different phases of the neurotoxic Cascade

Stem cells and Epo have actions that extend into the tertiary phase and thus may prove to be complementary to HT (27). Combination studies are needed where acute acting agents that target the early phase of injury (MEL, MgSO$_4$, AZI, or Noble gases) are given within 1−2 h at the initiation of cooling and long-term acting agents targeting regeneration and repair are given after rewarming (from 80 h onwards) (Epo, Stem cells). For these studies, longer term pre-clinical survival models are needed.

Recently, a pre-clinical piglet study assessed effects of 12 h HT &MEL, 12 h HT & EPO and combined 12 h HT, MEL & EPO (66) MEL and EPO were safe when administered with HT and had complementary effects on brain protection. HT+MEL *double therapy* showed modest but consistent beneficial effects across aEEG, Lac/NAA and immunohistochemistry; in future studies, an increase in the MEL dose to 30 mg/kg/24 h may increase exposure to therapeutic levels and further improve protection. HT + EPO *double therapy* had most effect on oligodendrocyte survival; this concurs with EPO's effect on regeneration, and indicates longer term studies are needed to assess its full potential. HT + MEL + EPO *triple therapy* did not augment brain protection further from that seen with *double therapies*. The data suggested that staggering the administration of therapies with early MEL and later EPO (after HT) may provide better protection; each therapy has complementary actions, which may be time-critical during the neurotoxic cascade after HI (66).

Nonomura et al. (67) reported on the feasibility of combination therapy with 300 U/kg EPO every other day for 2 weeks, 250 mg/kg magnesium sulfate for three days, and HT in NE; efficacy data are awaited.

Conclusion

Neurodevelopmental outcomes for babies with moderate to severe NE have improved with HT; the severity as well as the incidence of CP has reduced overall. However, adverse outcomes especially cognitive problems persist. Fine-tuning neuroprotection above that from HT will require targeted therapies in the acute and subacute (latent and secondary), and chronic (tertiary) phase. Understanding the events in each phase and targeting the right therapy for each phase will require collaboration across laboratories and preclinical models and across the clinical specialties of neonatology, pediatric neurology and developmental pediatrics. "Neuroprotection" can continue past the neonatal period into the tertiary phase. Clinically relevant surrogate outcome measures are needed to speed up therapies.

References

1. Lawn JE, et al. Lancet. 2014; 384(9938):189–205.
2. Lee AC, et al. Pediatr Res. 2013; 74:50–72.
3. NICE. Therapeutic hypothermia with intracorporeal temperature monitoring for hypoxic perinatal brain injury [IPG347]. 2010. https://www.nice.org.uk/guidance/ipg347.
4. Marlow N, et al. Pediatr Res. 2019; 86(5):567–572.
5. Jary S, et al. Acta Paediatr. 2015; 104(12):1241–1247.
6. Shalak L, et al. Early Hum Dev. 2004; 80(2):125–141.
7. Jensen EC, et al. J Physiol. 2006; 572(Pt 1):131–139.
8. Iwata O, et al. Brain Res. 2007; 1154:173–180.
9. Robertson NJ, et al. Ann Neurol. 2002; 52(6):732–742.
10. Mitra S, et al. Arch Dis Child Fetal Neonatal Ed. 2019; 104(4):F424–F32.
11. Fleiss B, et al. Lancet Neurol. 2012; 11(6):556–566.
12. Golden WC, et al. Brain Res Mol Brain Res. 2001; 88(1-2):94–102.
13. Northington FJ, et al. Ann Neurol. 2011; 69(5):743–758.
14. Klionsky DJ, et al. Science. 2000; 290(5497):1717–1721.
15. Koike M, et al. Am J Pathol. 2008; 172(2):454–469.
16. Lee CYZ, et al. Front Pharmacol. 2019; 10:1221.
17. Shankaran S. Curr Treat Options Neurol. 2012; 14(6):608–619.
18. Goswami I, et al. Semin Neurol. 2020; 40(3):322–334.
19. Jacobs SE, et al. Cochrane Database Syst Rev. 2013(1):CD003311.
20. Shankaran S, et al. N Engl J Med. 2012; 366(22):2085–2092.
21. Azzopardi D, et al. N Engl J Med. 2014; 371(2):140–149.
22. Guillet R, et al. Pediatr Res. 2012; 71(2):205–209.
23. Jull SE, et al. In *Avery's disease of the newborn*, 10th ed. Gleason C, Jull S, eds. Elsevier, 2017. pp. 910.e6–921.e6
24. Shankaran S, et al. JAMA. 2014; 312(24):2629–2639.
25. Shankaran S, et al. JAMA. 2017; 318(1):57–67.
26. Nair J, et al. Children (Basel). 2018; 5(7):99.
27. Robertson NJ, et al. J Pediatr. 2012; 160(4):544.e4–552.e4.
28. Thoresen M, et al. Neonatology. 2013; 104(3):228–233.
29. Laptook AR, et al. JAMA. 2017; 318(16):1550–1560.
30. Alonso-Alconada D, et al. Stroke. 2015; 46(1):275–278.
31. Davidson JO, et al. J Cereb Blood Flow Metab. 2018; 38(6):1047–1059.
32. Davidson JO, et al. J Cereb Blood Flow Metab. 2015; 35(5):751–758.
33. Wu Q, et al. Drug Discov Today. 2015; 20(11):1372–1381.
34. Robertson NJ, et al. Brain. 2013; 136(Pt 1):90–105.
35. Robertson NJ, et al. Sci Rep. 2020; 10(1):3898.
36. Robertson NJ, et al. Neurobiol Dis. 2019; 121:240–251.
37. Aly H, et al. J Perinatol. 2015; 35(3):186–191.
38. Galinsky R, et al. Front Neurol. 2020; 11:449.
39. Lingam I, et al. Pediatr Res. 2019; 86(6):699–708.
40. Rahman SU, et al. J Clin Neonatol. 2015; 4:158–163.
41. Tagin M, et al. J Perinatol. 2013; 33(9):663–669.
42. Amantea D, et al. Front Neurosci. 2019; 13:1256.
43. Barks JDE, et al. Pediatr Res. 2019; 86(4):444–451.
44. Maze M, et al. Mol Neurobiol. 2020; 57(1):118–124.
45. Broad KD, et al. Neurobiol Dis. 2016; 87:29–38.
46. Brucken A, et al. Resuscitation. 2014; 85(6):826–832.
47. Ruegger CM, et al. Cochrane Database Syst Rev. 2018; 8:CD012753.
48. Azzopardi D, et al. Lancet Neurol. 2016; 15(2):145–153.
49. Azzopardi D, et al. EBioMedicine. 2019; 47:484–491.
50. Hassell KJ, et al. Arch Dis Child Fetal Neonatal Ed. 2015; 100(6):F541–F552.
51. Juul SE, et al. Clin Perinatol. 2015; 42(3):469–481.
52. Huang R, et al. Neuroreport. 2019; 30(4):262–268.
53. Wassink G, et al. J Physiol. 2020; 598(5):999–1015.
54. Razak A, et al. J Perinat Med. 2019; 47(4):478–489.
55. Wu YW, et al. Pediatr Res. 2020; 87(5):879–884.
56. Juul SE, et al. Neonatology. 2018; 113(4):331–338.
57. Nitkin CR, et al. Pediatr Res. 2020; 87(2):265–276.
58. Islam MN, et al. Stem Cell Res Ther. 2019; 10(1):329.
59. Galeano C, et al. Cell Transplant. 2018; 27(3):501–514.
60. Vogel A, et al. EBioMedicine. 2018; 38:273–282.
61. Ludwig AK, et al. Int J Biochem Cell Biol. 2012; 44(1):11–15.
62. Ahn SY, et al. Sci Rep. 2018; 8(1):7665.
63. Herz J, et al. Brain Behav Immun. 2018; 70:118–130.
64. Robertson NJ, et al. Cytotherapy. 2020; S1465-3249(20)30930-0.
65. Bruschettini M, et al. Cochrane Database Syst Rev. 2020; 8:CD013202.
66. Pang R, et al. Brain Communications. 2020; 3(1):fcaa211.
67. Nonomura M, et al. BMC Pediatr. 2019; 19(1):13.

EFFECTS OF HYPOXIA ON CEREBRAL PERFUSION AND THE BLOOD-BRAIN BARRIER

Divyen K. Shah, W. L. Amelia Lee, David F. Wertheim and Stephen T. Kempley

Contents

Introduction

A normal birth produces a change from the relatively hypoxic intrauterine state of the fetus, to the better-oxygenated condition of the healthy newborn baby. Cerebral artery blood flow velocity is substantially reduced after birth but increases thereafter in healthy term infants. Oxygen delivery to the brain is prioritized as it is sensitive to hypoxic damage particularly around the time of birth. Reductions in cerebral oxygen delivery occur when hypoxia is severe, particularly when it is combined with brain ischemia. If the redistributory response is inadequate or if reductions in cardiac output are severe or repeated, then a combination of reduced brain blood flow and hypoxia may lead to brain injury.

This review also examines the relationship between hypoxic-ischemic encephalopathy (HIE) and the disruption of the blood-brain barrier (BBB). The extent of injury noted in HIE is not only determined by the biochemical cascades that trigger the apoptosis-necrosis continuum of cell death in the brain parenchyma but also by the breaching of the BBB by proinflammatory factors. The role of factors such as HIF-1α and VEGF are also explored.

Finally, the potential role of neurophysiology, near-infrared spectroscopy, cerebral magnetic resonance imaging (MRI), and blood biomarkers as tools for assessing neuronal injury are considered.

Cerebral perfusion during normal circulatory transition and following perinatal hypoxia-ischemia

Cerebral perfusion during normal circulatory transition

Cerebral oxygen delivery is prioritized to protect a vital organ, which is more sensitive to hypoxic damage than other human structures, particularly around the time of birth. Cerebral oxygen delivery is determined by cerebral blood flow and blood oxygen content. Before the onset of labor, the circulation responds to fetal hypoxia through circulatory redistribution, increasing cerebral blood flow (1) at the expense of blood flow to the viscera and placenta.

Normal labor and delivery result in a series of challenges to both cerebral oxygenation and perfusion. Uterine contractions increase intrauterine pressure, producing intermittent reductions in placental perfusion (2) and fetal oxygen saturation (3). In response to this stress, blood flow is centralized (4) to favor the brain, and there is an increase in circulating catecholamines (5).

In the minutes after birth, with aeration of the lungs, a complex set of circulatory changes take place including reduced pulmonary vascular resistance, increased systemic vascular resistance, and reversal in the direction of shunting through the ductus arteriosus and foramen ovale. Combined with the onset of regular breathing

DOI: 10.1201/9780367494018-23

and oxygen transfer from aerated alveoli, there is a substantial increase in blood oxygen content in the ascending aorta, carotid and vertebral arteries, increasing oxygen supply to the brain.

Using Doppler ultrasound, it has been possible to follow individual babies from intrauterine to extrauterine life. Cerebral artery blood flow velocity is substantially reduced in the hours after birth, compared with measurements taken before delivery (6, 7). During the following days, blood flow velocity gradually increases in healthy term infants (8), a finding mirrored in preterm infants using Doppler (9) and blood flow measured using near-infrared spectroscopy (NIRS) (10).

It is initially surprising that cerebral blood flow normally decreases after birth, especially as left ventricular output increases after birth (11). However, this reduction in cerebral blood flow is likely to be a response to increased arterial oxygen tension after birth. As arterial blood oxygen content increases, this offsets the reduction in blood flow, and perinatal cerebral oxygen delivery is maintained.

Cerebral perfusion with perinatal hypoxia

A normal labor will involve some degree of fetal hypoxia, but this does not cause problems as compensatory mechanisms, such as circulatory redistribution and increased oxygen extraction, preserve brain blood flow, and cerebral oxygenation. However, hazardous reductions in cerebral oxygen delivery may occur when hypoxia is more severe, and particularly when hypoxia is combined with brain ischemia. If the redistributory response is inadequate (e.g. with sepsis), or if reductions in cardiac output are severe or repeated, then a combination of reduced brain blood flow and hypoxia may be sufficient to cause brain injury. Within the brain, the redistributory response favors structures such as the brainstem, which is vital for basic functions of breathing and homeostasis. This has been shown in animal models of intrauterine asphyxia (12) and in hypoxic newborn lambs (13). In healthy human adults, hypoxia produces a preferential increase in vertebral artery blood flow supplying the brainstem and posterior brain structures (14). The hypoxic perfusion response in adults also varies between different areas of cerebral hemisphere gray matter (15).

This combination of hypoxia and ischemia is most likely to arise from disturbed utero-placenta function during labor, with the fetus completely dependent on the placenta for delivery of oxygen. Less commonly, insults before labor, or failed cardio-respiratory adaptation immediately after birth can cause or compound the insult.

Fetal hypoxia and circulatory compromise

The fetal circulation can be compromised directly from loss of circulating volume with hemorrhage at the utero-placental interface (placenta abruption), from the placental edge (in placenta praevia), or from umbilical cord rupture. This produces fetal hypovolaemia, reduced venous return, and ventricular stroke volume, with lowered cardiac output. Impaired placental perfusion may then reduce oxygen transfer, producing hypoxia.

However, it is more common for the fetal circulation to experience a secondary impairment due to fetal hypoxia. Failure of oxygen transfer through the utero-placental unit is particularly likely during labour, with contractions producing intermittent reduction in placental perfusion. Hypoxia is more likely if the placenta is already functioning poorly from disturbed vascularization (as in fetal growth restriction, pre-eclampsia, or post-maturity). Umbilical cord compression will also impair placental perfusion,

producing both hypoxia and loss of circulating volume into the placenta, and this will be particularly severe if the umbilical cord prolapses past the fetal head.

As hypoxia progresses, the fetus may exhibit a bradycardic response, similar to that seen in diving mammals. Combined with circulatory redistribution, this reduces oxygen consumption and preserves available oxyhemoglobin for the brain. Initially, these adaptive decelerations in heart rate will be short-lived (early decelerations) during contractions, but in more severe hypoxia, heart rate only recovers sometime after the end of the contraction (late decelerations). With prolonged severe hypoxia, sustained life-preserving bradycardia will result, and only recovers when oxygen delivery is restored, often expedited by obstetric delivery and active neonatal resuscitation. With anaerobic metabolism becoming necessary, lactic acidosis impairs cardiac contractility with further reductions in cardiac output and organ perfusion.

If there is a failure of cardio-respiratory adaptation after birth, systemic and tissue hypoxia or impaired cardiac output may continue. This may occur from meconium aspiration impairing alveolar function, from continuing pulmonary vasoconstriction, or from impaired myocardial contractility. In this case, cerebral hypoxia or ischemia can produce brain injury in the period immediately after delivery. Following delivery and effective resuscitation, arterial oxygen tension increases, and heart rate is the first circulatory parameter to recover. With increasing heart rate and stroke volume, cardiac output recovers and cerebral blood flow increases. As arterial oxygen saturations increase over the next 5–10 minutes, there is a restoration of cerebral blood flow and oxygen delivery. However, resuscitation using 80% oxygen may cause an excessive increase in oxygen tension, with prolonged vasocontriction and lower cerebral blood flow (16).

With insults severe enough to produce HIE, cerebral blood flow may be initially low on the first postnatal day, but it goes on to become significantly increased. This "luxury hyperperfusion" matches the time-course of secondary energy failure and the severity of cerebral injury (17). This has been demonstrated in studies using ^{133}Xe clearance, Doppler ultrasound (18), and MRI (19). The degree of cerebral vasodilatation is predictive of adverse outcome, as indicated by the Doppler waveform pulsatility (18) and by arterial spin labeling MRI (20). Impaired cerebral autoregulation has been shown in infants with HIE, using ^{133}Xe clearance (21) and NIRS (22). This pressure-passive cerebral circulation will place the brain at risk of further compromise.

Methods used to assess the perinatal cerebral circulation

Studies of human fetal and neonatal cerebral circulation around the time of birth have used a variety of methods. Studies for individual patients may be fixed-timepoint, repeated, or continuous. One of the earliest methods to measure neonatal cerebral blood flow, which is no longer used, was jugular occlusion plethymography (measuring the change in head circumference with bilateral occlusion of the jugular veins) (23). Early studies of neonatal cerebral blood flow were also made using the Fick principle with radioisotope indicator-dilution methods (particularly ^{133}Xe). More recently, positron-emission tomography (PET) also uses the Fick principle, but has limited use. These methods make fewer assumptions than NIRS or Doppler ultrasonography and have given important information, but are now rarely used, with preference given to less invasive methods, which minimise radiation exposure.

In obstetric studies before delivery, Doppler ultrasound has been used extensively to measure the velocity of blood flow and flow waveform pulsatility. With pulse-wave range-gated equipment, this can be performed from a specifically visualized segment of an artery supplying the brain (often the middle cerebral artery). Ultrasound has the advantage that it can be used repeatedly both before and after delivery. Its major disadvantage is that it is rarely possible to measure vessel diameter, so that volume flow is not computed, and it must be assumed that vessel diameter remains constant. This method has also been used extensively in the neonatal period. As the same equipment is used for echocardiography, simultaneous measurements of other aspects of the circulation can be acquired. Volumetric measurements that do measure vessel diameter have been obtained using Doppler ultrasound from the superior vena cava (SVC) (24), which includes blood flow from the brain, head, and upper limbs and from the common carotid artery (25). Low SVC flow in preterm neonates during the first 2 days of life is associated with an increased risk of developing periventricular hemorrhage (26).

NIRS passes near-infrared light through brain tissue, measuring its attenuation by oxy- and deoxy-hemoglobin. This can be used to measure total hemoglobin content and the oxygen saturation ratio in that tissue, calculating indices that correlate with perfusion. These methods have been used in the neonatal period and can be adapted for intrapartum use. In the neonate, a rapid-step-up in inspired oxygen can be used to produce an oxyhemoglobin tracer to calculate cerebral blood flow using the Fick principle. Depending on how many optodes are placed, neonatal measurements may indicate global, or spatially resolved perfusion. Although absolute values of NIRS measurement can be affected by optical path length algorithms, intracranial hemorrhage, and extracerebral blood flow (27), NIRS has a major advantage in its ability to provide continuous noninvasive measurements and trends.

Arterial spin-labeled (ASL) perfusion MRI can be used to measure cerebral blood flow (20). This tracer method uses magnetization of blood water during an MRI scan to provide accurate measurements of regional or global cerebral blood flow. Postnatal measurements of cerebral blood flow can be performed at fixed time points. Although the technique has been used to measure placental blood flow, the strong magnetic fields and bulky equipment required limit its application for intrapartum, repeated or continuous measurement of cerebral blood flow.

Hypoxic-ischemic encephalopathy and blood-brain barrier function

In the 1950s, Grontoft injected tryptan blue dye into newly aborted human fetuses and observed that the dye did not stain the brain as a whole but only those areas outside of the postulated BBB which include the choroid plexus and the circumventricular organs (28, 29). This was so for fetuses as early as 10 weeks gestation demonstrating the presence of a notional BBB from the early fetal period.

However, if the dye was injected after a period of up to half an hour after placental separation, then the dye permeated throughout the brain. This was postulated to be related to the effect of hypoxia rendering the BBB more permeable.

The unifying disturbance to neural tissue in HIE is a deficit in oxygen supply (30). This can occur because of hypoxemia, a diminished amount of oxygen in the blood supply as well as ischemia, which is a diminished amount of blood perfusing the brain. The resulting damage to the brain tissue continues to develop hours to days after the initial hypoxia-ischemia (HI) episode in term newborns (31). The BBB is an important functional and morphological organ maintaining homeostasis within the nervous system. In this section, we provide an overview of its relationship to HIE (32).

The blood-brain barrier

More than just being a physical barrier formed by tight junctions between the endothelial cells, the BBB is a dynamic physiological barrier that regulates the passage of hydrophilic molecules into the central nervous system (CNS) via transporters and enzymes (33). There is active communication between endothelial cells, pericytes, astrocytes, microglia, the structural basement membrane, and the extracellular matrix (ECM); the complex that makes up the neurovascular unit (34). The neurovascular unit is a morphological representation of the interface between the blood and CNS that underlies the BBB function (Figure 23.1). This communication is vital for the modulation and the maintenance of the selective permeability of the BBB. It enables the CNS environment to remain in stable homeostasis despite fluctuations in the composition of plasma and brain interstitial fluid, thus preventing interference with signal transmission.

The significant restriction of the passage of substances across the BBB is reflected in the transendothelial electrical resistance (TEER) across the endothelial cells of the BBB, which is fifty times higher than across peripheral endothelium (35). One of the main physical characteristics of the brain endothelial lining, underpinning its barrier function, lies in the complex tight junctions which limit intercellular movement of molecules (36).

The effects of HI injury on the BBB

Important effects of HI injury on the BBB include angiogenesis and changes in permeability. At a structural level, angiogenic sprouting whereby existing blood vessels are broken down to make way for new ones may contribute to BBB disruption though the relationship between hypoxia and this form of vascular remodeling has yet to be clearly established (37). There is an increased, early BBB permeability, peaking at between 2 and 4 hours post insult in neonatal models (38, 39). There is less compelling evidence of a delayed second phase of increased BBB permeability, which has been noted in the adult rat model (40). The BBB in human babies with HIE shows increased permeability as assessed by comparing the concentrations of albumin in cerebrospinal fluid versus plasma at 12–24 hours of age (41).

Whether or not the BBB experiences the second phase of increased permeability after HI injury, there is early activation of mechanisms leading to eventual restoration of BBB function after the insult; there is an upregulation in the transcription and expression of tight junction proteins (38, 39).

The effects of HI on the cellular components of the neurovascular unit

Endothelial cells are more susceptible to hypoxia-induced injury than pericytes and astrocytes; there is a disruption in the endothelial cytoskeleton structure, whereas pericytes and astrocytes retain the cytoskeleton arrangement even in the presence of prolonged hypoxia (42). In the normal brain environment, endothelial cells are exposed to higher concentrations of oxygen, whereas astrocytes and pericytes occupy areas exposed to lower oxygen

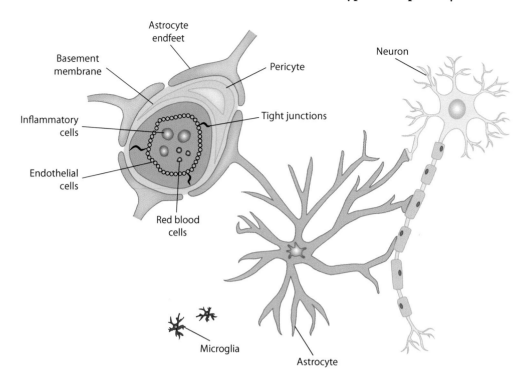

FIGURE 23.1 A cartoon (not to scale) representation of the components of the neurovascular unit that contribute to the blood-brain barrier.

concentrations (42). Also proliferation of astrocytes and pericytes is downregulated when exposed to hypoxia, whereas endothelial cells continue to proliferate despite this being counterproductive to the conservation of energy and ultimately, their survival. This is further associated with rapid induction of the HIF-1 (hypoxia-inducible factor), protein, and BBB disruption (42).

The role of VEGF and HIF-1α protein

Not only are the pericytes and astrocytes able to adapt better to the HI insult but they have also been shown to be vital in reducing injury through the secretion of protective factors, such as vascular endothelial growth factor (VEGF). VEGF proteins are important in coordinating the development and regulation of not only blood vessels but also that of neurons, earning them the classification of angioneurin (43). VEGF's protective effect is related to the increased survival of endothelial cells and reducing the volume of infarcted tissue via inhibition of apoptotic mechanisms (44).

However, simultaneously, VEGF increases BBB permeability via destabilization of junctional proteins, including the tight junctions and adherens junctions (45). This leads to vasogenic edema and may be a link between increased BBB permeability and the pathophysiological inflammation in HIE (46). The diversity of the VEGF family may explain their conflicting roles following HI brain injury.

HIF-1α protein is important in the upregulation of VEGF (47). Hypoxia initiates activation of HIF-1α, resulting in the expression of genes responsible for angiogenesis. However, conflicting effects of HIF-1α have been reported depending on the time period post-HI injury (37). Acutely, the absence of HIF-1α has been associated with a reduced degree of injury (48). Over a longer time course, however, mice unable to express HIF-1α were found to have a worse outcome compared to wild-type controls (49).

The impact of BBB dysfunction on the pathophysiology of HIE

Correlation between areas of BBB function disruption and regions of infarction in the brain has been demonstrated in the neonatal mouse model (39). Nedelcu et al. (50) noted that a moderate HI insult produced a first phase of cytotoxic edema in the brain of the P7 rat model, which was followed 4 h later by a second wave of cytotoxic edema and new development of vasogenic edema. Cerebral vasogenic edema develops in the presence of increased BBB permeability, allowing for an unregulated movement of plasma proteins and may ultimately lead to hemorrhagic transformation (51).

The increase in BBB permeability may contribute to HI injury of the brain through the increased exposure of brain tissue to inflammatory mediators and the peripheral immune system response. Neuroinflammation is postulated to play a major role in secondary energy failure and further chronic inflammation characteristic of the pathophysiology of HIE (52). Activated microglia release proinflammatory cytokines including tumor necrosis factor-alpha (TNF-α), which facilitates the activation of matrix metalloproteinases (MMP). These proteolytic enzymes, especially MMP-2 and MMP-9, have been implicated in BBB disruption due to proteolysis of extracellular matrix proteins and cleavage of tight junctions, resulting in edema and hemorrhage (53).

Mild therapeutic hypothermia (TH) is the only established clinical intervention that targets pathological mechanisms of HIE. At the BBB, therapeutic hypothermia has been shown to reduce the activity of enzymes, especially that of MMPs, as well as maintain ECM molecular and cellular integrity (54, 55). An improved understanding of the altered functioning of the BBB in response to HI may, in future, be used to advantage in allowing passage of therapeutic molecules access to the brain (32).

Tools for assessing neuronal injury

Tools for assessing neuronal injury directly in newborns are limited and arguably are most frequently indirectly assessed with neuro-imaging such as ultrasound and MRI. However, various tools may provide information about integrity of neuronal function at the bedside. In this section, we summarise and provide an overview about a few key modalities.

Electrophysiological tools: Conventional EEG

Electroencephalography (EEG) enables continuous bedside monitoring of cerebral function in newborn infants and hence is an important neurological assessment tool in babies who have been subjected to a hypoxic event. A single channel of EEG provides the voltage difference as detected between two electrodes on the scalp, representing the post-synaptic potentials from the underlying pyramidal cells in the cortex. The normal neonatal EEG has characteristic maturational changes such as increasing background continuity with increasing gestational age as well as exhibiting sleep state changes (56). Extensive research over many years has shown that EEG monitoring enables detection of seizures (57), can provide prognostic information (58–60), as well as helping assess the response to treatment, for example, in relation to anticonvulsants (61).

In interpreting EEG recordings, and particularly if short, it is important to consider factors that could affect the EEG in addition to sleep state and maturational changes; e.g. acidosis as well as administration of sedative drugs such as pethidine and morphine can be associated with reversible neonatal EEG changes. Limited channel EEG monitoring is straightforward to setup. However, potential problems include those arising from poor electrode contact or drying of electrode contact gel, an artifact from electrical interference, and movement artifact, for example, related to respiration.

Amplitude-integrated EEG (aEEG) and evoked responses

Prior and Maynard described the use of a cerebral function monitor at the London Hospital in the 1960s (62). The aEEG, as it is known today, was devised to monitor trends in electrical cerebral activity at periods when the cerebral perfusion may be vulnerable, for example, during open-heart surgery with cardiopulmonary bypass, a procedure that may last for several hours. The raw EEG signal is processed to produce the aEEG band; it is filtered so that very high and very low frequencies are excluded, the x-axis (time) is compressed, rectified, smoothed and plotted semi-logarithmically. In most modern digital machines, the aEEG is displayed side-by-side with the raw EEG.

Provided its limitations are understood, the aEEG is a useful tool for monitoring the electrocortical background and for seizures in newborns (63). Indirectly, it provides us with information about the presence of cerebral injury. The extent to which the aEEG is depressed correlates with severity of encephalopathy as well as extent of cerebral injury on MRI in babies with encephalopathy and/or seizures (64) (Figure 23.2). In turn, the more depressed the aEEG is within 6 h after birth, the worse the neurodevelopmental outcome in babies with HIE (65). This early predictive value of the aEEG has become very useful, as it remains the only objective tool for stratifying babies for brain-saving treatments such a therapeutic hypothermia, at the bedside. Additionally, the presence of seizures as noted on the aEEG monitors is associated with extent of brain injury on cerebral MRI, in babies who have undergone cooling treatment (57).

Evoked potentials (EPs) provide a means of investigating the visual, somatosensory, as well as auditory and brainstem pathways. These are typically carried out by recording electrical potentials on the scalp in response to appropriate stimuli in particular visual (VEP), median nerve somatosensory (SEP), or auditory brainstem responses (ABR) also known as brainstem auditory evoked responses (BAER). Studies have shown that VEPs (66), SEPs (67), as well as BAERs (68) could be of value in assessing pathways in newborn infants who may have been subjected to a hypoxic event.

Near-infrared spectroscopy (NIRS)

NIRS is a noninvasive method of obtaining measures of regional cerebral tissue oxygenation that represents a hemoglobin oxygen saturation value in brain tissue (69). This cerebral tissue oxygen saturation percent represents a ratio of oxygenated to total brain tissue hemoglobin. The technique makes use of the principle that biological tissue is relatively transparent to light in the near-infrared region wavelength (700–1000 nm), and this light is absorbed by hemoglobin, but differentially absorbed depending on whether the hemoglobin is oxygenated or deoxygenated. It would seem ideally suited for newborn babies who have relatively thin skin and skull thickness (70).

At a most basic level, the application of a sensor on the scalp allows continuous measurement of cerebral tissue oxygenation as a percentage. The fractional tissue oxygen extraction (FTOE) can be estimated from values of peripheral arterial oxygen saturation and cerebral oxygenation as a balance between oxygen delivery and consumption by the brain. This may be related to cerebral metabolism.

Hence although NIRS is not a tool for explicitly assessing neuronal injury, the technique is used in some neonatal units for ongoing neuromonitoring babies after HIE. Its exact role in monitoring these babies remains to be defined, but studies suggest that infants who have been more severely affected with HIE are more likely to have higher cerebral oxygen saturations within the first two days and conversely lower FTOE (70). This increased cerebral oxygenation in the adverse outcome groups has been interpreted as being related to decreased oxygen use due to mitochondrial dysfunction or injury as well as other hemodynamic changes.

Blood biomarker tools for neuronal injury

Global hypoxia and/or ischemia to the newborn brain results in neuronal injury and cell death by multiple mechanisms. Hence, products of neuronal injury and death are released, as well as substances representing responses of inflammation and repair. In the past, products of neuronal injury were only detectable in sufficient quantities in the cerebrospinal fluid. However, with more sensitive techniques available today, it is possible to detect and quantify very small concentrations of products in virtually any body fluids including plasma, urine and dried blood spots. Some biomarkers have been shown to be elevated in the cord blood of newborns with HIE, whereas others have been noted to rise in subsequent serial samples.

Products of neuronal damage that have been shown to be raised in relation to HIE include various proteins such as neurofilament light and heavy chains and UCH-L1 (ubiquitin C-terminal hydrolase L1) (71–73). Neurofilaments, a group of intermediate-sized filamentous proteins, are the most abundant cytoskeletal component, found predominantly in the myelinated axons of the central nervous system. Elevated levels of various cytokines (e.g. interleukins 1, 6, and 8, tumor necrosis factor-α, and interferon-γ)

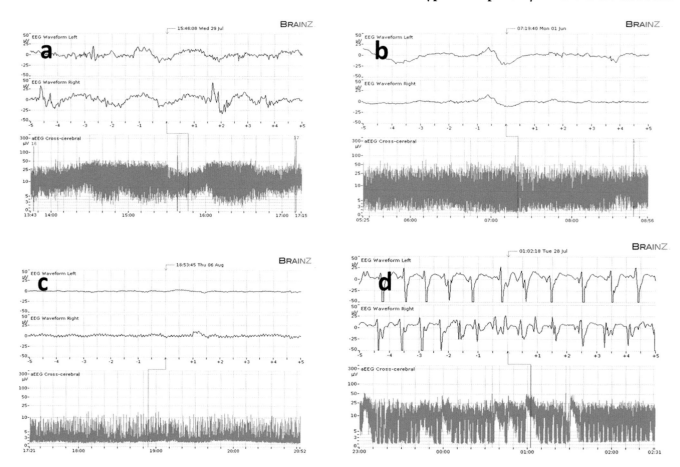

FIGURE 23.2 Amplitude-integrated EEG images. In each of the four panels (a–d), the upper part of the panel shows the two (left and right) channels of raw EEG (representing 10s) and the lower part shows the aEEG pattern (representing 3.5 h). (a) Normal aEEG background with sleep–wake cycling noted on the aEEG; (b) a moderately abnormal or discontinuous aEEG pattern showing a Broad aEEG band with a depressed lower margin; (c) a very depressed aEEG pattern (severely abnormal) with corresponding low-voltage raw EEG traces; and (d) frequent seizures (status epilepticus) noted on the aEEG with multiple rises in the lower and upper aEEG margin with corresponding rhythmic spike and wave activity present in the raw EEG.

and enzymes and proteins from glial cells (e.g. glial fibrillary acid protein (GFAP), neuron-specific enolase (NSE), S-100B) have been shown to be raised as part of the inflammatory response to HIE (74, 75). The studies of blood biomarkers of brain injury have been limited by small numbers and suboptimal sensitivity and specificity. Larger studies are required before these biomarkers become established for use in clinical practice.

Cerebral MRI techniques as tools for assessing neuronal injury after HIE

The signature brain injury associated with HIE involves basal ganglia and thalami. This is thought to be because these regions of the brain have a substantial blood supply and metabolic rate (76). Other areas of the brain that are affected by perinatal hypoxia-ischemia include the posterior limbs of the internal capsule, subcortical white matter, and the cerebral cortex (77). This pattern of brain injury is most clearly visualized using cerebral MRI (78). Injury may be noted as early as the second day with diffusion-weighted imaging (79) but generally later with conventional T1 and T2 weighted MRI. Infants treated with therapeutic hypothermia have fewer lesions noted on cerebral MRI, but when present, they are still predictive of adverse outcome (80), and in clinical practice, cerebral MRI remains highly predictive

of neurodevelopmental outcome in newborns who have received therapeutic hypothermia after HIE (81).

Acknowledgment

The authors are grateful to Ms Ammee AD Gala, University of St Andrews for the original artwork for Figure 23.1.

References

1. Vyas S, et al. Br J Obstet Gynaecol. 1990; 97(9):797–803.
2. Sato M, et al. Placenta. 2016; 45:32–36.
3. McNamara H, et al. Br J Obstet Gynaecol. 1995; 102(8):644–647.
4. Li H, et al. Early Hum Dev. 2006; 82(11):747–752.
5. Jones CM, et al. Am J Obstet Gynecol. 1982; 144(2):149–153.
6. Kempley ST, et al. Early Hum Dev. 1996; 46(1-2):165–174.
7. Meerman RJ, et al. Early Hum Dev. 1990; 24(3):209–217.
8. Fenton AC, et al. Early Hum Dev. 1990; 22(2):73–79.
9. Winberg P, et al. Acta Paediatr Scand. 1990; 79(12):1150–1155.
10. Meek JH, et al. Arch Dis Child Fetal Neonatal Ed. 1998; 78(1):F33–F37.
11. Agata Y, et al. J Pediatr. 1991; 119(3):441–445.
12. Johnson GN, et al. Am J Obstet Gynecol. 1979; 135(1):48–52.
13. Lou HC, et al. Eur J Pediatr. 1985; 144(3):225–227.
14. Ogoh S, et al. Exp Physiol. 2013; 98(3):692–698.
15. Nöth U, et al. J Magn Reson Imaging. 2006; 24(6):1229–1235.
16. Lundstrøm KE, et al. Arch Dis Child Fetal Neonatal Ed. 1995; 73(2):F81–F86.
17. Greisen G. Early Hum Dev. 2014; 90(10):703–705.

18. Levene MI, et al. Dev Med Child Neurol. 1989; 31(4):427–434.
19. Wintermark P, et al. Am J Neuroradiol. 2011; 32(11):2023–2029.
20. De Vis JB, et al. Eur Radiol. 2015; 25(1):113–121.
21. Pryds O, et al. J Pediatr. 1990; 117(1 Pt 1):119–125.
22. Massaro AN, et al. J Neurophysiol. 2015; 114(2):818–824.
23. Sankaran K, et al. Pediatr Res. 1981; 15(11):1415–1418.
24. Popat H, et al. Arch Dis Child Fetal Neonatal Ed. 2018; 103(3):F257–F263.
25. Sinha AK, et al. Arch Dis Child Fetal Neonatal Ed. 2006; 91(1):F31–F35.
26. Kluckow M, et al. Arch Dis Child Fetal Neonatal Ed. 2000; 82(3):F188–F194.
27. Murkin JM, et al. Br J Anaesth. 2009; 103 Suppl 1:i3–i13.
28. Grontoft O. Acta Pathol Microbiol Scand Suppl1954; 100:8–109.
29. Saunders NR, et al. Front Neurosci. 2014; 8:404.
30. Volpe JJ. *Hypoxic-Ischemic Encephalopathy: Biochemical and Physiological Aspects. Neurology of the Newborn.* 5th ed. Philadelphia: Saunders Elsevier; 2008. pp. 247–324.
31. Millar LJ, et al. Front Cell Neurosci. 2017; 11:78.
32. Lee WLA, et al. Dev Neurosci. 2017; 39(1–4):49–58.
33. Saunders NR, et al. J Physiol. 2018; 596(23):5723–5756.
34. Bell AH, et al. Front Neurosci. 2019; 13:1452.
35. Butt AMJ, et al. J Physiol. 1990; 429:47–62.
36. Wolburg H, et al. Vasc Pharmacol. 2002; 38(6):323–337.
37. Baburamani AA, et al. Front Physiol. 2012; 3:424.
38. Chen X, et al. Neuroscience. 2012; 226:89–100.
39. Ek CJ, et al. J Cereb Blood Flow Metab. 2015; 35(5):818–827.
40. Başkaya MK, et al. Neurosci Lett. 1997; 226(1):33–36.
41. Kumar A, et al. Pediatrics. 2008; 122(3):e722–e727.
42. Engelhardt S, et al. Fluids Barriers CNS. 2015; 12:4.
43. Zacchigna S, et al. Nat Rev Neurosci. 2008; 9(3):169–181.
44. Kunze R, et al. Prog Neurobiol. 2019; 178:101611.
45. Wang W, et al. Am J Physiol Heart Circ Physiol. 2001; 280(1):H434–H440.
46. Kaur C, et al. Glia. 2006; 54(8):826–839.
47. Fan X, et al. Brain Res Rev. 2009; 62(1):99–108.
48. Chen W, et al. Neurobiol Dis. 2008; 31(3):433–441.
49. Sheldon RA, et al. Dev Neurosci. 2009. pp. 452–458.
50. Nedelcu J, et al. Pediatr Res. 1999; 46(3):297–304.
51. Simard JM, et al. Lancet Neurol. 2007; 6(3):258–268.
52. Li B, et al. Prog Neurobiol. 2017; 159:50–68.
53. Rosenberg GA. Lancet Neurol. 2009; 8(2):205–216.
54. Baumann E, et al. Brain Res. 2009; 1269:185–197.
55. Jurkovich GJ, et al. J Surg Res. 1988; 44(5):514–521.
56. Pavlidis E, et al. Acta Paediatr. 2017; 106(9):1394–1408.
57. Shah DK, et al. Arch Dis Child Fetal Neonatal Ed. 2014; 99(3):F219–F224.
58. Connell J, et al. Arch Dis Child. 1989; 64(4 Spec No):452–458.
59. Dunne JM, et al. Arch Dis Child Fetal Neonatal Ed. 2017; 102(1):F58–F64.
60. Wertheim D, et al. Arch Dis Child Fetal Neonatal Ed. 1994; 71(2):F97–F102.
61. Pressler RM, et al. Lancet Neurol. 2015; 14(5):469–477.
62. Maynard D, et al. Br Med J. 1969; 4(5682):545–546
63. Shah DK, et al. Pediatrics. 2008; 122(4):863–865.
64. Shah DK, et al. Pediatrics. 2006; 118(1):47–55.
65. Toet MC, et al. Arch Dis Child Fetal Neonatal Ed. 1999; 81(1):F19–F23.
66. Mercuri E, et al. Arch Dis Child Fetal Neonatal Ed. 1999; 80(2):F99–F104.
67. Kontio T, et al. Clin Neurophysiol. 2013; 124(6):1089–1094.
68. Jiang ZD, et al. Clin Neurophysiol. 2009; 120(5):967–973.
69. la Cour A, et al. Neurophotonics. 2018; 5(4):040901.
70. Mitra S, et al. Front Neurol. 2020; 11:393.
71. Shah DK, et al. Front Neurol. 2018; 9:86.
72. Douglas-Escobar MV, et al. Front Neurol. 2014; 5:273.
73. Shah DK, et al. Front Neurol. 2020; 11:562510–562510.
74. Chalak LF, et al. J Pediatr. 2014; 164(3):468.e1–474.e1.
75. Roka A, et al. Acta Paediatr. 2012; 101(3):319–323.
76. Myers RE. Adv Neurol. 1975; 10:223–234.
77. Rutherford MA, et al. Pediatrics. 1998; 102(2 Pt 1):323–328.
78. Barkovich AJ, et al. Am J Neuroradiol. 1995; 16(3):427–438.
79. McKinstry RC, et al. Neurology. 2002; 59(6):824–833.
80. Rutherford M, et al. Lancet Neurol. 2010; 9(1):39–45.
81. Tharmapoopathy P, et al. Eur J Paediatr Neurol. 2020; 25:127–133.

EFFECTS OF HYPOXIA ON AIRWAY, ALVEOLAR FUNCTION, AND RESPIRATION

Y.S. Prakash, Christina M. Pabelick and Peter M. MacFarlane

Contents

Introduction

Premature birth predisposes infants to lung diseases such as bronchopulmonary dysplasia, wheezing, and asthma that contribute to significant morbidity and mortality in the pediatric population. Outcomes in these at-risk infants are influenced by perinatal exposures including prenatal and perinatal hypoxia and inflammation, postnatal intensive care unit interventions including hyperoxia (with or without mechanical ventilation), and subsequent environmental exposures. On the one hand, hypoxia is a natural aspect of development where the fetus grows in a hypoxic environment that promotes tissue patterning and growth including of the lung. However, premature birth has significant effects on pulmonary development and health where premature exposure to room air and furthermore perinatal supplemental oxygen administration represent a hyperoxic insult that causes harm at multiple levels of the lung. Preterm infants are also subject to increased episodes of hypoxia, given an immature respiratory control system superimposed on insufficient capacity of the lung to tolerate altered ventilation and perfusion, overall resulting in pulmonary damage and disease. Finally, exogenous insults such as perinatal inflammation and infection further superimpose detrimental changes in the context of hypoxia or hyperoxia. Here we summarize current understanding of the effects of oxygen, particularly hypoxia, on the developing lung and how low vs. high oxygen may predispose to disease that extends even into adulthood. Better understanding of mechanisms of hypoxic and hyperoxic action can help to identify novel therapies for improved care and outcomes in this vulnerable population.

Normal development

The details of embryonic lung development are described in detail in several recent reviews (1–4) and briefly summarized here. In the embryonic stage (<7 weeks gestation in humans), foregut endoderm cells become committed to form the primordial lung bud, a process orchestrated by a number of transcription factors. Arising from the ventral side of the foregut, the lung bud undergoes repeated elongation and branching into the surrounding mesenchyme. The buds are lined by endoderm, which gives rise to the epithelial cells of the future lung, while other elements of the airway wall arising from the mesenchyme. Early in gestation, the pulmonary vascular systems develop in parallel with the airways. Branching morphogenesis and elongation of the airways then occur, again modulated by several transcription factors and involving critical interactions between the epithelial and mesenchymal (future smooth muscle and fibroblast) layers. Substantial lung growth occurs during the pseudoglandular stage (5–17 weeks gestation in humans), such that the repeated centrifugal division of the airway buds into the surrounding mesenchyme results in all airway levels including terminal bronchioles forming by the end of this period. Here, airway elongation appears critically dependent on the epithelium, and less so on the mesenchyme; but airway branching is dependent on the presence of the mesenchyme. While the list and complexity of growth factors and signaling systems involved in embryonic lung growth are expanding, in general, airway growth and branching are stimulated by tyrosine kinase receptors, while transforming growth factor (TGF) family factors are inhibitory. During this period airway smooth muscle (ASM) is formed, along with cartilage in the larger airways, submucosal glands and the connective tissue within the airway wall. ASM cells are expressed in the larger airways early in the pseudoglandular phase with innervation also being evident. ASM cells in these early periods show spontaneous tone and peristalsis-like contractions that are transmitted to the airway and may contribute to airway elongation and growth, as well as the movement of fluid within the lung. Epithelial differentiation into multiple cell types (ciliated, goblet, and basal/stem cells) also occurs during this period. Parallel vasculogenesis occurs with the airway acting as an anatomical template. Interestingly, vascular smooth muscle cells in the newly formed pulmonary arteries derive from the ASM of adjacent airways. Overall, by 24 weeks, the adult airway wall structure becomes established. During the canalicular period (16–27 weeks gestation), there is growth of the pre-acinar airways with division of peripheral airways to form proximal branches of respiratory bronchioles and prospective alveolar ducts. These are accompanied by development of type I and type II alveolar epithelial cells

DOI: 10.1201/9780367494018-24

within saccular air spaces. By 24 weeks, type II cells form lamellar bodies for eventual secretion of surfactant by 27–28 weeks. A critical aspect of lung parenchymal growth is epithelial thinning and formation of the blood–gas barrier comparable to that in adults, and thus sufficient for oxygenation in premature infants. The alveolar stage occurs 27 weeks to term, with substantial growth of primitive alveoli, particularly closer to term, representing 30–50% of that in adults.

Hypoxia and fetal lung development

The fetal lung naturally grows in a hypoxic environment, with oxygen levels ~25% of that in adults (5). Even under these conditions, there is excess oxygen availability that provides a buffer for fetal survival and development, further facilitated by fetal hemoglobin with an equilibration curve that increases access of fetal tissues to any available oxygen (6). In turn, the hypoxic 20–30 mmHg range of oxygen tension is a critical driver for lung branching morphogenesis, angiogenesis, and deposition of collagen and other extracellular matrix proteins within the connective tissue layers during both pseudoglandular and canalicular stages (5). For example, in *ex vivo* rat lung explants, there is increased epithelial branching and proliferation of cells in both epithelial and mesenchymal layers following exposure to <5% O_2 compared to 21% O_2 (5). Studies in mice also find similar increases in epithelial and vascular branching. However, it is important to note that the comparison may be artificially increased given that 21% O_2 is substantially hyperoxic for early embryonic stages. Nonetheless, these data highlight the importance of an appropriately hypoxic environment during early fetal lung development and conversely demonstrate the impact of early exposure to much higher levels of O_2 as in premature birth. Indeed, postnatally, despite advances in medical care, exposure to chronic or intermittent hypoxia in premature infants occurs often, typically in the setting of apnea of prematurity or as a result of inability to adequately support oxygenation and ventilation in an extrauterine environment (7, 8). These abnormal hypoxic perinatal exposures may compromise alveolar, airway, and pulmonary vascular development, significantly contributing to the pathogenesis of multiple pulmonary diseases.

Despite a normally hypoxic environment and excess oxygen availability, fetal oxygen supply is a critical aspect to consider (8, 9). Fetal oxygen supply is influenced by placental oxygenation and blood flow and can be detrimentally affected by a number of maternal and fetal factors including reduced maternal oxygen supply *per se* in conditions such as high altitude or obstructive sleep apnea, impaired uterine blood flow due to uteroplacental insufficiency, maternal tobacco or cocaine use and fetal factors such as malformations (8, 9). Fetal hypoxia can also inhibit fetal breathing movements, increase airway resistance and pulmonary vascular pressure, thus impairing ongoing lengthening of the airways and parenchymal growth, and placing the postnatal lung at a disadvantage in terms of *ex utero* adaptations and subsequent lung growth (8, 9). Sustained maternal hypoxia in rat models show abnormal enlargement and impaired septation of saccules in the early postnatal period with an overall reduction in the number of alveoli, thus resembling an emphysema like pattern, which predisposes to detrimental postnatal lung growth (10). Sustained hypoxia particularly in later fetal stages can be detrimental to antioxidant pathways such as superoxide dismutase that remain diminished even after hypoxic recovery (11) – an effect relevant to premature birth, where iatrogenic interventions such as supplemental oxygen and/or mechanical

ventilation are likely to induce oxidant stress but the premature infant is disadvantaged by an immature, dysfunctional antioxidant systems. Interestingly, chronic hypoxia as occurs with altitude does not lead to substantial alveolar detriment at least *in utero*, although such data are derived from animal models such as guinea pig or sheep where most of the alveolar development occurs *in utero* (10). On the other hand, indirect hypoxia due to factors such as intrauterine growth retardation (IUGR) or maternal smoking leads to reductions in lung size proportionate to reductions in body weight, while reduced airway size and wall thickness involves decreased cartilage and epithelial growth: Effects that are fortunately reversible after birth and restoration of oxygen levels (12). However, more recent studies using a mouse model find that following IUGR, airways remain stiffer and more reactive to contractile agent that are sustained into adulthood (13). Similarly, with smoking, in humans, reduced lung size and reduced or abnormal alveolar growth are associated with reduced lung function that can be sustained for several months postnatally (14). Smoking also leads to increased fibrosis within the growing airway thus increasing airway resistance (14).

Mechanisms and targets of hypoxia effects in the developing lung

Cellular responses to hypoxia are now well-known to be mediated particularly by the highly conserved hypoxia-inducible factor (HIF) transcription factors that control a multitude of genes involved in cell growth, proliferation and apoptosis, metabolism, extracellular matrix formation, and angiogenesis (15–19). The HIF transcriptional complex is a heterodimer composed of one of the three oxygen-sensitive subunits (HIF-1α, HIF-2α, or HIF-3α) and a constitutive oxygen-insensitive HIF-β subunit. While the β-subunit is constitutively expressed in the nucleus, regulation of HIF by oxygen occurs through modifications of the HIF α-subunit such that in normoxia it is rapidly degraded by ubiquitination and proteasomal degradation via prolyl hydroxylases (PHD). With hypoxia, PHDs are degraded, facilitating stabilization of the HIF α-subunit which then accumulates in the nucleus to binds to the β-subunit, triggering hypoxia response elements (HRE) within promoter regions of hypoxia-responsive target genes. The most notable gene also relevant to lung development is vascular endothelial growth factor (VEGF). In the lung, in addition to the vasculature, VEGF is also expressed by airway epithelial cells while VEGF receptors are in the mesenchymal cells underlying the alveolar epithelium and vasculature (20–22). Furthermore, in the presence of hypoxia, human fetal lungs have a higher expression of VEGF permitting lung growth. Conversely, inhibition of HIF-1α or of VEGF disrupts pulmonary vascular development and interrupts epithelial branching morphogenesis in the fetal lung and disrupts postnatal alveolar growth (23). Deletion of HIF-2α also delays lung maturation and is dependent on VEGF. Converse to these knockdown effects, enhanced activity of HIF or VEGF pathways leads to interruptions in airway branching and vascular dsymorphogenesis (24).

Hypoxia and developing airways

There are multiple effects of hypoxia on both structural and inflammatory airway cells relevant to airway development as well as diseases of childhood (8, 25–28) (Figure 24.1). As in fetal lung, hypoxia can alter the extent of extracellular matrix (ECM) formation in proximal airways (5, 29) with effects relevant to the

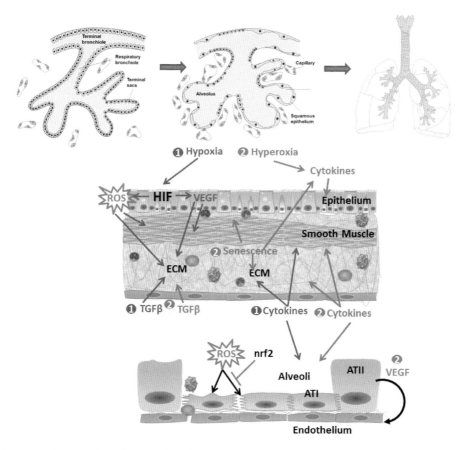

FIGURE 24.1 Schematic of potential mechanisms by which Hypoxia vs. Hyperoxia could influence the developing lung and the different cell types involved. Both hypoxia and hyperoxia can trigger multiple pathways such as HIF resulting in VEGF and downstream effects on epithelium, smooth muscle, and fibroblasts. They can also enhance cytokines (e.g. IL-6, IL-8) that have complex effects leading to airway hyperreactivity and remodeling in the bronchial airways. In the airways and particularly in the parenchyma, ROS induced by hypoxia or hyperoxia can promote multiple effects.

perinatal period, particularly in preterm infants where increased airway resistance and decreased compliance are detrimental. Postnatal hypoxia can also adversely affect the airway and contribute to structural and functional changes to such infants (30), who are already at risk of developing airway disease. For example, in human ASM, hypoxia stimulates cell proliferation and secretion of angiogenic mediators such as VEGF or IL-8 (30) and can contribute to airway remodeling (31). Hypoxia also induces reactive oxygen species (ROS) and mitochondrial fragmentation and dysfunction within human fetal ASM (31) mechanisms that promote cell proliferation. In airway epithelial cells, hypoxia decreases trans-epithelial Na+ transport and promotes mucus production (32) (Table 24.1), effects likely to be detrimental in a small, stiffer, and hyperreactive airway in the context of prematurity.

In addition to these "direct" effects of hypoxia, it is important to consider interactions between inflammation and oxygen. Intrauterine events such as chorioamnionitis or maternal inflammation can lead to elevated levels of inflammatory mediators in the developing lung. Furthermore, preterm infants can also be exposed to proinflammatory events that are further influenced by hypoxia. The relevance of these interactions between hypoxia and inflammation lies in perinatal conditions such as sudden infant death syndrome (SIDS). Autopsies show increases in a range of inflammatory cells within the lung including macrophages, eosinophils, and lymphocytes, with increased airway and

vascular thickening (33). There can be increased production of proinflammatory cytokines such as IL-1α, IL-1β, and IL-6 with downstream effects on tissue damage, altered metabolism, protein expression and lipid pathways, and ROS. In turn, cytokines can also influence hypoxia mechanisms. For example, proinflammatory cytokines such as tumor necrosis factor-alpha (TNFα) can increase HIF mRNA and protein expression but suppress HRE activity in human ASM (34), while TNF and interleukin-4 (IL-4) increase HIF transcription and VEGF expression in epithelial cells (35). These studies show the importance of interactions between hypoxia/HIF and inflammation, but there is more information needed to understand the extent to which hypoxia affects airway structure and function in newborns.

Hypoxia and developing alveoli

Given that alveolar development in humans primarily occurs postnatally (6, 36), the relevance of hypoxia is mostly in the context of prenatal events or premature birth where intermittent hypoxia might occur, and thus the effects of hypoxia on alveolar formation depend on the time period of exposure (10). Nonetheless, it is important to consider that the hypoxic environment in which fetal lung growth occurs is a critical factor in lung maturation and thus the production of surfactants. For example, deletion of HIF-2α delays maturation that is dependent on VEGF,

TABLE 24.1 Summary of Oxygen Effects in Different Lung Cell Types

	Cells	Effects
Hypoxia	Bronchial Epithelium	• ↑ Mucus secretion • ↓ Na^+ transport
	Smooth Muscle	• ↑ ASM thickness • ↑ Inflammation
	Alveolar Epithelium	• ↓ Alveolarization • Altered angiogenesis
Hyperoxia	Bronchial Epithelium	• ↑ Cytokines and chemokines • ↑ Epithelial thickness
	Smooth Muscle	• ↑ AHR • ↑ ASM proliferation • ↑ ECM remodeling • ↑ Immune cells
	Alveolar Epithelium	• ↓ Alveolarization • ↑ Interstitial fibrosis • ↑ Macrophage and PMN infiltration • ↑ Edema

thus increasing lung damage and decreasing survival at birth (24). Maternal hypoxic exposure results in progeny showing impaired alveolar development associated with reduced HIF-1α, HIF-2α, and VEGF (37) and thus longer-term influence. Postnatal hypoxia in newborns also impairs alveolarization (38), but the effects are mediated via TGFβ (39) (Table 24.1). In these effects, impaired alveolar vascular maturation is involved, and thus targeting pathways such as HIF, VEGF, or TGFβ to enhance postnatal angiogenesis and alveolarization becomes important. More recent evidence, albeit in model systems, suggests a role for HIF-induced changes in microRNAs (up-and downregulation), further complicating hypoxia effects (24). Hypoxia may affect these changes via transcription factors such as NFkB or p53 to induce miRNAs. While some miRNAs are protective via modulation of apoptosis, others modulate hypoxic effects on VEGF.

Hyperoxia and the developing lung

Even at term birth, the lung abruptly experiences relative hyperoxia following clearance of intraluminal fluid and inhalation of ambient oxygen (36). Accordingly, premature birth with associated interruption or impairment of lung morphogenesis results in a condition where the baby is not ready to cope with additional redox stress of a 21% O_2 environment. Intensive care interventions including supplemental oxygen while necessary and beneficial in the short term, are not without risk for long-term pulmonary health and are associated with significant morbidities (8, 40–45). Hyperoxia leads to altered structure of both airways and lung parenchyma (Table 24.1) with bronchopulmonary dysplasia (BPD) being a well-recognized problem.

Even in infants who do not develop BPD, long-term morbidities occur including susceptibility to respiratory infections, wheezing, and asthma (41, 46–49). In this regard, an emerging area of focus is the long-term impact of premature birth and hyperoxia on developing bronchial airways (25, 26, 28, 50, 51). For

example, there is a 30–90% increased risk of wheezing disorders in children born prematurely compared to term infants (49) with increased risk by the level of prematurity. Such symptoms can extend through childhood (51). While oxygen exposure in the intensive care unit likely plays a role, the underlying mechanisms for oxygen effect are still under investigation. Airway remodeling, characterized by hyperplasia and hypertrophy of ASM, enhanced ASM and airway reactivity, and greater ECM deposition has been observed (8, 25, 26, 31, 52). These changes result in a thicker, narrower, but more contractile airway. Such changes occur even with moderate hyperoxia (<60% O_2); for example, neonatal rat bronchial rings chronically exposed to 60% O_2 show increased ASM contraction (53). Human fetal ASM exposed to 50% O_2 show increased calcium responses to agonist and enhanced proliferation (31) as well ECM deposition (52). Hyperoxia effects may involve mechanisms such as disrupted nitric oxide cGMP signaling and increased arginase activity (54, 55), as well as growth factors such as neurotrophins (56). Remodeling changes can persist well beyond the neonatal and childhood years into adulthood (57). In addition to ASM, hyperoxia also detrimentally affects airway epithelium, disrupting the barrier, enhancing pulmonary permeability, and promoting inflammation (58). Hyperoxia can promote cytokines such as IL-8 and RANTES and chemokines. Most recently, there is evidence to suggest that hyperoxia effects can involve enhanced cellular senescence (59–61).

BPD involves abnormal alveolarization and interstitial fibrosis (21, 42, 44) and is usually due to oxygen with other concomitant risk factors including mechanical ventilation, infection, or nutrition. While BPD likely reflects a complex integration of multiple factors, hyperoxia itself can lead to alveolar simplification and decreased gas exchange (62, 63). Comparative clinical studies on the effects of targeting high or low oxygen saturation in extremely preterm neonates did not show a difference in BPD (64). While the mechanisms by which hyperoxia effects occur in the premature, developing airway are still under investigation, reduced

HIF-1α and VEGF may also be involved. Interruption in vascular formation due to inhibited VEGF blunts alveolar formation (65). Conversely, enhancing VEGF may be beneficial but can lead to pulmonary edema. Targeting HIF-1α might be an alternative target although studies to date have not been reassuring.

Developmental adaptations in respiratory control

Control of respiration during development undergoes multiple morphological and physiological changes *in utero* in order to prepare for transition to *ex utero* life (66–70). Postnatally, the respiratory system continues to develop and adapt to acute environmental stressors (70). The developing respiratory control system is in fact quite plastic in responding also to chronic environmental stimuli. In this regard, the late *in utero* and early perinatal periods are quite important with lifelong impact on breathing and respiratory control. While a number of prenatal and postnatal stimuli can lead to altered respiratory control, fluctuations in oxygen are considered an important player (66, 70). Much of the information to date derives from work in rodents and occasionally larger animal models such as sheep. Here it is important to note that prenatal hypoxia suppresses fetal breathing movements that can alter lung growth *per se*, and movement of fluid within the lung but obviously has no influence on fetal oxygenation given lack of a functioning lung. Thus, the effects of hypoxia in terms of respiratory control should be interpreted in terms of postnatal changes in multiple settings: Normal ventilatory patterns, responses to hypoxia, and responses to hypercapnia. Such changes likely involve structural and functional changes in the central nervous system as well as in the chemosensory pathways involving the carotid body (15, 18, 68). However, the detailed changes in neurotransmitters, neuronal structures, and sensitivities of the carotid body are not fully known. Interestingly, responses of the perinatal respiratory control systems are sensitive to the time window of exposures to altered oxygen levels, such that hypoxia later in life does not lead to alterations in the CNS or carotid body responses to hypoxia or hypercapnia for example (70). This likely reflects the progressive maturation of both brainstem and chemosensing systems and a greater resilience of the growing infant. Thus there are critical windows of vulnerability in terms of hypoxia and altered respiratory control.

Sustained hypoxia in the prenatal setting leads to persistent postnatal hyperpnea that can persist for several weeks although not into adulthood (70). Hypoxic ventilatory responses are initially increased suggesting at least initial sensitization of the carotid body which shows decreased dopamine content and of the brainstem that shows reduced noradrenaline (70). In contrast, sustained hypoxia in the immediate postnatal setting while also leading to persistent hyperpnea that lasts for several weeks, results in sustained reductions in the hypoxic ventilatory response particularly in males with no changes in ventilator responses to hypercapnia. Such changes appear to involve increased dopamine turnover in the carotid body (70). Interestingly, intermittent hypoxia as would occur in the setting of apnea of prematurity does not consistently lead to hyperpnea *per se* but is generally associated with a sensitized hypoxic ventilatory response with no changes in responses to hypercapnia (70).

In contrast to the changes with hypoxia, postnatal hyperoxia as would occur in the setting of prematurity leads to hypopnea and hypoventilation under normal conditions (although this does not

extend into adulthood) with initial increases in hypoxic ventilatory responses followed by reduced responses in adulthood (70). Hyperoxia can lead to reduced carotid body size and reductions in neurotransmitters and growth factors in the brainstem. However, intermittent hyperoxia again as could occur in the setting of prematurity with occasional exposure to supplemental oxygen does not substantially influence normal ventilatory patterns (70). Of note, postnatal hyperoxia in the resuscitation of hypoxic neonates with 100% oxygen resulted in a delayed onset of spontaneous respiratory efforts during the feto-neonatal transition (71).

Oxygen and injury to the developing lung

In the context of immaturity, it is important to recognize that hyperoxia is also associated with a robust inflammatory response (58, 62) with initial exposure leading to macrophage and polymorphonuclear cell infiltration that promotes interstitial edema as well as epithelial and endothelial cell injury (58). Inflammatory cells, particularly neutrophils, promote ROS within the immature lung that only furthers mitochondrial stress and apoptosis, resulting in cell death and lung remodeling. This becomes particularly important in premature infants at risk of developing BPD.

Although ROS with hyperoxia is more readily expected, hypoxia can also induce ROS via a superoxide burst that occurs rapidly with low oxygen exposure (72, 73) and contributes to lung injury. Such bursts are necessary for HIF-1α stabilization activation. ROS generated by hypoxia or hyperoxia can induce transcription factors such as HIF, Nrf2, and AP-1 (58, 74) that alter cellular proliferation and apoptosis. Lipid peroxides generated from hyperoxia can damage the mitochondrial membrane and promote apoptosis. In prematurity, these effects can impair postnatal alveolar development and enhance fibrosis (75). Oxidative stress can also activate inflammatory pathways such as MAPK, JNK and AP-1, and ER stress responses overall regulating multiple cellular functions (76). In turn, newborn mice treated with anti-inflammatory cyclooxygenase-2 inhibitors show blunted hyperoxia-induced lung injury, attributed to reduced ER stress response and improved alveolarization (77). As mentioned previously, there are emerging data for cellular senescence pathways that also promote inflammation and could contribute to lung injury (60).

Given the substantial impact of BPD, and the recognition of ROS as a contributory factor, antioxidant therapies have been a logical therapeutic avenue, but have largely been disappointing. However, there is also recognition that enhancing endogenous antioxidant pathways in the neonatal lung such as Nrf2 can be beneficial (78). Nrf2 is normally bound to and sequestered by Keap1, and increases in intracellular oxidation activate and degrades Keap1 permitting nuclear translocation of Keap1 and induction of antioxidant responses. Separately, there are data to support a beneficial role for vitamin A in extremely low birth weight infants in reducing oxygen dependency (79).

Oxygen, systemic inflammation and the developing lung

It is not uncommon for neonates to experience sequelae of maternal and intrauterine infections (including preterm birth itself and BPD) and postnatal infections that induce system inflammation (28). Given the medical need for supplemental oxygen in prematurity, and the higher likelihood of hypoxia due to increased apnea and bradycardia episodes in infected babies, both hypoxia and hyperoxia can synergize with infectious inflammatory processes to promote injury and remodeling in both airways and lung parenchyma. For example, a mouse model of systemic maternal inflammation leading to fetal inflammation *in utero* with superimposed postnatal hyperoxia shows increased TGFβ and profibrotic responses (80), while a similar model in rats leads to airway hyperreactivity (81). Maternal and fetal inflammation can also promote HIF-1α pathways within alveoli. Increased ROS in the setting of hypoxia or hyperoxia that initiate inflammatory cascades can synergize with infectious etiologies to depress respiratory activity (70).

Summary

Prematurity is a risk factor for perinatal and childhood lung diseases, with outcomes being influenced by perinatal exposures, particularly prenatal and postnatal changes in oxygen, and by infection and inflammation. While the fetus naturally grows in a hypoxic environment, the relative hyperoxia following premature birth, and the intermittent hypoxia from an immature respiratory system as well as any iatrogenic oxygen supplementation all lead to significant detrimental effects on respiratory control and lung development. Thus, understanding the effects of oxygen and inflammation on the developing respiratory system and the lung is critical to identify novel therapies for improved care and outcomes in this vulnerable population.

Acknowledgments

This study is supported by grants from US National Institutes of Health R01 HL056470 (Prakash, MacFarlane) and R01 HL138402 (MacFarlane, Pabelick).

References

1. Nikolic MZ, et al. Development. 2018; 145(16):dev163485.
2. Perl AK, et al. Clin Genet. 1999; 56(1):14–27.
3. Schittny JC. Cell Tissue Res. 2017; 367(3):427–444.
4. Whitsett JA, et al. Physiol Rev. 2019; 99(1):513–554.
5. Gebb SA, et al. Adv Exp Med Biol. 2003; 543:117–125.
6. Joshi S, et al. Early Hum Dev. 2007; 83(12):789–794.
7. Dylag AM, et al. Pediatr Res. 2017; 81(4):565–571.
8. Vogel ER, et al. Can J Physiol Pharmacol. 2015; 93(2):119–127.
9. Haworth SG, et al. Semin Neonatol. 2003; 8(1):1–8.
10. Massaro D, et al. Am J Physiol Lung Cell Mol Physiol. 2002; 282(3):L345–L358.
11. Giles BL, et al. Am J Physiol Lung Cell Mol Physiol. 2002; 283(3):L549–L554.
12. Wignarajah D, et al. Pediatr Res. 2002; 51(6):681–688.
13. Noble PB, et al. Front Physiol. 2019; 10:1073.
14. Hoo AF, et al. Am J Respir Crit Care Med. 1998; 158(3):700–705.
15. Prabhakar NR, et al. Physiology (Bethesda). 2015; 30(5):340–348.
16. Shimoda LA, et al. Am J Respir Crit Care Med. 2011; 183(2):152–156.
17. Samanta D, et al. Wiley Interdiscip Rev Syst Biol Med. 2017; 9(4):10.1002/wsbm.1382.
18. Semenza GL, et al. J Physiol. 2018; 596(15):2977–2983.
19. Wilson JW, et al. FEBS J. 2020. doi: 10.1111/febs.15374.
20. Laddha AP, et al. Respir Med. 2019; 156:33–46.
21. Mathew R. Children (Basel). 2020; 7(8):100.
22. Woik N, et al. Cell Mol Life Sci. 2015; 72(14):2709–2718.
23. McGrath-Morrow SA, et al. Am J Respir Cell Mol Biol. 2005; 32(5):420–427.
24. Tuder RM, et al. J Mol Med (Berl). 2007; 85(12):1317–1324.
25. Prakash YS. Am J Physiol Lung Cell Mol Physiol. 2013; 305(12):L912–L933.
26. Prakash YS. Am J Physiol Lung Cell Mol Physiol. 2016; 311(6):L1113–L1140.
27. Prakash YS, et al. Chest. 2017; 152(3):618–626.
28. Britt RD Jr., et al. Expert Rev Respir Med. 2013; 7(5):515–531.
29. Ryu J, et al. Thromb Haemost. 2005; 94(1):175–183.
30. Philippe C, et al. Sleep Breath. 2015; 19(1):297–306.
31. Hartman WR, et al. Am J Physiol Lung Cell Mol Physiol. 2012; 303(8):L711–L719.
32. Tan CD, et al. Br J Pharmacol. 2012; 167(2):368–382.
33. Prandota J. Am J Ther. 2004; 11(6):517–546.
34. Tsapournioti S, et al. J Cell Physiol. 2013; 228(8):1745–1753.
35. Jiang H, et al. Am J Physiol Lung Cell Mol Physiol. 2010; 298(5):L660–L669.
36. Davis RP, et al. Semin Pediatr Surg. 2013; 22(4):179–184.
37. Tsao PN, et al. Neonatology. 2013; 103(4):300–307.
38. Truog WE, et al. Pediatr Res. 2008; 64(1):56–62.
39. Ambalavanan N, et al. Am J Physiol Lung Cell Mol Physiol. 2008; 295(1):L86–L95.
40. Bancalari E, et al. Am J Perinatol. 2018; 35(6):534–536.
41. Domm W, et al. Front Med (Lausanne). 2015; 2:55.
42. Morty RE. Semin Perinatol. 2018; 42(7):404–412.
43. Perrone S, et al. Oxid Med Cell Longev. 2018; 2018:7483062.
44. Sahni M, et al. F1000Res. 2020; 9: F1000 Faculty Rev-703.
45. Vento M, et al. Clin Perinatol. 2019; 46(3):459–473.
46. Di Fiore JM, et al. Clin Perinatol. 2019; 46(3):553–565.
47. Maitre NL, et al. J Perinatol. 2015; 35(5):313–321.
48. Hibbs AM, et al. J Pediatr. 2008; 153(4):525–529.
49. Been JV, et al. PLoS Med. 2014;11(1):e1001596.
50. Holditch-Davis D, et al. J Obstet Gynecol Neonatal Nurs. 2008; 37(3):262–273.
51. Vrijlandt EJ, et al. Am J Respir Crit Care Med. 2013; 187(11):1234–1240.
52. Vogel ER, et al. Pediatr Res. 2017; 81(2):376–383.
53. Belik J, et al. J Appl Physiol (1985). 2003; 94(6):2303–2312.
54. Ali NK, et al. Neonatology. 2012; 101(2):106–115.
55. Britt RD Jr., et al. Am J Physiol Lung Cell Mol Physiol. 2015; 309(6):L537–L542.
56. Prakash YS, et al. Pharmacol Ther. 2014; 143(1):74–86.
57. O'Reilly M, et al. Anat Rec (Hoboken). 2014; 297(4):758–769.
58. Bhandari V. Front Biosci. 2008; 13: 6653–6661.
59. Parikh P, et al. Am J Respir Cell Mol Biol. 2019; 61(1):51–60.
60. Parikh P, et al. Am J Physiol Lung Cell Mol Physiol. 2019; 316(5):L826–L842.
61. You K, et al. Am J Physiol Lung Cell Mol Physiol. 2019; 317(5):L525–L536.
62. Bhandari V. Semin Fetal Neonatal Med. 2010; 15(4):223–229.
63. Velten M, et al. J Appl Physiol (1985). 2010; 108(5):1347–1356.
64. Manja V, et al. JAMA Pediatr. 2015; 169(4):332–340.
65. Vadivel A, et al. Am J Respir Cell Mol Biol. 2014; 50(1):96–105.
66. Bavis RW, et al. J Appl Physiol (1985). 2008; 104(4):1220–1229.
67. Mitchell L, et al. Respir Physiol Neurobiol. 2020; 273:103318.
68. MacFarlane PM, et al. Respir Physiol Neurobiol. 2013; 185(1):170–176.
69. Martin RJ, et al. Adv Exp Med Biol. 2012; 758:351–358.
70. Bavis RW, et al. Exp Neurol. 2017; 287(Pt 2):176–191.
71. Martin RJ, et al. Semin Perinatol. 2008; 32(5):355–366.
72. Kumar H, et al. Mediators Inflamm. 2015; 2015:584758.
73. Lee P, et al. Nat Rev Mol Cell Biol. 2020; 21(5):268–283.
74. Lee PJ, et al. Free Radic Biol Med. 2003; 35(4):341–350.
75. Hilgendorff A, et al. Am J Respir Cell Mol Biol. 2014; 50(2):233–245.
76. Chen AC, et al. Clin Transl Immunology. 2018; 7(6):e1019.
77. Choo-Wing R, et al. Am J Respir Cell Mol Biol. 2013; 48(6):749–757.
78. Cho HY, et al. Curr Opin Toxicol. 2016; 1:125–133.
79. Araki S, et al. PLoS One. 2018; 13(11):e0207730.
80. Velten M, et al. Am J Physiol Regul Integr Comp Physiol. 2012; 303(3):R279–R290.
81. Choi CW, et al. Pediatr Res. 2013; 74(1):11–18.

HYPOXIC RESPIRATORY FAILURE AND THE NEONATAL KIDNEY

Catherine Morgan and Po-Yin Cheung

Contents

Introduction

Early observations of edema, oliguria, and renal acidification defects during hypoxic respiratory failure and respiratory distress syndrome in neonates suggested impairment of renal function was a common course in these pathological states. Human and animal model observations and investigations have led to further characterization and understanding of the effect of hypoxia on the neonatal kidney, including the impact on renal perfusion and hemodynamics within the local microcirculation, glomerular filtration rate, free water excretion and diluting ability, and renal tubular transport function. Although hypoxemic neonates often present with derangements in renal physiology, with progressive severity or duration of hypoxia these processes become less likely to be reversible and the clinical picture progresses to acute tubular necrosis, acute kidney injury (AKI), and global dysfunction that may be irreversible. In addition, hypoxia, and hyperoxic resuscitation can have a long-standing impact on nephron development and long-term renal outcomes.

In the fourth week after conception, the nephrogenic cord is developed with the formation of pronephros, mesonephros, and metanephros. In the embryonic and fetal development, pronephric duct subsequently regresses, whereas there is sexual-dependent evolution or regression of mesonephros. Metanephric kidney begins at the fifth week and differentiates to form the permanent kidney with the continuation of nephrogenesis until 32 weeks gestation and functional maturation after birth to early childhood. Meanwhile the dorsal aorta develops branches to provide blood supply to the kidneys. The embryonic development of fetal kidneys is critically dependent on Hypoxia-Induced Factor 1β and Vascular Endothelial Growth Factors. However, these two factors are also related to the pathological (cellular and vascular) responses to hypoxia.

Hypoxic respiratory failure and acute kidney injury

Neonatal hypoxia often occurs simultaneously with significantly altered hemodynamics, resulting in hypoxic-ischemic injury to many organs, including the kidneys. Newborn kidneys are sensitive to oxygen deprivation and renal insufficiency may occur within 24 hours of hypoxic-ischemic episode, which, if prolonged, may even lead to irreversible acute tubular or cortical necrosis

with further parenchymal edema and sloughing of necrotic tubular epithelial cells into the tubular lumen. Identification and classification of AKI in this setting rely on a serial measurement of serum creatinine. In spite of all the limitations of using serum creatinine levels to define AKI in the neonate, it is still the most widely used marker. The Neonatal KDIGO (Kidney Diseases: Improving Global Outcomes) AKI definition, based on the degree of rise in serum creatinine level rather than a single absolute cut-off value, is currently widely accepted as a way to define AKI in the newborn (Table 25.1) (1).

AKI in hypoxic respiratory failure is common, affecting 47–72% of neonates with varying degrees of perinatal asphyxia and is associated with increased mortality independent of severity of illness (2–4). Growing evidence in animal models suggests that AKI is not an isolated event but leads to further remote organ dysfunction through neutrophil migration, cytokine expression, and increased oxidative stress; this organ cross-talk occurs between the injured kidneys and the lungs, heart, and brain (5, 6). Such sequences of escalating organ dysfunction could exacerbate pulmonary injury, further impair respiratory function and tissue oxygenation, and worsen encephalopathy. In human neonates, AKI is significantly associated with worsening hypoxic ischemic encephalopathy (HIE) and adverse long-term neurodevelopmental outcome (7–9). It has been shown in neonates that AKI is associated with hypoxic-ischemic lesions on brain MRI and that the severity of these lesions parallels worsening AKI, even after controlling for other risk factors, demographics, and interventions associated with perinatal asphyxia (10). Interestingly, observational studies have found the association of oliguria in the first 24 hours after birth and the occurrence of AKI in asphyxiated neonates with the subsequent neurodevelopmental outcomes (9).

In the lung, alveolar concentrations of pro-inflammatory cytokines and chemokines are increased, macrophage-mediated pulmonary vascular permeability is increased, apoptosis is upregulated, and T-cell trafficking of antigen is disrupted after isolated hypoxic kidney injury (11–13). In addition to organ cross-talk driving additional lung injury in AKI, respiratory physiology is further dysregulated through the disruption in the balance of nitrogenous waste, fluid and acid–base management. AKI with associated uremia affects gas exchange and lung mechanics (14, 15). Fluid overload due to AKI leads to a large difference between hydrostatic forces and oncotic forces, leading to fluid flux from the capillary bed into the alveolar space, with resulting pulmonary edema and impaired gas exchange. The management of acid–base balance by

DOI: 10.1201/9780367494018-25

TABLE 25.1 Neonatal KDIGO (Kidney Diseases: Improving Global Outcomes) Acute Kidney Injury Definition (1)

Stage	Serum Creatinine (SCr)
No AKI	No change in SCr or rise <0.3 mg/dL
1	SCr rise ≥0.3 mg/dL within 48 h or SCr rise ≥1.5 to 1.9 × reference SCr[a] within 7 days
2	SCr rise ≥2 to 2.9 × reference SCr[a]
3	SCr rise ≥3 × reference SCr[a] or SCr ≥2.5 mg/dL or receipt of dialysis

[a] Reference SCr is the lowest prior SCr measurement.

the kidney, specifically the equilibrium of bicarbonate, carbonic acid, and carbon dioxide, is critical to lung function; when the kidneys suffer injury, the ability to maintain this crucial balance is lost and the controls over acid–base regulation/buffering become compromised. AKI from hypoxic respiratory failure in the neonate exacerbates acute lung injury, leads to prolonged mechanical ventilation, and can contribute to the development of chronic lung disease (4, 16). Hypoxic respiratory failure associated AKI triggers a cascade of extra-renal responses, which exacerbates lung and brain injury and dysfunction.

Tubular dysfunction and injury during hypoxia

Although in its most severe or prolonged form, hypoxia can lead to renal cell death and irreversible renal injury, some defects seen with hypoxia are reversible upon restoring normoxia and the often associated abnormalities in extracellular fluid volume and cardiac output. Renal tubular epithelial cells are one of the major targets of hypoxia-induced injury. These cells are responsible for reabsorption of many substances filtered by the glomerulus, as well as regulation of water, electrolyte, acid–base balance. Proximal tubule cells are particularly sensitive to hypoxia as they rely predominantly on aerobic metabolism and the mitochondria within these cells are in a more oxidized state than in more distal segments (17). In addition, proximal tubule cells do not synthesize glutathione, a major cellular antioxidant, in response to hypoxia-induced reactive oxygen species (18). Unlike other segments of the nephron, proximal tubule cells need to take glutathione up from the blood (18). Thus, the proximal tubules are especially vulnerable to hypoxia. If a hypoxic state persists, cellular hypoxia leads to excessive reactive oxygen species production and overwhelming oxidative stress and inflammation induce compromise of the endothelial barrier, resulting in intensified hypoxia (19). Urine biomarkers of proximal tubular cell dysfunction and injury are elevated in asphyxiated neonates for 1–2 weeks after resuscitation, indicating that effects on the proximal tubular cell persist even after resuscitation and restoration of normoxemia (20).

The excretion rate of sodium increases during hypoxia, and remains elevated during recovery, due to a progressive fall in the fractional reabsorption of sodium. Hypoxia results in decreased sodium reabsorption by the proximal tubule (21, 22). Hypoxia causes a rapid fall in cellular ATP, resulting in disruption of the actin cytoskeleton (23). There is a dissociation of proximal tubular Na⁺-K⁺-ATPase from its cytoskeletal anchorage resulting in transient loss of Na⁺-K⁺-ATPase from the basolateral plasma membrane (23, 24); approximately 70% of renal oxygen consumption is related to Na⁺-K⁺-ATPase dependent transport across the renal tubular epithelial cell. The redistribution of Na⁺-K⁺-ATPase away from the basolateral membrane during hypoxia appears to be unique to proximal tubule cells and the Na⁺-K⁺-ATPase-cytoskeletal complex can be reestablished during cellular repair (25). This redistribution of Na⁺-K⁺-ATPase is in part responsible for reduced renal tubular sodium reabsorption, which occurs with hypoxia. There is also a decrease in the filtered load of bicarbonate during hypoxia, resulting in reduced $NaHCO_3$ reabsorption (22). An additional mechanism for natriuresis is related to peripheral O_2 chemosensitivity; isolated hypoxic perfusion of the carotid body causes hypoxic natriuresis by inhibition of renal tubular sodium reabsorption (26, 27). In response to the fall in proximal reabsorption of sodium, there is increased sodium reabsorption in the distal tubule; however, this is insufficient to fully compensate for the fall in proximal reabsorption, so sodium excretion is elevated.

Renal tubular water balance regulation is disturbed by hypoxic respiratory failure. Neonatal hypoxia induces an antidiuresis that is independent of alterations in cardiac output, mean arterial pressure, stroke volume, filtration fraction, renal nerves, or renal response to antidiuretic hormone (ADH) (18). Hypoxia (without an alteration in renal blood flow) in the neonate is associated with a fall in urine output and an increase in secretion ADH, with a fall in free water clearance (28). Hypoxia is a potent stimulus for ADH release and newborns with hypoxia have high circulating ADH (28–30), likely through stimulation of peripheral chemoreceptors (30). There is a decrease in free water clearance during hypoxia in newborns (11) due to increased release of ADH. In addition, mechanical ventilation itself can increase ADH release, further contributing to decreased free water clearance in hypoxic neonates (31, 32). The associated decreased free water clearance is associated with exacerbation of pulmonary problems and prolongation of respiratory support in neonates (31). Furthermore, acute onset of hyponatremia may be associated with cerebral edema. Recognition of increased ADH with cautious and thoughtful fluid administration is critical in the setting of hypoxia, with individualized fluid prescription to avoid fluid overload and its associated comorbidities.

Hypoxia, renal vascular function, and glomerular filtration

The effects of hypoxia on renal vascular function are induced in part by changes in the systemic circulation. Hypoxia leads to decreased mean arterial and, subsequently, renal perfusion pressure (33). Although kidneys are able to autoregulate relatively early in life, they do so with relatively lower efficiency in neonates (34, 35). At some point, as perfusion pressure decreases, there is a transition from autoregulated to pressure-dependent flow within the neonatal kidney; compared with the brain, the kidney is less well autoregulated and is subject to impaired or fluctuating perfusion if systemic hypotension occurs (21). Clinical studies have shown decreased renal blood flow velocities early in the course of neonates with hypoxic respiratory failure (36). In addition, resolution of renal blood flow disturbance in the kidney after resuscitation is prolonged relative to other organs. Indeed, the renal vasculature is the last to recover with the normalization of renal blood flow 1–2 hours after the reoxygenation of hypoxic newborn piglets (37). This contrasts to the immediate and early recovery of cerebral and mesenteric blood flows, respectively, following the reoxygenation.

The kidneys of newborn infants are particularly susceptible to hypoperfusion with resulting tissue hypoxia for several reasons. Neonates have high renal vascular resistance as well as high plasma renin activity (35); high plasma renin reduces the ability of the renal vessels to vasodilate. In addition, regional pO_2 pressures stay within a relatively narrow range within the kidney. Renal O_2 supply is utilized primarily to fuel transport processes that move various molecules across cellular membranes. Many of these processes are load-dependent, linking renal O_2 consumption and glomerular filtration rate. Given that renal blood flow and glomerular filtration rate predominantly change in parallel, an increase in renal blood flow and O_2 delivery is offset by increased consumption (28, 38). Thus, in the face of hypoxia, the kidney is unable to raise regional pO_2 by increasing blood flow and the susceptibility to hypoxic injury is high. It is important to note that mechanical ventilation can disrupt the coupling that occurs between renal blood flow, oxygen delivery, and oxygen utilization. Positive pressure ventilation causes a reduction in cardiac output by impeding venous return but at the same time results in release of neurohumoral mediators which lead to sodium reabsorption (39). Sodium reabsorption in the kidney requires high oxygen utilization; hence mechanical ventilation in the newborn may decrease oxygen delivery while subsequently increasing oxygen utilization, potentiating cellular injury.

There are direct renal microvascular effects of hypoxia, independent of hypocapnia and systemic hemodynamic changes, in neonatal respiratory failure (40). The renal vascular bed is very sensitive to decreased plasma oxygen tension. It is one of the first vascular beds that respond to hypoxia with vasoconstriction resulting in the redistribution of blood to vital organs including the brain (41). This response is mediated through several mechanisms. Michelakis et al. have shown high sensitivity to oxygen concentration of the mitochondria in the renal vascular smooth muscle cells (42). In addition, renal oxygen insufficiency reduces tubular transport and stimulates intrarenal adenosine release by ATP breakdown, inducing preglomerular vasoconstriction, post-glomerular vasodilatation, and decreased glomerular filtration rate (19, 43, 44). The resulting intra-renal hemodynamic shift represents a renoprotective mechanism that initially decreases oxygen expenditure and maintains post-glomerular tubular blood flow.

In addition to direct chemoreceptor-mediated reflex, tubuloglomerular feedback, and intra-renal adenosine, augmentation of the intrarenal activity of prostaglandins, angiotensin II, and nitric oxide by hypoxia plays a key role in the renal hemodynamic effects of hypoxia. Blockade of angiotensin II formation and adenosine antagonism both result in increased renal blood flow in the context of hypoxia, suggesting vasodilating agents are also activated during hypoxia (45). Nitric oxide is synthesized by the immature kidney and plays a role in the renal hemodynamics of the newborn. It is also thought to play a role during hypoxemic stress in the kidney. Hypoxia is a potent stimulus for the release of endothelium-derived relaxing factor in arterial structures and has a homeostatic counterregulatory role to prevent excessive vasoconstriction (33). Modulation of any of these mediators with therapeutic interventions has the potential to change the functional and injury response of the neonatal kidney to hypoxia. There is, however, a fine balance between hypoxia-induced mechanisms that protect the kidney from injury and those that amplify injurious processes. A far more detailed understanding of the effect of hypoxia on the human neonatal kidney, and prospective clinical trials based on this understanding are needed before standardized therapeutic recommendations can be made.

Measurement of renal oxygen supply-demand balance

Conventional hemodynamic monitoring techniques do not allow assessment of the microcirculation and the oxygen content in regional tissue beds. NIRS (near-infrared spectroscopy), which measures the differential changes in oxygenated and deoxygenated hemoglobin under a skin surface probe, is emerging as a noninvasive technology to assess renal oxygen supply-demand balance. There is little data on normative values for healthy newborns. In premature neonates, baseline physiological renal regional oxygen saturation (rSO_2) values average between 65 and 80 (33,46,47,48). This varies by gestational and postnatal age, although detailed normative values are not available. After birth, renal rSO_2 decreases with postnatal time until it stabilizes at approximately 2 weeks postnatal age; even though there is increased renal blood flow during this time, increased oxygen consumption likely outweighs delivery (33, 46–48).

A number of changes have been observed in renal NIRS measurements during or as a result of hypoxia. Hypoxia in neonates does not need to be prolonged to see renal effects. Even brief hypoxic events (less than 1 min), in the absence of significant systemic hemodynamic effects, are associated with decreased renal NIRS rSO_2 (46). This decrease occurs concurrent with the hypoxemia, which may reflect either a responsive change in renal blood flow or increased oxygen extraction. Importantly, more severe hypoxemia (SaO_2 75% or less), even for brief time periods, results in delayed/incomplete recovery of the renal rSO_2 (46). For more prolonged events of hypoxia with ischemia, such as in the setting with HIE, higher renal rSO_2 may be observed, as oxygen extraction is eventually significantly impaired due to cellular injury (7).

Hyperoxia

It is important to note that medical interventions for neonatal hypoxia may have negative renal consequences. Postnatal exposure to intermittent hypoxia followed by interventional hyperoxia induces oxidative stress and free radicals, which leads to direct cellular injury, oxidation of DNA, induction of cytokines, and cell death. In the setting of poorly developed, immature antioxidant systems, there is less capacity to scavenge reactive oxygen species; small for gestational age and premature neonates in particular demonstrate reduced kidney antioxidant capacity (49). In neonatal models of increased oxidative stress, adverse effects are seen, including enlarged renal corpuscles, renal tubular necrosis, interstitial inflammation, and abnormal tubular development (50). Preterm neonates less than 36 weeks gestational age show ongoing nephrogenesis. Not only is renal morphogenesis sensitive to hypoxia, which is a physiological trigger for the expression of vascular endothelial growth factor, but oxygen supplementation and hyperoxic exposure of the newborn have also been shown to result in impaired nephrogenesis (51). Thus, perturbation in oxygen exposure in the neonatal period has significant potential to alter long-term nephron development.

Hyperoxic resuscitation of asphyxiated neonates may also lead to increased risk of AKI. Studies including clinical trials have demonstrated that the use of 100% oxygen, given with positive pressure ventilation of the newborn infant during resuscitation, causes more oxidative stress than using air (52). The negative impact of this on overall mortality has been demonstrated (53, 54); however, less is known about the acute effects of hyperoxic resuscitation on the kidney. Neonates with asphyxia during the transition from fetal to extrauterine life have been shown to have elevated urine N-acetyl-beta-glucosaminidase (NAG) at 24 and 48 hours of life, relative to non-asphyxiated newborns (20) NAG is a lysosomal enzyme of the proximal tubule cell (a primary target of hypoxic injury) released into the urine with cell injury. In neonates resuscitated with high inspiratory fraction of oxygen (vs. room air), this biomarker of tubular injury is further increased, associated with markers indicating more prolonged oxidative stress (20). In addition, hyperoxic resuscitation appears to be associated with more prolonged renal tubular injury, with urine biomarkers remaining elevated for up to 2 weeks longer than room air resuscitated neonates. Although newborn resuscitation guidelines suggest avoiding hyperoxic resuscitation, there remains a large knowledge gap regarding the impact of these guidelines and avoidance of hyperoxia on clinically relevant renal injury outcomes.

Aminophylline and other novel therapeutic approaches

Aminophylline is an adenosine inhibitor and has been used in the treatment of apnea in preterm neonates (55). Hypoxia is associated with increased renal adenosine content and vasoconstriction (56). The prophylactic administration of aminophylline in asphyxiated neonates has been shown to reduce the incidence of AKI (57).

In addition to the use of 21% oxygen in the reoxygenation of hypoxic neonates, the renovascular protective effects of various interventions have been investigated in models of neonatal asphyxia. Anti-oxidative agents (N-acetylcysteine), matrix metalloproteinase inhibitor (doxycycline), and nitric oxide donor (L-arginine) have been examined (58–60). These agents were found to improve the renal vascular recovery with reduced renal tissue injury markers of oxidative stress and ischemia at different extents. Clinical studies are required to confirm if the renal protective effect of these agents can be translated to asphyxiated neonates. Improved renal recovery would help fluid and electrolytes homeostasis in these critically ill neonates, in addition to potential short- and long-term benefits in outcomes.

Summary

Hypoxic neonates commonly have impaired renal function and AKI. Related to the high sensitivity to hypoxic insult, the kidney tubules and renovascular bed are the first affected with deregulation of water, electrolytes and acid–base balance, perfusion deficits and reduced glomerular filtration rate, respectively. Upon the reoxygenation of hypoxic neonates, the renal tubular and vascular recovery is also affected by various therapeutic interventions

including hyperoxia, and other experimental medications (e.g. N-acetylcysteine and doxycycline). An adenosine inhibitor, aminophylline may be used prophylactically to reduce the incidence of AKI in asphyxiated neonates.

References

1. Nada A, et al. Semin Fetal Neonatal Med. 2017; 22(2):90–97.
2. Shah P, et al. Arch Dis Child Fetal Neonatal Ed. 2004; 89(2):F152–F155.
3. Hankins GDV, et al. Obstet Gynecol. 2002; 99(5 Pt 1):688–691.
4. Selewski DT, et al. J Pediatr. 2013 Apr; 162(4):725.e1–729.e1.
5. Yap SC, et al. Anesthesiology. 2012; 116:1139–1148.
6. Basu RK, et al. Pediatr Nephrol. 2013; 28(12):2239–2248.
7. Gupta BD, et al. Indian Pediatr. 2005; 42:928–934.
8. Martín-Ancel A, et al. J Pediatr. 1995; 127:786–793.
9. Perlman JM, et al. J Pediatr. 1988; 113:875–879.
10. Sarkar S, et al. Pediatr Res. 2014; 75(3):431–435.
11. Klein CL, et al. Kidney Int. 2008; 74:901–909.
12. Kramer AA, et al. Kidney Int. 1999; 55:2362–2367.
13. Hassoun HT, et al. Am J Physiol Renal Physiol. 2009; 297:F125–F137.
14. Daum S, et al. Cas Lek Cesk. 1965; 104(47):1285–1290.
15. Karacan O, et al. Ren Fail. 2004; 26(3):273–278.
16. Starr MC, et al. Am J Perinatol. 2020; 37(2):231–240.
17. Hall AM, et al. J Am Soc Nephrol. 2009; 20:1293–1302.
18. Anderson RJ, et al. J Clin Invest. 1978; 62(4):769–777.
19. Che R, et al. Am J Physiol Renal Physiol. 2014; 306(4):F367–F378
20. Vento M, et al. Am J Respir Crit Care Med. 2005; 172(11):1393–1398.
21. Chock V, et al. J Pediatr. 2018; 200:232–239.
22. Gibson KJ, et al. Clin Exp Pharmacol Physiol. 2000; 27(1-2):67–73.
23. Molitoris BA, et al. J Clin Invest. 1991; 88:462–469.
24. Adachi S, et al. Pediatr Res. 2004; 55(3):485–491.
25. Molitoris BA, et al. Am J Physiol Renal Physiol. 1992; 263(3):F488–F495
26. Swenson ER, et al. J. Appl Physiol. 1995; 78(2):377–383.
27. Honig A. Am J Physiol. 1989; 257(6 Pt 2):R1282–R1302.
28. Daniel SS, et al. Pediatr Res. 1984; 18(3):227–231.
29. Stegner H, et al. Pediatr Res. 1984; 18(2):188–191.
30. Rurak DW. J. Physiol.1978; 277:341–357.
31. Vuohelainen T, et al. PLoS One. 2011; 6(2):e16995.
32. Hemmer M, et al. Anesthesiology. 1980; 52(5):395–400.
33. McNeill S, et al. J Perinatol. 2010; 3:51–57.
34. Soni H, et al. Am J Physiol Renal Physiol. 2017; 313(5):F1136–F1148.
35. Sulemanji M, et al. Semin Pediatr Surg. 2013; 22(4):195–198.
36. Ilves P, et al. J Ultrasound Med. 2009 Nov; 28(11):1471–1480
37. Cheung PY, et al. J Vis Exp. 2011; (56):3166. doi:10.3791/3166.
38. Haase VH. J Am Soc Nephrol. 2013; 24(4):537–541.
39. Hepokoski ML, et al. Nephron. 2018; 140:90–93.
40. Ballèvre L, et al. Pediatr Res. 1996; 39(4 Pt 1):725–730.
41. Pichler G, et al. Nephrology (Carlton). 2015; 20(2):107–109.
42. Michelakis, et al. Circ Res. 2002; 90:1307–1315.
43. Gouyon JB, et al. Biol Neonate. 1988; 53(4):237–242.
44. Tóth-Heyn P, et al. Pedatr Nephrol. 1998; 12(5):377–380.
45. Prévot A, et al. Life Sci. 2002; 71:779–787.
46. Petrova A, et al. Pediatr Crit Care Med. 2006; 7:449–454.
47. Petrova A, et al. Arch Dis Child Fetal Neonatal Ed. 2010; 95(3):F213–F219
48. van der Laan M, et al. Neonatology. 2010; 110:141–147.
49. Soni H, et al. Redox Rep. 2019; 24(1):10–16.
50. Jiang JS, et al. Pediatr Neonatol. 2015; 56(4):235–241.
51. Sutherland MR, et al. Am J Physiol Renal Physiol. 2013; 304(10):F1308–F1316.
52. Torres-Cuevas I, et al. Redox Biol. 2017; 12:674–681.
53. Saugstad OD, et al. Neonatology. 2008; 94:176–182.
54. Perlman JM, et al. Circulation. 2010; 122(16 Suppl 2):S516–S538.
55. Bhatt-Mehta V, et al. Paediatr Drugs. 2003; 5:195–210.
56. Prévot A, et al. Pediatr Res. 2003; 54:400–405.
57. Bhatt GC, et al. Arch Dis Child. 2019; 104:670–679.
58. Lee TF, et al. Shock. 2011; 35:428–433.
59. Labossiere JR, et al. Shock. 2015; 43:99–105.
60. Basile DP, et al. Am J Physiol Renal Physiol. 2003; 284:F338–F348.

THE EFFECT OF HYPOXIA ON INTESTINAL FUNCTION

Eric B. Ortigoza and Josef Neu

Contents

Hypoxic-ischemic intestinal injury

The neonatal gastrointestinal (GI) system can be vulnerable to injury from hypoxic respiratory failure and birth asphyxia (1). Changes in intestinal hemodynamics occur during the transition from fetal to postnatal life as the newborn infant switches the source of nutrition from the placenta to the GI tract (2, 3). Intestinal vascular resistance is high in fetal life and rapidly decreases after birth. This postnatal decrease occurs in part because of increased endothelial production of nitric oxide, a vasodilator (3, 4). This low intestinal vascular resistance affects the ability of the neonatal intestinal vasculature to respond to systemic circulatory changes, such as hypotension, arterial hypoxemia, and hypoxia. Newborn infants have immature pressure-flow autoregulation in response to hypotension, resulting in decreased oxygen delivery to the intestines (5). In neonatal swine studies, severe hypoxemia causes newborns to respond with vasoconstriction, leading to intestinal ischemia (1). Hypoxia and ischemia occurring in the fetus and newborn can further reduce intestinal perfusion by eliciting a "diving reflex" that preferentially diverts blood flow away from organs such as the intestines to preserve blood flow to the brain, heart, and adrenals (6). It is unclear whether the diving reflex causes necrosis of the intestine, but developmental alterations in the microcirculation have been hypothesized to dispose to intestinal necrosis (3).

Hypoxic respiratory failure that results in hypoxic-ischemic injury to the GI tract can be a rare occurrence, except when it is associated with congenital heart defects. In fact, the risk of ischemia to the intestine is 10–100 times greater in term infants with a congenital heart defect than in term neonates without a cardiac defect (7, 8). The most common types of congenital heart defects that can increase the risk of intestinal injury are hypoplastic left heart syndrome, aortic arch obstruction, truncus arteriosus, and aortopulmonary window (9). All of these examples can lead to decreased blood flow to the descending aorta and can cause a lack of perfusion to the mesenteric arteries causing ischemia and necrosis. Because the mechanism of the intestinal injury seen with congenital heart defect differs from that seen in most preterm infants, this should not be termed "necrotizing enterocolitis (NEC)," but a term that is more descriptive of the real pathophysiology, such as "cardiogenic ischemic necrosis of the intestine" (10).

Hypoxic-ischemic intestinal injury vs. necrotizing enterocolitis

Hypoxic-ischemic intestinal injury has long been proposed as a key contributor to NEC. However, most preterm infants with NEC do not have a clear history of perinatal hypoxic-ischemic events (11, 12). Classic NEC is a disease that is primarily seen in preterm infants. The pathophysiology of classic NEC continues to be poorly defined; however, it is strongly associated with intestinal immaturity and it is likely related to an excessive inflammatory response and dysbiosis (13). In contrast, hypoxic-ischemic intestinal injury is more common in term infants, particularly those with congenital heart defects, without a clear link to inflammation or dysbiosis (14).

The confusion between hypoxic-ischemic intestinal injury and classic NEC may have caused a significant delay in our current understanding of the pathophysiology of classic NEC. Several animal models have been developed to study classic necrotizing enterocolitis. The original model (Figure 26.1) was first described in the 1970s, and its variations have been used in multiple studies (15). However, these models did not adequately represent classic NEC in human preterm infants because they addressed stressors that can occur at

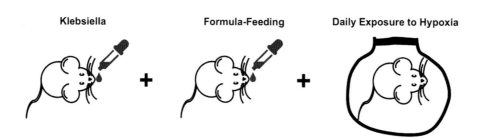

Klebsiella　　　　**Formula-Feeding**　　　　**Daily Exposure to Hypoxia**

FIGURE 26.1 Original rat model of "necrotizing enterocolitis." As described in Barlow et al. 1974, newborn rats were given inocula of *Klebsiella* either by mouth or by intrauterine administration. Formula feeds were administered via a dropper four times per day (0.5–2 mL per feeding). Hypoxia was induced by enclosing the animals in a plastic bag once a day until they were limp, cyanotic, and gasping (approximately 3–5 min) (44).

DOI: 10.1201/9780367494018-26

birth (asphyxia, hypothermia, hypoxia) in combination with gavage formula feeding and administration of proinflammatory agents. Stressors such as hypoxia and ischemia are not commonly seen in classic human NEC (14, 16). Thus, the intestinal injury in these animal models was not representative of the pathology seen in classic NEC in human preterm infants. Classic NEC is related to intestinal immaturity of barrier function, circulatory regulation, motility, digestion, and immunity. Immaturity can lead to the excessive inflammatory response that is seen with classic NEC. In addition, dysbiosis or intestinal microbial imbalance of the usual microbiome may contribute to the pathogenesis of classic NEC (13). This imbalance has been characterized as a predominance of bacteria belonging to the Proteobacteria phylum and a decrease in abundance of the Firmicutes and Bacterioidetes phyla (17). After decades of research, more investigators are starting to agree that hypoxic-ischemic injury to the intestine is a different disease process altogether and not a key contributor to classic NEC.

The role of hypoxia in barrier function, intestinal colonization, and the microbiome

The GI tract forms the largest barrier with the external environment (18). A monolayer of intestinal epithelial cells separates the lamina propria from the intestinal lumen. This epithelium allows translocation of nutrients, water, and electrolytes from the lumen and, at the same time, forms a tight barrier to prevent penetration of microorganisms (both commensal and potentially pathogenic) (18). Alterations in barrier functions can increase the risk of infection by pathogens from the GI tract and can lead to dysregulation of the mechanisms that allow for tolerance of the commensal organisms. Eventually, these events lead to inflammation of the GI tract (19, 20). To help separate the content of the intestinal lumen from the intestinal epithelial cells, goblet cells and Paneth cells secrete mucus and peptides with antimicrobial and antiviral properties (21). In addition, the intestinal epithelial cells have tightly juxtaposed adhesive junctional complexes between neighboring cells. This junctional complex is essential for establishing and maintaining the barrier function of the mucosal layer (22).

An important component of barrier function is the low oxygen level that is present in the lumen of the intestine. The relatively hypoxic lumen establishes the oxygen gradient of the intestinal epithelium as cells directly adjacent to the lumen are hypoxic relative to the cells at the base of the crypts (23). This hypoxic environment is essential for the survival of many commensal bacteria (24). The intestinal mucosa experiences profound fluctuations in the blood flow and oxygenation during normal physiological conditions, and intestinal epithelial cells are uniquely resistant to hypoxia (25). In this hypoxic environment, cells respond by regulating the expression of genes through the major hypoxic-induced transcription factor called hypoxia-inducible factor (HIF) (26). HIF plays an important role in the development of the intestinal microvasculature through regulation of vascular endothelial growth factor (VEGF), explained below (27). HIF can also function as a regulator of inflammation within the intestine. Induction of HIF-1α upregulates protective mechanisms along the intestinal mucosa that include increased expression of tight junction proteins and enhanced intestinal barrier functions (28). Thus, physiological levels of hypoxia and HIF signaling are essential for intestinal barrier regulation during homeostasis and active inflammation (29). Dysregulation of oxygen gradients and/or disruptions of the HIF mechanism can lead to inflammation and intestinal injury (28).

Anemia is a condition that can cause alterations in oxygen availability leading to dysregulation of oxygen gradients and intestinal injury (28, 30). Anemia can cause nonphysiologic hypoxia beyond the intestinal epithelium, inducing proinflammatory macrophages that reside in the lamina propria (30, 31). This anemia-induced hypoxia can increase HIF-1α expression inside these macrophages, resulting in release of proinflammatory cytokines such as interferon-gamma (IFNγ) and tumor necrosis factor-alpha (TNFα) (30). Proinflammatory cytokines can then impair gut barrier function and attenuate the protective impact of HIF activity in epithelial cells (32, 33).

Anemia itself has been associated with intestinal dysbiosis characterized by a dominance of Proteobacteria and decreased Firmicutes (34). Proteobacteria are Gram-negative bacteria that can produce lipopolysaccharide (LPS) that can promote inflammation and weaken epithelial barriers (35). The overgrowth of Proteobacteria (a facultative anaerobe) can suppress the growth of commensal obligate anaerobes such as Firmicutes (34). This reduction in commensal bacteria can reduce the production of short-chain fatty acids (SCFAs) such as butyrate that can promote maturation and proliferation of colonocytes and can mediate colonic inflammatory responses (Figure 26.2) (36, 37).

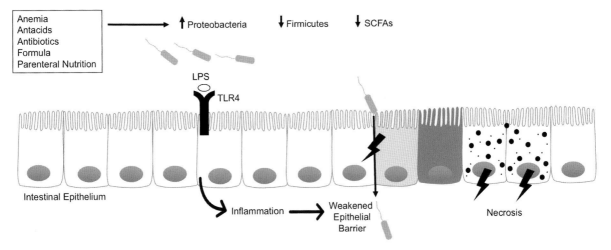

FIGURE 26.2 Pathogenic interactions are leading to intestinal necrosis in the preterm neonate. Intestinal dysbiosis, characterized by the overgrowth of Proteobacteria, can suppress the growth of commensal bacteria such as Firmicutes. Proteobacteria can promote inflammation via LPS. This inflammation weakens epithelial barriers leading to bacterial translocation, intestinal ischemia, and necrosis. The reduction in commensal bacteria can reduce the production of SCFAs that can enhance epithelial integrity.

The role of hypoxia in the development of the intestinal microvasculature

VEGF, a major regulator of angiogenesis, and its main receptor VEFG receptor-2 (VEGFR2), are strongly expressed during late fetal life (38). VEGF is an angiogenic protein that couples hypoxia sensing to angiogenesis and is necessary for the development and maintenance of capillary networks (3, 39, 40). Inhibition of VEGFR2 kinase activity decreases villous endothelial cell proliferation and can produce intestinal necrosis (41).

Transcription factor hypoxia-inducible factor-1 (HIF-1) regulates VEGF. HIF is the master regulator of the cellular response to hypoxia and ischemia (28). HIF-1α mediates angiogenesis in response to hypoxic injury by regulating the expression of growth factors including VEGF-A, which stimulates endothelial cell proliferation, promotes migration of endothelial cells and vascular smooth muscle cells, and inhibits apoptosis (27, 42, 43). Therapeutic oxygen supplementation to a preterm infant can increase intestinal oxygen levels to supraphysiologic levels, resulting in downregulation of HIF and its downstream targets (5). Decreased HIF-mediated signaling may contribute to the lack of VEGF production during intestinal vascular development, predisposing infants to intestinal injury (3).

Summary

Hypoxic-ischemic intestinal injury is rare in preterm infants, unless it is associated with congenital heart defects or other problems that can decrease blood flow to the descending aorta and mesenteric arteries, causing ischemia and necrosis. Hypoxic-ischemic intestinal injury is not the same as necrotizing enterocolitis. Classic NEC is multifactorial, strongly associated with intestinal immaturity, and likely related to an excessive inflammatory response and dysbiosis. In contrast, hypoxic-ischemic intestinal injury has no clear association with inflammation or dysbiosis. It is possible that the confusion between hypoxic-ischemic intestinal injury and classic NEC has caused a significant delay in our current understanding of the pathophysiology of classic NEC.

References

1. Nankervis CA, et al. Microcirculation. 2001; 8(6):377–387.
2. Nair J, et al. Pediatr Res. 2016; 79(4):575–582.
3. Bowker RM, et al. Semin Fetal Neonatal Med. 2018; 23(6):411–415.
4. Nair J, et al. Front Biosci (Schol Ed). 2019; 11:9–28.
5. Nowicki PT. Am J Physiol. 1998; 275(4):G758–G768.
6. Scholander PF. Sci Am.1963; 209:92.–106.
7. Ostlie DJ, et al. J Pediatr Surg. 2003; 38(7):1039–1042.
8. McElhinney DB, et al. Pediatrics. 2000; 106(5):1080–1087.
9. Spinner JA, et al. Pediatr Crit Care Med. 2020; 21(3):228–234.
10. Neu J. Neonatology. 2020; 117(2):240–244.
11. Nowicki P. J Pediatr. 1990; 117(1 Pt 2):S14–S19.
12. Neu J. Biol Neonate. 2005; 87(2):97–98.
13. Neu J, et al. N Engl J Med. 2011; 364(3):255–264.
14. Young CM, et al. J Pediatr. 2011; 158(2 Suppl):e25–e28.
15. Pitt J, et al. Pediatr Res. 1977; 11(8):906–909.
16. Stoll BJ. Clin Perinatol. 1994; 21(2):205–218.
17. Pammi M, et al. Microbiome. 2017; 5(1):31.
18. Konig J, et al. Clin Transl Gastroenterol. 2016; 7(10):e196.
19. Muenchau S, et al. Mol Cell Biol. 2019; 39(14):e00553–18.
20. Van Belkum M, et al. Cell Mol Life Sci. 2020; 77(7):1209–1227.
21. Pitman RS, et al. J Gastroenterol. 2000; 35(11):805–814.
22. Tsukita S, et al. Nat Rev Mol Cell Biol. 2001; 2(4):285–293.
23. Karhausen J, et al. J Clin Invest. 2004; 114(8):1098–1106.
24. Zheng L, et al. Am J Physiol Cell Physiol. 2015; 309(6):C350–C360.
25. Colgan SP, et al. Nat Rev Gastroenterol Hepatol. 2010; 7(5):281–287.
26. Dengler VL, et al. Crit Rev Biochem Mol Biol. 2014; 49(1):1–15.
27. Bowker RM, et al. Pediatr Res. 2018; 83(2):545–553.
28. Shah YM. Mol Cell Pediatr. 2016; 3(1):1.
29. Glover LE, et al. J Clin Invest. 2016; 126(10):3680–3688.
30. Arthur CM, et al. Transfusion. 2019; 59(4):1233–1245.
31. Palazon A, et al. Immunity. 2014; 41(4):518–528.
32. Wang F, et al. Am J Pathol. 2005; 166(2):409–419.
33. Capaldo CT, et al. Biochim Biophys Acta. 2009; 1788(4):864–871.
34. Ho TTB, et al. J Perinatol. 2020; 40(7):1066–1074.
35. Lindberg TP, et al. J Matern Fetal Neonatal Med. 2020; 33(3):349–358.
36. Couto MR, et al. Pharmacol Res. 2020; 159:104947.
37. Banasiewicz T, et al. Prz Gastroenterol. 2020; 15(2):119–125.
38. Yan X, et al. Am J Physiol Gastrointest Liver Physiol. 2016; 310(9):G716–G725.
39. Moonen RM, et al. Front Pediatr. 2020; 8:45.
40. Cuna A, et al. Semin Fetal Neonatal Med. 2018; 23(6):387–393.
41. Sabnis A, et al. Neonatology. 2015; 107(3):191–198.
42. Avraham-Davidi I, et al. J Exp Med. 2013; 210(12):2611–2625.
43. Grunewald M, et al. Cell. 2006; 124(1):175–189.
44. Barlow B, et al. J Pediatr Surg. 1974; 9(5):587–595.

EFFECTS OF HYPOXIA ON PERINATAL DRUG DISPOSITION

Karel Allegaert, Anne Smits and Pieter Annaert

Contents

Introduction

Clinical pharmacology intends to predict drug-related effects based on drug- and population-specific pharmacokinetics (PK, concentration-time, disposition), and pharmacodynamics (PD, concentration-effect), including intra- and interindividual variability. PK (*a*bsorption, *d*istribution, and elimination, through either *m*etabolism or primary renal *e*xcretion, *ADME*) aims to describe the relationship between a given drug concentration at a specific site (e.g. plasma, cerebrospinal fluid) and time (*"what the organism does to the drug"*). PD estimates the relationship between a concentration and its (side)-effects (*"what the drug does to the organism"*). These basic principles of clinical pharmacology also apply to the newborn and the placental-fetal compartment (linked to the maternal circulation) so that perinatal clinical pharmacology during asphyxia reflects the perinatal pathophysiology related to asphyxia (1). Effective and safe pharmacotherapy (*drug* and *dose* selection) following perinatal asphyxia necessitates integration of the available pieces of knowledge on (patho)physiology, further modulated by therapeutic interventions including whole-body hypothermia (WBH). As most hypoxic events in the newborn start at prenatal life or during delivery, it is also relevant to consider the placental-fetal compartment. In this chapter, we will not discuss the specific characteristics of maternal pharmacology but refer interested readers to recently published reviews (2, 3). Obviously, this is somewhat arbitrary, as the placental-fetal compartment is connected to the maternal compartments by blood flows to and from the placenta.

This review will start with an assessment of the impact of maternal-to-fetal blood pH and hypoxia on placental-fetal and neonatal PK/PD, respectively, with specific emphasis on the impact of asphyxia and its treatment (WBH). This will be followed by a discussion on how pathophysiological characteristics and PK datasets, respectively, serve to create prediction tools (physiology-based pharmacokinetics, PBPK) to subsequently explore their performance. Such PBPK tools are not only relevant to adapt dosing of currently used drugs but are also relevant to support drug development.

The placental-fetal compartment and fetal asphyxia

When deconstructed to its basics, the placenta is an active ("drug handling") barrier between two separated systems (maternal, fetal) with placental drug disposition driven by differences in concentration-time profiles between both systems, and the maternal and fetal blood flow to and from this interface. This "barrier" function of the placenta includes passive diffusion, facilitated diffusion, active transport, and pinocytosis. Passive diffusion is the most relevant mechanism, primarily determined (i) by the concentration gradient between maternal and fetal circulation and (ii) placental blood flow (4). Besides lipid solubility, molecular weight, and protein binding, the drug's ionization constant (pKa) can be determinants of placental transfer as only the nonionized form readily passes lipid membranes.

Interestingly, the fetal pH is 0.1–0.15 points lower than the maternal pH in late gestation (4). This gradient can affect the extent of transfer of acidic and basic drugs so that weakly basic drugs are ionized at the relatively lower (more acidic) pH of fetal blood to a higher degree than in maternal blood (5). This class of drugs may therefore accumulate in fetal blood (*ion trapping*) (Figure 27.1). Basic drugs such as amine-type local anesthetic agents are ionized to a greater degree in fetal blood than in maternal blood. Therefore, the *free* concentrations of drugs such as lidocaine, bupivacaine, 2-chlorprocaine, ropivacaine, and pethidine accumulate in fetal blood (by a factor of 1.5) even in the normal maternal-fetal pH setting (5). The reverse can be true for weak acidic drugs, as these compounds reach lower concentrations in fetal than in maternal blood. Relevant to this chapter, fetal asphyxia or maternal alkalosis (e.g. unintended hyperventilation) may further enlarge the maternal-fetal pH gradient and subsequent ion trapping of either basic drugs or acidic drugs, respectively (5).

Clinical pharmacology in neonates

Variability driven by maturational and nonmaturational covariates

The neonate is characterized by growth (size, weight increase) and maturation (organ function, neurodevelopment). Both affect ADME (disposition) resulting in extensive PK variability within the neonatal population: *Neonatal physiology determines neonatal pharmacology*. At the risk of oversimplification, metabolic, and renal clearances (CL) are low at birth as liver and kidney functions are immature to increase over neonatal life and beyond. The maturation of individual PK processes in early infancy is hereby driven by age (postnatal, gestational, or postmenstrual age) and/or weight as main covariates. However, it is important to realize that these maturational changes do not occur simultaneously,

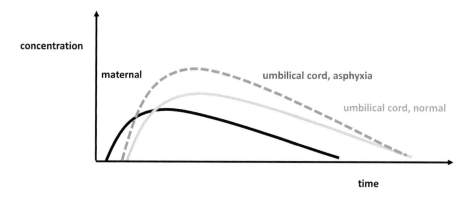

FIGURE 27.1 Potential impact of an increased pH gap between fetus and mother by ion trapping on the fetal and maternal concentration-time profiles for weakly basic drugs such as local anesthetics (dark gray to light gray) (5).

nor evolve at the same rate or linear. Figure 27.2 illustrates the isoenzyme specific maturational pattern over the pediatric age range for different cytochrome P450 (CYP) enzymes in human liver, and maturational patterns for the drug transporters have more recently been suggested (6, 7).

When we focus on the term newborn, glucuronidation activity will mature in early neonatal life (endogenous bilirubin conjugation, but also relevant to the metabolic clearance of drugs e.g. paracetamol, propofol, chloramphenicol). Similarly, CYP2D6 and CYP3A4 (which are the enzymes related to the metabolic clearance of tramadol, oxycodone, and midazolam, respectively) mature over the first weeks and 6–12 months of life, respectively. Interestingly, CYP3A7 activity decreases from birth onward. Glomerular filtration rate (expressed as mL/1.73 m^2) increases over the first 18–24 months of life. This is reflected, for example, in aminoglycoside clearance and subsequent dosing, with a dosing interval of 24 h in term cases, and a more prolonged interval in more immature cases (lower clearance, compensated by a longer time interval between doses (6). Knowledge on the isoenzyme or pathway-specific ontogeny and principles of PK in neonates increased over the last decades. Importantly, these pieces of mechanistic information can be put together to construct a

"prediction tool" on drug disposition in these neonates by constructing PBPK modeling and simulation tools (8).

Therapeutic hypothermia and neonatal hypoxic-ischemic encephalopathy affect pharmacokinetics

Besides maturational covariates (e.g. weight, age) as physiological properties, nonmaturational covariates such as disease (e.g. asphyxia, sepsis) and therapies (e.g. WBH) further contribute to the between- and within-patient variability in PK in neonates. This variability reaches the level that necessitates relevant dose modifications.

Data on enteral absorption and distribution are limited, but less relevant since the majority of drugs in these patients are administered by parenteral route. More relevant (renal) excretion and metabolic clearance are commonly reduced when compared to similar observations in term neonates (8, 9). However, similar to the maturational patterns, the impact of asphyxia and WBH neither displays a uniform pattern, as this will depend on drug (molecular weight, protein binding, biochemical characteristics, individual patient (extent of hepatic, circulatory or renal impairment, age, weight), and ADME (e.g. extraction ratio) characteristics (1, 8). For drugs primarily eliminated by the renal route (glomerular filtration), such as aminoglycosides, there is a decrease of −30 to −40% of clearance when compared to term controls. Consequently, the time interval should be extended from 24 to 30–36 h between consecutive doses (6, 8). In contrast, the CYP-mediated phenobarbital clearance is only marginally decreased by WBH, but more affected (−55%) by disease severity (pH ≤ 7.1 and Apgar score <5) (1). Along the same line, total midazolam clearance (CYP3A) is not affected by WBH, while renal midazolam elimination (1-hydroxy) is decreased (−26%) (10). Besides WBH, renal or hepatic impairment, drug-drug interactions can also be of relevance as phenobarbital is an inducer (factor 2.3 higher) of midazolam clearance (10, 11). Finally, the clearance of morphine by glucuronidation is 22% lower in asphyxiated neonates exposed to WBH when compared to those without hypothermia (12).

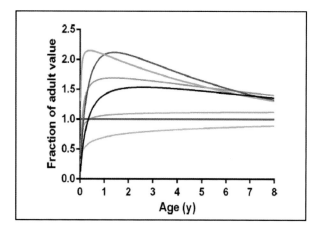

FIGURE 27.2 Summary of cytochrome P450 (CYP) isoenzyme specific *in vivo* ontogeny (fraction of adult value) for the major hepatic CYPs: CYP1A2 (black); CYP2A6 (gray); CYP2B6 CYP2D6 (purple); CYP2C9 (green); CYP2C19 (red); CYP1E2 (gold); and CYP3A (blue) (7).

Physiologically based pharmacokinetic models to enable precision pharmacotherapy

Precision medicine can be defined as a structured approach to treat or prevent specific diseases based on knowledge regarding known factors of interindividual variability (e.g. gender, polymorphisms), disease (e.g. asphyxia, hypoxic respiratory failure), or environment (e.g. drug-drug interaction, nutrition, WBH). Neonates undergoing and following WBH are a specific

TABLE 27.1 Overview on the Pharmacokinetic Data Reported for Anti-Epileptics in the Setting of Whole-Body Hypothermia (WBH) Following Moderate-to-Severe Hypoxic Ischemic Encephalopathy (8)

Drug	Study-Related Aspects and Findings
Phenobarbital	$N = 26$ neonates, clearance is lower (-15%), because disease severity affects clearance (-55%). WBH itself does not affect clearance
Phenobarbital	$N = 39$ asphyxia neonates, 20/39 underwent WBH, but this was not a significant covariate for clearance
Phenobarbital	$N = 31$ neonates, typical newborn (3.5 kg) 17.2 mL/h, not WBH, weight as covariate ($kg^{0.81}$, CYP activity correlates with weight)
Phenobarbital	$N = 19$ neonates, half-life 173.9, SD 62.5 h
Topiramate	$N = 13$ neonates, (oral), half-life 35.58, SD 19.3 h (deep vs. mild hypothermia, half-life prolonged $+ 38\%$)
Topiramate	$N = 52$ neonates, (oral), after cooling $+21\%$ higher compared to during cooling
Midazolam	$N = 9$ neonates, half-life 13 (2.75–50.52) h; clearance: 2.57 mL/kg/min, renal or hepatic impairment affects clearance
Midazolam + phenobarbital	$N = 68$ neonates, phenobarbital coexposure increases midazolam clearance (factor 2.3) during WBH (inducer effect)
Lidocaine	$N = 22$ neonates, compared to $N = 26$ historical noncooled asphyxia neonates, clearance -24%

Abbreviations: N, number; SD, standard deviation.

subpopulation in great need of precision medicine. This also relates to precision pharmacotherapy, covering both drug development programs (new drugs as adjunctive treatments in addition to WBH to further improve outcomes) as well as facilitating tailored dosing of currently available drugs.

PBPK is a knowledge-driven technique ("bottom-up") that applies mathematical approaches for mechanistic integration of pharmacology principles and can be part of such a structured approach. It hereby integrates different types of information, such as in vitro, in vivo, or in silico and clinical data (population-related). PBPK models will be used to conduct different simulations for "what-if" scenarios, including an estimate of (un)certainty and sensitivity testing of predicted PK profiles (7). PBPK hereby explicitly discriminates between drug characteristics and physiological properties of the population (6, 8, 13).

At present, such PBPK tools are already used to generate predictions up to the level to support pivotal decisions during drug development and acceptance by regulatory authorities (e.g. food-food interactions in adults, the impact of renal or hepatic impairment on drug dosing in adults). Consequently, the novelty is not the technique with an already proven track record, but in the integration of available pieces of knowledge, and unveiling knowledge gaps in this specific subgroup of neonates. PBPK serves as a tool to integrate data, test hypotheses, verify plausibility of underlying mechanisms, or even generate new insights (6, 8, 13). Furthermore, these tools enable to check data consistency obtained from different sources (in vitro, in vivo), to predict exposure, or enable study design optimization (6, 8, 13). Consequently, PBPK is a strong research tool to support neonatal drug development and to guide dosing for currently available drugs (6, 8, 13). At present, there are already several different PBPK platforms (e.g. Simcyp, PK-Sim). Using the same workflow, (patho)physiological data should be integrated into these PBPK models similar to renal or hepatic impairment in adults. However, to further develop such tools, input from the research community is crucial.

Contribution of the research community in the development of PBPK models

The workflow to develop and explore the performance of PBPK models is illustrated in Figure 27.3 (8, 14). We hereby highlight the need for both *PK datasets* as well as *population-specific system*

information to develop, explore, and improve such models in neonates.

PK datasets

As mentioned earlier in this chapter, data on compound specific observations have been reported with initiatives such as the PharmaCool project to boost the available knowledge (15). The PharmaCool project used an opportunistic sampling strategy on "any drug" administered to a cohort of neonates undergoing and following WBH and subsequently comparing these data to historical observations earlier published in "healthy" term neonates without asphyxia or in term asphyxia neonates before hypothermia was implemented in our practices. This approach resulted in data on e.g. β-lactam antibiotics, aminoglycosides, phenobarbital, midazolam, lidocaine, or morphine (15). Table 27.1 provides an overview on reported observations on PK of anti-epileptics in the setting of WBH. Subsequent data sharing with merging datasets from different populations of asphyxiated neonates is the key to explore the robustness of PBPK models (Figure 27.3, right). Such data sharing has been done to quantify the impact of asphyxia and WBH on the PK of aminoglycosides, phenobarbital, or lidocaine by comparing new data in WBH cases to historical controls (8, 15).

Population-specific system information

As you can see in Figure 27.3 (left), these PBPK models also need input on population-system information in this specific population, and similar data in nonasphyxia, nonhypothermia neonates to quantify differences. This covers both (patho)physiological parameters, as well as in vitro studies to assess the impact of hypoxia or hypothermia on isoenzyme metabolic or transport activity (8).

As WBH is restricted to (near)term neonates, this mainly refers to (patho)physiology parameters related to *cardiac output* (stroke volume, heart rate, blood flow), regional blood flow (e.g. pulmonary hypertension, cerebral blood flow, renal blood flow, hepatic blood flow), *renal function* (renal blood flow, glomerular filtration rate), as well as *plasma composition* (albumin, hematocrit, α-1 glycoprotein) or *hepato-biliary functions* (liver weight and function). Using a nonstructured search, we have summarized some pieces of the available information on pathophysiological characteristics in Table 27.2 (16–24).

The concept of in vitro studies to assess the impact of maturational changes in protein expression and activity of enzymes affecting metabolic clearance has a proven track record across

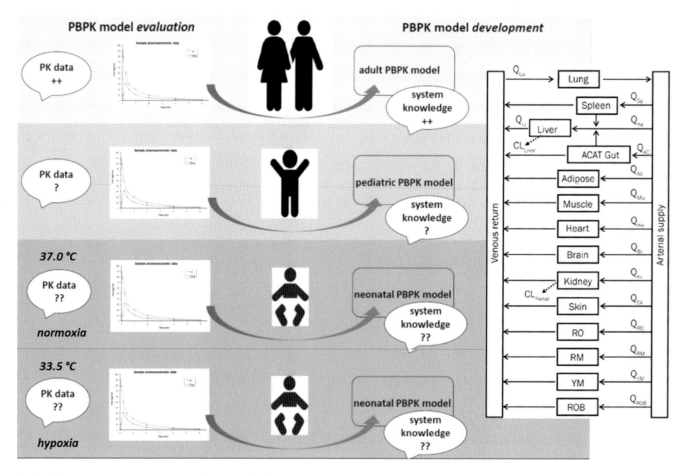

FIGURE 27.3 Consecutive steps and pieces of information needed to develop and evaluate a physiologically based pharmacokinetic (PBPK) model to neonates undergoing therapeutic hypothermia (Q, blood flow; PK, pharmacokinetics). Input is needed for compound specific PK datasets (*left*), and population-specific "system" knowledge (*right*) (14).

TABLE 27.2 Observations on the Impact of Asphyxia and/or Whole-Body Hypothermia on Specific Organ Functions (16–24)

Organ Function	Reported Findings
Cardiac output	Whole-body hypothermia ($n = 44$), compared to asphyxia ($n = 20$) and control term cases ($n = 20$), asphyxia was the main driver of impaired myocardial function (tissue Doppler deformation, strain rate about 50% slower), improving from day 4 (after rewarming) onward (16).
	Cardiac output is determined by disease state and whole-body hypothermia, with a right and left ventricular output pre-, during, and after rewarming of 136, 127 and 164 and 139, 130, and 172 mL/kg/min, respectively (17).
	Right and left ventricular output in asphyxiated whole-body hypothermia cases compared to normative values are 108 (−51%) and 107 (−52%) compared to 224 and 222 mL/kg/min (18).
Renal function	The incidence of oliguria (urine output <0.5 mL/kg/h) for >24 h after birth and rising serum creatinine (creatinine >0.9 mg/dL) was similar between whole-body hypothermia and selective head cooling (suggesting the relevance of disease severity) (19).
	Asphyxia results in increased creatinine values, but this is less pronounced in neonates during (24–24 h) whole-body hypothermia (20).
Plasma and blood	Hematocrit is lower in asphyxiated neonates (0.45–0.41 versus 0.53–0.50 on day 1 and day 5 of life) when compared to term healthy neonates (21).
	The mean albumin concentration (24 g/L) is decreased in the setting of asphyxia, and relates to its severity (grade 1, 2, and 3, 29, 24 versus 20 g/L, respectively) (22).
Intestinal	Decreased intestinal and hepatic blood flow, in addition to the reduced cardiac output, reflected in increased blood flow velocity (+20–25%) (23).
	The lactulose and renal lactulose/L-rhamnose excretion provide evidence for higher intestinal permeability up to at least day 9 in term neonates following perinatal asphyxia (24).
	In neonatal hypoxic-ischemic encephalopathy cases, whole-body hypothermia blunted the hepatic injury, reflected by lower liver enzymes and lower C-reactive protein (22).

the pediatric age range, with reported examples, e.g. propofol or tramadol, or incorporating developmental changes in membrane transporters (25–27). Along the same line, data on mRNA, protein expression, and especially abundance, as well as activity (isoenzyme-driven metabolic clearance; transporter activity) under hypoxia and/or hypothermia in target cells such as neonatal hepatocytes or renal tubular cells or cell layers are useful to further feed these PBPK models. At best, this should cover both immediate (during the event) as well as delayed (return to normalization after the event) effects.

Obviously, clinical pharmacology is not limited to PK, but also covers PD (concentration effect and concentration side effect relationship). At present, available observations in this specific setting are still limited and fragmented. However, there are observations that the antiepileptic effect of phenobarbital (same concentration) is more potent during WBH (28). Along the same line, the coadministration of bumetanide with gentamicin (NEMO trial) resulted in a significant increase in deafness in exposed cases. When considering the cardiovascular system, the QTc time interval is also prolonged by WBH (29, 30). Side effects of WBH also include persistent pulmonary hypertension of the newborn, a topic discussed elsewhere in the textbook. When this complication is treated with intravenous sildenafil, it is worth to consider how asphyxia and WBH will affect sildenafil clearance, as its metabolite (desmethyl sildenafil) has also pharmacodynamic effects and metabolites eliminated by renal route (31).

Acknowledgments

The activities related to the research line on the clinical pharmacology during whole-body hypothermia are supported by FWO Flanders (iPREDICT project, G0D0520N). The research activities of AS are supported by the Clinical Research and Education Council of the University Hospitals Leuven.

References

1. Pokorna P, et al. Curr Pharm Des. 2015; 21(39):5705–5724.
2. Dallmann A, et al. Curr Pharm Des. 2019; 25(5):483–495.
3. Kazma JM, et al. J Pharmacokinet Pharmacodyn. 2020; 47(4):271–285.
4. Bouazza N, et al. Curr Pharm Des. 2019; 25(5):496–504.
5. Ueki R, et al. J Anesth. 2009; 23(4):526–529.
6. Smits A, et al. Expert Opin Drug Metab Toxicol. 2019; 15(1):25–34.
7. Allegaert K, et al. J Clin Pharmacol. 2019; 59(Suppl 1):S33–S41.
8. Smits A, et al. Front Pharmacol. 2020; 11:587.
9. Lutz IC, et al. BMJ Pediatr Open. 2020; 4(1):e000685.
10. Favié LMA, et al. Neonatology 2019; 116(2):154–162.
11. Welzing L, et al. Klin Padiatr. 2013; 225(7):398–404.
12. Róka A, et al. Pediatrics 2008; 121(4):e844–e849.
13. Claassen K, et al. Curr Pharm Des. 2015; 21(39):5688–5698.
14. Allegaert K, et al. Neonatology 2019; 116(2):188–190.
15. de Haan TR, et al. BMC Pediatr. 2012; 12:45.
16. Nestaas E, et al. Early Hum Dev. 2014; 90(5):247–252.
17. Sehgal A, et al. J Neonatal Perinatal Med. 2019; 12(2):117–125.
18. Sehgal A, et al. Eur J Pediatr. 2012; 171(10):1511–1517.
19. Sarkar S, et al. J Perinatol. 2009; 29(8):558–563.
20. Róka A, et al. Acta Paediatr. 2007; 96(8):1118–1121.
21. Brucknerová I, et al. Interdiscip Toxicol. 2008; 1(3-4):211–213.
22. Muniraman H, et al. Eur J Pediatr. 2017; 176(10):1295–1303.
23. Ilves P, et al. J Ultrasound Med. 2009; 28(11):1471–1480.
24. Beach RC, et al. Arch Dis Child 1982; 57(2):141–145.
25. Michelet R, et al. J Pharmacokinet Pharmacodyn. 2018; 45(6):765–785.
26. T'jollyn H, et al. AAPS J. 2015; 17(6):1376–1387.
27. Cheung KWK, et al. J Clin Pharmacol. 2019; 59(Suppl 1):S56–S69.
28. van den Broek MP, et al. Clin Pharmacokinet. 2012; 51(10):671–679.
29. Pressler RM, et al. Nat Rev Neurol. 2015; 11(12):724.
30. Massaro AN, et al. Pediatr Crit Care Med. 2017; 18(4):349–354.
31. Cochius-den Otter SCM, et al. Eur J Clin Pharmacol. 2020; 76(2):219–227.

ANESTHETIC CONSIDERATIONS FOR THE NEONATE WITH HYPOXIC RESPIRATORY FAILURE

M. Ruth Graham

Contents

Introduction

Despite ongoing advances in anesthesia, surgery, and intensive care, neonates are at higher risk for perioperative morbidity and mortality, and present a management challenge for the perioperative care team (1). Neonates with preexisting hypoxic respiratory failure (HRF) comprise a subset of infants at particularly high risk as underlying respiratory compromise is associated with a serious perioperative complication rate of 23% (2), and a significant increase in the odds ratio (OR) for perioperative mortality to 2.7 (3). When assessing any individual patient, gestational age, surgical complexity, and comorbidities are additional factors that contribute to overall risk (3, 4). With low-risk procedures, mortality is estimated at 0.3% for a healthy term infant but increases to 2.7% with prematurity. Higher complexity surgery increases the risk of perioperative mortality to 17% in term neonates and alarmingly to 36% with prematurity (3). As such, perioperative management requires an understanding of the interplay between the proposed surgical procedure and anesthesia in the context of maturational age and underlying pathophysiology. This is best served by a multidisciplinary approach with the combined expertise of anesthesia, surgery, neonatology, cardiology, respiratory therapy, nursing, and the parents.

Neonatal HRF is not a single entity but may develop from diverse underlying etiologies with unique pathological features. These include parenchymal lung diseases arising from meconium aspiration, pneumonia, respiratory distress, or bronchopulmonary dysplasia (BPD), and hypoplastic conditions such as congenital diaphragmatic hernia (CDH). The advent of HRF is associated with significant morbidity and mortality (5), but clinical outcomes are impacted further if pulmonary hypertension (PH) develops (6). Well recognized in hypoplastic lung conditions, PH is increasingly diagnosed in infants with primary parenchymal abnormalities where secondary insults may induce remodeling of the underlying dysplastic vascular bed (5). In a retrospective cohort study of PH patients undergoing noncardiac surgery, BPD was the underlying abnormality in 46% of cases (7). Surgery in the neonate with BPD is associated with a 4-fold increased risk of mortality. Surgery plus PH further increases the risk of mortality by 10-fold (8), which correlates with PH severity (7). As such, a high index of suspicion for PH must accompany the perioperative assessment of an infant with HRF requiring surgery.

The goal of anesthesia is to maintain stable cardiorespiratory function and mitigate the pain and neurohumoral stress response to surgery. There is no unique anesthetic cocktail or technique that achieves this goal. An appropriate anesthetic plan requires careful consideration of the preoperative status and proposed operative intervention to inform decisions regarding patient optimization, preparation, and operative location. These, in turn, have implications regarding ventilator management, anesthetic options, and the need for adjuvant therapies to counter the alterations in cardiorespiratory dynamics anticipated to occur with surgical trespass.

Preop assessment

While the urgency of a planned procedure must be appreciated, safe perioperative management requires a thorough preoperative review of the history, physical findings, current medications, recent bloodwork, investigations, and ventilator management to allow for timely optimization and preparation of specific equipment and adjuncts. Recognition of sepsis and additional anomalies, particularly congenital heart lesions, have implications for intraoperative hemodynamic stability, fluid management, and drug handling.

The size, depth, and presence of a leak around the endotracheal tube (ETT) have implications for dislodgement/malposition and ventilation during transport and surgery. A tolerable leak under stable conditions in the neonatal intensive care unit (NICU) may become unacceptable intraoperatively when alterations in lung and chest wall compliance may be imposed on a compromised respiratory system. Compliance changes are anticipated with muscle relaxation, positioning, and distortion from retractors and packs that elevate the diaphragm or directly compress the lung. Reintubation with a larger or cuffed ETT may be beneficial, but risk must be balanced against any history of previous difficult airway attempts or current airway edema. The most recent chest X-ray provides information regarding ETT position, aeration, and regional parenchymal lung changes. New areas of consolidation or collapse require assessment to rule out a recent infectious process, atelectasis, pulmonary edema, or pneumothorax.

Review of ventilator management and stability of current settings is critical. Frequent titration of positive end-expiratory pressure (PEEP)/fraction of inspired oxygen (FiO_2) or escalation of inspiratory pressure (PIP), and intolerance of handling/position changes suggest pulmonary airway/parenchymal instability. Trends in arterial blood gas (ABG) analysis will help direct intraoperative CO_2 goals.

DOI: 10.1201/9780367494018-28

In any infant with unstable HRF, anatomic and functional echo-cardiography (ECHO) assessment is indicated to clarify anatomy, delineate congenital heart lesions, determine the presence and direction of ductal shunting, ascertain both left and right cardiac function, and diagnose the presence and severity of PH (9, 10). More sophisticated targeted ECHO is increasingly used to assess response when escalating therapy with pulmonary vasodilators, inotropes, or vasopressors are required for the management of PH and/or hemodynamic instability, providing invaluable direction for intraoperative cardiovascular management (11).

Inhaled nitric oxide (iNO) may be initiated for neonates with evidence of significantly elevated pulmonary pressures (12, 13), but efficacy should be determined by repeat ECHO as up to 30% of neonates with fixed PH will not respond to iNO (5). Second-line pulmonary vasodilators include intravenous sildenafil (a phosphodiesterase 5 inhibitor) and milrinone (a phosphodiesterase 3 inhibitor and inodilator) (14, 15). The addition of prostaglandin E1 in PH patients with a closing ductus arteriosus may help maintain systemic perfusion albeit at lower levels of oxygenation but indicates a subset of patients at higher risk for mortality (16).

Preoperative inotropes and vasopressors must be uninterrupted, anticipating the likelihood of increasing hemodynamic instability and escalating requirements. Correction of coagulation abnormalities and anemia is important to minimize bleeding risk and optimize oxygen-carrying capacity. Anticipation of significant blood loss mandates ordering age-appropriate cross-matched blood, plasma, and albumin, as indicated.

Transport

Adverse events are reported to occur in up to 75% of pediatric transports with increased risk in neonates with HRF (17). The potential for displacement/dislodgement of the ETT, loss of lung volume due to circuit disconnection and inadequate maintenance of PEEP are significant concerns. Periods of hypo- and hyperventilation and hypo/hyperoxia are well documented (18). Tobias et al. reported significant hyperventilation with potentially injurious low CO_2 levels in up to 40% of manually ventilated pediatric patients during transport (19). Hypothermia, loss of vascular access with discontinuation of vasopressors/inotropes, and acute hemodynamic deterioration leading to cardiac arrest are additional concerns (17, 20, 21). These issues justify a multidisciplinary discussion and prebriefing of the care plan regarding the risk, benefit, and alternatives to transport and the planned procedure for critically ill infants needing the highest levels of ventilatory and hemodynamic support. In such cases, the option for surgery at the bedside should also be considered. This in turn may mandate modification of the planned surgical approach: i.e. open versus minimally invasive, temporizing versus complete repair or palliation. Challenges associated with surgery at the bedside include unfamiliarity of the surgical team with the NICU environment, relocation of all required equipment and supplies, potentially inadequate air exchange, space, and lighting. Despite these concerns, numerous procedures including patent ductus arteriosus (PDA) ligations, laparotomies, and CDH repair, have been performed safely and effectively in the NICU (22–26).

Mechanical ventilation strategies

The neonatal resuscitation and intensive care literature provides compelling evidence that even brief exposure to injurious ventilation – excessive oxygen, pressure, hyperventilation, or large tidal volumes – may be detrimental to long-term pulmonary function (27, 28). Injurious ventilation may also cause deviations in arterial blood pressure, CO_2, and O_2 with associated perturbations in cerebral perfusion that increase the risk for intraventricular hemorrhage and periventricular leukomalacia (29). Until comparable perioperative outcome studies are available, extrapolation to the operative period is reasonable.

Following the principles of an open lung strategy (30), the challenge is to provide the least injurious ventilation that maintains lung volume and oxygenation at the lowest possible FiO_2 and airway pressure, with acceptable CO_2 and hemodynamics during the dynamically changing conditions that accompany all phases of perioperative care – transport, positioning, anesthesia, and the surgical procedure. Intraoperative oxygen and CO_2 targets have not been clearly defined, but recommended preoperative NICU goals – strict avoidance of hyperoxia and maintenance of preductal O_2 saturation at 89–95% with evidence of adequate organ perfusion and permissive hypercapnia – is a rational approach (31, 32).

Modern neonatal ventilators incorporate microprocessors and a flow sensor at the ETT connection, allowing precise measurement of flow and tidal volume (V_T), and continuous analysis of respiratory mechanics. This permits the use of volume-targeted ventilation (VTV) with precise maintenance of set V_T in the face of changing respiratory mechanics. VTV is currently the only neonatal ventilator mode to demonstrate an advantage in the composite outcome of BPD/mortality in a premature infant (33). By contrast, standard anesthesia ventilators are designed primarily for adult use with a flow meter positioned at the expiratory port. Although flow and compliance compensation ensure more accurate V_T delivery, the lower limit is typically 20 mL, which is excessive for many neonates (whose V_T is usually at 4–6 mL/kg) and lacks volume guarantee (34). The imposition of added equipment dead space (elbow connectors, end-tidal carbon dioxide (ETCO$_2$) lines, and humidvents) may also contribute to potential mismatch between desired and delivered V_T. Abouzeid et al. (35) used a dedicated respiratory monitor to measure delivered V_T in 26 neonates ventilated with a standard anesthesia ventilator in the operating room. They reported a mean expired V_T 3.2 mL/kg above that measured by the respiratory monitor and significant individual V_T variability, with more than 50% of individual breaths delivered outside the target range of 4–8 mL/kg. These data suggest that injurious ventilation may occur frequently if standard anesthesia ventilators are employed.

A dedicated neonatal ventilator in the OR offers the advantage of more precise maintenance of preoperative VTV settings and should be considered in any high-risk neonate. If unavailable, the option of bedside surgery permits continuation of current mechanical ventilation without the risks incurred with the use of a ventilator not designed for the vulnerable neonatal lung, but precludes the use of inhalational anesthetic agents that require a vaporizer in line.

Alternatively, high-frequency ventilation modes (HFV) may be considered under selected circumstances (36, 37). Purported advantages are maintenance of effective lung recruitment and avoidance of airway overdistension, limiting PIP and V_T excursions while providing effective CO_2 elimination (36). Although HFV has been traditionally used as a rescue mode in those infants unable to be managed safely with conventional ventilator settings (38), emerging literature offers evidence of potential utility during both abdominal and thoracic procedures, where it can provide a stable operative field with better control of intraoperative hypercarbia, particularly when a minimally invasive approach is contemplated (38–40). The disadvantages of HFV modes during surgery include an inability to visualize chest movements, auscultate the heart and lungs, or monitor $ETCO_2$. Concerns regarding potential negative hemodynamic effects of HFV are largely related to the use of excessive intrathoracic pressure and resultant decrease in preload and must be carefully monitored. At present, the major limiting factors are the lack of availability in many operating rooms, and anesthesia provider unfamiliarity. Increased training and/the presence of an experienced respiratory therapist may facilitate use.

Anesthetic agents

The foundation of modern neonatal anesthesia is based on the recognition that neonates mount a significant neurohumoral stress response to surgery, and that blunting of the response is associated with improved outcomes (41, 42).

A pure narcotic-based anesthetic regimen using fentanyl is common, but large doses (25–50 mcg/kg) are recommended to reliably blunt the stress response (42). Unfortunately, maturational changes in the volume of distribution, protein binding, hepatic function, and comorbidities result in 17-fold individual differences in narcotic clearance, making dosing unpredictable (43, 44). Although usually well-tolerated hemodynamically, higher doses may be associated with bradycardia and hypotension, and decreased clearance may result in prolonged ileus and respiratory depression mandating unnecessarily prolonged postoperative mechanical ventilation (44, 45).

Alternatively, remifentanil is an ultrashort-acting potent narcotic that is metabolized by plasma esterases present even in premature neonates. Remifentanil thus has a predictable, age-independent elimination with a half-life of 3.4–5.7 min (46). Pharmacokinetics of remifentanil dictate administration as a continuous infusion. Bolus doses may be associated with arterial hypotension, but titration can provide rapid increases in effect-site concentration during periods of intense surgical stress without prolonging elimination. While advantageous intraoperatively, the short half-life dictates the need for additional longer-acting analgesia postoperatively. The potential for chest wall rigidity must be considered with administration of any potent narcotic although muscle relaxation will mitigate this effect (45).

A balanced anesthetic approach incorporates a combination of agents to provide additive or synergistic anesthesia and minimize individual adverse effects. In stable neonates, lower dose narcotics may be balanced with a volatile anesthetic in the OR. The advantage afforded by inhalational anesthetics – attenuation of airway reactivity and lower narcotic requirements (47) – is countered by increased sensitivity to myocardial depressant effects (48), attenuation of hypoxic pulmonary vasoconstriction with increased ventilation–perfusion mismatch (49), and lack of availability with the use a dedicated neonatal ventilator. Additionally, a growing body of preclinical evidence links the administration of all commonly used inhalational anesthetic and sedative agents (propofol, ketamine, and midazolam) to increased neuroapoptosis and signaling damage that may be associated with long-term effects on learning and memory in immature animal models (50). Although clinical correlation is inconclusive (51, 52) and the largest randomized control trial to date demonstrates no long-term neurocognitive differences in infants undergoing inguinal hernia repair with either a spinal or inhalational anesthetic (53), the pediatric anesthesia community is actively seeking alternatives that minimize theoretical risk, particularly for longer duration procedures or when multiple exposures are anticipated.

Dexmedetomidine, a selective alpha-2-adrenergic agonist with sedative, analgesic, and anesthetic properties without respiratory depression is emerging as a viable alternative. Pre-clinical studies with dexmedetomidine suggest a neuroprotective effect – reduced hyperoxic neurodegeneration and some evidence for protection against the neuroapoptotic effect of inhalational anesthetics (54). In pediatric cardiac surgery, dexmedetomidine effectively attenuates hemodynamic and neurohumoral responses at incision, sternotomy, and postbypass (55). Adverse effects are primarily limited to bradycardia, which is usually well-tolerated. In neonates after surgery, dexmedetomidine is opioid-sparing (56, 57). In pediatric patients with PH, dexmedetomidine infusion is associated with bradycardia and hypertension but no change in pulmonary artery pressure (PAP) or right ventricular afterload, potentially affording better maintenance of coronary perfusion in this specific population (58). A large multicenter trial comparing neurodevelopmental outcomes in infants and children anesthetized for greater than 2 h with dexmedetomidine/remifentanil/low-dose sevoflurane versus standard sevoflurane is ongoing, and may better inform caregivers of a safe alternative (ClinicalTrials.gov NCT03089905).

The foregoing concerns promote an increasing interest in the incorporation of neonatal regional blocks and neuraxial techniques as part of a balanced approach (59). Regional analgesia combined with general anesthesia is more effective than general anesthesia with opioids at conventional doses in suppression of the stress response (60). The incorporation of ultrasound guidance provides increasing safety in performance of the blocks but experience and meticulous attention to needle placement and local anesthetic dosing is required to safely incorporate these techniques into neonatal practice (61). Although rigorous prospective evidence of the superiority of any particular technique is lacking, small case series support the use of a combined epidural/general anesthesia approach for procedures as diverse as laparotomies and thoracotomies, documenting shorter periods of postoperative ventilation and faster return of bowel function (62). Data from the general versus spinal anesthesia trial demonstrated greater hemodynamic stability in infants undergoing inguinal hernia repair with spinal anesthesia (63). In a pilot study, 87.5% of infants undergoing lower abdominal procedures could be effectively managed with a dexmedetomidine/remifentanil/neuraxial anesthetic regimen (64). Further work to determine safety and superiority in specific procedures and patient groups will be informative.

Intraoperative management

Standard American Society of Anesthesiologists (ASA) monitoring guidelines (ECG, noninvasive blood pressure (BP), arterial oxygen saturation (SaO_2), $ETCO_2$ and temperature) may be augmented with an invasive arterial pressure line for continuous BP measurement and arterial blood gas (ABG) analysis, pre- and postductal O_2 saturation monitors and a urinary catheter. Reliable peripheral venous and possible central access is crucial for anticipated fluid resuscitation and administration of vasoactive agents. While focus on noninjurious ventilation is paramount, hemodynamic stability must also be maintained. Historically, neonatal hemodynamic stability has been simplistically defined as mean arterial blood pressure above a threshold equivalent to gestational age (65). Intraoperative management is challenging due to lack of defined intraoperative thresholds and increasing evidence that BP targets alone are insufficient surrogates of adequate systemic blood flow, organ perfusion, and substrate delivery (66).

The introduction of near-infrared spectroscopy (NIRS) as a monitor of cerebral oxygenation in the NICU and OR may provide greater guidance to direct hemodynamic management, but interpretation of NIRS signals must include the composite influences of BP, CO_2, O_2, and temperature on cerebral vascular reactivity (67). While neonatal intraoperative hypotension is common (68), Olbrecht et al. (69) report significant cerebral desaturation occurring less frequently (67). The relevance of minor deviations in NIRS requires further study. Ideally, in high-risk neonates, some combination of NIRS, venous saturation, serum lactate, and urine output should be incorporated to provide more meaningful information. Correction of a single BP value may not be indicated but hypotension associated with evidence of inadequate organ perfusion requires treatment and should be directed by the underlying pathophysiology and intended response.

Recognizing the limited preload reserve of the immature myocardium and neonatal intolerance of fluid overload, hypovolemia requires treatment with blood products or crystalloid, depending on the underlying source of fluid loss (48). The addition of a vasoactive agent should be considered when hypotension and evidence of impaired organ perfusion persist, despite adequate fluid resuscitation. In neonates with HRF, and particularly in those with coexisting PH, selection of any cardiotropic agent must take into account potential undesirable effects on pulmonary vascular resistance (PVR) and maturational differences in adrenergic responses (11). When decreased systemic vascular resistance (SVR) is suspected, agents with a more favorable profile include those with relatively greater systemic versus pulmonary vasoconstriction. When primary myocardial dysfunction is suspected, an agent with positive inotropy should be considered. Dopamine, norepinephrine (NE), and vasopressin (VP) are predominantly vasopressors; dobutamine and milrinone are predominantly inotropes; epinephrine has dose-dependent dual effects (11).

Dopamine, often chosen as a first-line agent, demonstrates unpredictable responses echocardiographically, and unfavorably increases PVR to a greater extent than SVR (70). With moderate dose dopamine, some infants demonstrate a predominant vasoconstrictor effect with no change or a decrease in left ventricular (LV) output, while others demonstrate a significant increase in LV output and only modest vasoconstrictor response (71). Epinephrine may provide a more favorable response when pulmonary pressures or myocardial depression are of concern as it increases SVR and PVR proportionally, preserving the PVR: SVR ratio while also augmenting heart rate and LV output (72). NE and VP are both considered potent primary vasoconstrictors with limited inotropic actions, but neonatal pharmacological studies are extremely limited. Preclinical investigations with NE suggest a primary systemic vasoconstrictor response and some evidence for support of right ventricular function under hypoxic conditions (73). Extrapolation from adult and pediatric studies suggests VP may be beneficial in inotropic-resistant shock states, and use is expanding to other areas (74). Potent systemic vasoconstriction and some limited evidence suggesting a minimal vasoconstrictive effect on the pulmonary and cerebral vasculature provide a theoretical basis for use when PH is a concern (70, 75).

Management of pulmonary hypertension

The goals of anesthesia for the infant with PH do not differ from those outlined above, but prevention of a PH crisis – acute elevations in PVR, associated right ventricular failure, and impaired LV filling – is paramount. Intraoperative triggers include hypoxemia, hypercarbia, acidosis, hypothermia, and catecholamine surges

from noxious stimuli. Continuation of pulmonary vasodilators initiated preoperatively may mitigate the risk (76). Extracorporeal membrane oxygenation is a potential rescue modality, but availability and ability to institute emergently must be ascertained preoperatively.

Intraoperatively, the clinical signs of a PH crisis include arterial desaturation, decreased $ETCO_2$, sinus tachycardia followed by bradycardia and hypotension that can rapidly deteriorate to cardiac arrest. The degree of LV impairment may be underappreciated as increased R–L shunting via available pathways may maintain blood pressure at the expense of worsening hypoxemia.

The primary therapeutic goals are to decrease PVR, augment RV/LV function and improve systemic and coronary perfusion. Immediate treatment of PVR includes administration of 100% oxygen with the recognition that hyperoxia ($PaO_2 > 100$) does not promote further pulmonary vasodilation and may contribute to oxidative stress (76). SaO_2 targets are unknown but 92–95% may provide acceptable O_2 delivery provided perfusion is restored. Mild hyperventilation from the patient's baseline will also have salutary effects on pulmonary vascular resistance but overly aggressive reduction in CO_2 risks cerebral hypoperfusion.

Selective pulmonary vasodilators should be immediately available in line. Inhaled NO provides the most immediate direct acting pulmonary vasodilation with minimal systemic effect. Knowledge of preoperative iNO responsiveness from targeted ECHO assessment may guide titration. Consideration must be given for alternative treatments as infants with fixed PVR may not benefit from iNO and are at risk for profound hypoxemia and persistent low cardiac output in the setting of significantly elevated right ventricular afterload (9). The addition of an intravenous inodilator such as milrinone can be considered, but the slow onset of action and associated systemic hypotension limit any immediate benefit (77).

Concomitant support of SVR and RV/LV failure is more immediately relevant. Although definitive evidence to guide vasopressor management is lacking, options include epinephrine, norepinephrine, and VP. As discussed, VP or NE may provide greater systemic vasoconstriction with less pulmonary vascular effect, although careful titration of epinephrine may provide both positive inotropy and acceptable PVR: SVR balance. Ongoing RV/LV failure requires the addition of an inotrope. Epinephrine may be sufficient but dobutamine offers the additional advantage of a dose-dependent increase in CO with a salutary effect on pulmonary vascular resistance, (70), provided associated systemic hypotension is managed. Inotrope-associated tachycardia will increase myocardial oxygen demand and must be addressed with adequate systemic pressures to maintain coronary perfusion. Intraoperative targeted ECHO, if available, may provide guidance for ongoing management. Deterioration should prompt consideration for extracorporeal membrane oxygenation support as successful resuscitation is unlikely once cardiac arrest occurs (78).

Conclusions

Surgery in the neonate with HRF is a high risk and challenging undertaking. Collaboration between the entire perioperative care team is required to fully appreciate the complex pathophysiology and formulate a safe anesthetic plan. Current NICU insights regarding safer ventilation strategies, oxygenation, and CO_2 targets, neonatal pharmacology and cardiorespiratory function should be incorporated with an understanding of the physiological impact imposed by the chosen anesthetic technique and the surgical procedure. The neurotoxicity debate has promoted increased interest in research with a focus on the safe conduct of neonatal anesthesia, but current evidence regarding optimal anesthetic agent combinations, techniques, perioperative ventilation approaches, and cardiovascular support in the neonate remain limited. Ongoing research collaborations between NICU, surgery, and anesthesia will be needed to improve outcomes in this highly vulnerable population.

References

1. Bhananker SM, et al. Anesth Analg. 2007; 105(2):344–350.
2. Catré D, et al. Rev Col Bras Cir. 2013; 40(5):363–369.
3. Lillehei CW, et al. Pediatrics. 2012; 130(3):e538–e564.
4. Weinberg AC, et al. J Am Coll Surg. 2011; 212(5):768–778.
5. Lakshminrusimha S, et al. J Perinatol. 2016; 36:S12–S19.
6. Berkelhamer SK, et al. Semin Perinatol. 2018; 42:432–443.
7. Bernier ML, et al. Pulm Circ. 2018; 8(1):2045893217738143.
8. Devries LB, et al. J Perinatol. 2017; 37(9):1043–106.
9. Giesinger RE, et al. Pediatr Res. 2017; 82(4):901–914.
10. Tissot C, et al. Curr Opin Pediatr. 2020; 32(2):235–244.
11. Giesinger RE, et al. Semin Perinatol. 2016; 40:174–188.
12. Mourani PM, et al. Am J Respir Crit Care Med. 2004; 170(9):1006–1013.
13. Ballard RA, et al. NEJM. 2006; 355(4):343–353.
14. Lakshminrusimha S, et al. Semin Perinatol. 2015; 40(3):160–173.
15. Mourani PM, et al. J Pediatr. 2009; 153(4):379–384.
16. Inamura N, et al. Pediatr Surg Int. 2014; 30(9):889–894.
17. Haydar B, et al. Anesth Analg. 2020; 131(4):1135–1145
18. Costa JD, et al. J Perinatol. 2018; 38(12):1631–1635.
19. Tobias JD, et al. Pediatr Emerg Care. 1996; 12(4):249–251.
20. Bastug O, et al. J Matern Neonatal Med. 2016; 29(12):1993–1998.
21. Morehouse D, et al. Adv Neonatal Care. 2014; 14(3):154–164.
22. Gould DS, et al. Pediatrics. 2003; 112:1298–1301.
23. Lee LK, et al. BMC Anesthesiol. 2018; 18(1):1–11.
24. Altokhais T, et al. Am J Perinatol. 2016; 33(9):861–865.
25. Wang YL, et al. Pediatr Neonatol. 2015; 56(4):220–225.
26. He ZR, et al. Medicine. 2018; 97:36(e12257)
27. Saugstad OD, et al. Neonatology. 2008; 94(3):176–182.
28. Schmölzer GM, et al. J Pediatr. 2008; 153(6):741–745.
29. Fabres J, et al. Pediatrics. 2007; 119(2):299–305.
30. Dargaville PA, et al. J Paediatr Child Health. 2012; 48(9):740–746.
31. Reiss I, et al. Neonatology. 2010; 98(4):354–364.
32. Vali P, et al. Can J Physiol Pharmacol. 2019 March; 97(3):174–182.
33. Klingenberg C, et al. J Perinatol. 2011; 31(9):575–585.
34. Feldman JM. Anesth Analg. 2015; 120(1):165–175.
35. Abouzeid T, et al. J Pediatr. 2017; 184:51–56.
36. Morini F, et al. Semin Pediatr Surg. 2017 Jun 1; 26(3):159–165.
37. Ruzic A. Semin Pediatr Surg. 2019; 28(1):18–25.
38. Snoek KG, et al. Ann Surg. 2016; 263(5):867–874.
39. Bouchut J-C, et al. Anesthesiology. 2004; 100:1007–1012.
40. Noonan M, et al. World J Pediatr Congenit Heart Surg. 2017; 8(5):570–574.
41. Anand KJS, et al. Int Anesthesiol Clin. 1988; 26(3):218–222.
42. Anand KJS, et al. NEJM. 1992; 326(1):1–9.
43. Allegaert K, et al. Paediat Anaesth. 2014; 24:30–38.
44. Ziesenitz VC, et al. Clin Pharmacokinet. 2018; 57:125–149.
45. Pacifici GM et al. Pediatr Neonatol. 2015; 56(3):143–148.
46. Kamata M, et al. J Anesth. 2016; 30:449–460.
47. Trachsel D, et al. BJA. 2016; 117:151–163.
48. Baum VC, et al. Anesthesiology. 1997; 87:1529–1548.
49. Lumb AB, et al. Anesthesiology. 2015; 122:932–946.
50. Jevtovic-Todorovic V. Anesthesiol Clin. 2016; 34(3):439–451
51. O'Leary JD, et al. Br J Anaesth. 2017; 119(3):458–464.
52. MaCann ME, et al. BMJ. 2019; 367:l6459.
53. McCann ME, et al. Lancet. 2019; 393:664–677.
54. Mahmoud M, et al. BJA. 2015; 115:171–182.
55. Mukhtar AM, et al. Anesth Analg. 2006; 103(1):52–56.
56. Bellon M, et al. Pain Ther. 2016; 5(1):63–80.
57. Sellas MN, et al. J Pediatr Pharmacol Ther. 2019; 24(3):227–233.
58. Friesen RH, et al. Anesth Analg. 2013 Oct; 117(4):953–959.
59. Boretsky KR. Pediatr Drugs Adis. 2019; 21:439–449.
60. Wolf AR. Paediatr Anaesth. 2012; 22:19–24.
61. Marhofer P, et al. Acta Anaesthesiol Scand. 2014; 58:1049–1060.
62. Maitra S, et al. J Anesth. 2014; 28:768–779.
63. McCann ME, et al. Anesth Analg. 2017; 125(3):837–845.
64. Szmuk P, et al. Paediatr Anaesth. 2019; 29(1):59–67.
65. Lee J, et al. Arch Dis Child Fetal Neonatal Ed. 1999; 81(3):168–170.
66. Turner NMB. Curr Opin Anaesthesiol. 2015; 28(3):308–313.
67. Weber F, et al. Paediatr Anaesth. 2019; 29(10):993–1001.
68. Weber F, et al. Paediatr Anaesth. 2016; 26(8):815–822.
69. Olbrecht VA, et al. Anesthesiology. 2018; 128(1):85–96.
70. Joynt C, et al. Front Pediatr. 2018; 6:363.
71. Zhang J, et al. Arch Dis Child Fetal Neonatal Ed. 1999; 81(2):99–104.
72. Manouchehri N, et al. Pediatr Res. 2013; 73(4):435–442.
73. Hirsch LJ, et al. Chest. 1991; 100(3):796–801.
74. Bidegain M, et al. J Pediatr. 2010; 157(3):502–504.
75. Amer R, et al. Pediatr Pulmonol. 2019; 54(3):319–332
76. Latham GJ, et al. Paediatr Anaesth. 2019; 29:441–456.
77. James AT, et al. J Perinatol. 2015; 35(4):268–273.
78. Kaestner M, et al. Heart. 2016; 102(Suppl 2):ii57–ii66.

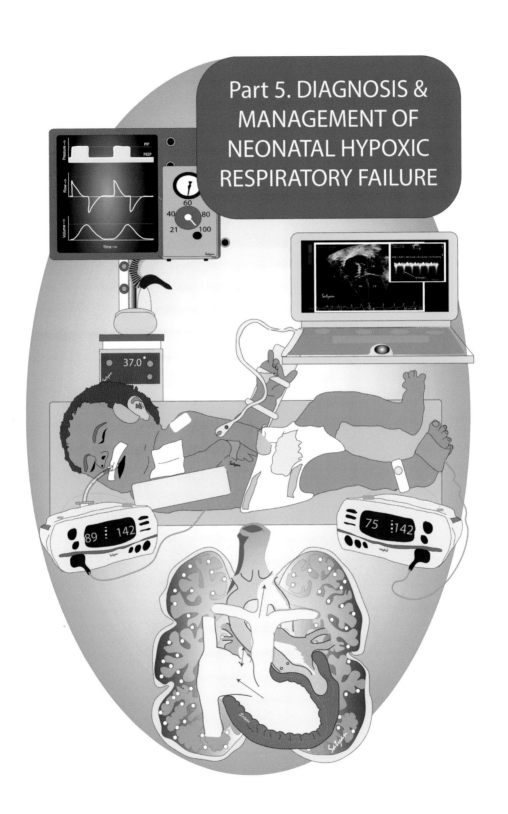

Part 5. DIAGNOSIS & MANAGEMENT OF NEONATAL HYPOXIC RESPIRATORY FAILURE

Part 5
Diagnosis and Management of Neonatal
Hypoxic Respiratory Failure

Edited by Patrick J. McNamara

EPIDEMIOLOGY AND OUTCOMES OF INFANTS WITH HYPOXEMIC RESPIRATORY FAILURE

Souvik Mitra, Roberta L. Keller and Prakesh S. Shah

Contents

Introduction

Acute hypoxemic respiratory failure (HRF) is a severe illness characterized by arterial hypoxemia refractory to supplemental oxygen therapy. Acute HRF is one of the most common reasons for admission to the neonatal intensive care unit (NICU) and is associated with high morbidity and mortality in preterm and term newborns. The etiology of HRF in neonates is multifactorial, and the underlying cause is often the primary determinant of outcome rather than the severity of respiratory failure (1). From a pathophysiologic perspective, HRF is caused by alveolar filling and intrapulmonary shunting of blood resulting from alveolar collapse or consolidation or by intracardiac shunting of blood from the right- to left-side of the circulation. Respiratory failure associated with the latter defines persistent pulmonary hypertension of the newborn (PPHN), which is a major contributing factor to hypoxemia, often resulting in prolonged hospitalization and even death (2).

Challenges with quantifying acute HRF and PPHN in neonates

The burden of HRF in the neonatal population is not well characterized in the literature. The likely reason is variability in definition of neonatal HRF. Acute HRF has been defined as a combination of

criteria that includes supplemental oxygen requirement (usually fraction of inspired oxygen; FiO_2), positive pressure requirement to recruit and maintain lung volume and partial pressure of arterial oxygen (PaO_2). For example, the Berlin definition of acute HRF, often used in adult intensive care settings, classifies HRF as mild (200 mmHg < PaO_2/FIO_2 ≤ 300 mmHg with PEEP or CPAP ≥ 5 cm H_2O), moderate (100 mmHg < PaO_2/FIO_2 ≤ 200 mmHg with PEEP ≥ 5 cm H_2O), and severe (PaO_2/FIO_2 ≤ 100 mmHg with PEEP ≥ 5 cm H_2O) (3). Bohn et al. had described neonatal respiratory failure (hypoxemic or hypercarbic) along similar lines as the presence of two or more of the following: $PaCO_2 > 60$ mmHg, $PaO_2 < 50$ mmHg or O_2 saturation < 80% with an FiO_2 of 1.0 and pH < 7.25 (4). As arterial blood gases may not be routinely performed for neonates, blood gas PaO_2 interpretation may differ depending on the site of sampling (e.g. due to right-to-left shunt at the level of a patent ductus arteriosus [PDA]). Additionally, these data are not often captured in neonatal clinical databases or clinical trials making it difficult to identify the incidence of neonatal acute HRF. Therefore, epidemiological data on HRF neonates may be variably extrapolated from three possible sources, although each of these carries its own limitations:

   a. *Randomized controlled trials* (RCT) on interventions for acute HRF. There are benefits of using pooled epidemiological data from RCTs. First, most studies provide precise

DOI: 10.1201/9780367494018-29

definitions of HRF that includes combination of MAP, FiO_2 and PaO_2. Second, the outcomes are precisely measured. Therefore, readers can obtain an estimate of the burden of clinical outcomes based on the severity of HRF. Limitations include bias due to nonrepresentative sampling from quaternary centers participating in research and additional recruitment issues. Thus, RCT-derived data provide an evaluation of treatment options but could lead to either under- or overestimation of the true burden of disease.

b. *Retrospective or prospective observational studies* in which HRF has been defined predominantly based on clinical features without concomitant blood gas values, with consequent substantial variation in classification. For example, a retrospective cohort study from Canada exploring outcomes of HRF in neonates at birth associated with previable rupture of membranes defined acute HRF as follows: need for $FiO_2 > 0.60$ for ≥2 hours during the first 72 hours of age despite the use of invasive ventilation and receipt of advanced therapy (5). In contrast, other studies in a similar population have used the definition "severe respiratory distress immediately after birth requiring ventilation with very high inflation pressures," or, more recently, lack of sufficient oxygenation despite FiO_2 of 1.0 and mean airway pressure >8 cmH_2O (6, 7). A considerable limitation of these definitions is the lack of specification and wide variations that may not be replicated at other centers or by different observers, limiting inference as to a population-wide estimate.

c. *Administrative datasets*, wherein HRF is defined by a combination of diagnostic codes (as there has not been a specific code for neonatal HRF). For example, a study to quantify the burden of HRF in preterm and term/near-term infants in the United States included data from the Vizient (formerly MedAssets) Health System Database, collected from member hospitals across the United States. The diagnosis of HRF/PPHN was based on the following ICD-codes (where ICD is International Classification of Diseases) (idiopathic PPHN (ICD-9-CM code: 747.83; ICD-10-CM code: P29.3) with or without meconium aspiration (ICD-9-CM codes 770.11, 770.12; ICD-10-CM codes: P24.00, P24.01) (2). Another study from population-based dataset of birth records in California used the ICD-9 PPHN code, as well as other pulmonary hypertension codes (primary pulmonary hypertension, ICD-9-CM 416.0, or other secondary pulmonary hypertension, ICD-9-CM 416.8), in combination with the exclusion of infants with codes for complex congenital heart disease to isolate the diagnoses of HRF/PPHN (8). A major limitation of administrative data is either over- or under-ascertainment through the diagnosis and coding process. Further, populations defined from these databases could be biased depending on the source of the dataset; multicenter data may be reported by only academic or community-based referral hospitals, in contrast to those population-based data collected by linkage to birth hospitals over a specified geographic area.

There are similar and overlapping issues in the consideration of PPHN in published literature. From a pathophysiological perspective, PPHN is characterized by hypoxemia refractory to supplemental oxygen therapy, often associated with a preductal-to-postductal oxygen saturation gradient of 5−10% in the absence of a congenital cyanotic heart disease (9). Echocardiography is therefore essential to confirm diagnosis, specifically to exclude congenital cyanotic heart disease. Neonatal databases seldom capture echocardiography data on a large scale to establish the true prevalence of PPHN. Therefore, epidemiological data on PPHN comes from pooled interventional RCTs, specific observational studies, and administrative datasets, with similar limitations described above.

With regard to epidemiological data obtained from RCTs for newborns with HRF/PPHN for instance, data are only available from those infants who have HRF severe enough to meet a predefined treatment threshold. These inclusions are often based on oxygenation index (mean airway pressure MAP (in cmH_2O) × $FiO_2 \times 100 \div PaO_2$) or postductal PaO_2, while receiving fraction of inspired oxygen (FiO_2) 1.0 and the documentation of right-to-left shunting via a patent ductus arteriosus (10−12). The latter may be absent in infants with a closed ductus and this criterion may even exclude patients with PPHN at the highest risk of right ventricular failure (13). Therefore, infants with PPHN included in clinical trials may only form a fraction of the entire spectrum of HRF or HRF/PPHN in a subset of population.

With respect to observational studies, the NICHD Neonatal Research Network (NRN) prospective study conducted across 12 NICUs between 1993 and 1994 reported high-quality data on the incidence of PPHN in late preterm and term neonates (14). In this study, neonates were defined as having PPHN if they met the following criteria: (i) mechanical ventilation and/or $FiO_2 > 0.50$ and (ii) documented PH as defined by either echocardiographic evidence of elevated pulmonary pressure (judged by right to left or bidirectional shunt), or a pre−post ductal oxygen gradient >20 mmHg (14). However, these data represent a more severely affected group, as mechanical ventilation is required, and again, are limited by collection only at quaternary centers.

Finally, as noted above, administrative datasets can be used for ascertainment of PPHN. Limitations include possible incorrect ascertainment, even when multiple ICD codes are used, and biased sampling, based on which institutions provide data for a particular dataset.

Thus, while the diagnosis of HRF may be based on both clinical and blood gas parameters, confirmation usually requires echocardiography. These limitations in definition should be kept in mind as we discuss the incidence and longitudinal outcomes in the following sections.

Epidemiology of acute HRF

Incidence and demographics

Acute HRF contributes to a substantial burden of NICU admissions. Substantial variability in the incidence of neonatal HRF is driven by both variation in HRF definitions (as discussed above) as well as the sampled population (Table 29.1). Many studies, however, have utilized criteria or coding specific to PPHN, it is difficult to broaden these data to estimate the full burden of HRF among newborns.

For example, from administrative data, Pandya et al. reported a prevalence of HRF/PPHN of 50.1% and 66.9% among preterm and term/near-term infants admitted to the NICU, respectively (2). Among preterm infants with HRF/PPHN, the distribution across gestational age strata seems to follow a U-shaped curve with the highest incidence in 27−28-week and 33−34-week age groups (gestational age groups: 27−28 weeks [29.6%]; 29−30 weeks (21.6%); 31−32 weeks [21.6%]; 33−34 weeks [27.6%]). Among late-preterm/term infants, the incidence of HRF/PPHN was significantly

TABLE 29.1 Incidence of Hypoxemic Respiratory Failure/PPHN in Neonates

Author, Year	Type of Study	Definition of HRF/PPHN		Reported Burden of HRF/PPHN	Comments
		Population Studied	Diagnosis of HRF/PPHN		
Walsh-Sukys 2000 (14)	Prospective observational study across 12 NICHD Neonatal Research Network sites, 1993–1994	Neonates with gestational age ≥ 34 weeks and <7 postnatal days of age	(1) mechanical ventilation and/or FiO$_2$ > 0.50 and (2) documented pulmonary artery hypertension as defined by either two-dimensional echocardiographic evidence of elevated pulmonary pressure (judged by right to left or bidirectional shunt), or a preductal to post ductal oxygen gradient > 20 mmHg	Prevalence of PPHN 1.9 per 1000 live births	Wide variation in prevalence among centers (0.43–6.82 per 1000 live births) noted
Chandrasekharan 2020 (18)	Prospective observational study across NICHD Neonatal Research Network sites, 2007–2015	Preterm neonates born ≤ 26 weeks gestational age	Maximal FiO$_2$ > 0.6 on either day 1 or day 3 of life	Incidence of early HRF was 22.7%	Infants with lower birth weight (<720 g), male sex, Small for gestational age (SGA), or delivery by cesarean were associated with increased risk of early HRF
Steurer 2017 (8)	Administrative data from California Office of Statewide Health Planning and Development database, 2007–2011	Neonates with gestational age ≥ 34 weeks	ICD-9-CM codes for PPHN as documented in the database (747.83 (persistent fetal circulation), 416.0 (primary pulmonary hypertension), or 416.8 (other secondary pulmonary hypertension)	Incidence of PPHN 1.8 per 1000 live births	PPHN incidence 5.4 per 1,000 live births at 34–36 weeks' GA and 1.6 per 1000 live births at term infants
Nakanishi 2018 (17)	Retrospective multicenter cohort study of preterm infants registered in the Neonatal Research Network of Japan (NRNJ). 2003–2012	Preterm infants born at a gestational age of < 28 weeks	Based on clinical and echocardiographic criteria as follows: A difference of > 10% between preductal and postductal SpO$_2$, despite optimal treatment of the patient's lung disease (mechanical ventilation and high concentration of oxygen); an estimated peak systolic pulmonary artery pressure > 35 mmHg, or more than two-thirds of the systemic systolic pressure, as indicated by the presence of a tricuspid regurgitation jet; and a right-to-left patent ductus arteriosus or atrial-level shunt	Prevalence of PPHN 8.1% (95% CI 7.7% to 8.6%)	Prevalence increased with decreasing gestational age: 18.5% (15.2%–22.4%) among infants born at 22 weeks; 13.1% (11.5–15.0%) among infants born at 23 weeks; 11.1% (9.8–12.5%) among infants born at 24 weeks; 8.1% (7.1–9.2%) among infants born at 25 weeks; 6.4% (5.6–7.3%) among infants born at 26 weeks and 4.4% (3.8–5.2%) among infants born at 27 weeks
Nakwan 2018 (15)	Multicenter retrospective study, involving seven level-III NICUs from six Asian countries, 2014–2016 (Nihon University School of Medicine of Japan, Kuwait University, Al-Sabah Maternity Hospital of Kuwait, Cloud nine Hospital and Govt. Medical College and Hospital of India, Aga Khan University of Pakistan, Singapore General Hospital of Singapore, and Hat Yai Hospital of Thailand)	Term and preterm infants	Presence of refractory hypoxemia plus one or more of the four following conditions: (i) echocardiographic evidence of elevated pulmonary pressure (right to left or bidirectional shunt at PDA and/or PFO level), (ii) a pre-to postductal partial pressure of oxygen gradient (PaO$_2$) equal to or greater than 20 mmHg, (iii) a pre to postductal pulse oximetry oxygen saturation (SpO$_2$) gradient equal to or greater than 10%, and/or (iv) a positive hyperoxia-hyperventilation test	Incidence of PPHN among live-birth inborn infants ranged between 1.2–4.6 per 1,000 live births	Incidence of PPHN per 1,000 live births: 1.2 (Kuwait), 2.5 (Japan), 2.6 (Thailand), 4.0 (Singapore), 4.4 (Pakistan), and 3.3 and 4.6 from 2 centers in India, respectively

TABLE 29.1 (*Continued*)

Author, Year	Type of Study	Definition of HRF/PPHN		Reported Burden of HRF/PPHN	Comments
		Population Studied	Diagnosis of HRF/PPHN		
Pandya 2019 (2)	Administrative data from multihospital database (Vizient), 2011–2015	Preterm (≤34 weeks of gestation) and term/near-terms (>34 weeks of gestation)	ICD-codes for HRF/PPHN as documented in the database (idiopathic PPHN [ICD-9-CM code: 747.83; ICD-10-CM code: P29.3] with or without meconium aspiration [ICD-9-CM codes 770.11, 770.12; ICD-10-CM codes: P24.00, P24.01])	Prevalence of HRF/PPHN was 50.1% in preterm and 66.9% in term/near-term infants	The study considered prevalence of HRF/PPHN only among infants admitted to the NICU
Sardar 2020 (16)	Retrospective single-center study conducted in a Level III NICU of a referral center in Kolkata, India	Term and preterm infants	Diagnosis based on clinical and echocardiographic criteria. Clinical criteria included: labile oxygen saturation (SpO$_2$), severe hypoxemia (SpO$_2$ < 85%), or differential cyanosis between preductal and postductal sites (more than 10% difference in SpO$_2$) Suggestive echocardiography findings included right ventricular hypertrophy, deviation of interventricular septum toward left, jet of tricuspid regurgitation, and right to left or bidirectional shunting through patent foramen ovale and/or patent ductus arteriosus	Incidence of PPHN 3.38/1000 live births (inborn infants)	Incidence of PPHN 5.49/1000 NICU admissions (including both inborn and outborn infants requiring admission)

higher in the 35–36-week group (69.3%) as compared to term infants born ≥37 weeks gestation (30.7%).

The population incidence of PPHN has been estimated as 1.9 per 1,000 live births (ranging 0.4–6.8 per 1000 live births for individual centers) in the United States, in a prospective cohort from the NICHD-NRN (14). A more recent study utilizing administrative data from the California Office of Statewide Health Planning and Development birth cohort database (2007–2011) estimated a similar incidence in near-term/term infants (1.8 per 1000 live births) (8). The incidence of PPHN was highest in late preterm infants (34–36 weeks) at 5.4 per 1000 live births (8).

A retrospective chart review of infants (preterm and term) with documented PPHN (by clinical and echocardiographic criteria, Table 29.1), from seven centers in six Asian countries (Japan, Kuwait, India, Pakistan, Singapore, and Thailand, 2014–2016), estimated an incidence of PPHN from 1.2 to 4.6 per 1000 live births (15). Another study from a tertiary care neonatal unit in Eastern India estimated the incidence of PPHN (by clinical and echocardiographic criteria, Table 29.1) at 3.38 per 1000 live births (16).

Acute HRF and PPHN are being increasingly recognized as a clinical entity in extremely preterm neonates (<28 weeks gestational age), although there is little epidemiology data in this gestational age group. A large cohort study conducted by the Neonatal Research Network of Japan (NRNJ) between 2003 and 2012 (n = 12 954) estimated the prevalence of PPHN (defined by clinical and echocardiographic criteria) at 8.1% (95% confidence intervals (CI) 7.7–8.6%) (17). In this cohort, there was a noticeable trend toward the increasing prevalence of PPHN with decreasing

gestational age: 18.5% (range, 15.2–22.4%) for infants born at 22 weeks compared with 4.4% (range, 3.8–5.2%) for those born at 27 weeks (17). Another study of preterm infants of ≤26 weeks' gestation born between 2007 and 2015 in the NICHD-NRN (n = 7639) centers reported incidence of early HRF (defined as maximal FiO$_2$ > 0.6 on either day 1 or day 3 of life) as 22.7% (18). Given that the burden of HRF/PPHN could be potentially higher in extremely preterm infants, future studies need to specifically describe the entity including incidence, risk factors, and outcomes in this high-risk group.

Etiology

Underlying etiologies of HRF/PPHN appear consistent across reported cohorts. In the NICHD-NRN cohort, the most common etiology for HRF in near-term/term infants was meconium aspiration syndrome (41%), followed by idiopathic pulmonary hypertension (17%), pneumonia (14%), and respiratory distress syndrome (13%) (14). In the California Birth cohort, infection/sepsis was noted to be the most common etiology for PPHN in near-term/term infants (30%), followed by meconium aspiration syndrome (MAS, 24.4%) (8). In the studies from Asia and India that included all infants with PPHN (preterm and term), meconium aspiration was the most common etiology overall (24.1% and 17.4%, respectively) (15, 16). Pandya et al. noted that while the incidence of HRF secondary to respiratory distress syndrome was significantly higher in preterm versus term infants (69.4% in preterm vs. 34.5% in term infants; $p < 0.001$), that due to sepsis was not different in the two groups (40.9% in preterm vs. 39.9% in term infants; $p = 0.75$) (2).

Perinatal risk factors
Several perinatal factors have been associated with increased incidence of HRF/PPHN. The most notable are as follows:

Sex
The incidence of HRF is significantly higher in males (59% vs. 40.9%; $p < 0.01$), across both preterm and term gestations (2). Similarly, among infants diagnosed with PPHN in the NICHD-NRN cohort of term infants, 58% were male (14). Sex differences in physiology, hormones, and growth factors have been postulated to play a role (19).

Race and ethnicity
Several studies have reported a higher incidence of PPHN among African American infants, even after adjusting for other perinatal factors, especially in late-preterm/term infants (8, 20, 21). Data from the NICHD-NRN cohort showed that among infants with PPHN, 33% were African American, 49% Caucasian, and 19% from other racial-ethnic groups (14). One study exploring the risk factors for PPHN among 1213 mothers from four metropolitan areas (Boston, Philadelphia, San Diego, and Toronto) between 1998 and 2003 reported an increased odds of PPHN among Asian infants (adjusted odds ratio (OR) 2.1; 95% CI 1.2–3.7) and African American infants (adjusted OR 2.3; 95% CI 1.4–3.7) (22). The effect of race and ethnicity on the prevalence of PPHN persisted even after adjustment for socioeconomic factors (e.g. maternal education, family income) or gestational age (22). Interestingly, the California birth cohort study, with a high proportion of Hispanic mothers, reported that Hispanic ethnicity was protective against PPHN (adjusted risk ratio (RR) 0.8; 95% CI 0.7–0.9), but incidence was higher among infants of Black mothers, compared to the reference race/ethnicity of White, non-Hispanic (8). The recent NICHD-NRN cohort of extremely preterm infants, however, showed that African American infants had a similar incidence of early HRF (21.7% vs. 23.3%) compared to other races (18).

Maternal body mass index
High maternal body mass index (BMI) has been shown to be associated with an increased risk of PPHN (adjusted OR: 2.2; 95% CI 1.4–3.5) (22). Whether this is related to a direct effect of obesity on fetal lung development (through endothelial dysfunction and inflammation) or an indirect effect of obesity on adverse pregnancy outcomes (such as increased C/S) remains unclear (23, 24). Steurer et al. reported an increased risk of PPHN with high maternal BMI, preexisting and gestational diabetes, and large for gestational age status in multivariable analyses, lending further credence to postulated effects of these pathways (8). Hernández-Díaz et al. demonstrated that compared with White women with BMI < 20, the odds of developing PPHN in infants of African American and Asian women with BMI > 27 were 6.1 (95% CI 2.9–13.2) and 7.0 (95% CI 2.0–24.8), respectively (22).

Mode of delivery
Multiple studies have demonstrated that infants born by Cesarean section (C/S) are at higher risk of developing HRF/PPHN (18, 22, 25–27). Adjusted odds for developing PPHN after C/S was found to be 7.4 (95% CI 5.2–10.4) and 4.9 (95% CI 1.7–14.0) in two separate retrospective cohort studies from the United States, although risk ratios were considerably lower in the population-based data from California (RR 2.6 (95% CI 2.4–2.8) for any PPHN by administrative coding, and RR 3.3 (95% CI 3.0–3.6) for severe (receiving positive pressure ventilation) PPHN) (8, 22, 25). It is unclear whether all C/S or those specifically in the absence of preceding labor were associated with increased risk of PPHN (22, 28, 29). Further, given the risk of residual confounding in most studies, it is also unclear if C/S itself or the underlying medical condition that prompted intervention increases the risk of PPHN.

Maternal chorioamnionitis
Presence of chorioamnionitis has been shown to be a risk factor for development of PPHN in both late-preterm/term (adjusted RR 2.3; 95% CI 1.9–2.7) as well as very preterm (<32 weeks gestation) infants (adjusted OR 2.80; 95% CI 1.01–7.73) (8, 30).

Antenatal drug exposure
Maternal use of selective serotonin reuptake inhibitors (SSRIs) during pregnancy has been associated with PPHN in preterm infants (31). Large population-based cohort studies from five Nordic countries ($n = 30\,000$; adjusted OR 2.1; 95% CI 1.5–3.0) and the United States ($n = 102\,179$; adjusted OR 1.10; 95% CI 0.94–1.29) have suggested such associations (32, 33). In a US-based administrative claims analysis from a predominantly White or non-Hispanic population, maternal SSRI use was associated with a dose-dependent increased risk of newborn respiratory distress (RR 2.19 and 2.39 for the highest level of SSRI exposure, compared to reference groups of maternal anxiety and depression without SSRI exposure); PPHN was not evaluated in these analyses (34). Finally, a systematic review and meta-analysis (9 studies; 7 540 265 subjects) reported a pooled OR of 1.5 (95% CI 1.04–1.99) with an absolute risk difference of 0.619 per 1000 live births (number needed to harm: 1615) (35). Thus, the absolute increase in risk of PPHN with antenatal SSRI exposure is likely to be outweighed by the potential benefits of treatment of maternal depression.

There are conflicting reports of the association of maternal use of aspirin and nonsteroidal anti-inflammatory drugs (NSAID) with PPHN. A case-control study by Van Marter et al. of 401 mothers (1985–1989) showed that *in utero* exposure to aspirin increased the odds of PPHN (adjusted OR 4.9; 95% CI 1.6–15.3), and NSAID exposure also increased the odds of PPHN (adjusted OR 6.2; 95% CI 1.8–21.8) (36). Another case-control study from Detroit, MI, reported a significant association between the presence of NSAIDs (i.e. aspirin, ibuprofen, indomethacin, naproxen) in meconium and odds of PPHN (OR 21.5; 95% CI 7.12–64.71) (37). A more recent multicenter epidemiological study reported no association of maternal aspirin or ibuprofen use with development of PPHN in the newborn (20). Surprisingly, they identified that among term infants, maternal ibuprofen consumption in the third trimester of pregnancy was associated with reduced odds of developing PPHN (OR 0.42; 95% CI 0.20–0.89). Thus, data on the association between maternal use of NSAID and neonatal PPHN remain inconclusive.

Smoking
There is conflicting evidence on the association of smoking with PPHN. Bearer et al., in a prospective observational study ($n = 70$), demonstrated that the proportion of infants with a detectable level of cotinine (a nicotine metabolite) was higher among infants with PPHN compared to control infants (64.5% vs. 28.2%; $p = 0.002$) (38). Data from the California birth cohort database also suggests maternal smoking as an independent risk factor for PPHN (adjusted RR 1.3; 95% CI 1.1–1.6) (8). Although biologically plausible, other epidemiologic studies have failed to confirm an association with maternal smoking (36, 39). Van Marter et al.

in their case-control study including 103 infants with PPHN and 298 controls, showed that when adjusted for perinatal confounders, smoking during pregnancy was not associated with increased odds of PPHN (adjusted OR 1.2; 95% CI 0.5–2.9) (36). Such conflicting evidence on the association of smoking with PPHN may relate to ascertainment of smoking or tobacco exposure.

Other factors

Pulmonary hypoplasia, secondary to preterm premature rupture of membranes (PPROM), and oligohydramnios is a risk factor for HRF/PPHN in preterm infants, especially in those who are born extremely preterm (40–43). A retrospective case-control study of 183 preterm infants (<37 weeks gestational age) showed that infants with PPHN had a higher incidence of PPROM (26.2% vs. 7.3%; $p < 0.05$) and oligohydramnios (18% vs. 2.4%; $p < 0.05$) compared to gestational age-matched controls (40). Being small for gestational age (adjusted RR 1.6, 95% CI 1.5–1.8) or large for gestational age (adjusted RR 1.6, 95% CI 1.5–1.8, and adjusted OR 1.8, 95% CI 1.3–2.7 in population-based and case-control studies, respectively) have also been implicated in the development of PPHN in near-term/term infants (8, 22).

Neonatal outcomes in acute HRF and PPHN

Clinical outcomes of neonates with HRF largely depend on the underlying etiology as well as gestational age at birth. There is substantial variability in documented outcomes, largely due to the variability in definition of HRF/PPHN across both observational studies as well as RCTs.

Outcomes in near-term/term infants
Mortality

Acute HRF/PPHN has been associated with high mortality, especially when inhaled nitric oxide was not available. Data from the NICHD-NRN cohort of 1993–94 reported an overall mortality rate for PPHN of 12% (14). Mortality rates varied significantly based on underlying etiology, ranging from 4 to 33%. Survival was 94% among those with MAS, 91% among those with respiratory distress syndrome (RDS) or pneumonia, but only 61% among those with congenital diaphragmatic hernia (CDH, $p < 0.0002$) (14). A population-based study from the California birth cohort demonstrated a PPHN mortality rate of 7.3% (571/7847) overall with a predischarge mortality of 6.5% and postdischarge mortality of 0.7% by 1 year of age (44). For infants receiving positive pressure ventilation (severe PPHN, comparable disease severity to infants in the NICHD-NRN cohort), mortality to 1 year was 10.1%, with 9.2% prior to discharge (44). Mortality from this population also varied significantly by etiology of PPHN, highest in infants with PPHN due to CDH or other pulmonary anomalies, and lowest in those with MAS or idiopathic PPHN (44). On the contrary, data from the Vizient Health System Database from the United States reported a much higher mortality rate for acute HRF (21.3%) (2).

The mortality statistics mentioned above partly corroborate with those documented in RCTs. To date, 17 RCTs have been conducted on use of iNO for HRF in near-term/term infants (45). Nine studies have compared iNO with control (placebo or standard care without iNO) (45). The pooled mortality rate excluding infants with CDH was 10.4% (9.6% in the iNO group vs. 11.5% in the control group) (45). In infants with CDH, the mortality rates were substantially higher at 42.9% (36/84) with no statistically significant difference between the iNO group versus controls

(45). Five RCTs have compared earlier initiation of iNO in infants with moderate HRF versus later initiation with severe HRF. The pooled mortality rate was 17.9% (16.7% in moderate HRF vs. 19.2% in severe HRF group) (45).

Five RCTs have explored the use of sildenafil in infants with HRF/PPHN (46). The pooled mortality rate in the three RCTs that compared sildenafil versus placebo in near-term/term neonates was 24.7% (7.5% in the sildenafil group vs. 43.2% in the placebo group). Detailed mortality data from RCTs that enrolled infants with HRF/PPHN are summarized in Table 29.2.

Need for extracorporeal membrane oxygenation

Data from RCTs show that 39.3% of infants with HRF without CDH (29.3% in the iNO group vs. 51.3% in the control group) and 75% of CDH infants with HRF (84.2% in the iNO group vs. 67.4% in the control group) required extracorporeal membrane oxygenation (ECMO) support (Table 29.2) (45).

Hospitalization and readmission

The average duration of hospitalization in the NICHD-NRN cohort was reported to be 19 ± 16 days with 18% of the infants staying > 28 days (14). Similarly, in the California birth cohort, infants with PPHN (MAS, infection, RDS, or idiopathic) were hospitalized for 18–20 days longer than near-term/term controls without PPHN; infants with CDH or other pulmonary anomalies and PPHN were hospitalized for an additional 60 days beyond the remainder of the cohort. Of the infants who survived until discharge, 28.6% were readmitted to the hospital at least once during their first year with a third of the readmission (10.4%) due to respiratory illness (44). The rehospitalization rate was higher compared with infants without PPHN (28.6% vs. 9.8%; $p < 0.001$) (44). In multivariate modeling, underlying etiology and severity of PPHN (aRR, 1.6; 95% CI 1.5–1.8 for severe vs. mild PPHN), conferred the greatest risks for postdischarge mortality or any hospital readmission by 1 year of age, with modest effects of Hispanic ethnicity (aRR, 1.2; 95% CI 1.1–1.4) and small for gestational age status (aRR, 1.2; 95% CI 1.1–1.3). As expected, CDH and other pulmonary anomalies conferred the highest risk for this adverse postdischarge outcome, as compared to other underlying causes of PPHN (44).

Neurodevelopmental outcomes

The incidence of neurodevelopmental delay is reported to be higher among infants with HRF. The pooled incidence of cerebral palsy without CDH was noted to be 9.4% in RCTs comparing iNO versus controls (Table 29.2) (45). The pooled incidence of cognitive delay (Mental Developmental Index [MDI] > 2 standard deviations below the mean) was 18.7%, and that of motor delay (Psychomotor Developmental Index [PDI] > 2 SD below the mean) was 15.5% (45). Of note, the incidence of motor delay was lower in the iNO group compared to controls (10% vs. 19.1%; RR 0.48; 95% CI 0.25–0.94) (45).

Increased incidence of sensorineural hearing loss has been reported in infants with PPHN in observational studies (47, 48). In a study of 51 infants with PPHN, Walton and Hendricks-Munoz demonstrated that the duration of hyperventilation was longer in infants who developed sensorineural hearing losses compared to normal-hearing children (48). Pooled incidence of hearing impairment among HRF survivors in RCTs comparing iNO versus control was noted to be as high as 32.6% with no difference between the iNO group versus controls (Table 29.2) (45). At the 7-year follow-up from the UK Collaborative ECMO Trial

TABLE 29.2 Reported Outcomes of Infants with HRF/PPHN in RCTs

Number of RCTs (Number of Infants Randomized)	Participant Characteristics	Proportion of Infants with Outcome in the Intervention Group	Proportion of Infants with Outcome in the Comparator Group	Overall Proportion of Enrolled Infants with Outcome
Mortality				
9 RCTs (12, 53–60) (*n* = 967)	Near-term/term infants with HRF	iNO: 9.6%	Control: 11.5%	10.4%
2 RCTs (54, 61) (*n* = 84)	Near-term/term infants with congenital diaphragmatic hernia and HRF	iNO: 21.1%	Control: 39.1%	42.9%
5 RCTs (62–66) (*n* = 495)	Near-term/term with HRF	iNO initiation with moderate HRF: 16.7%	iNO initiation with severe HRF: 19.2%	17.9%
3 RCTs (67–69)	Near-term/term with HRF	Sildenafil: 7.5%	Control: 43.2%	24.7%
1 RCT (70) (*n* = 65)	Near-term/term with HRF	Sildenafil: 3.2%	Magnesium sulfate: 5.9%	4.6%
1 RCT (71) (*n* = 24)	Near-term/term with HRF	Sildenafil plus iNO: 23.1%	Placebo plus iNO: 18.2%	20.8%
10 RCTs (59, 72–80) (*n* = 1066)	Preterm (<35 weeks gestational age) with HRF	iNO: 40.9%	Control: 39.4%	40.2%
Need for ECMO				
7 RCTs (12, 53–56, 58, 60) (*n* = 815)	Near-term/term infants with HRF	iNO: 29.3%	Control: 51.4%	39.3%
2 RCTs (54, 61) (*n* = 84)	Near-term/term infants with congenital diaphragmatic hernia and HRF	iNO: 84.2%	Control: 67.4%	75%
4 RCTs (62, 63, 65, 66) (*n* = 439)	Near-term/term with HRF	iNO initiation with moderate HRF: 14.3%	iNO initiation with severe HRF: 14.4%	14.4%
Chronic lung disease				
3 RCTs (64–66) (*n* = 437)	Near-term/term with HRF	iNO initiation with moderate HRF: 10.9%	iNO initiation with severe HRF: 12%	11.4%
8 RCTs (59, 72–75, 77, 78, 80) (*n* = 681)	Preterm (<35 weeks gestational age) with HRF	iNO: 42.2%	Control: 46.6%	44.5%
Intraventricular hemorrhage (all grades)				
4 RCTs (72, 73, 75, 79) (*n* = 314)	Preterm (<35 weeks gestational age) with HRF	iNO: 33.1%	Control: 33.6%	33.4%
Severe intraventricular hemorrhage (grades 3 and 4)				
6 RCTs (72, 73, 75–77, 80) (*n* = 773)	Preterm (<35 weeks gestational age) with HRF	iNO: 28.6%	Control: 23.1%	25.9%
Severe intraventricular hemorrhage (grades 3 and 4) or periventricular leukomalacia				
8 RCTs (59, 72–75, 77, 78, 80) (*n* = 901)	Preterm (<35 weeks gestational age) with HRF	iNO: 29.1%	Control: 26%	27.5%
Cerebral palsy among survivors				
2 RCTs (55, 60) (*n* = 299)	Near-term/term infants with HRF	iNO: 10%	Control: 8.9%	9.4%
1 RCT (61) (*n* = 22)	Near-term/term infants with congenital diaphragmatic hernia and HRF	iNO: 25%	Control: – (no events recorded)	9.1%
1 RCT (65) (*n* = 234)	Near-term/term with HRF	iNO initiation with moderate HRF: 8.3%	iNO initiation with severe HRF: 6.2%	7.3%
2 RCTs (77, 78) (*n* = 209)	Preterm (<35 weeks gestational age) with HRF	iNO: 18.2%	Control: 10%	13.9%
Cognitive delay (Mental Developmental Index [MDI] > 2 standard deviations below the mean) among survivors				
2 RCTs (55, 60) (*n* = 283)	Near-term/term with HRF	iNO: 15.4%	Control: 20.8%	18.7%
Motor delay (Psychomotor Developmental Index [PDI] > 2 standard deviations below the mean) among survivors				
2 RCTs (55, 60) (*n* = 283)	Near-term/term with HRF	iNO: 10%	Control: 19.1%	15.5%

TABLE 29.2 (*Continued*)

Number of RCTs (Number of Infants Randomized)	Participant Characteristics	Proportion of Infants with Outcome in the Intervention Group	Proportion of Infants with Outcome in the Comparator Group	Overall Proportion of Enrolled Infants with Outcome
Hearing impairment among survivors				
2 RCTs (60, 61) (*n* = 178)	Near-term/term with HRF (including infants with congenital diaphragmatic hernia)	iNO: 33.7%	Control: 31.6%	32.6%
1 RCT (65) (*n* = 234)	Near-term/term with HRF	iNO initiation with moderate HRF: 0.8%	iNO initiation with severe HRF: 2.7%	1.7%
Severe retinopathy of prematurity (≥ stage 3)				
3 RCTs (77, 78, 80) (*n* = 261)	Preterm (<35 weeks gestational age) with HRF	iNO: 24%	Control: 25%	24.5%
Retinopathy of prematurity requiring surgery				
4 RCTs (74, 75, 77, 80) (*n* = 673)	Preterm (<35 weeks gestational age) with HRF	iNO: 11.9%	Control: 14%	12.9%

for newborns with HRF with or without PPHN, 25/90 children (28%) had hearing impairment or disability, with similar rates for survivors in both the ECMO and conventional therapy groups (49). These data are consistent with the hypothesis that prolonged duration of hypoxia may compromise cochlear integrity leading to sensorineural hearing loss, though there may also be contributions from exposure to ototoxic medications and other insults (48, 50).

Outcomes in preterm infants
Mortality
Mortality in preterm infants with HRF is reported to be higher as compared to term infants (30.2% vs. 21.3%, $P = 0.002$) (2). Even within the preterm population, mortality is substantially higher in infants with HRF/PPHN (26.2% vs. 4.1%; $p < 0.0001$) (40). In Japan, the presence of PPHN was also found to be associated with higher mortality even after exclusion of infants with chronic lung disease (CLD) (29.9% (95% CI 26.1–34.0) compared to 8.4% (95% CI 7.8–9.1) in infants without PPHN (17). In the NICHD-NRN cohort of extremely preterm infants (≤26 weeks' gestation), early HRF was associated with a mortality of 51.3% (18). Lower birth weight and gestational age, male sex, Apgar scores <4 at 1 and 5 min, clinical chorioamnionitis, and C/S have been independently associated with increased risk of mortality in preterm infants with PPHN (17, 18, 40). There is conflicting evidence on whether PPROM per se increases the risk of death in the context of PPHN (5, 40, 42, 51).

Chronic lung disease
Chronic lung disease (CLD) data in the context of HRF/PPHN is highly variable and depends on the gestational age group as well as underlying comorbidities. Data from the Japanese cohort of extremely preterm infants (<28 weeks gestation) identified that the risk of CLD in infants with PPHN was 44.9%, while the NICHD-NRN cohort of preterm infants ≤26 weeks of gestation showed that about three-quarter of the infants with early HRF (741/977) developed CLD (18). In both instances, CLD rates were noted to be higher compared to those without HRF/PPHN (17, 18). Similarly, the risk of CLD in preterm infants developing HRF following previable rupture of membranes (pROM, <23 weeks' gestation and latency period ≥2 weeks) was reported to be 68% (5). Data from RCTs show a pooled CLD rate of 44.5% (303/681)

among survivors with HRF at birth with no difference between the iNO group versus controls (Table 29.2) (52).

Intraventricular hemorrhage and periventricular leukomalacia
Thirty-nine percent of extremely preterm infants with early HRF in the NICHD-NRN cohort developed severe intraventricular hemorrhage (IVH) and/or periventricular leukomalacia, as compared to 16.3% infants without early HRF ($p < 0.0001$) (18). Data from RCTs show a pooled incidence of 33.4% (105/314) for IVH (all grades), 25.9% (200/773) for severe IVH (grades 3 or 4) and 27.5% (248/901) for severe IVH or periventricular leukomalacia (Table 29.2) (52).

Hospitalization duration
The length of hospital stay for preterm infants with HRF/PPHN is longer than term infants, as per the Vizient Health System Database statistics (total duration of hospitalization: 54 days vs. 29 days, $p < 0.0001$; NICU stay: 34 days vs. 17 days, $p < 0.0001$) (2). Similarly, preterm infants were found to incur higher total hospitalization costs ($155,910 vs. $108,241, $p < 0.0001$) compared to term/near-term infants. Data from the NICHD-NRN cohort showed that surviving extremely preterm infants with early HRF had a longer length of hospital stay compared to those without early HRF (132.9 ± 55.8 117.1 ± 46.2; $p < 0.0001$) (18).

Neurodevelopmental outcomes
Surviving extremely preterm infants in the NICHD-NRN (≤26 weeks of gestation) cohort were found to have a higher incidence of moderate–severe neurodevelopmental impairment (41.2% vs. 32.3%, $p < 0.0001$) and cerebral palsy (22.1% vs. 12.8%; $p < 0.0001$) (18). The pooled incidence of cerebral palsy among preterm infants with HRF was noted to be 13.9% (29/209) from RCTs (52). The pooled incidence of motor or cognitive delay in preterm infants with HRF (Bayley MDI or PDI < −2 SD) was noted to be 8.2% (63/768) with a lower incidence among infants who received iNO (RR 0.57; 95% CI 0.36−0.9) (52).

Data from RCTs show a pooled incidence of 24.5% (64/261) for severe retinopathy of prematurity (ROP) (≥ stage 3) and 12.9% (87/673) for ROP requiring surgery (52). Furthermore, 3-year follow-up data from 5923 extremely preterm Japanese infants showed that PPHN was an independent risk factor for visual impairment (adjusted OR, 1.42, 95% CI 1.03–1.97) with an increase also documented with HRF in the NICHD-NRN cohort (2.8 vs. 1.3%, $p = 0.0019$) (17, 18). There is a lack of consistent reporting on neurodevelopmental outcomes among survivors of HRF and PPHN in the literature.

Summary and key points

- The burden of HRF is not well characterized in neonatal literature, primarily due to variability in the definition of HRF and variability in sample populations.
- There is a substantial overlap between the definitions of HRF and PPHN. This should be appreciated while considering the epidemiology of HRF and PPHN in neonates.
- The overall incidence of HRF/PPHN has substantial variability within and across geographical regions but is estimated at 1.8 per 1000 live births in recent US data.
- HRF/PPHN occurs more commonly in males and follows a U-shaped curve across gestational age strata, with highest incidence/prevalence described in extremely preterm and near-term infants.
- Meconium aspiration syndrome and infection appear to be the most common etiologies in term/near-term infants, while respiratory distress syndrome is the most common etiology in preterm infants.
- Risk factors include African American and Asian race, Cesarean section, maternal chorioamnionitis, exposure to SSRIs, maternal smoking, and pulmonary hypoplasia.
- Overall mortality varies from 10 to 20% in term/near-term infants and 30 to 50% in preterm infants, with substantial differences in survival based on etiology. Outcomes are significantly worse with CDH and congenital pulmonary anomalies.
- Rehospitalization rates are three times higher in term/near-term infants with PPHN compared to those without PPHN. Severity and etiology of PPHN are the primary risks for increased postdischarge mortality or hospital readmission in the first year after birth.
- PPHN significantly increases the risk of hearing impairment in term/near-term infants and visual impairment in preterm infants.
- There is a lack of inception cohort data on incidence, risk factors, and neonatal and childhood outcomes of neonates who had HRF/PPHN.

References

1. Peters MJ, et al. Intensive Care Med. 1998 Jul; 24(7):699–705.
2. Pandya S, et al. J Health Econ Outcomes Res. 2019 Jun 19; 6(3):130–141.
3. ARDS Definition Task Force, Ranieri VM, et al. JAMA. 2012; 307(23):2526–2533.
4. Bohn D, et al. In: *Pediatric and Neonatal Mechanical Ventilation: from Basics to Clinical Practice*. Rimensberger PC, ed. Berlin, Heidelberg: Springer; 2015. pp. 1185–1265.
5. Baczynski M, et al. J Perinatol. 2018 Aug; 38(8):1087–1092.
6. Uga N, et al. Pediatr Int. 2004 Feb; 46(1):10–14.
7. Losa M, et al. Eur J Pediatr. 1998 Nov; 157(11):935–938.
8. Steurer MA, et al. Pediatrics. 2017; 139(1):e20161165.
9. Lakshminrusimha S, et al. NeoReviews. 2015; 16(12):e680–e692.
10. Rawat M, et al. Neonatology. 2015; 107(3):161–166.
11. Kinsella JP, et al. J Pediatr. 1997; 131(1 Pt 1):55–62.
12. Roberts JD, et al. N Engl J Med. 1997; 336(9):605–610.
13. Jain A, et al. Semin Fetal Neonatal Med. 2015; 20(4):262–271.
14. Walsh-Sukys MC, et al. Pediatrics. 2000; 105(1 Pt 1):14–20.
15. Nakwan N, et al. J Matern Fetal Neonatal Med. 2020; 33(12):2032–2037.
16. Sardar S, et al. J Clin Neonatol. 2020; 9(1):18–26.
17. Nakanishi H, et al. Arch Dis Child Fetal Neonatal Ed. 2018; 103(6):F554–F561.
18. Chandrasekharan P, et al. Pediatrics. 2020; 146(4):e20193318.
19. Townsel CD, et al. Front Pediatr. 2017; 5:6.
20. Van Marter LJ, et al. Pediatrics. 2013; 131(1):79–87.
21. Reece EA, et al. Obstet Gynecol. 1987; 70(5):696–700.
22. Hernández-Díaz S, et al. Pediatrics. 2007; 120(2):e272–282.
23. Visser M, et al. JAMA. 1999; 282(22):2131–2135.
24. Anderson JL, et al. Epidemiology. 2005; 16(1):87–92.
25. Wilson KL, et al. Am J Perinatol. 2011; 28(1):19–24.
26. Heritage CK, et al. Am J Obstet Gynecol. 1985; 152(6 Pt 1):627–629.
27. Keszler M, et al. Pediatrics. 1992; 89(4 Pt 1):670–672.
28. Hales KA, et al. Int J Gynaecol Obstet. 1993; 43(1):35–40.
29. Hook B, et al. Pediatrics. 1997; 100(3 Pt 1):348–353.
30. Yum SK, et al. Pulm Circ. 2018; 8(2):2045894018760166.
31. Chambers CD, et al. N Engl J Med. 2006; 354(6):579–587.
32. Kieler H, et al. BMJ. 2012; 344:d8012.
33. Huybrechts KF, et al. JAMA. 2015; 313(21):2142–2151.
34. Bandoli G, et al. Pediatrics. 2020; 146(1):e20192493.
35. Ng QX, et al. J Womens Health (Larchmt). 2019; 28(3):331–338.
36. Van Marter LJ, et al. Pediatrics. 1996; 97(5):658–663.
37. Alano MA, et al. Pediatrics. 2001; 107(3):519–523.
38. Bearer C, et al. Environ Health Perspect. 1997; 105(2):202–206.
39. Delaney C, et al. Pulm Circ. 2012; 2(1):15–20.
40. Kumar VH, et al. J Perinatol. 2007; 27(4):214–219.
41. Aikio O, et al. J Pediatr. 2012; 161(3):397.e1–403.e1.
42. Williams O, et al. Early Hum Dev. 2009; 85(5):273–277.
43. Williams O, et al. Neonatology. 2012; 101(2):83–90.
44. Steurer MA, et al. J Pediatr. 2019; 213:58.e4–65.e4.
45. Barrington KJ, et al. Cochrane Database Syst Rev. 2017; 1(1):CD000399. doi:10.1002/14651858.CD000399.pub3.
46. Kelly LE, et al. Cochrane Database Syst Rev. 2017; 8(8):CD005494. doi:10.1002/14651858.CD005494.pub4.
47. Hosono S, et al. Pediatr Int. 2009; 51(1):79–83.
48. Walton JP, et al. J Speech Hear Res. 1991; 34(6):1362–1370.
49. McNally H, et al. Pediatrics. 2006; 117(5):e845–e854.
50. Fujikawa S, et al. J Am Acad Audiol. 1997; 8(4):263–268.
51. Shah DM, et al. J Paediatr Child Health. 2011; 47(6):340–345.
52. Barrington KJ, et al. Cochrane Database Syst Rev. 2017; 1(1):CD000509. doi:10.1002/14651858.CD000509.pub5.
53. Christou H, et al. Crit Care Med. 2000; 28(11):3722–3727.
54. Clark RH, et al. N Engl J Med. 2000; 342(7):469–474.
55. Davidson D, et al. Pediatrics. 1998; 101(3 Pt 1):325–334.
56. Field D, et al. Neonatology. 2007; 91(2):73–82.
57. Liu C, et al. Zhonghua Er Ke Za Zhi. 2008; 46(3):224–228.
58. Wessel DL, et al. Pediatrics. 1997; 100(5):E7.
59. The Franco-Belgium Collaborative NO Trial Group. Lancet. 1999; 354(9184):1066–1071.
60. Neonatal Inhaled Nitric Oxide Study Group. N Engl J Med. 1997; 336(9):597–604.
61. The Neonatal Inhaled Nitric Oxide Study Group (NINOS). Pediatrics. 1997; 99(6):838–845.
62. Barefield ES, et al. J Pediatr. 1996; 129(2):279–286.
63. Cornfield DN, et al. Pediatrics. 1999; 104(5 Pt 1):1089–1094.
64. González A, et al. J Perinatol. 2010; 30(6):420–424.
65. Konduri GG, et al. Pediatrics. 2004; 113(3):559–564.
66. Sadiq HF, et al. J Perinatol. 2003; 23(2):98–103.
67. Baquero H, et al. Pediatrics. 2006; 117(4):1077–1083.
68. Torres RH, et al. Rev Mex Pediatr. 2006; 73(4):159–163.
69. Vargas-Origel A, et al. Am J Perinatol. 2010; 27(3):225–230.
70. Uslu S, et al. J Trop Pediatr. 2011; 57(4):245–250.
71. Al Omar S, et al. J Neonatal Perinatal Med. 2016; 9(3):251–259.
72. Dani C, et al. Acta Paediatr. 2006; 95(9):1116–1123.
73. Hascoet JM, et al. J Pediatr. 2005; 146(3):318–323.
74. Field D, et al. Pediatrics. 2005; 115(4):926–936.
75. Kinsella JP, et al. Lancet. 1999; 354(9184):1061–1065.
76. Srisuparp P, et al. J Med Assoc Thai. 2002; 85 Suppl 2:S469–S478.
77. Van Meurs KP, et al. N Engl J Med. 2005; 353(1):13–22.
78. Van Meurs KP, et al. J Perinatol. 2007; 27(6):347–352.
79. Wei Q-F, et al. Zhongguo Dang Dai Er Ke Za Zhi. 2014; 16(8):805–809.
80. Su PH, et al. J Perinatol. 2008; 28(2):112–116.

CLINICAL EVALUATION OF HYPOXIC RESPIRATORY FAILURE

Yasser Elsayed and Shyamala Dakshinamurti

Contents

Introduction

The term "physioxia" is used to denote that desirable tissue environment where oxygen delivery (DO_2) is adequate to meet demand (VO_2) (1). Physioxia is sustained by the carriage of oxygen in the blood and the delivery of oxygenated blood to tissues according to their metabolic needs. To maintain physioxia, oxygen delivery requires a respiratory system with normal oxygen uptake and lung mechanics, a cardiovascular system with normal blood flow, and normal hemoglobin content together with normal performance of the oxygen dissociation curve. Simplified for clinical practice, the main components determining oxygen delivery to organs are blood flow, oxygen content, and hemoglobin saturation.

This chapter will classify hypoxia by its etiologies and diagnostic features, and review how oxygen exchange is perturbed in each, to describe a stepwise, physiology-based clinical approach to defining hypoxic respiratory failure.

Categorizing hypoxia

Colloquially, hypoxia means a PO_2 less than normal, whether in inspired air, arterial blood, or within a cell. An oxygen saturation <80% is used to define hypoxemia clinically (2). More precisely, an arterial PO_2 below normal, even if compensated by autoregulatory mechanisms, is defined as hypoxemia; while hypoxia, meaning a deficiency of oxygen falling below the threshold for compensation, suggests oxygen-limited cytochrome turnover. There are multiple intermediate compensatory mechanisms before development of anaerobic metabolism (3). Homeostatic mechanisms buffer the influence of FiO_2 and PaO_2 on intracellular PO_2, especially in muscle where myoglobin functions as an oxygen reserve cylinder; changes in mitochondrial redox and phosphorylation state may eke out more ATP per available molecule of oxygen, so even marked decreases in PaO_2 may not limit oxidative phosphorylation (4).

Alveolar ventilation and oxygen transport via the blood from pulmonary to systemic circulation are convective or "bulk flow" phases, relying on energy-utilizing work performed by respiratory and cardiac machinery; in contrast, the passage of oxygen from alveoli to pulmonary capillary, and from systemic capillary to intracellular mitochondria are passive, diffusive phases that depend on the gradient of oxygen partial pressures, the tissue capillary density, and the ability of cells to take up and use oxygen (5).

Tissue hypoxia can be classified by etiology, as (i) hypoxemic hypoxia, (ii) anemic hypoxia, (iii) circulatory hypoxia, and (iv) metabolic or histotoxic hypoxia.

Hypoxemic hypoxia

The composition of alveolar gas (and thus capillary blood) in each alveolar-capillary unit depends on four factors: Ventilation, the composition of inspired gas, blood flow, and the composition of mixed venous blood (6). Hypoxemia may arise from alveolar hypoxia, limited oxygen diffusion, inequality of ventilation to perfusion (V/Q), or shunt (7).

Alveolar hypoxia can occur during decreased availability of inspired oxygen, due to altitude or unpressurized transport, or as a result of hypercapnia. In both cases, the calculated PAO_2 is decreased but the A–a difference is normal. To evaluate the effectiveness of alveolar gas exchange, one can compare ideal alveolar gas concentrations to measured arterial concentrations, using A–a difference as an index of oxygenation. The alveolar gas equation, first calculated by Fehn, Rahn, and Otis in 1946 in order to solve the problem of wartime pilots breathing unpressurized air during flight (8), elegantly assembles the alveolar composition of gases at a specified altitude:

$$PAO_2 = FiO_2 \times (P_{ATM} - PH_2O) - PaCO_2 / RQ$$

where PAO_2 is the partial pressure of oxygen in alveolar gas, FiO_2 the fraction of inspired gas that is oxygen (0.21 in unadulterated air), P_{ATM} atmospheric pressure, PH_2O the partial pressure of water vapor when 100% saturated in air, $PaCO_2$ the partial pressure of carbon dioxide in arterial blood, and RQ the respiratory quotient or respiratory exchange ratio VCO_2/VO_2, where VCO_2 is the rate of CO_2 elimination from the blood and VO_2 is the rate of O_2 uptake from the alveolar gas (9). The space available for oxygen within the alveoli is thus determined in part by the space occupied by carbon dioxide; high altitude studies reveal the great extent to which alveolar hypoxia can be alleviated by hyperventilation, which lightens the right-hand side of the alveolar gas equation by blowing down CO_2 (10). On the other hand, acute CO_2

DOI: 10.1201/9780367494018-30

retention due to hypoventilation can result in hypercapneic alveolar hypoxia (11). Hypoxia due to high alveolar PCO_2 but normal A–a gradient, should respond to improved minute ventilation or increase in FiO_2 (12).

Oxygen diffusion limitation causes an increased A–a difference even with normal PAO_2. Thickening of the alveolar-capillary interface can be transient (e.g. pneumonia), fibrotic (bronchopulmonary dysplasia), or congenital (alveolar-capillary dysplasia). Hypoxemia is responsive to increased FiO_2, as oxygen diffusion is accelerated by the PO_2 gradient from alveolus to capillary (7). Nonpolar CO_2 crosses lipid bilayers 20× faster; O_2 is less hydrophobic, so its diffusion speed is limited by the distance traversed. Pulmonary interstitial thickening conditions such as edema or fibrosis prolong oxygen diffusion. Pulmonary congestion can be considered a subset of this category. A patent ductus arteriosus increases both arterial and venous pulmonary blood volume, while pulmonary venous stenosis or congestive heart failure engorge the venous compartment (13), spilling edema into alveoli and exacerbating oxygen diffusion limitation. Slower oxygen diffusion means more time is required to accomplish gas exchange. Pulmonary transit time scales linearly with body mass, as does the pulmonary diffusing capacity for oxygen, following allometric laws across mammals; only the smallest mammals reach a plateau in VO_2 during rising heart rate, as they are limited by the maximum speed of oxygen diffusion (14). While complete oxygen exchange usually takes 0.25–0.5 seconds in the healthy lung, diffusion impairment impedes oxygen (but not CO_2) exchange to take all the time available, while blood circulates through pulmonary capillaries (15). Under these conditions, tachycardia due to exercise, or in the neonatal intensive care unit (NICU), chronotropic agents decreasing pulmonary transit time, will reveal diffusion defects as oxygen exchange will not be completed by the time blood exits the pulmonary capillaries, so there will be an A–a difference, worsening as pulmonary transit speeds up (16).

In *disorders of V/Q inequality*, alveolar oxygenation may be impaired locally, not detectable by a PAO_2 calculation. Uptake of oxygen from alveoli requires perfusion of ventilated lung units. While the total volume of blood circulating through the lung per minute proves roughly equal to the total volume of air ventilating the lung per minute, the relative distribution of these volumes is critical (17). V/Q matching is distributed along a continuum of individual ascinar units: On one end, poorly ventilated alveoli receiving unneeded perfusion of blood (*shunted units* or unventilated lung, V/Q = 0), on the other well-ventilated alveoli robbed of their due perfusion by vasoconstriction or obstruction (*deadspace units* or unperfused lung, V/Q = ∞), and in the balance provided by hypoxic pulmonary vasoconstriction, the majority of ascinar units in a healthy lung approaching some ideal V = Q (18).

Physiological deadspace (V_D), or wasted ventilation, is calculated based on the $PACO_2$ from well-perfused lung units being diluted by the lack of CO_2 from deadspace units (7):

$$V_D / V_T = (PaCO_2 - PECO_2) / PaCO_2$$

where V_T is total minute ventilation, $PECO_2$ expired CO_2, and $PaCO_2$ is assumed the same as alveolar CO_2. Experimentally, absolute deadspace can be distinguished from poorly perfused lung, by testing exchange of multiple inert gases; gases of high solubility will still exchange in poorly perfused lung, while in deadspace they will not (18). Anatomic deadspace increases with minute ventilation; however, alveolar deadspace (the difference

between anatomic and physiologic deadspace) is affected only by V/Q matching; the proportion of alveolar volume that is deadspace increases as the proportion of the lung that is perfused decreases (17).

Pulmonary perfusion is sensitive to alveolar pressure, in a well-known U-shaped relationship. Derecruited alveoli have decreased perfusion due to local hypoxia and increased extra-alveolar (interstitial) pressure (19). Perfusion of dense pulmonary capillary networks is uniform at low mean airway pressure, with capillary recruitment even during abnormally low-flow states (20) but at high inflation pressures where alveolar pressure approaches or exceeds pulmonary artery pressure, alveolar overdistension directly compresses capillaries to increase pulmonary vascular resistance (19). Pulmonary perfusion is not normally sensitive to arterial flow. As cardiac output increases, pulmonary flow and hence gas diffusion capacity continue to increase without plateau, due to elastic distension of pulmonary vessels, and recruitment of the capillary network (21). In the neonatal period, however, alveolar hypoxia impedes pulmonary capillary recruitment, such that the pulmonary arterial pressure rises and gas exchange reserve is limited (22). Hypoxia markedly increases pulmonary arterial resistance as well as (modestly) venous resistance, rendering the pulmonary circuit pressure flow-sensitive (23).

Impaired ventilation relative to perfusion occurs in parenchymal lung diseases with suboptimal alveolar inflation or loss of functional residual capacity; specifically, the severity of hypoxemia corresponds with the degree of impairment in ventilation. Alveoli with a low V/Q ratio are on a steeper part of the hemoglobin dissociation curve than alveoli with a high V/Q, as they are also more acidic and poorly ventilated. Proportionally, more blood goes through areas of low V:Q. Therefore, the decrease in O_2 content associated with a decrease in PaO_2 is larger than the increase in O_2 content associated with an increase in PaO_2 of the same magnitude. Differing V/Q proportions yield characteristic PaO_2 curves during an oxygen reduction test, which can be used to diagnose degree of V/Q mismatch (24). Low V/Q increases the A–a difference, and improves with supplemental oxygen (7).

Low V/Q can also be detected by positioning changes, which temporarily alter the gravitational distribution of blood flow. The uniformity of V/Q matching is greatly improved while prone (25), as gravitational forces acting on blood flow while prone is balanced with dorsoventral differences in lung aeration (26). In injured lungs, the relative shunt fraction is also reduced by 30% when placed prone (27). Patients with V/Q mismatch are responsive to inhaled oxygen; decreasing FiO_2 will decrease arterial oxygen saturation. While single-photon emission computed tomography (SPECT) can definitively quantify V/Q matching in neonates (28), the use of a graded oxygen reduction test to derive V/Q mismatch is a validated diagnostic tool for which software calculators are available (29).

Intrapulmonary right-to-left shunt is the only category of hypoxemic hypoxia that is not responsive to supplemental oxygen. The shunted blood may travel via extrapulmonary right-to-left connections, as in congenital heart disease; or through intrapulmonary arteriovenous connections, bypassing the gas exchange surface. In the absence of shunt, the relationship between FiO_2 and PaO_2 is nearly linear; but as shunt fraction approaches 50%, the increment of PaO_2 with increasing FiO_2 flattens. A-a difference is increased (7). While fixed pulmonary oligemia due to obstructive hypoperfusion, vascular hypoplasia or right ventricular outflow obstruction cannot be relieved by oxygen, in shunt due to pulmonary hypertension (PH), ductal shunting arises as hypoxia increases pulmonary vascular resistance (30). Unlike other etiologies of shunt, pulmonary vasoconstriction is responsive to oxygen acting as a vasodilator, as well as to pharmacological pulmonary vasodilators (31).

As oxygen diffuses down its partial pressure gradient from alveolus to pulmonary capillary plasma, a small fraction remains dissolved in plasma, while 98% binds to hemoglobin. Each hemoglobin molecule binds up to four molecules of oxygen (giving 200 mL oxygen per 1 L blood). The oxygen content in arterial blood (CaO_2) is:

$$CaO_2 = (Hb \times 1.34 \times SaO_2) + (0.003 \times PaO_2),$$

where Hb is hemoglobin in g / dL

Calculations of the magnitude of intrapulmonary shunt reflect the degree to which the lung deviates from ideal as an oxygenator of pulmonary blood. The exact method uses the Fick equation, calculating deviation from a calculated ideal pulmonary capillary (pc) oxygen content when on 100% FiO_2:

$$Q_s / Q_t = (CpcO_2 - CaO_2) / (CpcO_2 - CvO_2)$$

This calculation requires mixed venous oxygen content, a figure difficult to obtain in neonates without pulmonary artery catheter. Central venous oxygen content has been proposed as a substitute, though it does not include myocardial oxygen consumption and may overestimate CvO_2 (32). Alternatively, intrapulmonary shunt fraction can be derived from iso-shunt graphs plotting the relationship between FiO_2 and PaO_2 during an oxygen reduction test (33) or distinguished by graphing measured SaO_2 against a range of inspired oxygen partial pressures, where decreasing V/Q right-shifts the x-intercept, while increasing shunt fraction decreases the slope of the curve (34).

Anemic hypoxia

Anemia is usually compensated by increased cardiac output, primarily by sympathetic tachycardia; systemic vascular resistance decreases due to decreased scavenging of endothelial nitric oxide by red blood cells, as well as decreased blood viscosity. The percentage of oxygen extracted by the tissues increases. These adaptations maintain oxygen delivery despite limited oxygen content of blood, such that, if euvolemic, anemia down to 50 g/L can be tolerated without metabolic derangement (35). The converse also holds: Induced polycythemia does not augment tissue oxygen delivery, as cardiac output decreases to keep DO_2 constant (36). During acute blood loss, compensatory mechanisms are limited by the inability to increase cardiac output; transfusion is required to avert hemodilution during volume resuscitation. Infants with anemia who also undergo perinatal asphyxia have the worst neurological outcomes, suggesting a more-than-additive impact on tissue oxygenation (37).

Conditions that right-shift hemoglobin oxygen affinity (increased hemoglobin P_{50}, or PO_2 for 50% saturation) including fever, acidosis, increased intracellular phosphate, or transfusion with adult hemoglobin, should theoretically improve tissue oxygen extraction; in addition, there are data that high P_{50} improves tissue oxygenation (38). However, despite some effects on tissue PO_2, there is no difference in tissue oxygen uptake or maximal VO_2 when perfused with low-P_{50} (39) or high-P_{50} blood (40).

Rare genetic variants of hemoglobin oxygen affinity (nearly 100 reported high-affinity variants, 70 low-affinity variants) can alter oxygen uptake or delivery (41, 42). Carbon monoxide poisoning, detailed elsewhere in this volume, also functions as an anemic hypoxia since the ability of hemoglobin to carry oxygen is lost.

Circulatory hypoxia

Low-flow states, termed "stagnant hypoxia," complicate heart failure by limiting oxygen delivery despite adequate oxygen content of blood. Increasing inspired oxygen is not helpful; perfusion must be addressed. The defect in blood flow can be systemic or localized. Changes in systemic hemodynamics following delivery in the very preterm infant may result in a systemic low-flow state with elevated vascular resistance (43). Asphyxial injury may also cause myocardial dysfunction and vasomotor dysregulation, while therapeutic hypothermia impairs capillary perfusion (44). Excessive vasoconstriction of extremities has been reported in neonates following use of pressors, particularly norepinephrine (44). Tissues distal to the circulatory compromise have curtailed oxygen delivery and anaerobic metabolism, sometimes followed by necrosis. Lactate from stagnant capillary beds may not find its way into central circulation, leading to underestimation of tissue hypoxia (45).

In neonates, four low-flow states are distinguished by clinical features:

Low preload: Decreased diastolic filling of left ventricle and/or diminished pulmonary venous filling of right ventricle can be expected in low-volume states (dehydration, hemorrhage, third space volume loss), severe pulmonary hypertension, or due to external venous compression e.g. high mean airway pressure or tension pneumothorax (46). Presence of a left-to-right shunt, as in patent ductus arteriosus or arterio-venous malformation, shifts significant blood volume from systemic to pulmonary circulation, stealing from systemic preload (47).

Low systemic vascular resistance: Peripheral loss of arteriolar muscle tone and systemic vasodilation is seen in systemic inflammatory response (distributive or septic shock), in severe hypoxemia, due to suprarenal dysfunction in preterm infants, or vasodilator medications including sedatives and anesthetic drugs. Imbalances of dilator versus constrictor forces may relate to autocrine, endocrine, paracrine, or neuronal factors. Low-resistance states may be managed with pressors, fluid infusion, or use of corticosteroids if evidence of adrenal dysfunction (48).

High systemic vascular resistance: Vasoconstrictive shock, arising from high systemic or pulmonary circuit resistance, features increased afterload and cardiac contractile work, impairing ventricular performance, and cardiac output. Typical examples include post-PDA ligation syndrome (left ventricle), acute pulmonary hypertension (mainly right ventricle), or hypoxemic ischemic encephalopathy (mainly right ventricle). Pulmonary and/or systemic afterload reduction may be indicated (46). In the preterm infant, as systemic vascular resistance rises faster than the adaptive ability of the myocardium, the transitional circulation can be complicated by a normal pressure, low-flow state, best managed by inotropy without augmenting afterload (49).

Myocardial performance: Circulatory shock can result from impaired ventricular contractility in the face of low or normal vascular resistance, due to systemic inflammatory response, cardiomyopathy, severe hypovolemia or prolonged arrhythmia, as well as severe pulmonary hypertension (50). Mean arterial pressure may be normal, pulse pressure normal, and calculated systemic vascular resistance high; impaired biventricular performance is ascertained by echocardiography, and addressed by inotropy (46).

Also falling within the category of circulatory hypoxia, tissue interstitial edema impairs oxygen diffusion from capillary beds toward cell mitochondria, by increasing the intercellular distance that oxygen must traverse. Tissue diffusion gradients are as critical as pulmonary diffusion gradients, and as limited by diffusion speed and time. The driving force for oxygen diffusion is PO_2; increasing the PaO_2 (even in well-saturated hemoglobin) accelerates diffusion. Diffusion is more impaired in edematous tissue that is hypoxemic, compared to anemic or low-flow states, as the latter have still driving pressure for diffusion, though all lack oxygen content (5). Various modalities now exist for monitoring tissue perfusion indices, regional tissue saturation, and oxygen extraction, including near-infrared spectroscopy (NIRS).

Histotoxic hypoxia

Oxygen reduction in the mitochondria normally depends on substrate abundance and energy requirements. Intracellular cytosolic oxygen rests at PO_2 3–10 mmHg; normally, mitochondrial cristae can produce ATP at 50% capacity, even down to PO_2 0.05 mmHg (51). Histotoxic or cytopathic hypoxia is defined as acquired intrinsic derangements in cellular respiration despite adequate cytosolic PO_2 and metabolic substrates (52). Uncoupling of mitochondria or toxic inhibition of cytochromes can occur in poisonings such as cyanide (53), or in severe sepsis (54). This causes a profound drop in tissue oxygen consumption, resulting in decreased oxygen extraction. Lactate rises due to tissue hypoxia, and also because accelerated catecholamine-induced aerobic glycolysis drives pyruvate production, exceeding the capacity of dysfunctional mitochondria to utilize pyruvate (51). Neither supplemental oxygen, nor other means of increasing oxygen delivery will improve tissue hypoxia; venous oxygen is high, as oxygen is not being metabolized by tissues despite adequate perfusion. Oxygen consumption measures including arteriovenous O_2 difference will be decreased (7).

Classifying hypoxia by oxygen delivery and uptake

Oxygen delivery to tissues (DO_2) is determined by oxygen content in arterial blood (CaO_2), multiplied by the cardiac output (CO × CaO_2).

By conservation of mass, every molecule of oxygen that is inhaled but not exhaled diffuses from alveolar gas to capillary blood, and could be obtained from that blood (24). Thus, *oxygen consumption* is the difference between arterial versus venous oxygen content (CvO_2), per unit blood flow (Q): $VO_2 = Q \times (CaO_2 - CvO_2)$.

VO_2 is not normally limited by DO_2, because fractional oxygen extraction increases proportionately. However, below a critical oxygen delivery threshold, extraction can no longer compensate, and VO_2 becomes supply-dependent (55). The biphasic relationships between oxygen delivery and consumption are not the same in healthy versus septic individuals, as consumption may increase even as delivery fails. Increasing DO_2 to supranormal levels can improve survival in the critically ill patient where mixed venous oxygen content is low due to increased extraction (56); however,

when consumption is decreased, boosting DO_2 does not improve outcome (57).

Measuring precise VO_2/DO_2-dependency relationships has been difficult in critically ill patients, especially where regional perfusion defects muddy the waters (58). Three elements are required: (i) VO_2; (ii) rate of oxygen extraction; and (iii) identification of the inflection point where VO_2 declines as DO_2 declines, resulting in anaerobic metabolism and lactate. Graphing these parameters, Siggaard-Andersen and colleagues (59) devised a classification rubric for hypoxia that distinguishes etiologies of hypoxia based on a critical mixed venous PO_2, above which the oxygen consumption rate is optimal and independent of the mixed venous PO_2, and below which the oxygen consumption rate decreases toward zero.

In *Class A hypoxia*, the primary observation is a decrease in mixed venous PO_2, with no change in optimal oxygen consumption rate and a normal inflection point. Oxygen delivery is the problem; etiologies include hypoxemic, anemic (including high-affinity hemoglobin) and ischemic hypoxia.

Class B hypoxia has an increased mixed venous PO_2, a normal oxygen consumption rate, and a right-shifted inflection point. Oxygen is delivered but remains unused, due to "dysperfusion" (arteriovenous shunt, constriction of regional circulation, or interstitial edema decreasing tissue diffusion) or histotoxic hypoxia.

Class C hypoxia, the rarest, is marked by an increased oxygen consumption rate, with decreased mixed venous PO_2 and a right-shifted inflection point. These include hypermetabolic states e.g. sepsis/burns or uncoupling of the respiratory chain.

Detecting compensatory mechanisms

Blood flow autoregulation is the first compensatory mechanism, acting within fractions of a second. When hemoglobin binds to oxygen in the lungs, the conformational change permits it to also react with nitric oxide, forming nitrosohemoglobin. Upon delivery of oxygen to hypoxic tissues, deoxygenation of hemoglobin is accompanied by release of its nitric oxide, causing vessels to dilate and blood flow to improve toward the demanding tissues (60). There is no clinical monitoring parameter to assess the effectiveness of flow autoregulation. Desaturation in nonessential capillary beds captured by NIRS has been used as a surrogate marker of "diving reflex" flow redistribution following hypoxia during cardiopulmonary bypass (61). Research trials in preterm neonates using spin-labeled perfusion MRI together with NIRS show promise (62, 63) but maybe impractical for routine practice.

In low blood flow states, anemia, or hypoxemia, where flow autoregulation is unable to compensate for the mismatch between oxygen supply and demand, then the tissues extract a greater proportion of delivered oxygen (normally fractional oxygen extraction is 15–30%) (64). This stage of compensation can be monitored by NIRS. The regional tissue oxygenation for any assessed organ reflects mainly the venous saturation in that organ, so an acceptable NIRS value ranges between 55% and 85%, depending on that tissue's metabolic activity (65, 66). Low tissue oxygen saturation with a high calculated fraction oxygen extraction signifies impaired oxygen delivery, and is an indicator that flow autoregulation has already been compromised (67).

The final threshold, when oxygen demand exceeds delivery and extraction is already maximized, is conversion to anaerobic

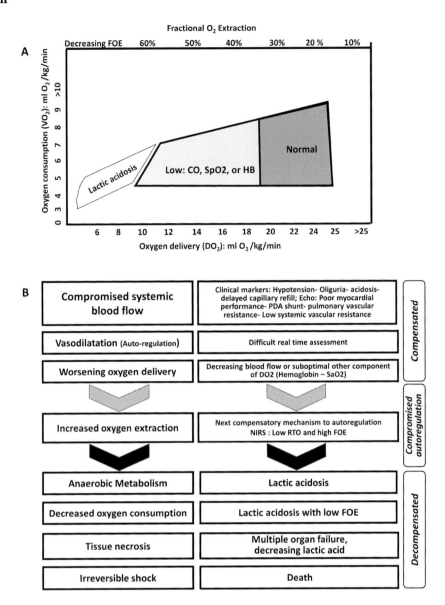

FIGURE 30.1 Oxygen delivery and consumption. (A) This three-dimensional graph presents oxygen delivery (mL/kg body weight/ minute) on the lower x-axis, percent oxygen extraction on the upper x-axis, and tissue oxygen consumption on the y-axis. While oxygen delivery decreases, if extraction increases, consumption remains acceptable. Once oxygen delivery reaches a critical level (<10 mL/kg/min), if extraction is maximized, then aerobic metabolism is detected. (B) Stages of compensation for hypoxia as monitored by integrated evaluation of hemodynamics. RTO, regional tissue oxygen; FOE, fractional oxygen extraction; both measured by NIRS.

metabolism, detectable as lactate. Glycolysis cannot sustain the ATP requirement of organs; end-organ dysfunction is a rapid consequence (68). Figure 30.1 illustrates relationships between oxygen delivery, extraction, and consumption, assessment of compensatory mechanisms, and the threshold of anaerobic metabolism (67).

Integrated assessment of hypoxia

We initiated an integrated NICU hemodynamics decision support program in 2014, aiming to optimize oxygen delivery and early detection of the mechanisms of hypoxia. This program has been shown to streamline hypoxia management and shorten time to clinical recovery (48). A typical multimodal assessment of hypoxia includes a detailed clinical assessment, calculation

of diffusion limitation, V/Q and shunt fractions, echocardiography for assessment of cardiac function and vascular resistances, calculation of oxygen indices including VO_2, DO_2, and regional tissue oxygen extraction by NIRS, and laboratory markers of end-organ function indicating compensated or decompensated tissue hypoxia. These parameters are integrated to recognize the dominant pathophysiologic mechanisms driving hypoxia, and to formulate a decision tree pertinent to that patient, with physiological recommendations for further medical interventions (67). A flow diagram (Figure 30.2) shows how the disambiguation of hypoxia physiology using the clinical measurements and calculations detailed in this chapter, can logically support the classification of hypoxia etiology and provide clarity for medical management. Equations for commonly calculated oxygen indices are collected in Table 30.1.

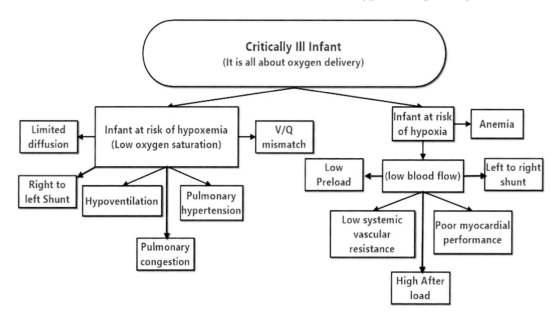

FIGURE 30.2 Decision tree for hypoxia analysis. Flow diagrams of etiologic classification of hypoxemia (left), and of tissue hypoxia (right).

TABLE 30.1 Quick Reference for the Most Important Oxygen Indices

Oxygenation indices	Parameter Captured	How Measured or Calculated
	Oxygen content CaO_2 (mL O_2/dL)	$(1.39 \times$ hemoglobin (g/dL) $\times SaO_2) + (0.0031 \times PaO_2)$
	Oxygen delivery DO_2 (mL O_2/kg/min)	LV cardiac output $\times CaO_2$
	Oxygen consumption VO_2 (mL O_2/kg/min)	LV cardiac output $\times (CaO_2 - CvO_2)$
	Fractional oxygen extraction ratio FOE	VO_2/DO_2
	Fractional oxygen extraction ratio FOE by pulse oximetry and NIRS	$(SpO_2 -$ regional tissue oxygen$)/SpO_2$

Abbreviations: CaO_2, oxygen content of arterial blood; LV, left ventricle; VO_2, oxygen consumption; DO_2, oxygen delivery; FOE, fractional oxygen extraction.

References

1. Carreau A, et al. J Cell Mol Med. 2011; 15(6):1239–1253.
2. Poets CF, et al. JAMA. 2015; 314(6):595–603.
3. Schwartz S, et al. Am J Physiol. 1981; 241(6):H864–H871.
4. Connett RJ, et al. J Appl Physiol (1985). 1990; 68(3):833–842.
5. Leach RM, et al. Thorax. 2002; 57(2):170–177.
6. West JB. J Appl Physiol (1985). 2004; 97(5):1603–1604.
7. Petersson J, et al. Eur Respir J. 2014; 44(4):1023–1041.
8. Fenn WO, et al. Am J Physiol. 1946; 146:637–653.
9. Curran-Everett D. Adv Physiol Educ. 2006; 30(2):58–62.
10. West JB. Ann Intern Med. 2004; 141(10):789–800.
11. Roussos C, et al. Eur Respir J Suppl. 2003; 47:3s–14s.
12. Lakshminrusimha S, et al. J Perinatol. 2016; 36 Suppl 2:S3–S11.
13. Elsayed YN, et al. Neonatal Netw. 2017; 36(5):265–272.
14. Lindstedt SL. Am J Physiol. 1984; 246(3 Pt 2):R384–R388.
15. Wagner PD, et al. J Appl Physiol. 1972; 33(1):62–71.
16. Agusti AG, et al. Thorax. 1994; 49(9):924–932.
17. West JB, et al. J Appl Physiol. 1965; 20(5):825–835.
18. West JB, et al. Am J Respir Crit Care Med. 1998; 157(4 Pt 2):S82–S87.
19. Vrancken SL, et al. Front Pediatr. 2018; 6:87.
20. Konig MF, et al. J Appl Physiol (1985). 1993; 75(4):1877–1883.
21. Carlin JI, et al. J Appl Physiol (1985). 1991; 70(1):135–142.
22. Means LJ, et al. Pediatr Res. 1993; 34(5):596–599.
23. Nelin LD, et al. Pediatr Res. 1994; 35(1):25–29.
24. Wagner PD. Eur Respir J. 2015; 45(1):227–243.
25. Henderson AC, et al. J Appl Physiol (1985). 2013; 115(3):313–324.
26. Treppo S, et al. J Appl Physiol (1985). 1997; 82(4):1163–1176.
27. Scholten EL, et al. Chest. 2017; 151(1):215–224.
28. Kjellberg M, et al. Pediatr Pulmonol. 2013; 48(12):1206–1213.
29. Elsayed YN, et al. Neonatal Netw. 2016; 35(4):192–203.
30. Lakshminrusimha S, et al. J Perinatol. 2016; 36 Suppl 2:S12–S19.
31. Lakshminrusimha S, et al. Semin Perinatol. 2016; 40(3):160–173.
32. Nebout S, et al. Cardiol Res Pract. 2012; 2012:370697.
33. Lawler PG, et al. Br J Anaesth. 1984; 56(12):1325–1335.
34. Smith HL, et al. Arch Dis Child Fetal Neonatal Ed. 2001; 85(2):F127–F132.
35. Salmen M, et al. Ann Am Thorac Soc. 2017; 14(7):1216–1220.
36. Lindenfeld J, et al. Am J Physiol Heart Circ Physiol. 2005; 289(5):H1821–H1825.
37. Kalteren WS, et al. Neonatology. 2018; 114(4):315–322.
38. Van Ameringen MR, et al. Pediatr Res. 1981; 15(12):1500–1503.
39. Schumacker PT, et al. J Appl Physiol (1985). 1987; 62(5):1801–1807.
40. Curtis SE, et al. J Appl Physiol (1985). 1997; 83(5):1681–1689.
41. Yudin J, et al. Am J Hematol. 2019; 94(5):597–603.
42. Shepherd JRA, et al. J Physiol. 2019; 597(16):4193–4202.
43. Andersen CC, et al. Pediatrics. 2017; 139(4):e20161117.
44. Joynt C, et al. Front Pediatr. 2018; 6:363.
45. Andersen LW, et al. Mayo Clinic Proc. 2013; 88(10):1127–1140.
46. Giesinger RE, et al. Semin Perinatol. 2016; 40(3):174–188.
47. Giesinger RE, et al. AJP reports. 2019; 9(2):e172–e176.
48. Amer R, et al. Am J Perinatol. 2017; 34(10):1011–1019.

49. Kluckow M. Front Pediatr2018; 6:29.
50. Giesinger RE, et al. Pediatr Res. 2017; 82(6):901–914.
51. Loiacono LA, et al. Crit Care Clin. 2010; 26(2):409–421.
52. Fink MP. Minerva Anestesiol. 2000; 66(5):337–342.
53. Pham JC, et al. Emergency Med J. 2007; 24(3):152–156.
54. Kohoutova M, et al. Physiol Res. 2018; 67(Suppl 4):S577–S592.
55. Schumacker PT, et al. J Appl Physiol. 1989; 67(3):1234–1244.
56. Kelly KM. Crit Care Clin. 1996; 12(3):635–644.
57. Ronco JJ, et al. Crit Care Clin. 1996; 12(3):645–659.
58. Vincent JL,et al. Intensive Care Med. 2004; 30(11):1990–1996.
59. Siggaard-Andersen O, et al. Acta Anaesthesiol Scand Suppl. 1995; 107:137–142.
60. Stamler JS, et al. Science. 1997; 276(5321):2034–2037.
61. Sanders J, et al. Am J Crit Care. 2011; 20(2):138–145.
62. Noori S, et al. J Pediatr. 2012; 160(6):943–948.
63. Wintermark P, et al. NeuroImage. 2014; 85 Pt 1:287–293.
64. Lister G, et al. Am J Physiol. 1979; 237(6):H668–H675.
65. Goff DA, et al. Semin Perinatol. 2010; 34(1):46–56.
66. Tweddell JS, et al. Semin Thorac Cardiovasc Surg Pediatr Card Surg Annu. 2010; 13(1):44–50.
67. Elsayed YN, et al. J Perinatol. 2018; 38(10):1337–1343.
68. Elsayed YN, et al. Neonatal Netw. 2016; 35(3):143–150.

DIAGNOSIS OF PULMONARY HYPERTENSION BY ECHOCARDIOGRAPHY

Danielle R. Rios, Patrick J. McNamara and Regan E. Giesinger

Contents

Pulmonary hypertension (PH) is characterized by high pulmonary artery pressure (PAP) which, in the neonatal population, may be either acute or chronic. In older infants, a mean (m)PAP >25 mmHg is considered abnormal; however, any level of mPAP sufficient to result in inadequate pulmonary blood flow (PBF) constitutes a diagnosis of acute PH (1). A numerical pressure-based definition is challenging in the neonatal population, particularly in the transitional period. Persistent pulmonary hypertension of the newborn (PPHN) is traditionally used to describe abnormal transition of the pulmonary vasculature after birth leading to hypoxemia. This terminology, however common, is technically inaccurate. It is typical for mPAP to remain elevated following delivery with a steep decline over the first 2–3 days followed by a more gradual decline over the ensuing 2 weeks (2), and many neonates have elevated PAP without clinically significant hypoxemia (3, 4). The term acute PH more accurately represents the disease entity in which high PAP results in oxygenation failure and/or increased RV afterload; hence for this chapter, we have used the terminology acute PH rather than PPHN. Demonstration of features of acute PH in preterm infants has been associated with a high rate of response to inhaled nitric oxide in the transitional period (5). Depending on degree of PAP elevation, consequences such as right ventricle (RV) dysfunction or dilation may be seen (6). In term infants, chronic PH is seen most often in the setting of congenital heart disease, neonatal lung diseases affecting the parenchyma, and abnormalities of the airways or pulmonary vasculature (7). In the premature population, it is most often seen in the setting of bronchopulmonary dysplasia which may include chronic vascular remodeling due to pulmonary over-circulation from shunts (7, 8).

Determining severity of PH

When assessing severity of PH, direct measurements of the relationship between pulmonary and systemic pressures should have a greater influence on overall assessment of relative pressure than those which are more distal to the location of interest (Table 31.1). For example, when present in the setting of normal left ventricle (LV) function, the direction of ductal flow provides the clearest assessment of this relationship as compared to, for example, septal position. It remains important to understand that every measurement has its own limitations that need to be considered in a holistic approach which will be discussed in further detail.

Interventricular septal wall motion

Normally, the crescentic RV wraps around the circular shaped LV with the septum in between the two chambers in the parasternal short axis. When right ventricular systolic pressure (RVSp), hence pulmonary artery systolic pressure (PASP), increases above half to 2/3 systemic level, flattening of the septum in end-systole may occur. When right and left ventricular systolic pressures are approximately equal, this results in a D-shaped pattern. As RVSp increases to supra-systemic level, paradoxical bowing of the septum into the LV may be seen. This relative measurement (to LV pressure) has low sensitivity in the presence of systemic hypertension. Flattening of the septum in end-diastole can be seen in

DOI: 10.1201/9780367494018-31

TABLE 31.1 Assessment of Severity of Pulmonary Hypertension and Cardiac Performance

Determination	Measurement	Image	Advantages	Limitations
Severity of PH	Septal wall motion Eccentricity index Peak TR jet velocity Shunt directionality	PSAX at level of papillary muscles Same as above Multiple planes evaluating tricuspid valve flow Multiple views (see shunt appraisal)	Direct assessment of relative RVSp and LVSp throughout the cardiac cycle Quantitative assessment of septal wall motion Allows calculation of RVSp with modified Bernoulli equation Easy to appraise percentage of right-to-left flow with Doppler	Systemic hypertension may underestimate RVSp Same as above Affected by signal quality, underestimated in RV dysfunction Lack of intra- or extra-cardiac shunt
RV systolic performance	FAC TAPSE TDI Strain and Strain Rate RVO	Apical 4-chamber or RV 3-chamber Apical 4-chamber Apical 4-chamber Apical 4-chamber or RV 3-chamber PLAX or PSAX PA view	Quantitative assessment of RV EF Quantitative, reproducible assessment of longitudinal motion of RV Easy image to obtain in most patients Allows for regional and global assessment of function Reflection of PBF in the absence of pulmonary to aortic shunt	Affected by image quality, influenced by septal wall motion in 4-chamber view Displacement of TV at single point, will not reflect other regional wall motion abnormalities Evaluates myocardial motion at single point, will not reflect other regional wall abnormalities Limited normative data Angle dependent, precise annulus measurement may be difficult due to image quality
Pulmonary vascular resistance	PA Doppler waveform RVET:PAAT	PLAX or PSAX PA view Same as above	Easily visualized measurement Semi-quantitative measure of PVR	Affected by RV performance, TR, PA dilation, presence of PDA Same as above, may occur in high flow states
LV systolic performance	EF by Simpson biplane Qualitative assessment of LV filling	Apical 4- and 2-chamber Multiple views evaluating LV	More accurate and reproducible measurement of EF Easy to visualize	Ability to trace endocardial border may be difficult due to image quality, requires 2 views for accurate assessment Imprecise
Systemic blood flow	LVO	Apical 5-chamber view for VTI and PLAX aortic valve view for annulus	Cursor almost parallel to the flow of blood in this view making accurate assessment easier	Angle dependent, requires precise sample volume placement, precise annulus measurement dependent on image quality and angle
Pulmonary blood flow	Pulmonary vein Doppler	Apical 4-chamber	Angle minimized for right lower vein	Affected by atrial and ventricular pressure and function
Shunt appraisal	PDA PFO VSD	High parasternal ductal view or PSAX Subcostal atrial view PLAX and PSAX VSD sweep views	Direct assessment of pressure differential between aorta and pulmonary artery Direct assessment of pressure differential between left and right atria Direct assessment of RVSp and LVSp	Absence of PDA Absence of PFO, Doppler angle may be difficult Absence of VSD, Doppler angle may be difficult

Abbreviations: EF, ejection fraction; FAC, fractional area change; LV, left ventricle; LVO, left ventricular output; LVSp, left ventricle systolic pressure; PBF, pulmonary blood flow; PDA, patent ductus arteriosus; PFO, patent foramen ovale; PH, pulmonary hypertension; PLAX, parasternal long-axis; PSAX, parasternal short-axis; PA, pulmonary artery; PAAT, pulmonary artery acceleration time; PVR, pulmonary vascular resistance; RV, right ventricle; RVET, right ventricular ejection time; RVO, right ventricular output; RVSp, right ventricle systolic pressure; TAPSE, tricuspid annular plane systolic excursion; TDI, tissue Doppler imaging; TR, tricuspid regurgitant; TV, tricuspid valve; VSD, ventricular septal defect; VTI, velocity time integral.

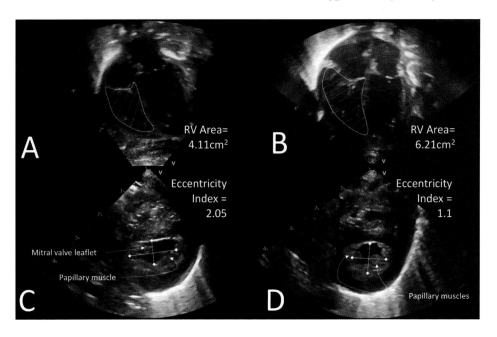

FIGURE 31.1 Optimal visualization is essential for accurate measurements. Apical 4-chamber (A/B) and parasternal short axis (C/D) of the same patient <1-minute between images. Off-axis imaging (A/C) underestimates right ventricle (RV) size and overestimates the degree of septal flattening (eccentricity index [EI]) compared to well-aligned imaging (B/D). EI measurement involves recording the smallest diameters of the left ventricle (LV) perpendicular (D1) and parallel (D2) to the septum. EI = D2 ÷ D1 care should be taken to use the endocardial border, ignoring the papillary muscles and ensuring the intersection of both axis diameters are perpendicular at the center of the LV.

volume loading situations (i.e. due to large atrial level shunt) (9). It is important to note that qualitative assessment of septal flattening may be inaccurate (10), whereas the LV eccentricity index is an objective measure of septal configuration (11) (Figure 31.1D). An eccentricity index of ≥1.3 in end-systole is indicative of an estimated RVSp of more than half systemic (12).

Estimation of RVSp through tricuspid regurgitant jet velocity (TRJV)

Measurement of RVSp continues to be a standard for estimating PASP. RVSp can be estimated from the TRJV using the modified Bernoulli equation:

$$RVSp = RAp + 4 \times V_{max}^2$$

where RAp is the estimated Right Atrial Pressure and V_{max} is the peak TRJV. Accurate measurement of the TRJV is imperative. To obtain TRJV, continuous wave (CW) Doppler is utilized in multiple views to obtain the cleanest jet with a minimal angle of insonation.

There are important limitations to measuring TRJV which can result in over or underestimation of the maximum TRJV. Overestimation is often related to modal frequency, which is the frequency at which most of the red blood cells are moving (depicted by the brightest signal representing laminar flow). Measurement of TRJV should only be obtained when modal frequency is clearly demonstrated. Underestimation usually relates to poor signal quality, the presence of an incomplete jet or no identifiable envelope. In the setting of an incomplete or unidentifiable envelope, accurate PASP estimation is not possible; however, this does not rule out significant PH. Another potential source of underestimation is seen in the setting of severe RV dysfunction,

where the force required to elicit a complete TRJV envelope is not generated. In the modified Bernoulli equation, RAp is estimated to be 5–7 mmHg, which may not always be accurate. A significantly increased RAp that is not accurately accounted for can also lead to underestimation of RVSp. Anatomic limitations to the use of TRJV to estimate RVSp include abnormal valve physiology (e.g. tricuspid valve stenosis or tethered leaflets) and ruptured chordae.

Right ventricle ejection time to pulmonary artery acceleration time (RVET:PAAT)

As blood traverses from the RV into the main pulmonary artery (PA), the resistance encountered may alter the envelope of the normally laminar blood flow (Figure 31.2A). In the absence of elevated PAP, the envelope of flow should be in the shape of an isosceles triangle or bullet-shaped with gradual acceleration and deceleration. The time to the peak velocity of the Doppler envelope is the PAAT, which in this situation, will be directly in the middle of the envelope. When pulmonary vascular resistance (PVR) is elevated, the RV must pump against higher resistance resulting in more rapid acceleration of blood flow leaving the RV. The envelope will approximate the shape of a right-angle triangle with rapid flow acceleration followed by more gradual deceleration; therefore, the peak velocity will be closer to the beginning of the envelope (Figure 31.2B). Notching of the PA envelope in the deceleration phase may also occur due to high PVR. This occurs because equilibration of pressure briefly occurs during mid- to late-systole resulting in rapid deceleration until the continued generation of force by the still-contracting RV propels blood forward to generate a second peak (Figure 31.2C). To account for heart rate variability, PAAT is indexed to RVET. This ratio can provide a semi-quantitative measure of the severity of increased

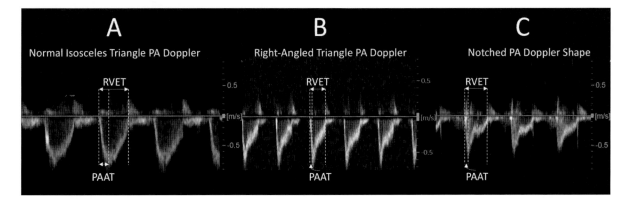

FIGURE 31.2 Assessment of right ventricular ejection time (RVET) to pulmonary artery acceleration time ratio (PAAT) to calculate the pulmonary vascular resistance index (PVRi) and evaluate Doppler shape. Pulse wave (PW) Doppler at the level of the pulmonary artery (PA) leaflets is utilized. In long-axis or short-axis at the aortic level, the Doppler sample volume should be at the level of the tips of the PA leaflets when maximally open. Normal (A) can be compared with increased RVET:PAAT (B) and notched PA Doppler (C).

PVR (13). RVET:PAAT is considered normal when <4 (some commentators report inverse PAAT:RVET ratio, considered normal if >0.25). In adults, mPAP can be calculated from PAAT (14). This method, however, may be inaccurate when heart rate is >100 and has not been validated in neonates.

Assessment of RV performance

Morphology
The RV is normally a thin-walled crescentic structure that wraps around the LV, and is coupled to systemic venous return on one side and the pulmonary circulation on the other. Pressure overload on the RV, as is seen in PH, leads to RV hypertrophy, predominantly end-systolic and early-diastolic flattening of the interventricular septum, progressive RV dilation, and dysfunction (15). The RV may respond with "adaptive" remodeling characterized by relatively preserved volumes and function, and concentric hypertrophy often referred to as homeometric adaptation. When this adaptation is exhausted and contractility can no longer increase to match afterload, "maladaptive" remodeling commences with "eccentric" hypertrophy and progressive RV dilatation or heterometric adaptation ultimately resulting in RV failure (15).

Fractional area change (FAC)
FAC of the right ventricle may be used as a surrogate measurement of RV ejection fraction (Figure 31.3). It can be measured in the apical 4-chamber view or in the RV 3-chamber view. The RV 3-chamber view is an RV-centric view that may be less influenced by interventricular septal motion and more reflective of the systolic function of the RV infundibulum (16). To calculate RV-FAC, the following equation is used:

$$RV - FAC = \frac{(End - diastolic\ RV\ area) - (End - systolic\ RV\ area)}{(End - diastolic\ RV\ area)}$$

Values for RV-FAC ≥0.35 are considered normal, although it has been shown that normative data varies based on gestational and postnatal age (16, 17).

Tricuspid annular plane systolic excursion (TAPSE)
TAPSE is an m-mode measurement of the downward vertical distance that the tricuspid annulus moves during systole (in millimeters) (Figure 31.4). More specifically, it describes the apex-to-base shortening of the RV or, in other words, the longitudinal motion of the RV which represents the main component of RV systolic

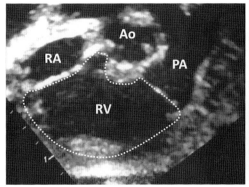
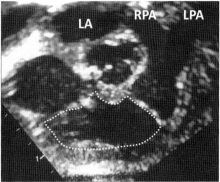

FIGURE 31.3 Measurement of right ventricle (RV) fractional area change from the RV 3-chamber view. To obtain the RV-3 chamber, rotate clockwise, slide medially and tilt anteriorly from the apical 4-chamber. The desired image has the left heart out of view, the aorta round and in the center with the tricuspid and pulmonary valves seen and with simultaneous visualization of the inferior wall. The RV end-diastolic (left) and end-systolic (right) area are measured by tracing the endocardial borders, including the RV trabeculations within the area. RA, right atrium; Ao, aorta; PA, main pulmonary artery; RPA, right pulmonary artery; LPA, left pulmonary artery.

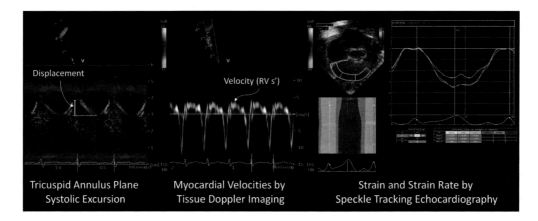

FIGURE 31.4 Tricuspid annular plane systolic excursion (TAPSE), tissue Doppler imaging (TDI) and strain imaging for pulmonary hypertension (PH). TAPSE is the longitudinal displacement of the apex to the base (in centimeters/millimeters). Right ventricular (RV) s' is a measure of peak systolic velocity. RV strain is the deformation of the RV as measured, in this case as the movement of speckles and strain rate is the speed at which this deformation occurs.

performance (18). The line of interrogation should be placed perpendicular to the lateral aspect of the tricuspid annulus while maintaining vertical alignment with the apex (16). Normal values for TAPSE will vary based on gestational age, birth weight, and postnatal age (16, 19, 20). Some limitations to this method are that it assumes the displacement of a single segment represents the function of a complex 3D structure, is angle-dependent, and maybe load-dependent (21).

Myocardial velocities

Tissue Doppler imaging (TDI) relies on the detection of the shift in frequency of ultrasound signals reflected off moving objects, similar to conventional Doppler techniques (Figure 31.4). Unlike conventional Doppler, which assesses the velocity of blood flow by measuring high-frequency, low-amplitude signals from small, fast-moving red blood cells, TDI is used to measure the higher amplitude, lower velocity signals of myocardial tissue motion. Myocardial velocities are most commonly measured in the apical 4-chamber view because the longitudinally oriented endocardial fibers are mostly parallel to the angle of insonation in this view. To measure myocardial velocities, the pulse wave (PW) sample volume is placed in the wall of the RV just below the lateral tricuspid annulus, with the TDI mode applied, at the attachment of the anterior leaflet of the tricuspid valve. The peak systolic (s'), early diastolic (e'), late diastolic (a'), and peak isovolumetric contraction velocities may be used (16). TDI s' has been shown to be a reliable and reproducible measurement of RV longitudinal performance (6, 22); normative data is available for neonates according to gestational age and birth weight (23, 24). TDI has the same limitations as TAPSE.

Strain and strain rate

Strain and strain rate are measures of deformation that may help describe the nature and function of cardiac tissue (Figure 31.4). Strain analysis refers to the absolute tissue deformation of the ventricle during systole. It is expressed as a percentage of change compared to its length at baseline. Strain rate measures the time taken for the deformation to occur. Strain rate is thought to be less related to loading conditions, making it a more reliable measure of contractility (25). Strain and strain rate can be measured either via Tissue Doppler-derived strain imaging or speckle tracking techniques. With these modalities, it is possible to quantify global and regional ventricular function. Normative values for strain in infants and children have been reported (26); normative longitudinal reference ranges for neonates are increasing (27).

Right ventricular output (RVO)

RVO (ml/kg/min) represents the amount of blood ejected from the RV into the main PA. The equation for calculating RVO is:

$$RVO = \left[\Pi (PAr)^2 \times VTI \times HR \right] \div weight(kg)$$

where PAr is the radius of the pulmonary valve annulus, VTI is the velocity-time integral of the pulmonary artery outflow, and HR is heart rate. RVO can be assumed to provide an estimate of PBF if there is no pulmonary-to-aortic shunt or significant pulmonary regurgitation. Limitations include: (i) Dependence on obtaining a Doppler signal perfectly aligned with the RV outflow tract (Figure 31.5); (ii) precise measurement of the pulmonary valve annulus may be difficult or may skew the results in the presence of dilation of the outflow tract; and (iii) the presence of turbulent flow in the PA resulting from left-to-right PDA flow near the main PA can make the tracing of the VTI envelope unreliable. Serial assessments may help overcome some of these limitations as it will provide correlation to changes in stroke volume (13).

RV-PA coupling

An important concept in the evaluation of PH is that of RV-PA coupling. To remain hemodynamically coupled to the pulmonary circulation, the RV must adapt to the increasing pulmonary vascular load. In the early phase of disease, coupling is maintained by an up to 4- to 5-fold increase in RV contractility (28). The increase in contractility may be obtained by muscular hypertrophy. As the disease progresses, the RV will dilate, and heart rate will increase to maintain cardiac output. Wall stress will increase with a subsequent increase in oxygen consumption and eventually, the septum will bow into the LV. With continued progression of disease, the RV will become uncoupled from the pulmonary vasculature and cardiac output will be reduced with high metabolic demand. Once the RV has uncoupled, the influence of RV motion on the LV via ventriculo–ventricular interaction becomes more apparent, and it is of the utmost importance to monitor closely for LV failure. RV-PA coupling may be monitored with echocardiography. PAAT has been shown to correlate with PAP and pulmonary

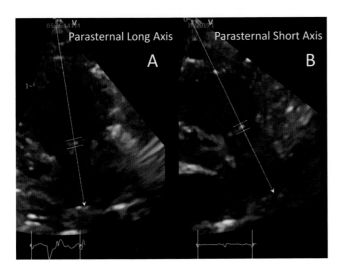

FIGURE 31.5 Ideal angle of insonation is required to calculate right ventricular output. The pulmonary artery (PA) velocity time integral (VTI), is obtained from either the parasternal long- (a) or short-axis (B) (aortic level). The pulse wave (PW) Doppler sample volume must be at the leaflet level the cursor parallel to the direction of blood flow and bifurcated by the valve when closed. The annulus (inner edge to inner edge of the leaflet hinge points) must be measured in the same view used to obtain the VTI.

vascular compliance (29), with some correlation to disease processes in neonates and infants (30). TAPSE indexed to PAAT has been shown to be inversely correlated with PASP and PVR and positively correlated to pulmonary arterial compliance and RV strain in children (31).

Assessment of LV performance

Morphology
The changes in the RV that are seen in the setting of PH affect the LV as well, due to the two ventricles sharing the interventricular septum. This becomes more apparent in the setting of a pressure-loaded RV contributing to decreased LV volume by hampering filling with bowing of the septum into the LV cavity, or decreased filling from generally poor pulmonary venous return. In contrast to the hypertrophy seen in RV myocytes, underfilling of the LV may lead to atrophy. Once the RV becomes uncoupled from the pulmonary vasculature with progressive dilation and decreased function, LV failure may be induced.

Measurement of LV systolic function
Fractional Shortening (FS) and Ejection Fraction (EF) may be used to assess LV systolic function. To obtain FS, the left ventricular end-diastolic (LVEDD) and end-systolic (LVESD) diameters by m-mode are measured from the parasternal long-axis or short-axis views. FS is determined by the equation:

$$FS\;(\%) = \frac{(End-diastolic\;diameter)-(End-systolic\;diameter)}{(End-diastolic\;diameter)} \times 100$$

Normal values range between 0.25 and 0.4. M-mode measurements of LV function are, however, of limited value in patients with acute PH because of the assumption that the LV is circular in cross-section. When mPAP is elevated, the shape of the LV cavity may be significantly altered by interventricular septal motion. EF using Simpson's Biplane method, therefore, is recommended in the presence of septal flattening. This method utilizes LV end-diastolic and end-systolic volumes that are obtained by tracing the endocardium of the LV in the apical 4- and 2-chamber views. The total LV volume is calculated from the summation of a stack of elliptical disks, providing a more reliable estimate of the volume of the LV, which is a 3-dimensional structure. EF is determined utilizing LV end-diastolic volume and end-systolic volume with the equation:

$$EF\;(\%) = \frac{(End-diastolic\;volume)-(End-systolic\;volume)}{(End-diastolic\;volume)} \times 100$$

Similar to the RV, TDI may be used to measure myocardial velocities of the LV free wall and septum. Both strain and strain rate may be measured and may provide more load-independent measures of LV contractility.

Left ventricular output (LVO)
LVO (mL/min/kg) is a reliable surrogate estimate of systemic blood flow in the absence of a PDA (32) (Figure 31.6). LVO is calculated using the aortic annulus radius (Aor) measured at the hinge points of the aortic valve, aortic VTI, and HR in the following equation:

$$LVO = \left[\Pi(Aor)^2 \times VTI \times HR\right] \div weight\,(kg)$$

When a PDA is present with bidirectional or right-to-left shunt, the effective post-ductal systemic blood flow is a combination of LVO and net right-to-left transductal flow.

Superior vena cava (SVC) flow
SVC flow has been proposed as a marker of systemic blood flow in neonates that is not influenced by the presence of intra- or extracardiac shunts (33). It should be recognized that SVC flow represents head and neck perfusion only, so is not reflective of whole-body perfusion. SVC flow is measured in the subcostal and parasternal long-axis views with PW Doppler as it enters the right atrium. Diameter measurements are assessed with M-mode tracing and are prone to inaccurate calculations, as the SVC is consistently oval-shaped. Validation of echocardiography SVC flow measurements compared to phase-contrast MRI has been shown to have poor correlation (34). For these reasons, caution should be exercised when using this measurement to guide clinical therapy.

Preload
Left heart filling can be assessed by using pulmonary vein Doppler and mitral valve inflow. For pulmonary vein Doppler flow, from an apical four-chamber view, the PW sample volume is placed in the right lower pulmonary vein at the opening to the left atrium. It is important for the cursor to be aligned with the blood flow to minimize the angle of insonation. Low peak pulmonary vein velocity can be an indication of decreased pulmonary venous return as a result of low PBF in the setting of PH. Low peak velocity may also be seen in the setting of dilated pulmonary veins. High pulmonary vein velocity may be seen in flow-mediated PH and pulmonary vein stenosis. To evaluate mitral valve flow, PW Doppler sample volume should be placed within the mitral valve annulus. The VTI can be traced to provide a semi-quantitative assessment of effective LV preload including pulmonary venous return and the amount of blood from right-to-left shunting

---

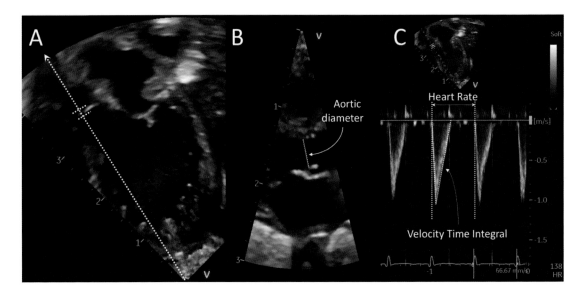

FIGURE 31.6 Calculation of left ventricular output. The LV five-chamber view should be optimized to attain a zero angle of insonation with the left ventricular outflow tract (LVOT). The pulse-wave Doppler sample volume is placed at the hinge points of the aortic valve with the angle parallel to the LVOT (left). The Doppler is traced (tight to the laminar envelope) to measure the velocity time integral (right). The aortic annulus is measured between each hinge-point inner-edge in long-axis (middle).

across a patent foramen ovale (PFO). Left heart filling can be affected adversely by high mean airway pressure (P_{aw}) leading to decreased pulmonary venous return. Hypoxic respiratory failure among patients with PH may prompt clinicians to increase P_{aw} as an attempt to improve oxygenation; however, excess Paw may inadvertently contribute to elevated PVR, impaired left heart filling, and poor cardiac output. Serial echocardiography may aid in determining optimal Paw.

Appraisal of intra- and extracardiac shunts

Patent ductus arteriosus
Flow direction across the PDA provides the most direct method of evaluating the relationship between PAP and systemic arterial pressure. Direction and peak velocity of PDA flow are measured by combining color Doppler with either PW or CW Doppler. The presence of an exclusive right-to-left shunt is always abnormal. In fact, the presence of right-to-left shunt of ≥60% indicates suprasystemic PASP (35). A bidirectional shunt <60% is seen when PASP is near systemic level or less while a left-to-right shunt is seen when systemic pressure is higher than PASP. Pre- and post-ductal oxygen saturation gradient will only be present if there is exclusive or almost exclusive right-to-left transductal shunt; therefore, an absent gradient should not be interpreted as PASP is not pathologically elevated. Similarly, some neonates will have a closed or restrictive PDA in the first hours after birth, and many will be closed in evaluations of chronic PH. Importantly, in situations where the systemic arterial pressure is very low (i.e. in patients with severe vasodilator shock), right-to-left shunt may be present without a clinically relevant elevation in PASP. In addition to its diagnostic role, the presence of a PDA may be clinically desirable in the setting of acute PH. Elevated mPAP may precipitate RV failure. Right-to-left ductal flow reduces effective afterload on the RV, unless systemic pressure is also very elevated (e.g. with exogenous vasoconstrictors). The presence of a PDA may also provide supplemental post-ductal systemic blood flow. In the setting of moderate to severe PH with closing or functionally

closed PDA, the clinical team may need to consider initiation of prostaglandin to reopen the ductus to provide an outlet for the RV until PASP declines.

Patent foramen ovale
In the normal transitional circulation, the transatrial shunt changes from exclusively right-to-left to bidirectional shortly after birth. Therefore, the presence of an exclusive right-to-left atrial level shunt in the assessment of acute or chronic PH is always abnormal and should prompt evaluation for abnormal pulmonary venous drainage. The presence of an atrial communication can be assessed from the subcostal view and confirmed in the other views. The directionality of the atrial level shunt is assessed with a combination of Color and PW Doppler. The presence of a right-to-left transatrial shunt can exacerbate the severity of hypoxemia in severe acute PH when PBF is critically low and deoxygenated blood traverses the PFO to the systemic circulation contributing to a lower pre-ductal saturation. On the other hand, this phenomenon might be beneficial in patients with severe RV systolic dysfunction and critically low PBF through the ability to augment preductal cardiac output (though with more pronounced hypoxemia).

Fundamental principles of neonatal hemodynamic-focused echocardiography

There are several key features of quantitative echocardiography, which are essential both to produce an accurate impression of physiology and to optimize reproducibility. First, several forms of duct-dependant congenital heart defects may have a similar clinical appearance; therefore, the first echocardiography evaluation must include all images/sweeps sufficient to define normal cardiac anatomy. Second, it is important to produce images that are straight and optimally visualize the desired landmarks and structures (Figure 31.1). Over- or under-rotation, misalignment, and lack of precision imaging may result in missing important details. Specifically, it is essential that Doppler measurements have as

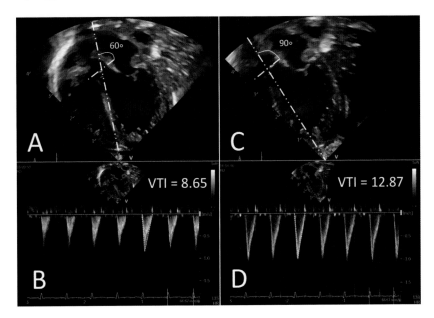

FIGURE 31.7 Zero angle of insonation is essential for accurate calculation of ventricular output. Apical 5-chamber (A/C) and aortic pulse-wave Doppler (B/D) with the aortic leaflets bifurcating the cursor between the sample volume taken in the same patient with <1-minute between comparators. A 60° angle of insonation (A) underestimates the velocity time integral (VTI) (B). Solely by correcting the angle of insonation (C), the VTI increases by ~50% (D).

close to zero angle of insonation as possible (Figure 31.7). Also, the position of the sample volume should be precise. For example, when measuring the LVO, the sample volume should straddle the aortic annulus, because either too high (in the aortic root) or too low (in the ventricle) will result in a smaller VTI due to a larger chamber diameter. High-quality training with an emphasis on methodology and sufficient volume of echocardiograms to maintain the skill of the operator is important. Finally, the patient should be at their physiologic baseline. Echocardiography performed under non-optimized conditions (e.g. hypothermia, hypoxia, correctible blood gas abnormalities) may not accurately represent the physiology, which is often dynamic. Similarly, "out of keeping" physiologic status (such as tachycardia) may modify time-based measurements and lead to inaccurate impressions.

Pitfalls in assessment of patients with presumed PH

Diagnosis and follow-up of patients with PH require a holistic, comprehensive echocardiography approach. Cardiac Point of Care Ultrasound, or other types of limited assessment, presents myriad risks for incorrect diagnostic ascertainment. For example, RV dysfunction could lead to an underestimation of TRJV (6) the presence of a right-to-left PDA shunt is commonly seen both in the setting of severe PH and LV dysfunction. The presence of TRJV, PA dilation, and PDA shunt can all affect the ability to measure RVET:PAAT (6). Additionally, notching of the PA Doppler can be seen in high flow states unrelated to PH (36). Because each measurement has intrinsic limitations, it is essential to understand the method and background of each test. The comprehensive assessment of multiple quantitative variables will contribute to a more accurate appraisal of the severity of acute or chronic PH. Therapeutic strategies used to reduce PVR in acute PH may be destabilizing for lesions associated with excessive PBF (e.g. anomalous pulmonary venous return) or lesions with left-sided outflow tract obstruction (e.g. hypoplastic left heart syndrome). The main components of assessment of PH are quantification of mPAP, evaluation of RV and LV performance, and appraisal

of intra- and extracardiac shunts. Comprehensive echocardiography may be instrumental in facilitating diagnosis, informing treatment decisions, and determining response to therapy in this potentially complex physiology.

Role of cardiac catheterization

Cardiac catheterization is considered the gold standard for the diagnosis of PH. It is more commonly used in children and adults than in neonates. Catheterization enables direct measurement of pulmonary hemodynamics, but it is an invasive procedure (typically requiring general anesthesia) and should only be performed at centers proficient with care of the infant with PH, to minimize complications. As echocardiography is a non-invasive method of obtaining serial measurements of severity of PH at the bedside and with the patient in their normal awake or asleep physiological state, it is used more frequently in the neonatal population for diagnosis and longitudinal follow-up. Cardiac catheterization should be considered for infants with prolonged, severe, or refractory PH, to rule out pulmonary vein stenosis in compatible clinical situations and in those patients where physiology may be complex including neonates suspected to have left heart disease or shunt physiology.

In conclusion, echocardiography is an essential tool in the diagnosis, stratification, and longitudinal care of patients with PH. It is essential that high-quality imaging is obtained in order to maximize the accuracy of the physiologic information. Comprehensive imaging with quantitative evaluation is important to ensure phenotypic precision and select the appropriate management trajectory.

References

1. Abman SH, et al. Circulation. 2015; 132(21):2037–2099.
2. Rudolph AM. Circulation. 1970; 41(2):343–359.
3. Kumar VH, et al. J Perinatol. 2007; 27(4):214–219.
4. Rudolph AM, et al. Pediatrics. 1961; 28(1):28–34.

5. Ahmed MS, et al. J Paediatr Child Health. 2019; 55(7):753–761.
6. Giesinger RE, et al. Pediatr Res. 2017; 82:901.
7. Rosenzweig EB, et al. Eur Respir J. 2019; 53(1):1801916.
8. Varghese N, et al. Pediatr Allergy Immunol Pulmonol. 2019; 32(4):140–148.
9. Kingma I, et al. Circulation. 1983; 68(6):1304–1314.
10. Smith A, et al. Echocardiography. 2019; 36(7):1346–1352.
11. Ryan T, et al. J Am Coll Cardiol. 1985; 5(4):918–924.
12. Abraham S, et al. Echocardiography. 2016; 33(6):910–915.
13. Jain A, et al. Curr Pediatr Rev. 2013; 9(1):55–66.
14. Parasuraman S, et al. Int J Cardiol Heart Vasc. 2016; 12:45–51.
15. Sanz J, et al. J Am Coll Cardiol. 2019; 73(12):1463–1482.
16. Jain A, et al. J Am Soc Echocardiogr. 2014; 27(12):1293–1304.
17. Levy PT, et al. J Am Soc Echocardiogr. 2015; 28(5):559–569.
18. Brown SB, et al. Chest. 2011; 140(1):27–33.
19. Koestenberger M, et al. Neonatology. 2011; 100(1):85–92.
20. Koestenberger M, et al. J Am Soc Echocardiogr. 2009; 22(6):715–719.
21. Aloia E, et al. Int J Cardiol. 2016; 225:177–183.
22. Alp H, et al. Early Hum Dev. 2012; 88(11):853–859.
23. Mori K, et al. Heart. 2004; 90(2):175–180.
24. Nestaas E, et al. Pediatr Res. 2018; 84(Suppl 1):18–29.
25. Sutherland GR, et al. J Am Soc Echocardiogr. 2004; 17(7):788–802.
26. Cantinotti M, et al. J Am Soc Echocardiogr. 2018; 31(6):712.e6–720.e6.
27. El-Khuffash A, et al. Pediatr Res. 2018; 84(Suppl 1):30–45.
28. Vonk Noordegraaf A, et al. J Am Coll Cardiol. 2017; 69(2):236–243.
29. Levy PT, et al. J Am Soc Echocardiogr. 2016; 29(11):1056–1065.
30. Patel MD, et al. J Am Soc Echocardiogr. 2019; 32(7):884.e4–894.e4.
31. Levy PT, et al. J Am Soc Echocardiogr. 2018; 31(8):962–964.
32. Slama M, et al. Am J Physiol Heart Circ Physiol. 2003; 284(2):H691–H697.
33. Kluckow M, et al. Arch Dis Child Fetal Neonatal Ed. 2000; 82(3):F182–F187.
34. Ficial B, et al. J Am Soc Echocardiogr. 2013; 26(12):1365–1371.
35. Musewe NN, et al. J Am Coll Cardiol. 1990; 15(2):446–456.
36. Kitabatake A, et al. Circulation. 1983; 68(2):302–309.

RIGHT VENTRICULAR PERFORMANCE AND VENTRICULAR INTERDEPENDENCE IN HYPOXIA

Afif El Khuffash and Philip T. Levy

Contents

Introduction

Pulmonary hypertension in neonates has many underlying etiologies. The clinical presentation depends on the onset and severity of the disease process, characterized by hypoxic respiratory failure and driven via an elevation in pulmonary artery pressure and a sustained exposure to increased afterload by the right ventricle (RV). The degree of RV failure is the major determinant of morbidity and mortality associated with pulmonary hypertension in the neonatal population. The RV and pulmonary arterial (PA) circulation function as one unit, referred to as the RV-PA axis (1). Since the RV is a pulsatile pump, the challenge in neonatal pulmonary hypertension is for the RV to remain hemodynamically coupled to a compliant PA circulation. A comprehensive understanding of the determinants and tools to characterize the RV-PA axis offers a pathway to define causes and optimally manage neonatal pulmonary hypertension. In this chapter, we discuss the pulmonary circulation and the right/left ventricular (LV) remodeling associated with progressing pulmonary hypertension. The concept of RV-PA coupling will be introduced with a focus on the perturbations that lead to abnormal RV-PA interactions. Finally, we will discuss up-to-date echocardiography methods used in the comprehensive assessment of RV systolic and diastolic function in addition to RV morphology.

Pulmonary circulation and right ventricle development: Right and left ventricular remodeling

Galen (130–199 C.E.) was the first to describe the relationship between the right and left side of the heart and conceptualized the right heart as passive conduit through which part of the circulating volume of blood passes to the lungs with the remainder seeping through invisible pores in the interventricular septum to reach the left side of the heart (2). Ibn Nafis (1213–1288 C.E.) suggested that for blood to reach the LV, it did not pass through invisible pores, but traveled from the RV to the lungs and back to the left side of the heart (3). William Harvey (1578–1657 C.E.) proposed a closed vascular system where blood is constantly recirculated from the right side of the heart through the pulmonary vasculature, to the left side of the heart, and onto the systemic circulation (4, 5). Although historically the RV was thought of as a chamber that only provided capacitance to the pulmonary circulation (6), or a ventricle that caused problems confined to congenital heart disease, several neonatal complications (e.g. pulmonary hypertension) are now recognized as diseases of altered RV-PA vasculature interactions where the main determinant of the clinical course and prognosis is the response of the RV to changes in its afterload (7).

Cardiac morphogenesis precedes airway development during the embryonic stage. Critical components of the pulmonary system actually arise from the primitive heart tube (8). The genetic investigation of cardiac morphogenesis has shown that the 1st heart field cells gives rise to the LV and parts of the right and left atria. The second heart field progenitor cells mature into the RV forming the main PA trunk, parts of the atria, septum, and the base of the aorta during the looping process (9, 10). The pulmonary circulation arises through temporal and spatially controlled signaling pathways linked to both the cardiac and airway development (10), and consists of thin, elastic vessels that accompany the arborization of the bronchial airway, but remains constricted by vasoactive mediators (11). A continuous circulation between the RV and lungs is present by the fifth week of gestation as the PA precursors form a multilayered vascular network linking the arterial and venous poles of the heart. The RV and PA circulation are separated from the LV and systemic circulation by atrial and ventricular septation, although they remain a parallel circulation during fetal life through a patent foramen ovale and ductus arteriosus. The RV matures into a thin-walled crescent shaped tripartite structure composed of an inflow portion with a trabeculated apex and smooth outlet infundibulum running into the PA circulation.

In utero, the RV is the dominant chamber close to 60% of the total cardiac output with 15–25% of the total cardiac output circulating through the pulmonary vasculature. The remaining RV output is redirected through the ductus arteriosus into the systemic circulation (12). At birth, inflation of the lungs, increased oxygen tension, and appropriate reduction in pulmonary vascular resistance (PVR) lead to increased pulmonary blood flow to the

DOI: 10.1201/9780367494018-32

left side of the heart. The natural physiological changes may fail to progress, resulting in the failure of RV afterload to decrease after birth. The thin-walled RV structure and the coarse trabeculations provide the substrate for the RV to accommodate increases in volume and afterload. Therefore, it is imperative to consider the developmental biology of the pulmonary vasculature, the RV, and the effects of injury during the perinatal transition, to aid in classification and management of neonatal pulmonary hypertension (13).

The intrinsic characteristics of the developing myocardium also place it at risk of hemodynamic compromise soon after birth. The neonatal myocardium is comprised of an underdeveloped contractile system with disordered myofibrils, an inefficient calcium handling system, and a noncompliant collagen, predisposing it to poor tolerance to increased afterload, lack of reserve to cope with states of reduced preload, and diastolic dysfunction (14). Furthermore, when the neonatal myocardium is exposed to hypoxia, as in neonatal pulmonary hypertension, the outcomes relate to alterations in cardiac function and morphometry associated with developmental programming of the heart.

Since the RV and LV myocardium are structurally distinct, their functional roles change in the postnatal period. With the increased awareness of the impact that LV dysfunction has on the RV-PA axis, it is important to understand how these ventricular-ventricular interactions are intimately related to the embryological development of the myocardium. The RV and LV are built upon a shared framework of collagenous fibers. The RV myofiber architecture is composed of superficial oblique and dominant deep longitudinal layers (15). The superficial oblique fibers of the RV are arranged in parallel with the AV groove and turn obliquely toward the cardiac apex and continue into the superficial myofibers of the LV. The LV also consists a midwall layer of circumferential fibers and deep longitudinal fibers. The middle layer of circumferential fibers, which occupies approximately 60% of the ventricular wall thickness, provides the main driving force of the LV by reducing ventricular diameter. These three layers (superficial oblique, midwall circumferential, and deep longitudinal) contribute to the complex movement of the LV, which contains torsion, translation, rotation, and thickening (16). In contrast, the RV lacks a middle layer of circumferential fibers, and the deep longitudinal layer makes up 80% of the RV wall thickness and provides the major contribution to ejection fraction (EF) and stroke volume during systole.

Ventricular mechanics begin to undergo maturational changes in the early and late postnatal periods that are specific to each ventricle, and can have a long-term impact on cardiac function beyond the first year of age, especially in preterm infants (17). The exposure of a neonatal heart to a sustained increase in hemodynamic load of postnatal circulation, at a time in the development when the heart primarily supports a low resistance circulation, induces myoarchitectural adaptation that may lead to ventricular remodeling (18). The complex three-dimensional structure of the RV, with thin wall and high compliance, is evolutionally different from the thick-walled and highly contractile LV. RV function increases over the first year of age in term and preterm infants with distinct regional changes, but LV function remains relatively preserved through the neonatal period and infancy (19). Some common morbidities following premature birth (e.g. bronchopulmonary dysplasia and late pulmonary hypertension) leave a negative impact on RV mechanics with unchanged LV performance, suggesting a less developed intrinsic

RV myocardial function response following preterm birth (20). Important morphological differences likely explain the relative dysfunction that is exacerbated as prematurity exposes the RV to the stress of postnatal cardiovascular performance before development is concluded (19).

Hemodynamic profiles of abnormal RV-PA interactions: Ventricular interdependence; right ventricle pulmonary arterial vascular coupling

The efficiency of the RV-PA axis depends on proper hemodynamic coupling of the RV with its compliant pulmonary arterial circulation (21). RV-PA coupling depicts the physical change in energy between the two entities, and is mathematically equal to the work expended by a force through displacement (22). Although RV performance is determined by an intricate balance between its preload, afterload, contractility, and ventricular-ventricular interactions, RV-PA coupling principally offers a clinically useful understanding of how RV contractility adapts to changes in afterload, and can serve as a comprehensive measure of RV pump function associated with outcome in PH patients (23).

Despite the underlying etiopathology of pulmonary hypertension, persistently high PVR and/or pulmonary venous congestion from increased pulmonary blood flow or pulmonary capillary wedge pressure (PCWP) will result in a direct increase in RV afterload resulting in pulmonary hypertension (24). There are three distinct stages of RV coupling (and uncoupling) that may offer another avenue for risk assessment and tailoring potential therapeutic interventions in neonatal pulmonary hypertension with decreased RV performance (Figure 32.1). In Stage 1, under normal circumstances and within a certain physiological range, the RV remains coupled to the pulmonary circulation with preservation of the RV-PA axis. In Stage 2, the RV adapts to the increasing vascular load by enhancing contractility to maintain pulmonary blood flow (1). Additionally, the contractile capabilities of the RV are further enhanced by muscle hypertrophy and increased wall thickness. Prolonged exposure to increased PVR and progressive pressure loading on the RV will, however, perpetuate the progressive burden on the RV-PA axis, leading to further maladaptive ventricular remodeling with RV dilation, decreased stroke volume, and increased heart rate to maintain cardiac output. Unfortunately, the neonatal myocardium is sensitive to changes in loading conditions and often incapable of rapid adaptation (this is even more evident in premature infants), preventing it from properly handling all of these complex hemodynamic changes (25). Beyond a certain afterload threshold, or in a suboptimal physiologic state, the RV exhausts all of its adaptive capabilities as it enters into Stage 3. The poor myocardial tolerance to the progressive rise in afterload ultimately leads to uncoupling of the RV from the PA circulation reflected by a decrease in RV performance, efficiency (work), and overt RV failure (25).

There are multiple contributors that can lead to abnormal RV-PA coupling responses during this early transitional period, including causes related to pulmonary vasculature, lung parenchyma, and cardiac diseases (26). Pulmonary vascular etiologies (e.g. delayed or failed transition) and lung parenchymal etiologies (e.g. respiratory distress syndrome) have been well studied, and recent evidence has shown that LV diastolic dysfunction (resulting in an increase in PCWP) is associated with a higher risk for

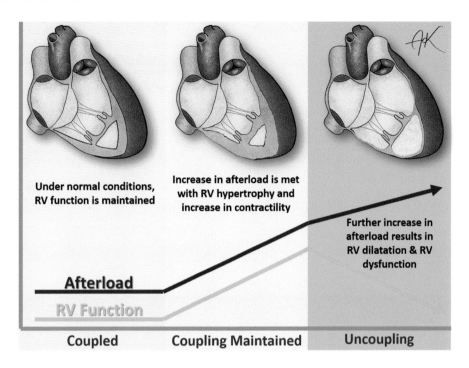

FIGURE 32.1 Stages of right ventricle – pulmonary arterial coupling.

invasive ventilation and pulmonary hemorrhage (14) with a direct correlation to abnormal coupling of the RV to its afterload during the transitional period (27).

Rising RV afterload without compensatory increases in contractility leads to alterations in RV-PA coupling that appear more pronounced based on gestational age at birth (28, 29). Comparisons between term-born and preterm-born infants over the first year of age have demonstrated a similar blunted gestational age-dependent contractility response to increases in afterload (20). A recent meta-analysis showed that preterm-born individuals have RV systolic impairment from birth through adulthood (30). Knowing that even slight elevations in PA pressure have been associated with a rise in mortality in adults born preterm (31), further studies are needed to evaluate the physiological response of the RV to increased afterload in the setting of hypoxic respiratory failure in preterm born infants throughout the lifespan.

Advanced cardiac imaging and methods of assessing right ventricle morphology, systolic, and diastolic function: Deformation and strain in neonatal pulmonary hypertension

Sustained elevation of pulmonary artery pressures secondary to elevated pulmonary vascular resistance leads to a reduction in pulmonary blood flow and a failure of gas exchange in the lungs. This results in cyanosis and oxygenation failure of varying degrees (32). Crucially, elevated pulmonary artery pressures contribute to increased RV afterload. Due to the developmental and maturational challenges described above, in addition to the impaired RV-PA coupling relationship that it ubiquitous in neonates (especially premature infants), the neonatal myocardium is generally incapable of adapting to the increased afterload resulting in

progressive RV dilatation and dysfunction (27). RV dysfunction in the setting of elevated pulmonary arterial pressure (PAP) leads to both intracardiac (at the level of atrial shunt) and extracardiac (at the level of ductus arteriosus) mixing of deoxygenated blood and oxygenated blood resulting in cyanosis and hypoxemia. Lower pulmonary blood flow and progressive RV dilatation resulting in septal bowing into the LV cavity will impair pulmonary venous return, thereby reducing LV filling with a subsequent decline in LV output. This will eventually lead to clinical manifestations of low systemic blood flow including hypotension, shock, and at the end organ dysfunction.

RV function plays an important role in disease progression and prognostication in the setting of pulmonary hypertension in neonates. Depressed RV function is an independent risk factor for death or the need for extracorporeal membrane oxygenation (ECMO) in neonates with pulmonary hypertension. In addition, RV dysfunction is an independent risk factor for adverse outcomes including mortality when associated with pulmonary hypertension in specific disease states including bronchopulmonary dysplasia (33), congenital diaphragmatic hernia (34), hypoxic ischemic encephalopathy (35) and Down syndrome (36). Therefore, accurate characterization of RV function, in addition to thorough appraisal of RV afterload and pulmonary hemodynamics, is an essential component of the holistic approach to the management of infants with hypoxic respiratory failure secondary to elevated PAP. Although cardiac catheterization remains the gold standard for assessment of RV performance and pulmonary hemodynamics, its invasive nature and the difficulty in obtaining serial assessments limits its applicability in the neonatal population (37). Therefore, transthoracic echocardiography remains the ideal modality for the assessment of pulmonary haemodynamics and RV performance to facilitate the integration of hemodynamic information relevant to the etiology and clinical situation. This, in turn, offers a vehicle to enable formulation of a scientifically based diagnostic impression, determine a pathophysiological choice for support, and evaluate the response to therapeutic intervention (25).

The use of echocardiography in the setting of hypoxic respiratory failure falls under three broad categories: (i) Estimation of PAP and PVR (including an estimation of RV-PA coupling); (ii) assessment of right (and left) myocardial function and morphology; and (iii) assessment of intra- and extracardiac shunts (Figure 32.2).

Assessment of pulmonary artery pressure and PVR

Systolic PAP can be assessed in the presence of a tricuspid valve regurgitant jet using the modified Bernoulli equation ($p = 4V^2 +$ RAP, where p is the pressure gradient between the RV and the RA, V is the velocity of the tricuspid regurgitant (TR) jet in m/s, and RAP is the right atrial pressure usually estimated to be between 3 and 5 mmHg). This method is generally reliable and correlates with invasive measures of right heart pressure (32). Accurate

and reliable assessment is dependent on obtaining a clear TR jet with a minimal angle of insonation. This measurement has several disadvantages including the potential for underestimation of systolic pulmonary artery pressure in the presence of RV failure or RV outflow obstruction; in addition, TV regurgitation may be absent in up to 50% of infants with pulmonary hypertension (38–42). Diastolic PAP (DPAP) can be estimated in the presence of pulmonary valve regurgitation (PR) using the following equation (DPAP = 4 V_{max} PR^2 + RVdP, where V_{max} PR is the peak velocity of the PR jet in m/s, and RVdP is the RV diastolic pressure estimated to be between 2 and 5 mmHg).

Assessment of the intraventricular septal shape during systole can provide a subjective assessment of RV pressure. In normal circumstances (PVR < systemic vascular resistance, SVR), the septum bows into the RV, giving the LV a round shape from the parasternal short-axis view at the level of the papillary muscles. With increasing RV pressure, the septum becomes flattened

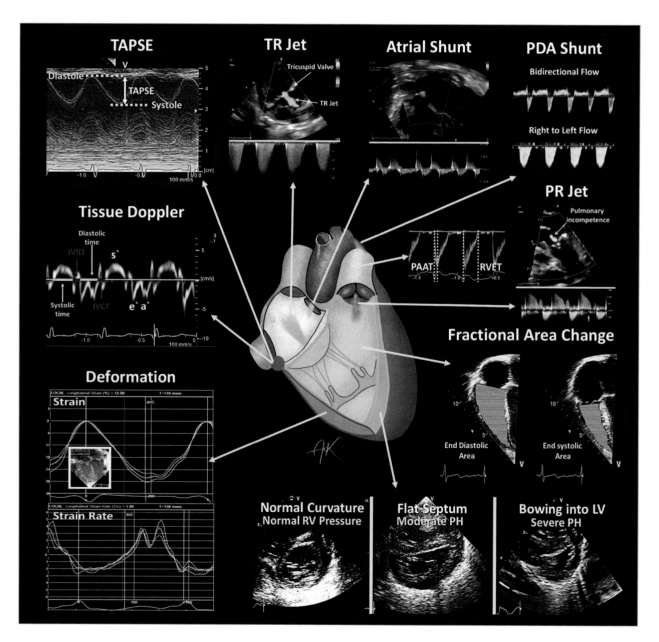

FIGURE 32.2 Comprehensive echocardiographic assessment of RV performance.

(PVR = SVR) or bowed into the LV (PVR > SVR) with increasing severity of RV pressure (43, 44). The LV systolic eccentricity index (LV EI), provides a more objective assessment of septal wall morphology in the setting of elevated PAP. LV EI is a measure that quantifies the ratio of the LV anteroposterior and septolateral diameters indicating an elevated RV pressure when the ratio > 1.0 (45).

Recent advances in echocardiography methods in the neonatal field have facilitated a more comprehensive assessment of pulmonary hemodynamics. The ratio of pulmonary artery acceleration time (PAAT), to right ventricular ejection time (RVET), referred to as PAATi can be used as a reliable and valid quantitative estimate of invasive measures of PVR (37). Those measurements are derived from the pulmonary artery pulsed-wave Doppler signal usually obtained from the parasternal long-axis view. Recent studies have demonstrated the ability of this measurement to identify the presence of pulmonary hypertension in the setting of bronchopulmonary dysplasia in premature infants (46), and in term infants.

Assessment of right ventricular function and morphology

The RV has complex geometry comprised of an inflow area, a trabeculated ventricular chamber and a smooth infundibular outlet leading to the pulmonary artery. This unique morphology has traditionally made assessment of RV performance difficult. Newer echocardiography functional measurements have facilitated enhanced assessment of systolic and diastolic RV function, including tissue Doppler imaging (TDI), tricuspid annular plane systolic excursion (TAPSE), fractional area change (FAC), and deformation imaging using speckle-tracking echocardiography (STE).

TDI facilitates measurement of peak systolic (s'), early diastolic (e') and late diastolic (a') velocities from the base of the RV free wall. This technique (due to its high temporal resolution) can also be used to measure event timings within the cardiac cycle including systolic (S) time, diastolic (D), time and isovolumic contraction and relaxation times. Normative values in premature and term infants are now established (47). TDI can be used to assess RV function to provide important clinical prognostic information in infants with congenital diaphragmatic hernia and may be used to monitor treatment response in infants with early presentation of pulmonary hypertension at birth (commonly referred to as acute pulmonary hypertension) (48). Similarly, the ratio of systolic to diastolic times (S:D ratio) can be used to detect global RV dysfunction secondary to increased RV afterload with an increasing ratio being associated with death or the need for ECMO in the setting of pulmonary hypertension (42).

Fractional area of change (FAC) is a measure of the change in RV cavity area from diastole to systole in the four-chamber view. Recent studies have demonstrated its utility in characterizing function in the setting of pulmonary hypertension in both premature and term infants with low values being associated with mortality and/or the need for ECMO (49). TAPSE is a measure of the displacement of the tricuspid valve annulus toward the apex during systole. It is obtained from the apical four-chamber view at the level of the lateral TV annulus using M-Mode. TAPSE provides useful information about longitudinal fiber shortening and it has shown good correlation with techniques estimating RV global systolic function. TAPSE may have an important prognostic role in various scenarios in the presence of pulmonary hypertension, with low values predicting the need for ECMO and/or death in infants with PPHN (49), and severe brain injury in the setting of hypoxic-ischemic encephalopathy (35).

Deformation analysis using STE measures the change in shape of the RV free wall in the longitudinal plane (shortening) during systole as a measurement of RV systolic function (termed strain). In addition, the speed of this deformation (systolic strain rate) and the speed at which the RV free wall resumes its baseline diastolic shape (early and late diastolic strain rates) can be derived (50). Infants with pulmonary hypertension demonstrate reduced RV peak systolic strain values, with even lower values indicating progression to death or ECMO in neonates with pulmonary hypertension (49, 51). Similarly, preterm infants with late onset pulmonary hypertension occurring at around 36 weeks gestation also exhibit lower values of RV free wall longitudinal strain when compared to preterm infants without pulmonary hypertension (19).

RV morphology measurements enable objective assessment of RV shape and size to provide an accurate appraisal of evolving RV hypertrophy or dilatation in the face of increasing afterload. These measurements are generally obtained from a RV-focused four-chamber view and include: end systolic and diastolic areas (52), annular, basal, mid-cavity and RV length dimensions, and RV outflow dimensions obtained from either the parasternal long axis or short axis view (53).

Assessment of intra- and extracardiac shunts

The presence of intracardiac shunts (patent foramen ovale) and extracardiac shunts (patent ductus arteriosus) is common in neonates in the setting of pulmonary hypertension. Increased RV systolic and diastolic pressure can lead to right-to-left shunting at atrial level leading to intracardiac mixing of deoxygenated blood with blood returning to the left atrium. Increased PAP will lead to right-to-left shunting across the ductus arteriosus. The presence of those shunts can facilitate the diagnosis of pulmonary hypertension. In addition, these shunts may play a vital role in augmenting the systemic circulation in the face of low LV output (38, 39, 42). Right-left shunting across at the atrial level can augment LV output and therefore cerebral blood flow, whereas right-left shunting across the PDA can augment blood flow to the body and to some extent to the brain. The shunt across the ductus can be used to estimate PAP and determine disease severity in the absence of a TR jet; specifically, bidirectional shunting indicating PVR to be equivalent to SVR, or exclusive right-to-left shunting indicating PVR to be higher than SVR. An exclusive right-to-left transductal shunt in patients with PPHN is associated with an increased risk of mortality (39). However, this does not imply that shunting is the primary problem; it is merely a marker of disease severity.

Assessment of RV-PA coupling

Echocardiography can be used to estimate RV-PA coupling. Recent work has demonstrated that TAPSE can be used as a surrogate marker for contractile state, and PAAT can be used as a measure of the developed force (afterload) (21); therefore, the ratio of TAPSE/PAAT may represent RV-PA coupling (21). Recent work has demonstrated that TAPSE/PAAT (and TAPSE/PAATi, corrected for heart rate) significantly correlates with invasive catheterization-derived measures of pulmonary vascular resistance, PA compliance, and RV strain in addition to invasive right-heart catheter-derived measures of RV-PA coupling, namely ventricular elastance (E_{es}, contractility) to arterial elastance (E_a, afterload) ratio (21), thereby serving as a useful non-invasive measure of RV-PA coupling (54). Further work is needed to assess the utility of this measurement in the clinical setting.

Conclusions

Neonatal pulmonary hypertension is a disorder characterized by elevated PAP that is usually associated with RV dysfunction. The neonate is particularly vulnerable to adverse outcomes associated with pulmonary hypertension due to the impaired RV-PA coupling interactions ubiquitous in the population. The degree of RV dysfunction generally determines the degree of adverse outcomes associated with this condition. A thorough assessment of RV performance and integrating the findings with the clinical condition is the cornerstone of the holistic approach to managing this condition, to improve survival and reduce morbidity.

References

1. Vonk-Noordegraaf A, et al. J Am Coll Cardiol. 2017; 69:236–243.
2. Greyson CR. Rev Esp Cardiol. 2010; 63:81–95.
3. West JB. J Appl Physiol. 2008; 105:1877–1880.
4. Schultz SG. News Physiol Sci. 2002; 1:175–180.
5. Cattermole GN. J R Soc Med. 1997; 90(11):640–644.
6. Kagan A. Circulation. 1952; 5:816–823.
7. Ghio S, et al. Ital Heart J. 2005; 6:852–855.
8. Haddad F, et al. Circulation. 2008; 11:1436–1448.
9. Wu M. Pediatr Cardiol. 2018; 39:1082–1089.
10. Paige SL, et al. Circ Res. 2015; 116:341–353.
11. Lau EM, et al. Eur Heart J. 2011; 32:2489–2498.
12. Brezinka C. J Perinat Med. 2001; 29:371–380.
13. Goss KN, et al. Pulm Circ. 2017; 7:7–19.
14. Bussmann N, et al. J Perinatol. 2018; 38:1205–1211.
15. Greenbaum RA, et al. Br Heart J. 1981; 45:248–263.
16. Buckberg G, et al. Circulation. 2008; 118:2571–2587.
17. Lewandowski AJ, et al. Circulation. 2013; 127:197–206.
18. Kluckow M, et al. Early Hum Dev. 2005; 81:429–437.
19. Levy PT, et al. J Am Soc Echocardiogr. 2018; 31:962–964.
20. Levy PT, et al. J Pediatr. 2018; 197:48–56.
21. Levy PT, et al. J Am Soc Echocardiogr. 2017; 30:685–698.
22. Guazzi M, et al. Am J Physiol Heart Circ Physiol. 2013; 305(9):H1373–H1381.
23. Jone PN, et al. Eur Heart J Cardiovasc Imaging. 2018; 19:1026–1033.
24. Jain A, et al. Semin Fetal Neonatal Med. 2015; 20:262–271.
25. El-Khuffash A, et al. Clin Perinatol. 2017; 44:377–393.
26. Giesinger RE, et al. Pediatr Res. 2017; 82:901–914.
27. Bussmann N, et al. Early Hum Dev. 2018; 128:35–40.
28. Mulchrone A, et al. Am J Respir Crit Care Med. 2020; 201:615–618.
29. Mohamed A, et al. JACC Cardiovasc Imaging. 2020; 13(9):2046–2048
30. Telles F, et al. Pediatrics. 2020; 146(2):e20200146.
31. Douschan P, et al. Am J Respir Crit Care Med. 2018; 197:509–516.
32. de Boode WP, et al. Pediatr Res. 2018; 84:68–77.
33. Altit G, et al. Pulm Circ. 2019; 9(3):2045894019878598.
34. Patel N, et al. Am J Respir Crit Care Med. 2019; 200:1522–1530.
35. Giesinger RE, et al. Am J Respir Crit Care Med. 2019; 200:1294–1305.
36. Martin T, et al. J Pediatr. 2018; 193:21–26.
37. Levy PT, et al. J Am Soc Echocardiogr. 2016; 29:1056–1065.
38. Skinner JR, et al. Arch Dis Child Fetal Neonatal Ed. 1996; 74:F26–F32.
39. Fraisse A, et al. Cardiol Young. 2004; 14:277–283.
40. Peterson AL, et al. Pediatr Cardiol. 2009; 30:160–165.
41. Sehgal A, et al. Acta Paediatr. 2012; 101:410–413.
42. Aggarwal S, et al. Early Hum Dev. 2015; 91:285–289.
43. Bendapudi P, et al. Paediatr Respir Rev. 2015; 16:157–161.
44. King ME, et al. Circulation. 1983; 68:68–75.
45. Ehrmann DE, et al. J Pediatr. 2018; 203:210–217.
46. Patel MD, et al. J Am Soc Echocardiogr. 2019; 32:884.e4–894.e4.
47. Nestaas E, et al. Pediatr Res. 2018; 84:18–29.
48. Patel N, et al. Neonatology. 2009; 96:193–199.
49. Malowitz JR, et al. Eur Heart J Cardiovasc Imaging. 2015; 16:1224–1231.
50. El-Khuffash A, et al. Pediatr Res. 2018; 84:30–45.
51. Jain A, et al. Eur J Pediatr. 2016; 175:1464–1465.
52. Levy PT, et al. Am Soc Echocardiogr. 2015; 28:559–569
53. Lang RM, et al. J Am Soc Echocardiogr. 2015; 28:1–39.
54. Levy PT, et al. JACC Cardiovasc Imaging. 2018; 2019; 12(4):761–763.

VENTILATION STRATEGIES IN NEONATAL HYPOXEMIC RESPIRATORY FAILURE

Bradley A. Yoder, Michelle J. Yang, Nicholas R. Carr and Martin Keszler

Contents

Introduction

The goal of the cardiopulmonary system is to provide an adequate supply of oxygen at the tissue level to support organ function and adequate elimination of CO_2 to maintain acceptable pH (1). Severe lung disease leads to altered oxygen uptake and delivery, necessitating assisted respiratory support. In this chapter we will focus on the use of mechanical support systems, specifically mechanical ventilation and extracorporeal life support (ECLS), to support oxygenation.

Oxygenation

Optimizing gas exchange and oxygenation is more complicated than simply measuring partial pressures of arterial carbon dioxide ($PaCO_2$), oxygen (PaO_2) or arterial saturations (SaO_2). Oxygen delivery (DaO_2) is determined by cardiac output (CO) and oxygen content (CaO_2), where CaO_2 is determined predominantly by hemoglobin (Hgb) content and its saturation profile. [$CaO_2 = (1.34\ ml\ O_2/g\ Hgb * Hgb\ g/100\ ml * SaO_2) + PaO_2 * 0.003\ ml/mmHg$)] (Figure 33.1). The most important factors for DaO_2 are CO, Hgb content and SaO_2. Except for how it affects SaO_2, dissolved O_2 contributes minimally to overall oxygen delivery (Figure 33.1). Supraphysiologic PaO_2 values (>100 mmHg) indicate relatively good gas exchange across the lung alveolar-capillary interface, which still may be associated with inadequate tissue oxygenation if there is severe anemia and/or CO is compromised. Optimizing ventilator support for the neonate with hypoxemic respiratory failure (HRF) requires careful balancing of the beneficial effects of mean airway pressure (PAW) on lung volume and adverse effect on blood flow/CO, both pulmonary and systemic.

"Optimal" ventilatory support would be that associated with the lowest PAW necessary to establish and maintain a normal functional residual volume. This level of support will theoretically be associated with optimal lung perfusion via low pulmonary vascular resistance (PVR) and minimal intra-pulmonary shunt, as well as minimal adverse effect on systemic venous return and CO (Figure 33.2A, B). Determining the optimal PAW and lung volume is critical to optimizing cardiorespiratory function and DaO_2. The ventilatory approach employed should include consideration of factors contributing to ventilator-associated lung injury, the suspected underlying developmental and pathological features of lung injury, and how these factors may change over time.

Estimating lung volume

Lung recruitment strategies

In the absence of extrapulmonary shunts, oxygenation is closely linked to end-expiratory lung volume (EELV) (2–5). Optimizing EELV plays a key role in the ventilatory management of HRF, since both low and high lung volume is associated with increased PVR (3, 5–8) (Figure 33.3). As shown in Table 33.1, several approaches may aid the establishment and assessment of EELV. Among these, the lung recruitment maneuver is the best studied and most cost-effective approach; in addition, it is readily available to all clinicians with access to basic physiologic monitoring. It is unclear, however, how often this technique is actually employed in clinical practice. Importantly, most lung recruitment studies have been done in animal models or infants whose predominant pathophysiology is diffuse alveolar disease, rather than more complicated diseases such as pneumonia, aspiration syndromes, and disorders of impaired lung growth, where aggressive lung volume recruitment may not be feasible and could even be detrimental. Additionally, most reports related to lung recruitment have been done in the context of high-frequency ventilation (2–8).

As described in Table 33.1 and pictured in Figure 33.2A, the process of lung recruitment is based on 1–2 cmH_2O (most studies

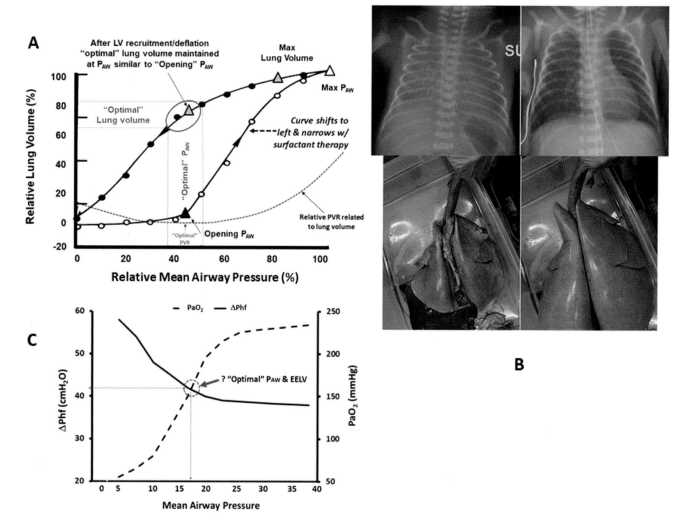

FIGURE 33.1 Key factors in oxygenation and systemic oxygen delivery. PaO_2, partial arterial pressure of oxygen; SaO_2, arterial oxygen saturation; HgB, hemoglobin; CaO_2, arterial oxygen content; Qp, pulmonary blood flow; SVR, systemic venous return; CO, cardiac output; DaO_2, arterial oxygen delivery.

FIGURE 33.2 Airway pressure relationships. (A) hysteresis curve overlaid on curve showing relationship of pulmonary vascular resistance (PVR) lung volume; "optimal" PVR, lung volume and mean airway pressure (PAW) intersections are shown. (B) externalized lung to radiographic representations of under-inflated versus adequately inflated lung. (C) overlaid curves showing relationship of delta Phf (change in oscillator pressure amplitude with set tidal volume) and PaO_2 to increasing mean airway pressure during lung recruitment. [Figures modified from (1, 7, 11).]

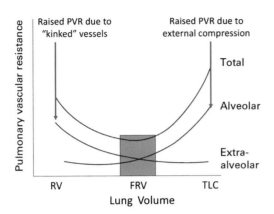

FIGURE 33.3 Relationship between lung inflation and pulmonary vascular resistance (PVR). PVR is typically lowest in the range of normal functional residual volume (FRV) and increases with atelectasis (i.e. RV or residual volume) and excessive lung inflation (i.e. TLC or total lung capacity).

suggest 2 cmH$_2$O increases) serial escalations in either PAW or positive end-expiratory pressure (PEEP), typically increased at 2–3 minute interval, until a significant improvement in oxygenation occurs (9, 10). Several key points are to be noted: (i) The initial assumption is that oxygenation measures are low, FiO$_2$ is high and EELV is inadequate (chest radiograph or lung US); (ii) as PAW is gradually increased, so does EELV; (iii) at some pressure level, oxygenation increases; this is commonly referred to as the "opening" pressure (i.e. SpO$_2$ increases from 86 to 93%); (iv) at this opening pressure EELV begins to improve, but still remains sub-optimal and well below both normal functional residual volume and maximum lung volume, as seen in Figure 33.1; (v) typically PAW continues to be increased and FiO$_2$ reduced until a targeted FiO$_2$ value is achieved and oxygenation stability is sustained, or until there is no further improvement in oxygenation after two increments of PAW; and (vi) once target FiO$_2$ (typically ≤0.30) is achieved, PAW is reduced by 2 cmH$_2$O every 2–3 minutes until SpO$_2$ drops below desired low range (i.e. <92%); this pressure has been termed the "closing" pressure. PAW is then raised back by 2 cmH$_2$O, a level termed "optimal PAW." Different approaches have been suggested for this re-escalation of PAW, just above the closing pressure, but the end goal is to achieve an

TABLE 33.1 Approaches or Tools for Optimizing Lung Recruitment in Hypoxic Respiratory Failure

Approach	Comments
Lung recruitment adjusting paw (HFOV)	Step-wise increase PAW ~ 2 cmH$_2$O q 2–5 minutes → Increase SpO$_2$ target Maintain SpO$_2$ target → Wean FiO$_2$ to target (<0.50 vs. <0.30, or lower)[a]
	May need to further increase PAW if SpO$_2$ falls w/ weaning FiO$_2$
	When stable at target FiO$_2$ → wean PAW ~ 1–2 cmH$_2$O q 5–10 minutes
	When SpO$_2$ begins to fall → Increase PAW by 2–3 cmH$_2$O
	See Figure 33.2A
Adjusting PEEP (MV, Jet)	Similar approach to above using PEEP (increase PEEP 1–2 cmH$_2$O q 2–5 minutes) to increase PAW & promote increasing resting lung volume
	See Figure 33.2A
Clinical measures	Changes in SpO$_2$ and or SpO$_2$/FiO$_2$
	Changes in Transcutaneous pCO$_2$
	Change in tidal volume on pressure-limited support
	Change in amplitude (HFOV) or PIP (MV) on volume-targeted support
	Change in Servo Pressure on HFJV
	See Figure 33.2C
Radiograph	Chest x-ray to assess resting lung volume
	Background density, diaphragm position relative to anterior (6th rib meets diaphragm in mid-clavicular line) or posterior rib (diaphragm dome at ~ 9th rib mid-clavicular line), flattened versus domed diaphragm
	See Figure 33.2B
Impedance tomography	Relative measures of V$_T$ and changes in EELV correlate with gas exchange
	EIT (electrical impedance tomography)
	• developing technology with stand-alone and in-machine systems
	• used in several lung recruitment studies
	• likely to be incorporated into practice over next 10 years
	RIP (respiratory inductance plethysmography)
	• available for over two decades but mostly limited to research use
	• unable to distinguish between changes in lung and blood volume
Lung US	Lung US score correlates to oxygenation measures
	Lung US score predicts chest x-ray consolidation/aeration

Abbreviations: PAW, mean airway pressure; HFOV, high-frequency oscillatory ventilation; SpO$_2$, oxygen saturation; PEEP, positive end-expiratory pressure; MV, mechanical ventilation; V$_T$, tidal volume; EELV, end-expiratory lung volume.

[a] Miedema et al. (5), "High" vs. "Medium" lung volume approach → target FiO$_2$ to < 0.30 vs. ~0.60 before moving to deflation steps.

EELV that supports oxygenation and ventilation on the descending limb of the pressure-volume curve using a pressure well below that needed for maximum lung volume. The studies by Tingay and colleagues suggest "optimal" EELV is approximately 50% of maximal lung volume and supported at a PAW about 40% of PAW needed to achieve maximum EELV (7). An animal model study suggests that stepwise approach to lung recruitment is more effective than a single or multiple sustained inflations (3). A recent study by Miedema compared two different approaches to lung recruitment in a surfactant deficient preterm lamb model; one that escalated PAW to an EELV needed to reduce FiO_2 below 0.30 compared to an approach that targeted a reduction in FiO_2 to 0.60 (5). After 2 hours, the high EELV-low FiO_2 group had better oxygenation indices, but similar ventilation and postmortem markers of lung injury. Given the very short time interval of this study, it is unclear what the long-term effects on lung injury might be between these different approaches on lung recruitment; thus, we currently recommend lung recruitment to an FiO_2 closer to 0.30.

Recently, another potential approach to identify optimal EELV during lung recruitment using volume-targeted high-frequency oscillatory ventilation (HFOV) (Draeger VN500) was reported (11). In an animal model of RDS the authors noted that ΔPhf, a measure of the amplitude needed to deliver the targeted tidal volume, decreased during the stepwise lung recruitment maneuver, reflecting improved lung compliance (Figure 33.2C). They showed a ΔPhf inflexion point that closely intersected with the PAW at which PaO_2 also began to markedly increase, suggestive of an "optimal" lung volume (Figure 33.2C). Their finding is consistent with the report by Tingay and colleagues in a small cohort of infants with EELV monitoring by respiratory inductive plethysmography (RIP) and tidal volume (V_T) measured via hotwire anemometry at the airway opening during lung recruitment maneuvers while on the Sensormedic 3100A oscillator (7). They noted a bell-shaped relationship between EELV, transcutaneous CO_2 and measured tidal volume. As recruitment improves lung volume, compliance also improves until near-maximum lung volume is reached (Figure 33.2A). Weaning PAW from peak lung volume is again accompanied by improved lung compliance, and both ΔPhf/delta peak pressure and transcutaneous CO_2 will again reflect better lung compliance (Figure 33.2A–C). The clinical application of lung volume optimization approaches remains inadequately studied. A recent trial by de Jagere et al. suggests poor sensitivity for any one marker related to "optimal" lung volume as measured by inductance plethysmography (12).

Few centers/clinicians have the technology to measure (V_T) during HFV with the Sensormedics 3100A, outside of research studies. During lung recruitment with this device one should consider incorporating monitoring of both transcutaneous CO_2 and SpO_2. Overall, SpO_2 is a good marker of improving lung volume, but alone may not adequately reflect optimal EELV compared to inadequate/excessive lung EELV (5, 6, 10). With the Life Pulse High-Frequency Jet Ventilator (HFJV), lung recruitment can be performed via step-wise escalation in PEEP (13). In a preterm lamb study by Musk et al., as EELV improved, measures of oxygenation increased, $PaCO_2$ fell and peak inspiratory pressure was decreased. In theory, monitoring the Servo Pressure might be a technique to identify when EELV improves. As lung compliance improves with increasing EELV, Servo Pressure should increase in a fashion analogous (but opposite) to changes in ΔPhf as reported with "volume-targeted" HFOV. This was not noted in the study by Musk et al., however; they lowered peak inspiratory pressure with

improvement in EELV and Servo Pressure drops as set peak pressure is decreased (13). Potentially, if peak pressure is kept constant as lung recruitment is performed, then an increase in Servo Pressure could be shown. The addition of a low rate of intermittent tidal inflations (sighs) is another widely used approach to optimizing lung inflation during HFJV, but it has not been well studied (14). However, we are not aware of any clinical studies assessing changes in Servo Pressure as a potential aid to determine optimal EELV during HFJV, nor changes in PIP as a marker of optimal EELV during conventional mechanical ventilation.

Impedance/inductance technology
All of the previously referenced studies assessed EELV via a variety of tools including respiratory inductance plethysmography (RIP) and electrical impedance tomography (EIT). RIP has been available for almost two decades, used almost exclusively in a research capacity. EIT is a newer technology with the potential for increasing clinical application due to improvements in band technology and software/interface development. A more robust discussion of these and other technologies are available in other publications (15–18).

Lung ultrasound
The use of ultrasound to assess for lung disease is a rapidly expanding technology with increasing applications in the neonate (19, 20). Though most studies have focused on identification of neonatal lung disease in preterm infants to facilitate earlier indicated surfactant therapy, studies have also used gray scale analysis to assess relative lung inflation (21). Again, there is limited clinical evidence to provide recommendations for the application of lung US to optimizing EELV, but that may change in the future.

Mechanical ventilation

Many devices and approaches other than those described here can be employed in the management of neonates with HRF. The single most important factor associated with safe and successful ventilator management of the ill neonate is the device *operator*, not the device itself. Recognition of the specific pathophysiology is essential to success in managing HRF in critically ill neonates. Therefore, the approach to ventilation for various lung diseases is described below.

Diffuse alveolar disease
Despite the increasing success with noninvasive respiratory support, many neonates still require mechanical ventilator support for RDS, particularly those at the lowest gestational ages. The indications for and approach to surfactant replacement therapy for neonatal RDS continues to be an area of very active investigation but will not be addressed in this chapter (22–24). Relative immaturity of the neonatal lung, particularly those of extremely low gestation, may increase the risk of ventilator induced lung injury (VILI) (25–27). As noted above, establishing optimal lung volume and avoiding excessive (V_T) are key to lung-protective ventilation strategies in neonates (Tables 33.2 and 33.3).

An active lung recruitment approach is recommended to establish optimal lung volume (Table 33.1, Figure 33.2). Most clinicians typically provide early surfactant replacement therapy to all preterm infants intubated for RDS, then begin the process of optimizing lung inflation. We do not usually reduce PAW to "closing pressure," but more commonly will gradually reduce PAW by 2–3 cmH$_2$O once FiO_2 has been reduced to <0.25. "Optimal" lung

TABLE 33.2 Keys to Managing Neonatal Hypoxic Respiratory Failure

Optimize end-expiratory lung volume (EELV)

PEEP/PAW (recruitment technique)

Minimize oxygen toxicity (lower FiO_2)

Minimize ventilator-induced lung injury (VILI)

High-frequency ventilation (lowest tidal volumes)

Volume-targeted modes (5–6 ml/kg)

Tolerance to relative hypercapnia (45–60 mmHg)

Tolerance to relative hypoxemia

   Target SpO_2 rather than PaO_2

   Target SpO_2 88–95 in absence of acute PH

   Target SpO_2 93–98 if also has acute PH

   Use preductal SPO_2/blood gas to monitor oxygenation

Limit adverse effects of lung volume on CV function

Increase PVR (related to pathophysiology and low/excess lung inflation)

Impaired venous return, CO (lung over-inflation)

Abbreviations: PEEP, positive end-expiratory pressure; PAW, mean airway pressure; SpO_2, pulse oximetry saturations; PaO_2, arterial oxygen tension.

inflation by chest radiograph may be suggested by the relative position of the diaphragm and appearance of the lung parenchyma (Table 33.1, Figure 33.2B). A flattened diaphragm profile should be avoided. Determining optimal lung volume/inflation can be challenging with heterogeneous lung diseases such as meconium aspiration syndrome, pneumonia and severe BPD. It is also more complex with lung hypoplasia disorders where optimum volume may occur at volumes that appear quite low on radiographs. During HFOV, ventilation is dependent on V_T and rate. During HFOV, V_T has a relatively greater effect on minute ventilation than rate. Factors affecting V_T during HFOV include lung compliance and airway resistance, inspiratory time, and the amplitude or power of the oscillatory breath. It is critical to remember that changes in frequency during HFOV can markedly affect V_T (higher as frequency decreases, and lower as frequency increases). Dynamic changes in lung volume and compliance, that accompany increased lung inflation, can significantly impact not only oxygenation but ventilation through effects on V_T (28). Either frequent blood gas assessment or transcutaneous monitoring during the initial implementation of HFOV is recommended. Mild permissive hypercarbia is acceptable to minimize VILI at all gestational and post-natal ages (29).

TABLE 33.3 Ventilation in HRF

	Diffuse Alveolar Disease	Airway Disease	Lung Hypoplasia	Bronchopulmonary Dysplasia
Pathophysiology	Low lung volume ↓ Surfactant function ↓ Lung compliance ↑ V/Q shunt	Obstruction/Local-Diffuse Lung over-expansion ↑ Airway resistance ↑ Time constant	Impaired lung growth ↑ PVR ↓ Lung surface area Hypoxemia, hypercarbia	Multicompartmental lung with largetime constant variations ↑ Airway resistance Airway collapse ↑ Alveolar dead space
High Frequency				
Oscillator	P_{aw} as needed; ~9 rib inflation Lung recruitment	Use lower Hz; 6–8 ΔP vibrate chest/abdomen P_{aw} to support good LV, but not over-expansion	Hz 8–12 range; lower P_{aw} P_{aw} – limit over-inflation; Wean P_{aw} rather than increase for hypoxemia	Rarely indicated due to long time constants, active exhalation collapsing airways
Jet	PEEP as needed; ~9 rib inflation Consider back-up rate 3–5	Lower HF Rate; 240-320 Minimal to no back-up rate	Jet may be preferred mode Limit PEEP as above	Limited data suggest that Jet may be better than oscillator. Low rate (240–320) and high PEEP (10–14)
Conventional				
Volume-targeted	V_T 4–6 ml/kg; AC or SIMV with PS < set PIP *PEEP 5–8* cmH$_2$O; lung recruitment as above Monitor lung graphics	V_T 5–6 ml/kg; rate < 30; PEEP 4–6 cmH$_2$O; with PS < set PIP Monitor lung graphics	V_T 4–4.5 ml/kg AC preferred *PEEP 3–5* cmH$_2$O Faster rate, short I-time Monitor lung graphics	V_T 8–12 ml/kg; rate < 20; long I-time *PEEP 8–15* cmH$_2$O Volume-controlled ventilation may be appropriate Monitor lung graphics
Pressure-controlled	PIP to move chest; Target V_T 4–6 ml/kg PEEP 5–8 cmH$_2$O; PS < set PIP	PIP to move chest; longer I-time Target V_T 5–6 ml/kg PEEP 4–6 cmH$_2$O; PS < set PIP	PIP to move chest; short I-time Target V_T 4–4.5 ml/kg PEEP 3–5 cmH$_2$O;	PIP to move chest, Target V_T 8–12 ml/kg; rate < 20; long I-time PEEP 8–15 cmH$_2$O;
Surfactant	Indicated if radiograph consistent w/ RDS, FiO_2 ≥0.30	May be useful for MAS; may require 2 doses	Indicated if radiograph consistent w/ RDS	No evidence of benefit
Inhaled NO	As indicated by ECHO, OI	As indicated by ECHO, OI	As indicated by ECHO, OI	As indicated by ECHO; transition to sildenafil

In patients with neonatal RDS, the preferred mode for conventional mandatory ventilation (CMV) support is volume-targeted, unless a large (>50%) air leak occurs around the endotracheal tube, in which case a pressure-limited mode may be necessary (30). In general, we prefer slightly higher PEEP values (6–8 cm H_2O) to optimize lung recruitment. Tidal volumes should be set in the 4-6 ml/kg range using clinical assessment of adequacy of support as well as analysis of ventilator graphics to assure V_T is appropriate. If a pressure-limited mode is used the goal is targeting measured tidal volumes of around 5 ml/kg (inaccurate if large leak is present). Assist control mode is preferred by many; pressure support is commonly employed if using SIMV to minimize work of breathing, yet encourage diaphragmatic activity, while intubated (30, 31).

There is no convincing evidence from randomized controlled trials (RCT) in the era of surfactant availability that an "open-lung" approach to HFOV results in improved outcomes compared to conventional ventilation via a "lung-protective," volume-targeted approach (32). Despite this lack of evidence, many centers employ HFV for "rescue" of neonates with severe HRF.

Meconium aspiration syndrome

Infants with severe meconium aspiration syndrome (MAS) often require ventilator support (33–35). MAS has a complex, multifactorial pathophysiology that may include surfactant dysfunction, airway obstruction, and pulmonary hypertension (PH). The clinical features of MAS may be variable between infants and change during the course of management; thus, the ventilatory approach must be individualized and reassessed often (Tables 33.2 and 33.3).

Disturbances in surfactant metabolism and function lead to atelectasis and intrapulmonary shunt (36–38). Establishing an optimal EELV via lung recruitment techniques remains a primary goal, however this approach is not well studied. With severe MAS there needs to be a balance between the benefits of an open lung approach improving areas of atelectasis versus over-expansion of those lung areas with airway obstruction. Evidence for surfactant therapy in MAS is less compelling than for neonatal RDS. Nonetheless, studies do suggest that early use in babies with significant alveolar disease may reduce the need for ECMO (39). Beyond the use of surfactant replacement therapy in an effort to improve lung compliance, lung inflation should be optimized through judicious application of PEEP and/or PAW using clinical tools such as blood pressure, gas exchange and chest radiographs. Acute PH is a common and significant problem in infants with severe MAS (40, 41) and makes oxygenation-guided lung volume recruitment difficult. Adjunct therapy with inhaled nitric oxide (iNO), other pulmonary vasodilators, as well as inotropic support of the right ventricle, may be required for management of the PH if optimization of lung volume and hemodynamics fail.

The key to ventilator management in MAS is recognition of the predominant underlying pathophysiology (42). Given the relative infrequency of MAS, there are no randomized trials to suggest the best ventilator approach or mode (Table 33.3). It is important to recognize the impact of increased airway resistance and potential lung over-distention when using HFV. Due to increased time constants, initial rates of 6–8 Hz may be indicated with HFOV, and 300–340 with HFJV. For infants with poor lung inflation, PAW is typically started at least 3 cmH_2O above that on conventional ventilation and then adjusted based on FiO_2 response and radiographic assessment of lung inflation. With significant air-trapping, a frequency of 6Hz via HFOV or a rate

of ≤320 via HFJV may minimize inadvertent air trapping. A volume-targeted approach should generally be used for conventional mechanical ventilation (Table 33.3). The same guiding principles should be used for initiating and adjusting support as described above. When air trapping is the predominant pathology, it may be related to inadvertent (dynamic) PEEP with inadequate expiratory time in the face of long expiratory time constant. Set PEEP may need to be limited (≤6 cmH_2O) with lower set rates (≤30 bpm), to allow adequate expiratory time and minimize gas trapping. As inspiratory time constants may be prolonged, attention must be paid to ensure that the I-time is long enough to complete V_T delivery. The flow waveform of the ventilator display needs to be inspected to ensure that both inspiratory and expiratory flow is completed. For infants with predominantly alveolar disease and low lung volumes, PEEP should set at higher levels (6–8 cm H_2O) and adjusted as needed to achieve an acceptable EELV. As alveolar dead space may be higher with MAS, infants with severe disease may require larger V_T (6 ml/kg) than infants with more homogeneous lung disease (43).

Lung hypoplasia disorders

HRF due to disorders of lung hypoplasia remains one of the most challenging neonatal lung disorders to manage (Table 33.3). Although evidence from RCTs are limited, adoption of a "gentle" approach to ventilator support has been associated with improvements in morbidity and mortality in congenital diaphragmatic hernia (CDH) and other etiologies of lung hypoplasia (44–47). It remains unclear, however, what the best ventilation mode is to provide "gentle" support (48, 49). The only RCT to date is the VICI trial comparing HFOV to CMV (48). Although there was no difference in the primary outcome of survival without BPD, the CMV group, which was managed with significantly lower airway pressures than the HFOV group, had less inotrope use and decreased need of extracorporeal membrane oxygenation. Excessive PAW as used in the VICI trial contributes to lung over-inflation and cardiopulmonary dysfunction in several ways including altered lung mechanics, compression of pulmonary vasculature, and limited ventricular preload due to impaired venous return (44, 50–52).

The most obvious pathophysiologic problem is impaired lung growth, with severity linked to how early in gestation lung growth is affected. The specific mechanisms for impaired lung development in the context of processes promoting lung hypoplasia are beyond the scope of this chapter; the reader is referred to other reviews for more information (53–55).

Over 30 years ago Wung et al. published their seminal work describing a "lung-sparing" or "gentle" approach to mechanical ventilation of neonates with severe HRF, including lung hypoplasia (46, 47). There are several key principles to the management of babies with lung hypoplasia including: (a) Start at a lower PEEP/PAW than typically used with normally grown lungs, (b) recognize that lung over-inflation may occur with radiographic lung volumes well below expected and "flattening" of the diaphragm may be a better marker, and (c) PH or impaired right ventricular performance are important factors contributing to hypoxemia. Again, there is no evidence that one specific mode of ventilation is superior to another. There is limited clinical evidence that suggests HFJV may be the optimal ventilatory approach in babies with lung hypoplasia related to the use of small tidal volumes and a lower PAW while minimizing adverse cardiovascular effects (50–52, 56, 57).

Irrespective of the ventilatory approach used for managing lung hypoplasia, several key concepts must be kept in mind. First, the lung is small, with a functional residual capacity considerably less than normal (58). Given the effects that both atelectasis and hyperinflation have on pulmonary microvasculature and PVR, careful attention must be paid to optimizing lung inflation (59–61). In that regard, the PAW needed to achieve optimal lung inflation may be less than that required for a normal-sized lung, even with surfactant dysfunction as in preterm infants. It is also much more difficult to determine optimal PAW and lung inflation under conditions of lung hypoplasia. Attempting to employ the stepwise increase in PAW as with RDS is not currently recommended with lung hypoplasia. This may be especially problematic with underlying PH. An alternate, but unproven, approach is to start at a lower PAW and assess radiographic lung inflation; if classic features of diffuse airway disease are present, then PAW should be increased, but if the lungs are relatively clear, a reduction in PAW may be more appropriate. The minute ventilation necessary to achieve normocarbia should be the same as for infants with normal lungs, thus with smaller number of alveoli the risk of volutrauma is increased. This would suggest a theoretical advantage for HFV and/or higher rates (i.e. 60 bpm) and lower V_T (4 mL/kg) (62). Those infants with the greatest degree of lung hypoplasia have increased dead space-to-V_T ratios, suggesting that more of the applied V_T is "lost" as ineffective dead space ventilation (63). Oxygenation is dependent as much on the impaired pulmonary vascular bed as it is on relative lung volumes. Adjustments in ventilator support must be made with the recognition that altered oxygenation could be due to increased PVR related to factors other than changes in lung inflation/volume.

Bronchopulmonary dysplasia (BPD)

The prominent feature of BPD pathophysiology is heterogeneity of parenchymal and airway involvement, resulting in marked regional variability in time constants resulting in multi-compartmental lung physiology (64). This heterogeneity results in increased alveolar dead space and makes it difficult to ventilate the lungs optimally. Areas with relatively low airway resistance, referred to as "fast compartments," fill and empty relatively rapidly, but the regions that have high airway resistance ("slow compartments") require more time to inflate and even longer to deflate. Consequently, much slower respiratory rates and longer inspiratory and expiratory times are required to optimize ventilation in infants with established BPD. The increased alveolar and anatomical dead space result in a great deal of wasted ventilation. This coupled with the slower ventilator rate requires leads to a need for much larger (V_T) than acute RDS – V_T of 8-12mL/kg, or higher, may be needed with set ventilator rate of ≤20/min. SIMV with PS is the preferred mode; the slow rate large V_T inflations of SIMV ventilate the slow compartments while the more rapid spontaneous breaths with PS ventilate the fast compartments. Higher than usual PEEP is needed to maintain airway patency of the poorly-supported small airways that tend to collapse as the lung empties, as well as the large airways that are often susceptible to collapse due to trachea-bronchomalacia. The focus of respiratory support in established BPD shifts from a push to extubate, to a chronic care model that emphasizes optimal support while allowing for growth and developmentally appropriate activities. Adequacy of support is better judged by resting respiratory rate and ability to be interactive, than by blood gas measurement. Permissive hypercarbia (as long as well compensated) and generous SpO_2 targets are recommended. Chronic PH is a feared complication of severe BPD and should be actively sought by regular echocardiograms to appraise PVR, severity of PH and the

adaptive response of the right ventricle. If present it may require treatment with iNO (to establish responsiveness) followed by transition to other approaches for treatment of PH.

Extracorporeal membrane oxygenation

Extracorporeal membrane oxygenation (ECMO) remains an alternative life-saving therapy to manage neonates with HRF (65). ECMO is a complex form of ECLS utilizing external oxygenation and ventilation to support patient organ dysfunction refractory to conventional treatment. First reported in 1975 for a newborn with meconium aspiration, neonatal HRF remains the most common indication for ECMO despite increasing utilization in the adult, pediatric, and neonatal cardiac populations since 2005 (66–68). As of 2020, over 30,000 infants have received ECMO for neonatal HRF, with a reported survival rate to decannulation of 87%. Despite overall high survivability to decannulation and reduction in patient and mechanical complications over time, there remains a high rate of morbidities and risks associated with ECMO and ultimate survival to discharge is now around 70% (68).

Patient candidacy

Most ECMO facilities have standardized criteria for ECMO consideration based on clinical course, respiratory support needs, physiologic and laboratory parameters, and risk of estimated mortality. Common physiologic criteria for ECMO support include reversible cardiorespiratory failure, an oxygenation index of >40, PaO_2/FiO_2 ratios of <80, lack of response to optimal mechanical ventilation and other rescue therapies, and need for high ventilator pressures or evidence VILI (67, 68). Cardiac decompensation manifested as poor oxygen delivery, organ hypoperfusion, hypotension despite use of two medications, oxygen saturations <50%, or persistent lactate >4.0 are important but less well standardized indications for ECLS.

Commonly reported exclusion considerations for ECMO include significant prematurity (<34 weeks), birth weight below 1800g, suspected lethal genetic conditions, existing or evolving severe brain damage, or ongoing bleeding (67, 68). However, recent trends in patient case reports and outcomes have made these relative contraindications as gestational age, patient size thresholds, and genetic diagnoses have reported improved survival (69, 70). Additionally, as anticoagulation strategies become more refined, the management of bleeding, including intracranial intraventricular hemorrhage should not exclude all candidates (67–72).

Cannulation approaches and types of ECMO

Neonates may be placed on veno-venous (VV) ECMO which diverts blood back to the venous system or veno-arterial (VA) ECMO which diverts blood back to the arterial circulation, bypassing pulmonary circulation (73, 74). Like older patients, neonates may undergo extracorporeal cardiopulmonary resuscitation (ECPR) in which VA ECMO is initiated in the setting of cardiopulmonary arrest (73). VA ECMO is commonly accomplished through separate cannulation of the right carotid artery and internal jugular vein. VV ECMO utilizes single venous cannulation of the jugular vein using a specialized dual lumen catheter providing drainage of the superior and inferior vena cava with oxygenated blood directed toward the tricuspid valve.

Decision for type of cannulation is often dependent on primary indication, ventricular performance, facility clinical preference, availability of appropriate equipment, and the size of the patient and great vessels at cannulation site in the neonate. Both VV and VA ECMO share risks inherent of surgical/percutaneous instrumentation, systemic anticoagulation, endothelial injury, and perfusion issues related to manipulation of blood vessels. The potential benefits of VV over VA ECMO include preservation of intact carotid artery, decreasing the risk of myocardial stun, maintaining native pulsatile blood flows, potentially shorter cannulation times, and the use of the lungs as filter for thromboemboli as opposed to direct access to the systemic and cerebral circulation (73, 74). VA ECMO on the other hand, provides the benefit of direct cardiac output support for systemic perfusion and greater efficiency. Additionally, VA cannulation can be achieved with a smaller diameter cannula, utilizing smaller great vessels than a dual-lumen VV cannula. Long-term outcomes in mortality and development tend to favor VV cannulation, but this may reflect selection bias (73, 74). According to the ELSO registry (2015–2020), approximately 75% of neonatal respiratory cases were supported with VA ECMO, with decreasing use of VV ECMO due to clinical challenges with obtaining appropriate equipment (68).

Circuit pump and oxygenator choice

Circuit flow is generated through a pump incorporated into the ECMO circuit. Currently, both roller-head and centrifugal pumps are used in neonates, with both techniques having theoretical advantages in terms of complications. Roller-head pumps generate propulsion through semi-occlusion of circuit tubing, with circuit flow a product of revolutions per minute (rpm) of the pump head, the degree of occlusion produced by the rollers, and the internal diameter of the tubing. Roller pumps may induce high arterial pressure levels, thereby leading to disruption of connections, as well as negative venous pressure levels, with the risk of endothelial damage in the cannulated veins (75, 76). Centrifugal pumps act through a spinning rotor to generate blood flow. This technique avoids high pressures in the case of distal circuit occlusion, but it may induce shear stress and turbulence to blood cells that may lead to increased hemolysis and thromboembolic complications. A recent survey of ELSO-registered ECMO centers worldwide demonstrated that 53% of neonatal and pediatric centers continue to use roller pumps (77). The use of roller-head and centrifugal pumps remains controversial as clinicians balance conflicting reports of risk of hemolysis, hyperbilirubinemia, hypertension, acute renal failure, and overall survival between groups (75–78).

Gas exchange occurs through the circuit oxygenator, an artificial lung that adds oxygen and removes carbon dioxide. Initially, ECMO utilized spirally-wound silicone membrane oxygenators, which were effective, but prone to clot formation because of stagnant flow and a very large surface area in contact with blood. Recent advances in membrane oxygenator technology solved the problem of plasma leak, so that now most programs utilize polymethyl pentene, nonporous hollow fiber oxygenators to provide efficient gas exchange (78). Gas exchange occurs via diffusion across the semipermeable membrane, without direct contact between blood and ventilating gas, with low resistance to flow and small priming volumes that are important for neonates (65, 67, 73).

Anticoagulation and its related complications

Anticoagulation is generally required to prevent circuit and patient-related thrombotic events. Regardless of indication and type of ECMO employed, there is a fine balance between the complications of thrombosis and bleeding, complicated by the developmental hemostasis of neonates compared to adults (71). According to the ELSO registry, 35% of patients require a circuit change or change of components due to thrombotic issues; intracranial hemorrhage (ICH) occurred in 10% of neonates with a respiratory indication, representing the most common patient-related complication associated with mortality (39% associated survival).

Anticoagulation strategies vary between institutions, and there is currently no consensus on the best method to manage anticoagulation and blood product administration in patients supported with ECMO (71, 79). Unfractionated heparin is the most widely used systemic anticoagulant in the initiation and maintenance of ECMO (68–72). Bivalirudin, a direct thrombin inhibitor, is a useful alternative to heparin for anticoagulation in neonates (72, 80). Bivalirudin, unlike heparin, does not require antithrombin to be effective, and as a result, has the potential to provide more consistent anticoagulation (72, 80). Limited clinical studies suggest that bivalirudin is as effective as heparin at reaching target-activated clotting times or activated partial thromboplastin times, with equivalent or the lower rates of bleeding or thromboembolic complications. Only recently has bivalirudin use begun to be validated with large group studies in the neonatal population despite successful utilization in many ECMO centers (72, 80).

Recent trends and controversies

Along with changing trends for ECMO indication, the overall survival for neonatal ECMO has recently decreased since 2000 (75%), with a 69% overall survival rate reported in 2019 (68). Historically, MAS, CDH, and refractory PH were the most common indications for ECMO consideration, representing over 75% of cases (67, 68). As of 2020, the ELSO registry now reports "other" conditions as the primary indication for neonatal respiratory ECMO, suggesting expanded patient candidacy and indications. This likely reflects increasingly complex neonatal patients deemed candidates for ECMO along with the decreased utilization for conditions like MAS, a condition with greater than 90% ECMO survival (68). Declines in MAS cases are attributed to improved medical strategies for HRF including adjunct therapies like iNO, exogenous surfactant, high frequency and other "gentle lung" strategies and refined selection of cardiovascular drugs using targeted neonatal echocardiography (67, 68). However, use for CDH and PH has remained consistent, despite these interventions (67, 68). Additionally, use of ECMO for RDS continues to increase as the prematurity threshold for inclusion continues to be pushed.69 Most current clinical guidelines suggest ECMO is contraindicated in neonates < 34–35 weeks, attributed to early reports of increased ICH and poor overall survival (69, 70). However, recent studies support consideration at lower gestational ages approaching a threshold of 29 weeks, citing similar rates of ICH despite inherent higher mortality and risk of thrombotic injury (70). Current limitation for this population is reflected in the size of cannula placement with some centers advocating for utilization of smaller 6Fr arterial cannulas (67–70).

Finally, neonatal ECMO is increasingly utilized for conditions other than bridge to recovery from a primary diagnosis. ECLS can additionally be utilized as organ support for ECPR, renal recovery, long-term cardiac support, bridge to surgical intervention, organ transplant, organ donation, and ultimately bridge to decision making for families (67).

Summary

A variety of respiratory disorders may be encountered in the neonatal period, the most common of which have been discussed in this chapter. A firm understanding of the underlying pathophysiology, and how it may change over time, is necessary to optimally apply any approach to mechanical ventilation. A variety of ventilatory modes are available although there is limited evidence to strongly support one mode or approach over another for most conditions. Given the limited evidence base for much of the care we provide, there is much to be gained through controlled interventional trials within collaborative networks. It is critical to recognize that the lungs of all newborns are not developmentally complete (not just the most premature) and may be more susceptible to VILI. Protocols for weaning and extubation are also strongly recommended. The most important factor associated with safe and successful ventilator management of the sick neonate is the person operating the ventilator rather than the ventilator itself.

References

1. Cheifetz IM. Respir Care. 2014; 59(12):1937–4195.
2. Rimensberger PC, et al. Intensive Care Med. 2000; 26(6):745–755.
3. Pellicano A, et al. Intensive Care Med. 2009; 35(11):1990–1998.
4. Burkhardt W, et al. Neonatology. 2013; 103(3):218–223.
5. Miedema M, et al. Front Pediatr. 2019; 6:436.
6. De Jaegere A, et al. Am J Respir Crit Care Med. 2006; 174(6):639–645.
7. Tingay DG, et al. Crit Care Med. 2013; 41(1):237–244.
8. Zannin E, et al. Pediatr Res. 2014; 75(4):493–499.
9. Weber K, et al. J Appl Physiol (1985). 2000; 89(1):364–372.
10. Miedema M, et al. Intensive Care Med. 2012; 38(2):294–299.
11. Rodríguez Sánchez de la Blanca A, et al. Pediatr Pulmonol. 2020; 55(12):3525–3531.
12. de Jager P, et al. Ann Intensive Care. 2020; 10(1):153.
13. Musk GC, et al. Pediatr Res. 2011; 69(4):319–324.
14. Keszler M, et al. Crit Care Med. 1986; 14(1):34–38.
15. Bhatia R, et al. J Pediatr. 2017; 187:80.e2–88.e2.
16. Frerichs I, et al. Thorax. 2017; 72(1):83–93.
17. Gaertner VD, et al. Am J Respir Crit Care Med. 2020, in publication. doi:10.1164/rccm.202007-2701OC.
18. King A, et al. Acta Paediatr. 2020; 109(4):667–678.
19. Bello G, et al. J Ultrasound Med. 2019; 38(1):27–37.
20. Sharma D, et al. J Matern Fetal Neonatal Med. 2019; 32(2):310–316.
21. Raimondi F, et al. PLoS One. 2018; 13(10):e0202397.
22. Polin RA, et al. Pediatrics. 2014 Jan; 133(1):156–163.
23. Brix N, et al. BMC Pediatr. 2014; 14:155.
24. Herting E. Early Hum Dev. 2013; 89(11):875–880.
25. Clark RH, et al. J Pediatr. 2001; 139(4):478–486.
26. Dargaville PA, et al. J Paediatr Child Health. 2012; 48(9):740–746.
27. van Kaam AH, et al. Crit Care Med. 2007; 35(3):925–931.
28. Miedema M, et al. Am J Respir Crit Care Med. 2011; 184(1):100–105.
29. Ryu J, et al. Clin Perinatol. 2012; 39(3):603–612.
30. Keszler M. Arch Dis Child Fetal Neonatal Ed. 2019; 104(1):F108–F112.
31. Patel DS, et al. Arch Dis Child. 2009; 94(6):434–436.
32. Cools F, et al. Cochrane Database Syst Rev. 2005; 19(3):CD000104.
33. Wiswell TE et al. Pediatrics. 2000; 105(1 Pt 1):1–7.
34. Vain NE, et al. Lancet. 2004; 364(9434):597–602.
35. Yoder BA. Obstet Gynecol. 1994; 83(1):77–84.
36. Hofer N, et al. Pediatr Pulmonol. 2016; 51(6):601–606.
37. Janssen DJ, et al. J Pediatr. 2006; 149(5):634–639.
38. Lopez-Rodriguez E, et al. Biophys J. 2011; 100(3):646–655.
39. Dargaville PA, et al. J Pediatr. 2011; 158(3):383–389.
40. Choudhary M, et al. J Matern Fetal Neonatal Med. 2016; 29(2):324–327.
41. Hsieh TK, et al. Acta Paediatr Taiwan. 2004; 45(4):203–207.
42. Dargaville PA. Int J Pediatr 2012; 2012:965159.
43. Sharma S, et al. Am J Perinatol. 2015; 32(10):916–919.
44. Williams O, et al. Neonatology. 2012; 101(2):83–90.
45. de Waal K, et al. J Pediatr. 2015; 166(5):1113–1120.
46. Wung JT, et al. Pediatrics. 1985; 76(4):488–494.
47. Wung JT, et al. J Pediatr Surg. 1995; 30:406–409.
48. Snoek KG, et al. Ann Surg. 2016; 263:867–874.
49. Yang MJ, et al. J Perinatol. 2020; 40(6):935–942.
50. Otto CW, et al. Anesth Analg. 1983; 62:298–304.
51. Boros SJ, et al. Pediatr Pulmonol. 1989; 7(1):35–41.
52. Meliones JN, et al. Circulation. 1991; 84(5 Suppl):III 364–368.
53. Muehlethaler V, et al. Am J Physiol Lung Cell Mol Physiol. 2008; 294(1):L110–L120.
54. Boucherat O, et al. Am J Physiol Lung Cell Mol Physiol. 2010; 298(6):L849–L856.
55. Solari V, et al. J Pediatr Surg. 2003; 38(5):808–813.
56. Zobel G, et al. Crit Care Med. 1994; 22:1624–1630.
57. Engle WA, et al. J Perinatol. 1997; 17(1):3–9.
58. Landolfo F, et al. J Pediatr Surg. 2013; 48(7):1459–1462.
59. Shekerdemian L, et al. Arch Dis Child. 1999; 80(5):475–480.
60. Gattinoni L, et al. Crit Care. 2018; 22(1):264.
61. Guevorkian D, et al. J Pediatr. 2018; 200:38–43.
62. Sharma S, et al. Am J Perinatol. 2015; 32(6):577–582.
63. Arnold JH, et al. Crit Care Med. 1995; 23(2):371–375.
64. Abman SH, et al. J Pediatr. 2017; 181:12.e1–28.e1.
65. Brogan TV, et al. *Extracorporeal Life Support: The ELSO Red Book*, 5th ed. Ann Arbor, Michigan: Extracorporeal Life Support Organization; 2017.
66. Bartlett RH. ASAIO J. 2017; 63(6):832–843.
67. Mahmood B, et al. Semin Perinatol. 2018; 42(2):80–88.
68. Wild KT, et al. ASAIO Journal. 2020; 66(5):463–470.
69. Wild KT, et al. Fetal Diagn Ther. 2020; 47(12):927–932.
70. Rozmiarek AJ, et al. J Pediatr Surg. 2004; 39(6):845–847.
71. Cashen K, et al. Front Pediatr. 2019; 7:366.
72. Hamzah M, et al. Pediatr Crit Care Med. 2020; 21(9):827–834.
73. Rais-Bahrami K, et al. Semin Perinaatol. 2014; 38(2):71–77.
74. Keckler SJ, et al. Eur J Pediatr Surg. 2010; 20(1):1–4.
75. Green TP, et al. ASAIO Trans. 1991; 37(4):572–576.
76. Barrett CS, et al. Ann Thorac Surg. 2012; 94(5):1635–1641.
77. O'Halloran CP, et al. Pediatr Crit Care Med. 2019; 20(12):1177–1184.
78. Dalton HJ, et al. Pediatr Crit Care. 2019; 20(12):1195–1196.
79. Bembea MM, et al. Pediatr Crit Care Med. 2013; 14(2):e77–e84.
80. Buck ML. J Pediatr Pharmacol Ther. 2015; 20(6):408–417.

PULMONARY HYPERTENSION PHENOTYPES IN THE NEWBORN

Regan E. Giesinger, John P. Kinsella, Steven H. Abman and Patrick J. McNamara

Contents

Pulmonary hypertension is defined as a pathological elevation in pressure in the pulmonary vascular bed. It has numerous consequences which have been detailed extensively in this textbook and may include right ventricular dilation, hypertrophy and dysfunction due to afterload and impaired pulmonary blood flow with systemic consequences such as low cardiac output, hypoxemia and abnormal LV mechanics. Although most commonly thought of as a primary disorder of elevated resistance of the arterial side of the pulmonary circulation, neonates may also experience elevated pulmonary artery pressure (PAP) for a variety of other reasons. Understanding the fundamental biologic nature of elevated PAP, and relevant confounding variables, are essential determinants of a physiology-based approach to treatment. Mean PAP (mPAP) depends on flow (cardiac output and shunts), pulmonary vascular resistance (PVR) and downstream pressure in the left atrium. It may be calculated using the following formula where pulmonary capillary wedge pressure (PCWP) is a surrogate for left atrial pressure:

$$mPAP = [PVR \times CO] + PCWP$$

It is therefore important to consider pathological changes in each variable, as potential contributors to disease. In this chapter we will review the phenotypic variance of both acute and chronic pulmonary hypertension, and the unique relationship between lung compliance, PVR and heart function of each phenotype. All of these variables need consideration when formulating an approach to clinical treatment.

Biological phenotypes contributing to acute pulmonary hypertension (aPH) in neonates

Both cardiovascular and lung parenchymal disease may present with hypoxemic respiratory failure in the perinatal period. It is common for elements of more than one lung parenchymal pathology (e.g. atelectasis, edema, local hyper-expansion) and more than one contributor to pulmonary vascular pathology

(e.g. pulmonary arterial remodeling, hypoxic vasoconstriction, alveolar compression of intra-acinar vessels) to be present simultaneously. It is also important to note that after identification of a presumptive or definitive diagnosis, treatment aimed at optimizing gas exchange may have significant impact on the cardiovascular system and vice versa. Clinical assessment is often challenging as there is significant overlap between disease phenotypes; therefore, a high index of suspicion for cardiac/pulmonary vascular disease is important. While the potential contributors to lung parenchymal disease are commonly discussed, there is less emphasis on the spectrum of physiology that may play a role in the cardiovascular contributors to hypoxemia (Table 34.1)

Acute pulmonary hypertension (PH) phenotype of arterial (classic) origin

In the early postnatal period, a rapid decline in PVR is essential for the transition from the placenta to the lungs as the primary organ of gas exchange. This is accomplished by labor-induced changes in the fetal lung from a fluid-secreting to fluid-absorbing phenotype (1), compression of the fetus thereby increasing abdominal pressure to aid in fluid expulsion (2) and finally a large negative inspiratory pressure generated by neonatal breathing that forces the remaining fluid into the interstitial space (3). The aeration of alveoli prompts vascular dilation and blood flow to the lungs and the establishment of functional residual capacity (FRC) lowers PVR (4). Factors that may interfere with this process may include failure of the initiation of spontaneous neonatal respirations, failure to achieve FRC, inadequate clearance of fetal lung water, primary parenchymal lung disease, and other factors. Regardless of etiology, either diffuse or localized areas of hypoxic vasoconstriction, which is a normal adaption to optimize ventilation to perfusion (V/Q) matching, occurs. If a large portion of the pulmonary vascular bed is involved, this may manifest as the clinical phenotype most commonly associated with neonatal aPH. Although in all cases the most important first management step is to establish alveolar aeration and recruitment, it is important to remember that normally compliant lungs may

DOI: 10.1201/9780367494018-34

TABLE 34.1 Phenotypic Contributors to Elevated Main Pulmonary Artery Pressure with Associated Pathophysiology, Echocardiography Features and Treatment Approach

Subtype	Pathophysiology	Characteristic ECHO Features	Physiologic Approach to Treatment
Acute PH Phenotype			
Classic	Hypoxic pulmonary vasoconstriction, V/Q mismatch	Dilated RV, ↓LVO, septal flattening in systole, predominantly R→L shunts, ↑PVRi, PA Doppler notching	Optimal lung parenchyma and recruitment, pulmonary vasodilators, systemic vasoconstrictors which do not ↑PVR
Shunt mediated	High volume of blood in a circuit with limited compliance, endothelial damage, oxidative stress	Dilated RV or LV, discrepant ventricular outputs with either ↑RVO, ↑LVO or both septal flattening in diastole if ASD/VSD	Manage shunt; maintain ↑PVR, avoid selective pulmonary vasodilators
Left heart mediated	Impaired flow through pulmonary circuit due to poor LV compliance and high LVEDP	Dilated LV, LV systolic and diastolic dysfunction (↓MVE, ↑IVRT, ↓PV velocities), MR and/or AI, ↓LVO	↓ LV afterload, (+) inotropy, maintenance of R→L ductal shunt if ↓SBF, maintain ↑PVR, diuretics (pulmonary edema)
Chronic PH Phenotype			
Classic	Pulmonary vascular remodeling, intermittent hypoxia	Dilated RV, ↓LVO, septal flattening in systole, predominantly R→L shunts, ↑PVRi, PA Doppler notching	Optimal lung parenchyma and recruitment, pulmonary vasodilators
Shunt mediated	High volume of blood in a circuit with limited compliance, vascular remodeling, interstitial edema	Dilated RV or LV, discrepant ventricular outputs with either ↑RVO, ↑LVO or both septal flattening in diastole if ASD/VSD	Manage shunt; maintain ↑PVR, avoid selective pulmonary vasodilators
Systemic hypertension	High LV afterload leads to ↑LVEDP, LA hypertension, pulmonary venous congestion	Dilated LV, LV diastolic dysfunction (↓MVE, ↑IVRT, ↓PV velocities), MR and/or AI	Antihypertensive therapy, potential role specifically for ACE inhibitors/ARBs

Abbreviations: V/Q, ventilation/perfusion; LV, left ventricle; LVEDP, left ventricular end-diastolic pressure; LA, left atrium; RV, right ventricle; LVO, left ventricular output; R, right; L, left; PVRi, pulmonary vascular resistance index; PA, pulmonary artery; RVO, right ventricular output; ASD, atrial septal defect; VSD, ventricular septal defect; MVE, mitral valve early wave; IVRT, isovolumetric relaxation time; PV, pulmonary vein; MR, mitral regurgitation; AI, aortic insufficiency; PVR, pulmonary vascular resistance; SBF, systemic blood flow; ACE, angiotensin converting enzyme; ARB, angiotensin II receptor blocker.

appear phenotypically similar to diseased lungs at the outset. Assessment of compliance and avoidance of overdistension is essential. It is possible to generate intra-alveolar pressures that are greater than pulmonary venous pressure using standard hand-bagging or ventilator settings. Compromised pulmonary venous flow secondary to over-distension may be clinically difficult to distinguish from progressive PH. This is particularly important in the patient population with hypoxic ischemic encephalopathy (HIE). It is common for patients with HIE to have high mPAP with very little or no lung disease, and therefore no issue with lung compliance. Added afterload imposed by overdistension has the potential to be detrimental to already compromised RV systolic performance. Low cardiac output further results in poor aortic root pressure and impaired RV perfusion via the coronary circulation. RV dysfunction, both related to and/or independent of the fundamental disturbance in the pulmonary vascular bed, is a common problem among patients with HIE and has been associated with the degree of subsequent brain injury (5). The most appropriate management strategy of patients with this phenotype is to focus first on appropriate lung recruitment followed by a pulmonary vasodilator strategy, with blood pressure support as needed by vasopressors which do not vasoconstrict the pulmonary vascular bed.

Acute PH phenotype related to excessive pulmonary blood flow

Even in the presence of normal PVR, a high volume of flow through the pulmonary vascular circuit may result in elevated mPAP for the following reasons. *First*, a greater amount of blood is forced through a circulation with a limited vascular capacity to expand to accommodate it creates higher pressure against vascular walls. Animal models, however, suggest less obvious consequences of pulmonary over-circulation that further complicate the relationship of shunt to pulmonary hypertension. Unlike the systemic circulation, which adapts to increased flow by dilating to normalize shear stress (6) and increasing expression of nitric oxide synthase (NOS) to increase relaxation capacity (7), the pulmonary circulation may respond negatively to elevated blood flow. Compared to unexposed mature dogs, pulmonary artery rings isolated from animals with an arterial-to-venous shunt (creating a 3:1 Qp:Qs) exhibit lower vasorelaxation both through endothelium-dependent and -independent pathways (8). Although under normal circumstances, the fetal endothelium readily releases nitric oxide (NO) in response to sheer stress, PH impairs endothelium-dependent pulmonary vasodilation, possibly through attenuation of inducible NO synthase in a lamb experimental model (9, 10). Neonatal swine exposed to shunt demonstrate paradoxical vasoconstriction

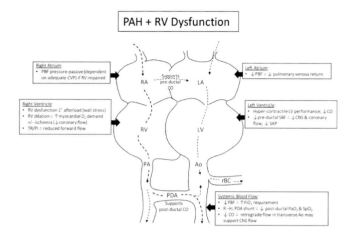

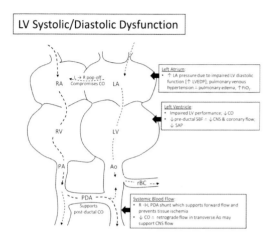

FIGURE 34.1 Physiological changes in blood flow and heart function for patients with classic acute pulmonary hypertension compared with left ventricular systolic/diastolic dysfunction-mediated pulmonary venous hypertension. PBF, pulmonary blood flow; RV, right ventricle; O_2, oxygen; TR, tricuspid regurgitation; PI, pulmonary insufficiency; RA, right atrium; PA, pulmonary artery; PDA, patent ductus arteriosus; CO, cardiac output; LA, left atrium; LV, left ventricle; Ao, aorta; rBC, right brachiocephalic; SBF, systemic blood flow; CNS, central nervous system; SAP, systolic arterial pressure; FiO_2, fraction of inspired oxygen; R, right; L, left; PaO_2, arterial partial pressure of oxygen; SpO_2, oxygen saturation; LVEDP, left ventricular end diastolic pressure; PAH, pulmonary arterial hypertension; CVP, central venous pressure

in response to acetylcholine, supporting the hypothesis of endothelial dysfunction in immature animals (11). Neonatal lambs exposed to shunt demonstrate uncoupling of endothelial NOS (eNOS) from nicotinamide adenine dinucleotide phosphate (NADPH), which results in lower production of NO and instead, generation of superoxide, which in turn binds any available NO to create vasoconstricting peroxynitrite (12). In the setting of inhibited NO generation, late-gestation fetal lambs demonstrate a linear increase in PVR when partial ductal occlusion is used to increase PBF. This phenomenon may be related to an exaggerated myogenic response which may become an important regulatory mechanism when NO-dependent vasoreactivity is impaired (13). It is biologically plausible that these changes represent an innate attempt to limit over-circulation by reducing the systemic vascular resistance (SVR):PVR ratio, however, that speculation remains to be evaluated. An extreme example of this phenomenon may be the patient with Vein of Galen Aneurysmal Malformation (VGAM). These patients, who have a large systemic to venous connection in the preductal circulation, may present with dilated right heart structures and exclusively right to left ductal shunt consistent with PH. However, treatment with pulmonary vasodilator therapy to manage perceived PAH may be disadvantageous. In these patients, right to left ductal shunt may be used to supply post-ductal organ perfusion in a similar manner to the treatment of aortic coarctation. Treatment which lowers PVR may reduce the right-to-left pressure gradient and thereby compromise post-ductal perfusion. Among patients with chronic PDA which is not managed to limit excessive flow, prolonged shunt exposure has been associated with the development of BPD and chronic PH (14, 15). In all cases of shunt-mediated PH, shunt control is of primary importance as the bedrock of management.

Acute PH phenotype due to left ventricular dysfunction

While external compression with excessive positive pressure ventilation is one avenue to develop pulmonary venous flow obstruction, so too is left heart disease. With each cardiac cycle, a failing left ventricle ejects a less than optimal proportion of its end-diastolic volume resulting in a gradual escalation of left ventricular

end-diastolic pressure (LVEDP). This increased pressure is transmitted backwards through the circuit, resulting in left atrial and pulmonary venous congestion. High pressure in the pulmonary veins leads to a hydrostatic gradient to the interstitium and pulmonary edema (Figure 34.1). Similar to shunt physiology, neonatal piglets exposed to pulmonary venous hypertension due to partial obstruction to pulmonary venous drainage develop endothelial dysfunction with loss of endothelium dependent vasodilation (16). The effects of post-capillary pulmonary hypertension on the right-sided circulation are similar to classic PH; however, the treatment may be different. Administration of pulmonary vasodilator therapy to neonates with pulmonary venous disease has been associated with flash pulmonary edema (17), which is hypothesized to be due to reduction in pre-capillary driving pressure in the setting of downstream obstruction. This may lead to a buildup of relatively static blood in the small pulmonary vessels and a further increase in hydrostatic pressure relative to the interstitial space. Newborns with congenital diaphragmatic hernia (CDH) represent an important population in which this phenomenon is accentuated, and if not considered by the clinician may lead to an incorrect approach to treatment. Both left (LV) and right (RV) ventricular dysfunction may be present in the transitional period, and while a component of LV disease may be associated with interventricular interaction, several investigators have demonstrated that hypoxemia may relate to LV dysfunction that is independent of RV disease (18, 19). This may be due to abnormal LV growth, development and structure due to disturbed fetal patterns of blood flow, hypoxia and metabolism, which is further exacerbated by increased afterload following loss of the low resistance placental circuit (19).

Biological phenotypes contributing to chronic pulmonary hypertension (cPH) in neonates

The correlation between pulmonary parenchymal and pulmonary vascular maldevelopment among neonates born extremely preterm exists on a spectrum as they mature (Table 34.1). In some infants, lung parenchymal disease, characterized by fibrosis with large and simplified alveolar development (20, 21) leads to reduced lung surface area for gas exchange, and may on its own present with respiratory failure and chronic dependence on mechanical support. For infants with severe BPD, however, the reported incidence of contemporaneous chronic PH is between 15–58% (22–25). The optimal approach to diagnosis and screening in this patient population is not yet established (26). There is evidence to suggest that even patients with mild BPD (23, 25, 27, 28) may have increased risk of chronic PH; and there are several other disease entities with a similar presentation. This suggests a role for screening convalescent extremely preterm infants on respiratory support to evaluate for modifiable contributors to lung disease severity. Pulmonary vein stenosis, an uncommon but important developmental anomaly that may be encountered among patients with BPD, should be considered in all patients with the BPD phenotype; Doppler studies of the pulmonary veins should be included as a routine part of screening for chronic PH. A pulmonary venous velocity of ≥1 m/s measured by Doppler studies should be a red flag for further echocardiography and/or cardiac catheterization (29).

Chronic PH phenotype related to bronchopulmonary dysplasia (BPD)

The pathophysiology of cPH among extremely preterm infants is multifactorial. It is primarily thought to be related to abnormal vascular growth which parallels abnormal parenchymal development by several mechanisms. *First*, large, simplified alveoli are fewer in number than in normal lung and have correspondingly lower numbers of intra-acinar arteries (30). *Second*, disruption of normal cellular signaling via both the vascular endothelial growth factor (VEGF) and NO pathways have been implicated in abnormal vascular growth (31). *Third*, inflammation such as from chorioamnionitis, postnatal infection or ventilator-induced lung injury, precipitates invasion by dendritic cells, a high concentration of which are associated with dysangiogenesis (32). In combination, this leads to a substantial reduction in the alveolar-capillary surface area available for gas exchange. Prolonged vasoconstricting stimuli, such as due to chronic or intermittent hypoxemia, has been associated with disruption in the nitric oxide pathway in a piglet model (33). Oxidative stress may play an additional role. Endothelial cells are particularly vulnerable to damage, including fragmentation of mitochondria, by reactive oxygen species (34). Exposure to chronic hypoxemia causes upregulation of redox-sensitive transcription factors with downstream gene targets that modify vascular proliferation, differentiation, matrix deposition and chemokine production (35). *Finally*, smooth muscle cell proliferation occurs. Small peripheral vessels mature early and incorporate immature mesenchymal ells, fibroblasts and myofibrils into vessel walls, which further contributes to elevated PVR by causing a widespread reduction of small caliber vessel radius (36). Risk factors may include younger gestation, intrauterine growth restriction, chorioamnionitis and genetic predisposition (25, 37–39). Management of this condition includes a combination of optimization of oxygenation and ventilation to minimize progression of disease and pulmonary vasodilator therapy (e.g. sildenafil). Diuretics may be considered to optimize RV conformation if there is evidence of RV dilation.

Chronic PH phenotype secondary to excessive pulmonary blood flow

Sustained left-to-right flow leading to pulmonary over-circulation may commonly occur at the level of an atrial communication (e.g. patent foramen ovale [PFO] or atrial septal defect [ASD]) or, particularly in centers where a tolerant approach to the persistent ductus arteriosus (PDA) has evolved, at the level of a ductal communication. Over-circulation has the potential to modify the pulmonary circulation both by precipitating chronic pulmonary edema and by fundamentally modifying the growth of the pulmonary vasculature. Similar to patients with a flow-driven acute PH phenotype, excessive volume in the pulmonary circulation creates a hypertensive phenotype by virtue of excess blood in a vascular system with limited compliance. In an ovine model, this phenomenon has been associated with impaired vascular growth, abnormal alveolarization and upregulation of endothelin-1 which has potently anti-angiogenic effects in addition to vasoconstriction in the immature lung (40, 41). Endothelin-1 levels are typically further elevated in human infants with BPD, suggesting a potential role of chronic left-right shunt as a contributor to BPD-associated PH. In a neonatal porcine model, chronic exposure to left-to-right shunt resulted in a significant decrease in lung compliance, hypertrophy of the pulmonary arteries extending from hilum to periphery, muscular extension into smaller intra-acinar arteries and ventricular hypertrophy (42). Younger animals exhibited the greatest change in vessel caliber, which may relate to the stage of development of the pulmonary vasculature at the time of exposure to shunt. Human neonates exposed to PDA shunt for <4 weeks compared to >8 weeks demonstrated lower PVR by cardiac catheterization, better growth and more rapid reduction in respiratory illness severity suggesting a similar phenomenon (43). Finally, upregulation of the renin-angiotensin system (RAS) has been identified in infants exposed to left to right shunt in the setting of congenital heart disease, particularly those with lower arterial pressure implicating renal perfusion pressure as the driver (44). As will be described in detail below, the RAS may have an important role to play in remodeling and oxidative damage among patients with chronic shunt (45). Patients with both ASD and PDA, or other multi-level shunt are at greatest risk of abnormal pulmonary outcomes due to the presence of over-circulation from two distinct sources. The use of pulmonary vasodilators in this phenotype may be harmful both due to increasing SVR:PVR ratio and the potential contribution to oxidative stress. Shunt management is the hallmark of therapy, which for PDA may include medical, surgical or interventional closure. Symptom control with diuretics could be considered after exhaustion of medical therapy; however, furosemide upregulates the production of prostaglandin and may be counter-productive in conjunction with non-steroidals (46, 47). Fluid restriction below 140 ml/kg/d is not recommended, based on ineffectiveness and due to the risk of under-perfusion of post-ductal circulation (48). For patients with ASD, diuretics are a mainstay of therapy and device closure has been reported for patients 2–2.5 kg (49).

Chronic PH phenotype related to left heart mal-compliance

Neonates with BPD are at increased risk of systemic hypertension with reported rates between 6.8–43% (50–52). The mechanism of this association is not well understood; whether BPD contributes to the development of systemic hypertension, systemic hypertension contributes to the development of BPD, or both arise via a shared common origin, likely varies. Although some authors suggest that angiotensin converting enzyme (ACE) may be protective against fibrosis in experimental models (53), neurohormonal stimuli including activation of the renin-angiotensin system have been implicated in pulmonary vascular smooth muscle proliferation, migration, oxidative stress, fibrosis, inflammation and impaired endothelial function among patients with pulmonary hypertension across a variety of human and experimental models (54–57). Additionally, polymorphisms in ACE genes have been associated with acute PH among neonatal patients with CDH (58), and modulation of the pathway by stimulating the angiotensin II receptor has been associated with attenuated cardiopulmonary disease in a neonatal rat model (59). Angiotensin II plays an important role in the modulation of blood pressure via increases in SVR and stimulation of vasopressin and norepinephrine release. It is therefore biologically plausible that neonatal hypertension and BPD may both relate to abnormal activity of this pathway. Arterial stiffness, as measured by high-resolution echocardiography, has also been implicated as a contributor to systemic hypertension among neonatal patients with BPD (52). It is likely that multiple contributors to disease are present among individual patients and that a spectrum of disease exists with a hypertension-predominant phenotype as one end of the spectrum (50). It is well-established in the adult literature that chronic exposure to systemic hypertension may be associated with LV diastolic dysfunction (60). Although neonatal evidence is limited, the biological principle is similar to adults. High end-diastolic pressure in the aortic root is transmitted to the LV, resulting in failure to sufficiently empty, gradual left ventricular and left atrial dilation followed by elevated pulmonary venous pressure and pulmonary edema. Sustained exposure to poorly controlled systemic afterload may result in a very similar clinical phenotype to chronic PH. Anti-hypertensive therapy, such as with ACE inhibitors, is the recommended treatment along with careful monitoring for acute kidney injury, especially in the setting of concurrent diuretic therapy. The use of PH-targeted drugs to selectively lower PVR should generally be avoided. Patients with left-heart malcompliance are at risk for acute or chronic pulmonary edema if treated with pulmonary vasodilation (17).

Approach to phenotypic delineation

Clinical differentiation of these phenotypes is challenging. Acute cyanotic episodes (or "spells"), hypoxemia, increased pre- and post- ductal saturation gradients, systolic hypotension and evidence of poor systemic perfusion may be typical of acute PH regardless of etiology. Similarly, dependence on respiratory support is the hallmark feature of chronic PH, regardless of etiology. Echocardiography is the most commonly used tool to delineate physiology in this and other neonatal cardiopulmonary presentations. Comprehensive quantitative hemodynamic evaluation, such as is performed by practitioners trained in Targeted Neonatal Echocardiography (TnECHO) (61, 62) may provide valuable insights into disease physiology.

Echocardiography-guided management of acute PH
The fundamental considerations in the initial assessment of a patient suspected to have acute pulmonary hypertension are to confirm the diagnosis of elevated mPAP, evaluate PVR and the impact on RV health, assess for potential contribution by LV disease, evaluate the adequacy of systemic blood flow, document shunt status and capture images of sufficient quality to rule out potentially subtle but critical anatomic cardiac disease (e.g. anomalous venous drainage, coarctation). Qualitative evaluation of, in particular RV, performance is unreliable (63) and, therefore quantitative techniques which document objective metrics of both RV and LV performance are recommended.

In cases of biventricular dysfunction, it may be difficult to determine the relative contributions of each ventricle to the overall physiology. This is, however, of paramount importance because management strategies may be dramatically different in situations of primary LV vs. primary PAH and RV disease. When RV disease is dominant, with LV disease secondary to interventricular interaction, a pulmonary vasodilator strategy which may include iNO and/or milrinone combined with a vasopressor that does not increase PVR (i.e. Vasopressin) may be the most appropriate choice of therapy. In contrast, pulmonary vasodilators are relatively contraindicated among patients with severe LV disease in part because right-to-left ductal shunt may be imperative to maintain systemic perfusion, such as it is in hypoplastic left heart physiology. Vasopressors, similarly, are of little value in the management of severe primary LV disease unless severely low diastolic arterial pressure is compromising coronary perfusion pressure, because LV afterload reduction is a mainstay of therapy. One population in which this dichotomy is particularly well documented is neonates with CDH in whom both PAH and LV dysfunction-mediated pulmonary venous hypertension may occur. Atrial shunt direction prior to initiation of pulmonary vasodilator therapy has been proposed as one method of discerning the likely dominant physiology (19). The combination of high mPAP transmitted to the right atrium and low pulmonary venous return to the left atrium should result in right-to-left atrial shunt in the former situation (PAH); whereas LV disease is characterized by high left atrial pressure, which should manifest as a left-to-right atrial shunt even in patients with clear right-to-left shunt across the ductus arteriosus.

Shunt-mediated acute PH should be considered in any patient where significant dilation of any cardiac chamber is identified. Preductal arteriovenous malformations, for example, may present with severe right heart dilation and classically a dilated superior vena cava and innominate artery with retrograde flow in the pre-ductal aortic arch. Identification of these findings on echocardiography should prompt a head ultrasound. Similarly, especially among extremely preterm infants, a high-volume ductal shunt may generate sufficient left-to-right flow to manifest as severe dilation of the left heart and pulmonary veins. The measurement of cardiac output may be especially valuable in distinguishing dilation due to shunt from dilation due to afterload, such as may occur in the setting of classic PH of arterial origin. Afterload-mediated dilation should be associated with normal or low ventricular output, whereas high cardiac output is typical in patients with shunt physiology unless concurrent cardiac dysfunction is present. The phase of the cardiac cycle in which septal flattening is present may also provide a clue. Neonates with PAH have septal flattening in systole because, when the aortic valve is open, the RV systolic pressure needed to eject blood (i.e. develop a pressure gradient) is determined by the pressure in the pulmonary vascular bed. Patients with RV volume loading as the reason for septal flattening primarily develop a flat septum in diastole, which is when the RV overfilling is reflected as the end-diastolic pressure. The use of the ratio of right ventricular ejection time (RVET) to pulmonary artery acceleration time (PAAT) may also be a helpful tool to quantify resistance; however it may be difficult to measure, and reflective of both PVR and SVR among patients with a large PDA (64), and may be underestimated in patients with RV dysfunction. In addition, one study found that eccentricity index, but not abnormal PAAT, was associated with the severity of BPD at 36 weeks postmenstrual age (65).

Echocardiography-guided management of chronic PH
The optimal approach to screening for chronic PH in patients with BPD is unknown. Its presenting features are often subtle, the timing of onset is insidious and also likely variable, with findings reported as early as 28 weeks postmenstrual age in some patients (23). Recently, three expert consensus guidelines on the assessment and management of chronic PH have been published (66–68). Recommendations include routine echocardiography screening at the time of BPD diagnosis, and approaches to medical therapy and thresholds for cardiac catheterization or advanced imaging (e.g. MRI) when chronic PH is diagnosed. Although quantification of mPAP and classification of severity of chronic PH is recommended, the threshold to define disease among this patient population remains unclear. On echocardiography, important findings among patients with BPD-associated chronic PH may include bidirectionality or predominantly right to left flow at any residual shunts, septal flattening in systole which may be quantified using the eccentricity index (69, 70), doppler interrogation of any tricuspid (for RVSp) or pulmonary (for mPAP) valvular regurgitation and evaluation of RV size, wall thickness and systolic function. The use of RVET: PAAT to evaluate PVR may be useful, particularly as a tool to trend response to pulmonary vasodilator therapy. As previously mentioned, pulmonary vein Doppler interrogation is important to screen for pulmonary vein stenosis, with any concerns followed up by cardiac catheterization. However, PVS often occurs late during the course of preterm infants with BPD, and it is not unusual to have no signs of PVS on multiple serial echocardiograms (71). These findings suggest the need to maintain high suspicion for PVS, especially with late echocardiographic signs of PH during follow-up. In addition, PVS may be diagnosed by cardiac catheterization without clear echocardiographic evidence (72).

The treatment approach for chronic PH among patients with BPD also remains in evolution. It is in the choice of therapy that physiological delineation may provide the most value and echocardiography may provide valuable clues. Biomarkers such as B-type natriuretic peptide (BNP) and related peptides including N-terminal fragment of BNP (NT-proBNP) have been associated with chronic pulmonary hypertension in this patient population (73, 74). BNP is synthesized by the ventricles in response to pressure and volume overload, however, thus these biomarkers should not be used to discriminate causality. Because a source of pressure upstream in the circulation may be transmitted back to generate elevated pressure at any point before it in the circuit, evaluation of LV systolic and diastolic performance and high-quality measurement of systemic arterial pressure are of paramount importance. Convalescent extremely preterm neonates in the chronic phase of illness may have few measurements of systemic blood pressure in a nursing shift, and there is a tendency for bedside care providers to present more normal vital signs than would be recorded if all measures were systematically collected by a computer (75). This may reflect a tendency to portray their patient as the 'best version' of their clinical condition, or knowledge of outside factors that may contribute to derangement in arterial pressure measurements (e.g. agitation, motion). Systemic hypertension is a common comorbidity, and care should be taken to measure arterial pressure optimally and report it accurately. Echocardiography features of LV diastolic dysfunction may include low early wave of mitral valve flow as compared to the atrial phase, a prolonged isovolumetric relaxation time and the presence of a wave reversal in the pulmonary veins. Other less load-dependent echocardiography features in use in adult patients (i.e. E/e' ratio of the septal

or lateral wall of the LV using conventional and tissue Doppler imaging) are emerging as research tools, however, are yet to be used in routine clinical practice. Among patients with systemic hypertension and LV diastolic dysfunction, antihypertensive therapy may be a treatment strategy for pulmonary hypertension. A case report in the neonatal population, for example, describes two patients with catheter-proven LV diastolic dysfunction whose pulmonary symptoms improved with ACE inhibition (76). Accurate measurement and reporting of systemic blood pressure are important for the interpretation of echocardiography findings. Unlike cardiac catheterization, echocardiography is dependent on the relationship between systemic and pulmonary circulatory pressures. This means, for example, that a patient with a systolic arterial pressure of 80 mmHg could have clinically relevant chronic PH with a round interventricular septum because of the limited sensitivity of septal flattening in the detection of abnormal pressures <½ systemic level. Both in clinical care and when designing academic endeavors in this field, systemic hypertension should always be considered. Cardiac catheterization should be considered when echocardiography is unclear.

As in a situation of acute shunt, chronic shunt produces dilation and imbalance in cardiac output. For example, chronic large ASD shunt will precipitate RA and RV dilation and a right ventricular output that is greater than the left ventricular output. There is no conclusive evidence for specific medical therapy to manage chronic atrial-level shunts among BPD patients; however, persistent ASD shunts have been associated with higher risk of late PH. Pulmonary over-circulation in these patients may also lead to pulmonary edema and worsen the need for respiratory support. Short-term diuretic therapy, usually with furosemide, a potent and rapid acting loop diuretic, may improve cardiorespiratory symptoms by reducing cardiac volume loading and pulmonary interstitial edema. Over time, however, furosemide is often associated with deranged electrolytes and decreased intravascular volume, which can lower cardiac output and further increase neurohumoral mediator production, including ADH, aldosterone, and others. In addition, furosemide is associated with increased renal prostaglandin production which may lower PVR. These adverse effects, in addition to a tendency to produce tolerance, suggest cautious use of furosemide in the management of BPD-associated PH, particularly for extended periods. The use of spironolactone, either alone or in combination with a thiazide diuretic, may be advantageous to reduce the adverse effects of chronic furosemide therapy. As previously described, the renin-angiotensin system is involved in pulmonary vascular remodeling and spironolactone, an aldosterone antagonist, has a theoretical biological advantage.

Patients with chronic PDA shunt, in contrast to atrial level, will develop dilated left heart structures and with elevated left ventricular output. Importantly, chronic left atrial dilation may be associated with stretching of the PFO such that PDA shunt exacerbates left-to-right atrial shunt and both left and right ventricular outputs become higher as does the degree of pulmonary over-circulation. If left unchecked, chronic shunt may produce pulmonary vascular remodeling which may make it challenging to identify the primary issue with a single time-point measurement. Patients with chronic PDA shunt who develop elevated PVR may make treatment decisions difficult because it may be challenging to separate flow from resistance mediated PH. Most patients with flow-mediated PH continue to have markers of left heart volume loading including high pulmonary vein and mitral valve flow velocities, short isovolumetric relaxation time and dilated left heart structures (77) (Table 34.2). LV output may

TABLE 34.2 Echocardiography Markers to Aid in Differentiation of Flow (PDA Driven) vs. Resistance (PDA Supportive) Phenotype

	PDA Driven	PDA Supportive
FiO$_2$	<50%	>50%
PDA shunt (R-L component)	<10%	>10%
Relevance of shunt (echo)	Left heart volume loading (e.g. PVd ≥0.5 m/s, MVE ≥0.8 m/s, IVRT ≤40 ms) LVO ≥1.5 RVO Left-Right atrial shunt Diastolic flow reversal dAo	Right heart volume loading Normal/low LVO Right-Left atrial shunt Forward dAo diastolic flow
RV function	Normal	Abnormal
Evolution	Serial evidence of moderate/high volume Left-Right shunt	Serial evidence of Right-Left shunt
Pulmonary vasodilator response	Reversal of ductal shunt (most)	Ductal shunt irreversible (most)

Abbreviations: PVd, pulmonary vein D wave velocity; MVE, mitral valve E wave velocity; IVRT, isovolumetric relaxation time; LVO, left ventricular output; RVO, right ventricular output; dAo, descending, post-ductal thoracic aorta.

be substantially larger than RV output unless there is a large atrial left to right shunt which may increase the RV output also. Evidence of diastolic flow reversal in the descending aorta has been shown by cardiac magnetic resonance imaging to be a good surrogate marker of PDA shunt volume (78). Resistance-mediated PH among patients with PDA should be absent of those findings, and may have elevated RVET:PAAT ratio, RV dilation, dysfunction and/or hypertrophy (Table 34.2). Serial evaluation may be beneficial. Avoidance of high-volume chronic level shunt by early intervention, prior to the development of pulmonary vascular damage, is recommended if the clinical situation is amenable. PDA closure for patients with features of high volume shunt and PH may be beneficial and may improve both PH findings and respiratory status; however, care should be taken to avoid closure of the PDA for patients with resistance-mediated PH, as this could lead to pulmonary hypertensive crisis and escalation of RV afterload, resulting in rapid onset of severe RV dysfunction.

Although cardiac catheterization is the gold standard test for evaluation of pulmonary hemodynamics in adults, echocardiography is the preferred and most commonly used method in neonatology due to its non-invasive nature, safety and feasibility in small patients. Echocardiography is documented to be approximately 85% sensitive as a diagnostic test for chronic PH among neonates (25, 79). Echocardiography has the added advantage that it may more accurately reflect the baby's baseline hemodynamics, because it can be done awake and under normal ambient conditions. In contrast, the degree of chronic PH may be underestimated among patients with a significant dynamic component to their pulmonary vascular disease because cardiac catheterization is typically performed sedated and muscle relaxed. Among patients with severe, multifactorial, complex or refractory disease, such as those with all of chronic shunt, markers of PVR and systemic hypertension, cardiac catheterization may be an important tool. In particular, catheterization is essential if pulmonary vein stenosis is suspected, and may be useful to assess the relative contribution of ductal or atrial level shunt of pulmonary venous hypertension to PH in infants who are not showing clinical improvement on medical management.

Conclusion

The biological contributors to neonatal pulmonary hypertension are complex, during the acute and chronic phases. Careful delineation of the phenotype is essential to enable physiologically

appropriate selection of therapy that optimizes blood flow and tissue oxygenation. Standardized TnECHO evaluations which are comprehensive, quantitative and thorough may be a valuable tool in identification of physiology and monitoring therapeutic response. It is incumbent of neonatal and adult clinical researchers, physiologists, and developmental scientists to build academic bridges that enable the identification of important modulators of abnormal cardiopulmonary development and opportunities for therapeutic intervention. Health surveillance of survivors of neonatal PH from childhood to adulthood, which includes a standardized and multidisciplinary approach to the evaluation of cardiovascular performance, is needed to guide preventative strategies.

Key points

- Classic acute pulmonary hypertension is related to failure of normal decline in pulmonary vascular resistance after birth. Shunt lesions (e.g. patent ductus arteriosus, ventricular septal defect) may lead to excessive pulmonary blood flow which both increases pressure due to a greater blood volume in a physically limited circuit and by negatively impacting the pulmonary vascular to sheer stress. Left heart disease may lead to elevated left-ventricular end diastolic pressure which may be transmitted backwards in the pulmonary circuit and raise pulmonary artery pressure.
- Bronchopulmonary dysplasia associated pulmonary hypertension is related to abnormal development of the pulmonary parenchyma and its associated vascular surface. Chronic over-circulation may contribute to impaired lung compliance, abnormal muscularization and biochemical abnormalities such as of the renin-angiotensin system, which mediate vasoconstriction and remodeling. Left heart disease and/or systemic hypertension may also be mediated by the renin-angiotensin system and other neurohormonal stimuli. Similar to in the acute phase, both systemic hypertension and LV disease result in high LVEDP and therefore, pulmonary edema and pulmonary venous hypertension.
- Comprehensive, quantitative echocardiography may help distinguish the etiology. In the acute phase, measures of systolic function of both ventricles may be useful in determining whether the right or left ventricle has the greater degree of dysfunction. Shunt lesions should always be

suspected in the presence of significant dilation of any chamber. In the chronic patient, measurements of resistance (i.e. the ratio of pulmonary artery acceleration time to right ventricular ejection time) may help to identify arterial-side remodeling or vasoconstriction. It is essential to remember that all echocardiography measurements are relative and careful attention should be paid to systemic arterial pressure.

- Several biomarkers are being used, however as non-specific measures of cardiac stretch, they do not convey etiology. Cardiac catheterization should be considered in complex or unclear cases and to evaluate for pulmonary vein stenosis in the appropriate setting.

References

1. Olver RE, et al. J Physiol. 1974; 241(2):327–357.
2. Brown MJ, et al. J Physiol. 1983; 344:137–152.
3. Hooper SB, et al. Paediatr Respir Rev. 2015; 16(3):147–150.
4. Creamer KM, et al. Am J Respir Crit Care Med. 1998; 158(4):1114–1119.
5. Giesinger RE, et al. Am J Respir Crit Care Med. 2019; 200(10):1294–1305.
6. Kamiya A, et al. Am J Physiol. 1980; 239(1):H14–H21.
7. Nadaud S, et al. Circ Res. 1996; 79(4):857–863.
8. Fullerton DA, et al. J Thorac Cardiovasc Surg. 1996; 111(1):190–197.
9. Storme L, et al. Pediatr Res. 1999; 45(4 Pt 1):575–581.
10. Rairigh RL, et al. Am J Physiol. 1999; 276(3):L513–L521.
11. Vitvitsky EV, et al. Ann Thorac Surg. 1998; 66(4):1372–1377.
12. Aggarwal S, et al. Trends Cardiovasc Med. 2010; 20(7):238–246.
13. Storme L, et al. Pediatr Res. 1999; 45(3):425–431.
14. Clyman RI, et al. Am J Perinatol. 2020; 37(2):216–223.
15. Kaempf JW, et al. J Perinatol. 2012; 32(5):344–348.
16. Serraf A, et al. Ann Thorac Surg. 1995; 59(5):1155–1161.
17. von Schnakenburg C, et al. Pediatr Crit Care Med. 2003; 4(1):111–114.
18. Massolo AC, et al. Neonatology. 2019; 116(1):68–75.
19. Kinsella JP, et al. J Pediatr. 2018; 197:17–22.
20. Bonikos DS, et al. Hum Pathol. 1976; 7(6):643–666.
21. Husain AN, et al. Hum Pathol. 1998; 29(7):710–717.
22. An HS, et al. Korean Circ J. 2010; 40(3):131–136.
23. Bhat R, et al. Pediatrics. 2012; 129(3):e682–e689.
24. Khemani E, et al. Pediatrics. 2007; 120(6):1260–1269.
25. Mourani PM, et al. Am J Respir Crit Care Med. 2015; 191(1):87–95.
26. Levy PT, et al. J Pediatr. 2020; 217:199.e4–209.e4.
27. Weismann CG, et al. J Perinatol. 2017; 37(5):572–577.
28. Mirza H, et al. J Pediatr. 2014; 165(5):909.e1–914.e1.
29. Laux D, et al. Pediatr Cardiol. 2016; 37(2):313–321.
30. Gorenflo M, et al. Pediatr Pathol. 1991; 11(6):851–866.
31. Abman SH. Adv Exp Med Biol. 2010; 661:323–335.
32. De Paepe ME, et al. Pediatr Dev Pathol. 2011; 14(1):20–27.
33. Berkenbosch JW, et al. Am J Physiol Lung Cell Mol Physiol. 2000; 278(2):L276–L283.
34. Ma C, et al. Arterioscler Thromb Vasc Biol. 2018; 38(3):622–635.
35. Nozik-Grayck E, et al. Adv Exp Med Biol. 2007; 618:101–112.
36. Jones R, et al. Am J Pathol. 1984; 117(2):273–285.
37. Bhandari V, et al. Pediatrics. 2006; 117(6):1901–1906.
38. Yum SK, et al. Pulm Circ. 2018; 8(2):2045894018760166.
39. Trittmann JK, et al. Acta Paediatr. 2018; 107(12):2158–2164.
40. Grover TR, et al. Am J Physiol Lung Cell Mol Physiol. 2005; 288(4):L648–L54.
41. Gien J, et al. Pediatr Res. 2013; 73(3):252–262.
42. Rendas A, et al. J Thorac Cardiovasc Surg. 1979; 77(1):109–118.
43. Philip R, et al. J Perinatol. 2020. doi: 10.1038/s41372-020-00772-2.
44. Buchhorn R, et al. Int J Cardiol. 2001; 78(3):225–230.
45. Segar JL. Pediatr Pulmonol. 2020; 55(5):1100–1103.
46. Green TP, et al. NEJM. 1983; 308(13):743–748.
47. Sulyok E, et al. Pediatr Res. 1980; 14(5):765–768.
48. De Buyst J, et al. J Pediatr. 2012; 161(3):404–408.
49. Bishnoi RN, et al. Pediatr Cardiol. 2014; 35(7):1124–1131.
50. Abman SH, et al. J Pediatr. 1984; 104(6):928–931.
51. Alagappan A, et al. Am J Perinatol. 1998; 15(1):3–8.
52. Sehgal A, et al. J Perinatol. 2016; 36(7):564–569.
53. Gandhi C, et al. JSM Atherosclerosis. 2016; 1(3):1014.
54. Jiang JS, et al. Neonatology. 2012; 101(1):47–54.
55. de Man FS, et al. Am J Respir Crit Care Med. 2012; 186(8):780–789.
56. Maron BA, et al. Pulm Circ. 2014; 4(2):200–210.
57. Sehgal A, et al. Physiol Rep. 2018; 6(17):e13821.
58. Solari V, et al. J Pediatr Surg. 2004; 39(3):302–306.
59. Wagenaar GT, et al. Am J Physiol Lung Cell Mol Physiol. 2013; 305(5):L341–L351.
60. Graettinger WF, et al. Cardiol Clin. 1995; 13(4):559–567.
61. Mertens L, et al. J Am Soc Echocardiogr. 2011; 24(10):1057–1078.
62. Hebert A, et al. J Am Soc Echocardiogr. 2019; 32(6):785–790.
63. Smith A, et al. Echocardiography. 2019; 36(7):1346–1352.
64. Gaulton JS, et al. Echocardiography. 2019; 36(8):1524–1531.
65. Ehrmann DE, et al. J Pediatr. 2018; 203: 210.e1–217.e1.
66. Abman SH, et al. Circulation. 2015; 132(21):2037–2099.
67. Hansmann G, et al. J Heart Lung Transplant. 2019; 38(9):879–901.
68. Krishnan U, et al. J Pediatr. 2017; 188:24.e1–34.e1.
69. McCrary AW, et al. Am J Perinatol. 2016; 33(1):57–62.
70. Ryan T, et al. J Am Coll Cardiol. 1985; 5(4):918–927.
71. Mahgoub L, et al. Pediatr Pulmonol. 2017; 52(8):1063–1070.
72. Frank BS, et al. Pediatr Res. 2019; 208:127–133.
73. Behere S, et al. Pediatr Cardiol. 2019; 40(5):973–979.
74. Avitabile CM, et al. Neonatology. 2019; 116(2):147–153.
75. Cunningham S, et al. Int J Clin Monit Comput. 1996; 13(4):235–241.
76. Mourani PM, et al. J Pediatr. 2008; 152(2):291–293.
77. de Freitas Martins F, et al. J Pediatr. 2018; 202:50.e3–55.e3.
78. Broadhouse KM, et al. NMR Biomed. 2013; 26(9):1135–1141.
79. Mourani PM, et al. Pediatrics. 2008; 121(2):317–325.

SPECIAL CONSIDERATION
HRF in Congenital Diaphragmatic Hernia

Gabriel Altit, Jason Gien, Nolan DeLeon and Richard Keijzer

Contents

Predicting the severity of pulmonary hypoplasia in congenital diaphragmatic hernia

In the last 10 years, prenatal ascertainment of congenital diaphragmatic hernia (CDH) severity has markedly improved with high volume centers able to differentiate high risk from low risk cases with relative certainty. This has allowed for more accurate prenatal counseling, with providers able to predict risk for extracorporeal membrane oxygenation (ECMO), prolonged hospitalization and mortality. In addition, high risk fetuses can be referred to a tertiary care center, and suitable candidates enrolled in fetal intervention studies. Fundamental to determining the severity of the defect is identifying the position of the liver, estimating fetal lung volumes, and detecting associated abnormalities. Utilizing detailed ultrasonography and ultrafast fetal magnetic resonance imaging (MRI) one can estimate the severity of lung hypoplasia as well as rule out associated fetal anomalies. To complete the evaluation, fetal echocardiography should be performed to rule out associated cardiac anomalies and evaluate for left ventricular (LV) hypoplasia. Identification of associated fetal anomalies raises concern for the presence of a chromosomal defect and identifies fetuses who will benefit from amniocentesis for detailed genetic analysis (1) with chromosomal analysis and high-resolution microarray. Chromosomal abnormalities including aneuploidies, chromosomal deletions/duplications, and complex chromosome rearrangements are identified in 10–35% of non-isolated, prenatally diagnosed CDH cases (2). Trisomy 13, 18, 21 and 45X are the most common aneuploidies associated with CDH. In addition to karyotype abnormalities, copy number variants (CNV) (e.g. microdeletions, microduplications) have been diagnosed in 3.5–13% of isolated CDH cases using microarray analysis (2). As the presence of a significant chromosomal defect impacts outcome greater than any predictor of lung hypoplasia, amniocentesis is recommended in all cases of CDH with associated anomalies.

Approximately 60% of CDH cases are diagnosed prenatally either on routine ultrasound or as part of workup for maternal polyhydramnios (3). Direct signs include the presence of abdominal organs within the thoracic cavity, and indirect signs include polyhydramnios, abnormal cardiac axis, or mediastinal shift (4). Left-sided CDH (Figure 35.1) is characterized by the presence of fluid-filled stomach and small bowel in the chest cavity, adjacent to the heart. Herniated liver appears as a homogeneous mass in the chest at the level of the heart that is continuous with the intra-abdominal liver. Right sided CDH is more difficult to diagnose because the herniated liver and lung have similar echogenicity (4). Identifying the gallbladder in the chest is diagnostic of right-sided CDH. Once the diagnosis of CDH is confirmed, more detailed anatomic evaluation can determine the severity of the lung hypoplasia.

Liver herniation

Liver herniation into the thoracic cavity remains one of the most reliable predictors of CDH severity (5–7) with a meta-analysis in 2010 demonstrating 45% survival and 80% ECMO utilization with liver herniation versus 74% survival and 25% ECMO utilization without liver herniation (5–8). A more recent report has described similar survival in liver up CDH (45%) but 94% survival when liver was down (8). While ultrasound can accurately detect the presence of liver herniation, fetal MRI allows for quantification of liver herniation. A recent report quantified % liver herniation (%LH) into the chest and demonstrated that patients with greater than 20% liver herniation had an increased risk for long term pulmonary sequalae, specifically chronic lung disease (9). In another report, liver/thoracic volume ratio (LiTR) and %LH were measured and correlated with mortality and need for ECMO (10). The presence of a %LH greater than 21% predicted mortality and need for ECMO with an accuracy of 77% and 75%, respectively. LiTR greater than 14 predicted mortality and need for ECMO with an accuracy of 77% and 70%, respectively. When combined with MRI measurements of lung volume, observed-to-expected total lung volume (O/E-TLV), %LH had the highest accuracy in predicting mortality and the need for ECMO. The combination of o/e-TLV and %LH improved accuracy in predicting either mortality or the need for ECMO to 83% and 82%, respectively.

DOI: 10.1201/9780367494018-35

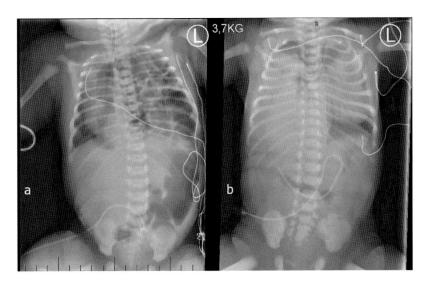

FIGURE 35.1 Radiography of two newborns with CDH. Panel (a) demonstrates a left-sided CDH with a shift of the cardiac axis towards the right side of the chest and bowels herniated on the left side of the chest. Panel (b) demonstrates a right-sided CDH with a shift of the cardiac axis towards the left of the chest.

Lung area/Head circumference ratio (LHR)

One of the oldest modalities for quantifying lung volume in infants with CDH is the lung area/head circumference ratio (LHR) (4). LHR is calculated by dividing the 2-dimensional area of the contralateral lung taken at the level of the 4-chamber view of the heart by the head circumference. While earlier studies used an LHR of 1.4 as a cutoff for poor prognosis (11, 12), more recent studies have demonstrated an LHR of <1.0 to be a predictor of poor outcomes (13, 14). The original description of LHR by Lipshultz et al. in 1997 was calculated between 24 and 26 weeks of gestation and did not take the gestational age (GA) into consideration (12). However, studies on normal fetuses have shown that between 12 and 32 weeks of gestation, there is a 16-fold increase in lung area versus a 4-fold increase in head circumference (15). To correct for GA, LHR is now expressed as a percentage of what can be expected in a normal fetus or O/E LHR (16, 17). For left-sided CDH, O/E LHR has been classified as extreme (<15%), severe (15–25%), moderate (26–35%), and mild (36–45%) (18). Based on O/E LHR and liver herniation, data from an antenatal CDH registry in Europe, the overall survival rates for isolated left-sided CDH were approximately 0%, 20%, 30-60% and >75% for extreme, severe, moderate, or mild O/E LHR (18). Due to the mortality associated with O/E LHR in the extreme and severe range, infants with an O/E LHR <25% are candidates for fetal intervention with fetoscopic endoluminal tracheal occlusion (FETO) in the context of a trial and should be referred to a center capable of performing this procedure. More recently, a trial assessing the effect of FETO on outcomes in infants with moderate CDH (O/E LHR 26–35% irrespective of liver herniation, O/E LHR 35–45% with liver herniation) has been initiated, to assess if FETO can decrease mortality, length of hospital stay and the development of bronchopulmonary dysplasia. For infants with right-sided CDH, data is more limited but to date O/E LHR < 45% is associated with > 90% mortality, with mortality decreasing to 40% with O/E LHR 45–55% and 30% with O/E LHR >55% (17). Based on these outcome data (Figure 35.2), infants with right-sided CDH and O/E LHR <45%, are also candidates for FETO under compassionate use and should be referred to a center capable of performing this procedure.

MRI (percent predicted lung volume, total lung volume, observed/expected)

Fetal MRI has added significantly to predicting severity of lung hypoplasia in fetuses with CDH (8, 19, 20). Parameters utilized to estimate fetal lung volumes include percent predicted lung volume (PPLV), late gestation TVL and O/E TLV. PPLV is calculated by subtracting mediastinal volume from total thoracic volume and is expressed as a percentage of the predicted lung volume (PPLV). Fetuses with a PPLV <15% required ECMO 100% of the time, versus 10% (PPLV>15%), had significantly longer hospital stays (102 vs. 37 days) and increased mortality (60% vs. 0%) (21). Another measure of severity of pulmonary hypoplasia is TLV, calculated in late gestation (34 week). TLV is quantified by measuring the tissue volume of the right and left lung, excluding hernia contents and mediastinal structures on each coronal image. Patients with higher lung volumes had better survival and less need for ECMO support. Patients with a TLV of greater than 40 mL had a 90% versus 35% survival, 10% need for ECMO versus 86% and an average stay of 146.3 ± 56.2 days versus 50.1 ± 34.3 days when compared to patients with TLV of less than 20 mL (22). Extrapolating from the O/E LHR, MRI has been utilized to calculate the O/E TLV, which is a percentage of the measured TLV/the expected TLV based on the initial description by Rypens et al. (23). When utilizing a cutoff of 0.3, the accuracy of O/E TLV alone in predicting survival and need for ECMO is 77% and 76%, respectively (10), however as mentioned above when combined with %LH, reliability increases with accuracy for predicting survival improving to 80–82% and need for ECMO to 83%. The potential value of O/E TLV is is subject of several studies. In one multicenter study retrospectively comparing O/E TLV with O/E-LHR with no standardization of postnatal care, MRI measurement of the O/E-TLV was found to be a more accurate predictor of postnatal survival than was the O/E-LHR (24). Single center studies have questioned the utility of O/E TLV when compared to other more established measurements. In a small single-center study, Madenci et al. demonstrated PPLV, to be a better predictor of survival compared with O/E-TLV, O/E-LHR or the LHR (25). Schaible et al. did not find that O/E-TLV improved prediction of early mortality over O/E-LHR alone (26).

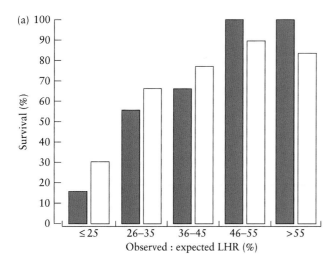
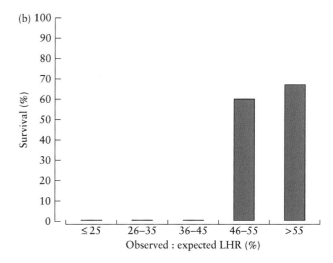

FIGURE 35.2 Survival rate according to the fetal observed to expected lung area to head circumference ratio (LHR) in fetuses with isolated left-sided (a), and right-sided (b), diaphragmatic hernia. The filled bars represent fetuses with intrathoracic herniation of the liver and the open bars represent those without herniation (21).

In summary, there are several antenatal parameters that can be utilized to assess severity of lung hypoplasia in CDH, the validity of each only relevant to each institution and their specific ECMO utilization and mortality. This was highlighted by Victoria et al. who described their experience at the Center for Fetal Diagnosis and Treatment at the Children's Hospital of Philadelphia (CHOP) with 85 patients who had underwent fetal MRI evaluation. In this report, they describe the utility of MRI performed between 18 and 39 weeks, (mean 25^6/7 weeks) and their institutional cutoffs for survival based on several parameters. As an example, right and left lung volume and TLV were compared between survivors and non-survivors (right lung volume 8.2 cc (5.7–16.8), versus 6.5 cc (3.6–9.7), left lung volume, 2.4 cc (1.8–3.9), versus 1.0 (0.6–2.1) and TLV 11.6 (7.7–21.9) versus 7.6 cc (4–11.9). They also describe outcomes for other parameters, stressing the importance of each institution's tracking and continually assessing their specific cutoffs for relevant clinical outcomes (11). As a general guideline, the following parameters can be utilized to stratify high from low risk infants with CDH, LHR <1, O/E LHR <25%, PPLV <15%, TLV <20ml, O/E TLV <30% and %LH >21% and LiTR greater than 14.

Pulmonary hypertension and cardiovascular management in CDH

Varying degrees of pulmonary hypoplasia in the context of CDH are associated with decreased pulmonary vascular capacity, abnormal structural pulmonary vasculature, disturbed transition to extra-uterine life and altered responsiveness to endogenous and exogenous pulmonary vasodilating substances (27–29). The natural fall in pulmonary vascular resistance (PVR) following birth is further altered by the often concomitant cardio-respiratory and metabolic disturbances (such as respiratory distress, hypoxia, acidosis, hyperlactatemia, intubation and other noxious stimuli, as well as reactive oxygen species). Studies have shown that pulmonary vessels of CDH newborns have increased muscular content, reduced total cross-sectional area and the abnormal muscularization of intra-acinar arterioles (27). Furthermore, expression of endothelin and prostacyclin pathway receptors was aberrant in lung tissues obtained from CDH newborns who did not survive the first hours of life (29).

Newborns with CDH often present with a clinical picture consistent with severe pulmonary hypertension (PH): Pre- and post-ductal saturation differences, hypoxic respiratory failure, hepatomegaly, altered perfusion, end-organ injury and, eventually, cardiovascular collapse. PH is often secondary to a combination of persistently increased PVR, decreased pulmonary vascular capacity and post-capillary obstruction. Newborns with isolated CDH have a reported survival of 75%, with 20–39% requiring ECMO during the neonatal period (30, 31).

Recently, depressed LV performance, as well as decreased LV dimensions (Figure 35.3) have been reported as a determinant of adverse outcomes (ECMO use and mortality) in multiple CDH cohorts (32–35). LV hypoplasia is thought to be secondary to various factors, including: Compression of the fetal heart by the herniated abdominal organs preventing optimal growth, left-sided

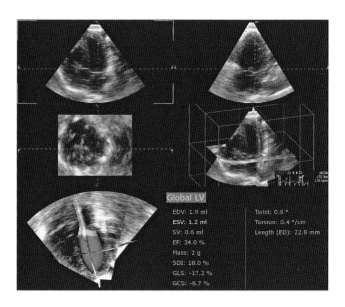

FIGURE 35.3 3D echocardiography of apical view obtained on a 2.5 kg CDH newborn in the first day of post-natal life. Patient was found to have decreased LV estimated end-diastolic volume (1.9 mL) and reduced ejection fraction.

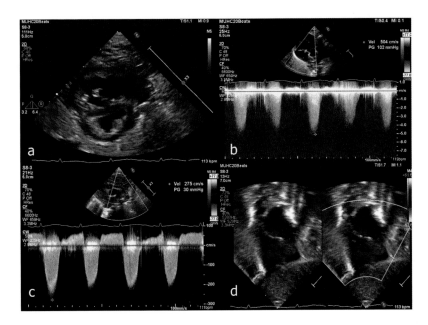

FIGURE 35.4   Echocardiography views obtained on a CDH newborn in the first post-natal day of life. Panel (a) demonstrates a parasternal-short axis view at papillary muscle level with RV dilation and bowing inter-ventricular septum towards LV cavity at end of systole, suggestion RV pressure overload. Panel (b) is the continuous-wave (CW). Doppler spectral profile of the tricuspid regurgitant jet estimating systolic pulmonary arterial pressure at 102 mmHg (for systolic blood pressure of 70 mmHg). Panel (c) is the CW Doppler spectral profile of the patent ductus arteriosus demonstrating bidirectional shunting with right to left systolic gradient of 30 mmHg. Panel (d) is a subcostal view demonstrating a left-to-right inter-atrial shunt, suggesting increased LV end-diastolic pressures despite significant increase in RV afterload.

mesenchymal migration anomalies, distorted fetal flow through the ductus venosus preferentially filling the right ventricle (RV) and disturbed fetal cardiac axis (35, 36). Additionally, decreased LV capacity in post-natal life may occur secondary to under-filling due to decreased LV preload (decreased pulmonary venous return from increased PVR), as well as compression by the hypertensive RV (RV-LV crosstalk) (37). Indeed, left-to-right inter-atrial shunting has been reported in a majority of CDH newborns, even in the presence of supra-systemic pulmonary pressures, indicating increased LV end-diastolic pressures (Figure 35.4) (32, 33, 35). However, interpretation of these findings is limited by the lack of information regarding the concomitant use of pulmonary vasodilators at the time of echocardiography. The persistence of LV hypoplasia/dysfunction during pediatric and adolescent life has also been reported (38).

The complex inter-play between pulmonary vasculature and cardiac performance is unique to CDH newborns, and a deep understanding of their post-natal physiological adaptation is critical to ensure adequate care. As such, the judicious use of a multi-modal therapeutic approach, targeting the underlying mechanisms of disease, is likely key in improving outcomes. Since hemodynamic instability and PH are critical for prognosis, an adequate understanding of underlying cardiovascular physiology is critical when choosing therapeutic agents to support cardiac function and address PH.

Inhaled nitric oxide (iNO)

Hemodynamics management has traditionally focused on addressing the high PVR. Inhaled nitric oxide (iNO), a selective pulmonary vasodilator leading to increased cyclic guanosine monophosphate (cGMP) production in vascular smooth muscle cells by the activation of guanylate cyclase (39), is effective in term and near-term infants with acute PH in the immediate post-natal

life (40). These benefits, however, were not reproduced in the CDH population; specifically, iNO was not associated with a reduction in the combined outcome of need for ECMO and mortality (40). Altered LV mechanics in CDH newborns possibly explain the non-response to this pulmonary vasodilator. Indeed, decreased LV size and performance may lead to left atrial hypertension and, consequently, pulmonary venous congestion. In this context, initiation of a pulmonary vasodilator (such as iNO) may lead to pulmonary vascular congestion (and pulmonary edema and/or hemorrhage), decreased LV preload, and impaired LV cardiac output (Table 35.1). Pulmonary edema leads to abnormal pulmonary mechanics, perfusion to ventilation mismatch, gas exchange and surfactant inactivation. Newborns with abnormal LV function or filling may be dependent on the right to left ductal shunt to provide systemic output. By initiating pulmonary vasodilators, one may decrease systemic perfusion by favoring increasing blood flow to the pulmonary vasculature at the expense of systemic organs. Nonetheless, iNO use has been described in those with acute PH to address the concomitant abnormally increased PVR and certain authors have noted an increasing exposure despite the publication of negative results (41). Recent guidelines have advocated for judicious use of iNO and careful phenotypic profiling based on underlying physiological assessment and in those with adequate LV function and size (42).

Milrinone

Diastolic dysfunction has been described in CDH newborns (43) and is associated with prolonged respiratory support and longer length of hospital stay (44). Milrinone, a phosphodiesterase type 3 inhibitor, increases intracellular smooth muscle cyclic adenosine monophosphate (cAMP) and calcium levels, leading to vasodilation and improved cardiac relaxation (45). Milrinone has been used in the neonatal population for its afterload reduction,

TABLE 35.1 Bimodal Nature of Altered Left Ventricular (LV) Performance in the Context of Neonatal Pulmonary Hypertension

	Primary LV Dysfunction Leading to Post-Capillary Pulmonary Venous Congestion	LV Dysfunction Secondary to Acute PH, Increased PVR, Hypoxia and Acidosis
Increased RV afterload	+ Impaired LV diastolic function leading to left atrial hypertension with insufficient decompression by inter-atrial septal defect.	+++ Abnormally high PVR and/or a decrease in pulmonary vascular cross-sectional area
RV to pulmonary circulation coupling	+ LV dysfunction is hallmark of clinical picture with poor systemic output. RV dysfunction may occur as a late finding.	+++ Significant right ventricular failure (systolic and diastolic). Usually associated with neonatal right to left inter-atrial shunting.
Inter-ventricular crosstalk	+	+++ RV pressure overload impedes on LV cavity, due to bowing interventricular septum.
Coronary artery hypoperfusion	May occur to varying degree in both clinical situations. Hypoperfusion and/or hypoxia may further impair biventricular myocardial contraction and relaxation, especially in the setting of increased myocardial oxygen consumption (such as with: tachycardia or chronotropic medication).	
Decreased LV preload	– Preload is usually preserved until late stages of disease. Diastolic dysfunction may be associated with LV dilation in the context of inadequate LV contraction and emptying.	+++ Pulmonary venous return is significantly lower than expected. Underfilling of left atrium promotes right to left inter-atrial shunting. LV is under-filled, systemic cardiac output may be impaired and dependent on ductal shunting.
Decreased LV structural capacity	+++ Filling may be impaired, and systemic output may be sub-optimal. May also be associated with left atrial hypertension, left to right (or bidirectional) inter-atrial shunt.	– Preserved LV ventricular dimensions.
Increased LV afterload	+++ Inability of LV to adequately perform in the context of rising SVR, compensating for inadequate perfusing pressure. Other clinical situations involve anatomical obstruction (example: small aortic arch, aortic stenosis, coarctation)	–
iNO/pulmonary vasodilators responsiveness	– Pulmonary vasodilators should be avoided in post-capillary pulmonary hypertension and may lead to pulmonary edema.	++ Pulmonary vasodilators act by vasodilating pulmonary arterioles, decreasing RV afterload and promoting pulmonary forward flow.

Abbreviations: iNO, inhaled nitric oxide; LV, left ventricle; PH, pulmonary hypertension; PVR, pulmonary vascular resistance; RV, right ventricle; SVR, systemic vascular resistance.

positive inotropic and lusitropic effects (46). Milrinone has been proposed as an agent potentially addressing the LV involvement in the PH pathophysiology specific to CDH. Off-label use has been described in various cohorts, and up to 50% of CDH newborns are exposed during initial hospitalization (41, 47, 48). In a retrospective study matching patients with mild-to-moderate CDH based on oxygenation index (OI) (47), milrinone use was not associated with improvement in OI, estimated pulmonary pressures and LV dimensions, nor to the occurrence of adverse effects such as nonoperative bleeding, dysrhythmia, hypokalemia, thrombocytopenia, hypotension or change in inotropic scores. Other CDH case series have anecdotally reported improved RV function, LV ejection fraction and OI in association with milrinone (49). Nonetheless, milrinone is currently under investigation in a multi-centric randomized-control trial specifically addressing CDH-related cardiovascular management (50).

Prostaglandin (PGE1) and prostacyclin analogs (prostaglandin I2)

Maintaining ductal patency has been advocated in those with impaired LV output to promote systemic forward flow and/or in those with supra-systemic pulmonary pressures, as a way to decompress the failing RV (37, 51). PGE1 may also have a pulmonary vasodilator effect. Its use in CDH newborns was associated with improved echocardiography PH indices (52) and oxygenation (53). A single retrospective study has described increased hospital stay in association with PGE1 use in CDH, without any survival advantage (54). Other prostacyclin analogs (Treprostinil, Epoprostenol, Iloprost, Beraprost sodium) vasodilate by increasing intracellular cAMP in smooth muscle cells and may be administered by intravenous, subcutaneous, inhaled or oral routes. Although data is limited, PGI2 use has been described in newborns with acute PH in immediate post-natal life or CDH (41, 55).

Sildenafil

Sildenafil, a phosphodiesterase type 5 inhibitor, leads to pulmonary vasodilation by increasing smooth muscle intra-cellular cGMP. In the absence of iNO use, it has been associated with improvement in OI and mortality in non-CDH patients with acute PH (56). In a CDH case series, oral sildenafil was associated with improved echocardiographic PH indices (57). CDH newborns exposed to intravenous sildenafil had improved oxygenation (58) but increased exposure to vasopressor support (59). The effect on PH in CDH of intravenous sildenafil is currently being investigated in a prospective randomized control trial (56).

Hydrocortisone and inotropic support

Adrenal insufficiency has been described in CDH newborns and supplementation may be considered in those with catecholamine-resistant shock (60). Hydrocortisone increased cGMP levels and improved oxygenation in a neonatal lamb model of increased PVR, possibly by promoting pulmonary vasodilation (61). However, one hydrocortisone study in CDH newborns with shock refractory to vasopressors reported increased risk of sepsis with no improvement in survival (62). In a CDH case series, vasopressin was associated with a rise in arterial pressure and a decline in the pulmonary to systemic pressure ratio (63). Finally, other agents commonly used for their inotropic, chronotropic and/or vasoactive properties, such as epinephrine, dobutamine, dopamine and norepinephrine, may be used based on their hypothetical physiological effects, but without specific evidence in the CDH population (64). Norepinephrine (65) and vasopressin (66) have been described to decrease the pulmonary to systemic pressure ratio. As such, these agents are of interest in the management of acute neonatal PH with adequate LV function. Epinephrine is postulated to improve myocardial contractility and increase the systemic vascular resistance, as well as the mean arterial pressure, with an increase in pulmonary vascular resistances only at higher dosages. Finally, dopamine has been associated with an increase in pulmonary to systemic pressure ratio in neonatal animal models (67). As such, this effect may theoretically worsen pulmonary perfusion in CDH newborns with acute PH and, in this situation, may deteriorate their hemodynamics.

Extracorporeal life support

The past decades have been marked by an increase in the use of a protocolized approach to care (42, 68, 69) and lung protective ventilation strategies leading to improvement in survival rates and a decreased use of ECMO (70). Indeed, adoption of a standardized protocol of care (including: Specific minimization of stimulation, use of pre-ductal saturation for saturation targets, gentle ventilation and a step-wise (less aggressive) approach to pulmonary vasodilators and inotropic support), has led to decreased ECMO use and improved survival (71). CDH remains the most frequent indication for neonatal respiratory extra-corporeal support (72), even though available evidence has not shown a survival benefit for ECMO in CDH (42). Veno-venous (VV; respiratory) or veno-arterial (VA; cardio-respiratory) ECMO both have been used, but VA is often the mode of choice in the context of concomitant severe cardiac dysfunction. The choice of ECMO mode (VV or VA) has not been associated with significant effect on mortality or severe neurologic injury (73).

Determinants of surgical timing for diaphragmatic hernia repair

The optimal timing for surgical repair of the diaphragmatic defect in CDH is under debate. Traditionally, repair of the diaphragmatic defect was performed in the immediate neonatal phase as reduction of the intrathoracic herniated abdominal organs was believed to be required to improve the physiology of the newborn. This practice changed when a protocol of permissive hypercapnia/spontaneous respiration/elective surgery demonstrated improved survival in 2002 (74). The surgical closure of the diaphragmatic defect is now commonly delayed until physiological stability is achieved. The Canadian CDH Collaborative and the CDH Euro Consortium have both published consensus clinical criteria guidelines for readiness to proceed with surgical diaphragmatic defect repair (Table 35.2) (42, 69, 75). Typically, if these criteria are not met after the first two weeks of life, a discussion between the treatment team and parents is warranted to discuss next steps, such as proceeding with the surgery or palliative care. Even within the two-week timeframe after birth, there is controversy surrounding the timing of diaphragmatic defect repair – early versus late – and how this affects patient outcomes. On the one hand, late repair may provide a period of respiratory stabilization which allows for the development of hypoplastic lungs; reducing the chance of prolonged PH (76). Other studies demonstrate no difference in survival when early and late repair are compared (42). A randomized controlled trial compared the survival rates of 54 infants who underwent early repair (≤4 hours) or late repair (>24 hours after birth) and reported survival rates of 57% and 46%, respectively (P = 0.42) (77). These

TABLE 35.2 Comparison of the Physiologic and Treatment Criteria as Stated by the Canadian Congenital Diaphragmatic Hernia Collaborative and the CDH EURO Consortium

Physiologic and Treatment Criteria	Canadian Congenital Diaphragmatic Hernia Collaborative	CDH EURO Consortium
	Required Values	
Urine output	>1 mL/kg/h	>1 mL/kg/h
FiO$_2$	>0.5	>0.5
Preductal oxygen saturation	Between 85% and 95%	Between 85% and 95%
Mean arterial pressure	Normal for gestational age	Normal for gestational age
Lactate	<3 mmol/L	<3 mmol/L
Estimated pulmonary artery pressures	Less than systemic pressure	N/A
Postoperative chest tube placement	N/A	None
Relationship with ECMO	Delay until successfully weaned off of ECMO	Repair can be performed on ECMO

Abbreviations: CDH, congenital diaphragmatic hernia; FiO$_2$, oxygen supplementation; ECMO, extracorporeal membrane oxygenation.

results corroborated results from an earlier study by Nio et al., who reported 75% survival in the early repair (≤6 hours) group and 73% in the late repair (≥96 hours) group (78). A review by Puligandla et al. (79) summarizes many of these studies in detail and concludes that there is currently no evidence to favor early or late repair. Though the timing of repair may not affect survival, early repair in moderate cases of CDH may contribute to shorter treatment duration (80). Variable definition of "early-repair" and "late-repair" hampers interpretation and comparison of the reported studies.

The uncertainty around optimal timing for surgical repair becomes even more prominent when discussed in the context of CDH infants treated with ECMO. The Canadian CDH Collaborative and the Congenital Diaphragmatic Hernia Study Group (CDHSG) both recommend to delay surgical repair until successful weaning of ECMO (35). A recent study demonstrated that repair on-ECMO might increase the duration of ECMO runs to last longer than 2 weeks. This increased duration is likely due to the addition of physiological recovery time on ECMO following surgery (81). A study examining a limited, de-identified data set from the CDHSG registry found that repair post-ECMO, as well as other covariates (right-sided defect, lower birth weight, patch repair, longer duration of ECMO run, and lower Apgar score at 5 minutes), were all associated with higher mortality (82). When correcting for all other covariates, death was 1.41 times more likely over a given time period when repair was performed on-ECMO compared to post-ECMO. Another retrospective cases series also reported improved outcomes in patients who received surgical repair post-ECMO, compared to patients who were repaired pre-ECMO and on-ECMO (83). In this study, patients had no difference in "side" of the CDH defect, liver herniation, birth weight, or gestational age and were repaired pre-ECMO (n = 3), on-ECMO (n = 41), or post-ECMO (n = 17). The authors reported survival rates of 60%, 44%, and 100%, respectively (p < 0.01). This study also demonstrated differences between the post-ECMO repair group compared to the on-ECMO group in the median duration of ECMO therapy (311 hours and 452 hours, respectively [p = 0.02]) and surgical site bleeding (0% and 29%, respectively [p < 0.01]).

In contrast to the aforementioned studies, benefits of early repair during ECMO have been highlighted by the CDH Euro Consortium (75). A retrospective study of CDH infants placed on ECMO (n = 46) at the Texas Children's Hospital compared early repair on-ECMO (<72 hours after cannulation), late repair on-ECMO (>72 hours after cannulation), and post-ECMO repair (84). Compared to the late repair on-ECMO and post-ECMO groups, patients who underwent early repair on-ECMO showed a trend towards improved survival (64%, 50%, and 74%, respectively). Compared to late on-ECMO repair, the early on-ECMO repair group also showed a decrease in mean duration of ECMO treatment (18 ± 6.1 days and 12 ± 7.5 days, respectively [p = 0.01]), and in circuit complications (72% and 27%, respectively [p = 0.03]). Another retrospective study of patients undergoing early repair on-ECMO (n = 48) reported acceptable morbidity (surgical site bleeding rates of 8.8%) and mortality rates (survival rates of 71%) (30). When all other surgical readiness criteria are met, benefits of early repair on-ECMO may include improved venous return, decreased mass effect, greater chance of developing normal thoracic anatomy, and fewer days on ECMO (47, 48). Finally, a recent study from the CDHSG reported that in a group of 136 patients undergoing repair on-ECMO or post-ECMO, the patients repaired on-ECMO had better survival (hazard ratio

0.54 (0.38, 0.77) (p < 0.05) and lower incidence of no repair of the diaphragmatic defect, 5.9% versus 33.8% (p < 0.05) (85). In another subgroup analysis of 77 patients the authors demonstrated that patients repaired early on-ECMO had a lower mortality HR 0.51 (0.33, 0.77) (p = 0.002) as well as a lower incidence of non-repair, 9.1% versus 44.2% (p < 0.001) than patients repaired later on-ECMO. As discussed, many controversies remain surrounding the timing of surgical diaphragmatic defect repair in CDH. This is true for both early or late repair after birth as well early or late repair on-ECMO and post-ECMO. Ongoing studies from the CDHSG will hopefully provide more answers in the near future. It is incumbent of researchers engaged in CDH science to strive for sufficiently powered, multicentre, prospective, randomized controlled trials to definitively determine what the best time is to repair a diaphragmatic defect in CDH. In the interim, clinicians should incorporate best practice evidence within the context of the unique cardiopulmonary physiologic status to optimize the clinical decision-making process.

References

1. Thebaud B, et al. Intensive Care Med. 1997; 23(10):1062–1069.
2. Wynn J, et al. Semin Fetal Neonatal Med. 2014; 19(6):324–330
3. Garne E, et al. Ultrasound Obstet Gynecol. 2002; 19(4):329–333.
4. Graham G, et al. Semin Perinatol. 2005; 29(2):69–76.
5. Cannie M, et al. Ultrasound Obstet Gynecol. 2008; 32(5):627–632.
6. Lazar DA, et al. J Pediatr Surg. 2012; 47(6):1058–1062.
7. Mullassery D, et al. Ultrasound Obstet Gynecol. 2010; 35(5):609–614.
8. Victoria T, et al. Prenatal diagnosis. 2012; 32(8):715–723.
9. Zamora IJ, et al. J Pediatr Surg. 2014; 49(5):688–693.
10. Ruano R, et al. J Pediatr Surg. 2014; 43(6):662–669.
11. Sbragia L, et al. J Ultrasound Med. 2000; 19(12):845–848.
12. Lipshutz GS, et al. J Pediatr Surg. 1997; 32(11):1634–1636.
13. Keller R, et al. Ultrasound Obstet Gynecol. 2003; 21(3):244–249.
14. Jani JC, et al. Am J Obstet Gynecol. 2006; 195(6):1646–1650.
15. Peralta C, et al. Ultrasound Obstet Gynecol. 2005; 26(7):718–724.
16. Benachi A, et al. Semin Fetal Neonatal Med. 2014; 19(6):331–337.
17. Jani J, et al. Ultrasound Obstet Gynecol. 2007; 30(1):67–71.
18. Deprest JA, et al. Semin Fetal Neonatal Med. 2009; 14(1):8–13.
19. Hedrick HL, et al. Am J Obstet Gynecol. 2007; 197(4):422.e1–424.e1.
20. Büsing KA, et al. Radiology. 2008; 248(1):240–246.
21. Barnewolt CE, et al. J Pediatr Surg. 2007; 42(1):193–197.
22. Lee TC, et al. J Pediatr Surg. 2011; 46(6):1165–1171.
23. Rypens F, et al. Radiology. 2001; 219(1):236–241.
24. Jani J, et al. Ultrasound Obstet Gynecol. 2008; 32(6):793–799.
25. Madenci AL, et al. J Pediatr Surg. 2013; 48(6):1190–1197.
26. Schaible T, et al. Eur J Radiol. 2012; 81(5):1076–1082.
27. Au-Fliegner M, et al. J Pediatr Surg. 1998; 33(9):1366–1370.
28. Kumar VHS, et al. Pediatr Surg Int. 2018; 34(7):735–742.
29. Mous DS, et al. Respir Res. 2017; 18(1):187.
30. Dassinger MS, et al. J Pediatr Surg. 2010; 45(4):693–697.
31. Kays DW, et al. J Am Coll Surg. 2014; 218(4):808–817.
32. Altit G, et al. J Pediatr. 2017; 191:28.e1–34.e1.
33. Altit G, et al. Pediatr Cardiol. 2018; 39(5):993–1000.
34. Patel N, et al. J Pediatr. 2018; 203:400.e1–407.e1.
35. Wehrmann M, et al. J Pediatr. 2020; 219:43–47.
36. DeKoninck P, et al. Prenatal diagnosis. 2014; 34(13):1262–1267.
37. Kinsella JP, et al. J Pediatr. 2018 Jun; 197:17–22.
38. Abolmaali N, et al. Eur Radiol. 2010; 20(7):1580–1589.
39. Archer SL, et al. Proc Natl Acad Sci USA 1994; 91(16):7583–7587.
40. Barrington KJ, et al. Cochrane Database Syst Rev. 2017; 1(1):CD000399.
41. Zalla JM, et al. J Pediatr Surg. 2015; 50(4):524–527.
42. Puligandla PS, et al. CMAJ. 2018; 190(4):E103–E112.
43. Tanaka T, et al. Pediatr Surg Int. 2015; 31(10):905–910.
44. Moenkemeyer F, et al. Pediatr Crit Care Med. 2014; 15(1):49–55.
45. McNamara PJ, et al. J Crit Care. 2006; 21(2):217–222.
46. Lakshminrusimha S, et al. Pediatr Crit Care Med. 2013; 14(1):107–109.
47. Mears M, et al. Am J Perinatol. 2020; 37(3):258–263.
48. Malowitz JR, et al. Am J Perinatol. 2015; 32(9):887–894.
49. Patel N. Neonatology. 2012; 102(2):130–136.
50. Lakshminrusimha S, et al. Matern Health Neonatol Perinatol. 2017; 3:27.
51. Aljohani OA, et al. World J Pediatr Congenit Heart Surg. 2020; 11(4):525–527.
52. Lawrence KM, et al. J Pediatr Surg. 2019; 54(1):55–59.
53. Duc L K, et al. J Pediatr Surg. 2020; 55(9):1872–1878.
54. Shiyanagi S, et al. Pediatr Surg Int. 2008; 24(10):1101–1104.
55. Carpentier E, et al. J Pediatr Surg. 2017; 52(9):1480–1483.
56. Cochius-den Otter S, et al. BMJ Open. 2019; 9(11):e032122.

57. Noori S, et al. Neonatology. 2007; 91(2):92–100.
58. Eur J Pediatr Surg. 2015; 25(2):171–176.
59. Kipfmueller F, et al. Pediatr Pulmonol. 2018; 53(4):452–460.
60. Kamath BD, et al. J Pediatr. 2010; 156(3):495.e1–497.e1.
61. Perez M, et al. Am J Physiol Lung Cell Mol Physiol. 2012; 302(6):L595–L603.
62. Robertson JO, et al. Pediatr Surg Int. 2017; 33(9):981–987.
63. Acker SN, et al. J Pediatr. 2014; 165(1):53.e1–58.e1.
64. Buijs EA, et al. Pediatr Crit Care Med. 2014; 15(4):343–354.
65. Tourneux P, et al. J Pediatr. 2008; 153(3):345–349.
66. Mohamed AA, et al. J Matern Fetal Neonatal Med. 2020:1–9.
67. Barrington KJ, et al. Crit Care Med. 1995; 23(4):740–748.
68. Zalla JM, et al. J Pediatr Surg. 2015; 50(4):524–527.
69. Reiss I, et al. Neonatology. 2010; 98(4):354–364.
70. Harting MT, et al. Semin Fetal Neonatal Med. 2014; 19(6):370–375.
71. Yang MJ, et al. J Perinatol. 2020; 40(6):935–942.
72. Maslach-Hubbard A, et al. World J Crit Care Med. 2013; 2(4):29–39.
73. Guner YS, et al. J Pediatr Surg. 2018; 53(11):2092–2099.
74. Boloker J, et al. J Pediatr Surg. 2002; 37(3):357–366.
75. Snoek KG, et al. Neonatology. 2016; 110(1):66–74.
76. Chatziioannidis I, et al. Hippokratia. 2014; 18(4):381.
77. de la Hunt MN, et al. J Pediatr Surg. 1996; 31(11):1554–1556.
78. Nio M, et al. J Pediatr Surg. 1994; 29(5):618–621.
79. Puligandla PS, et al. J Pediatr Surg. 2015; 50(11):1958–1970.
80. Okuyama H, et al. Pediatr Surg Int. 2017; 33(2):133–138.
81. Delaplain PT, et al. J Pediatr Surg. 2020; 55(6):993–997.
82. Bryner BS, et al. J Pediatr Surg. 2009; 44(6):1165–1171.
83. Partridge EA, et al. J Pediatr Surg. 2015; 50(2):260–262.
84. Fallon SC, et al. J Pediatr Surg. 2013; 48(6):1172–1176.
85. Dao DT, et al. Ann Surg. 2019. doi:10.1097/SLA.0000000000003386.

SPECIAL CONSIDERATION

Hypoxemic Respiratory Failure among Patients with Hypoxic Ischemic Encephalopathy

Arvind Sehgal, Satyan Lakshminrusimha and Regan E Giesinger

Contents

Introduction

Neonatal encephalopathy related to perinatal asphyxia is a clinical syndrome presenting as abnormal neurologic function following birth (1). Among neonates where hypoxia-ischemia is the predominant mechanism, low Apgar scores, umbilical artery acidemia and the presence of multiorgan failure are typical (1). Hypoxic-Ischemic Encephalopathy (HIE) carries affects approximately 1–2/1000 to 26/1000 live births in developed (2) and low-resource countries, respectively (3). Birth asphyxia, defined as lack of blood flow and/or gas exchange immediately before, during or after delivery (4), accounts for ~1 million deaths per year (5) and is a leading cause of infant mortality. The ~1 million children who survive birth asphyxia yearly may have chronic neurodevelopmental morbidities, including cerebral palsy, intellectual, and learning disabilities (6).

The fetal brain is relatively more resilient to hypoxia-ischemia than the older child or adult due to utilization of alternative energy sources (e.g. lactate, ketones), fetal and placental mechanisms to optimize gas exchange and fetal circulatory adaptation. Fetal asphyxia precipitates adaptation aimed at preserving blood flow to essential organs (7). A catecholamine surge produces vasoconstriction thereby centralizing blood flow, and hypoxemia increases pulmonary vascular resistance (PVR). Increased PVR reduces the 10% of combined cardiac output (CO) that normally flows to the lungs, to divert further blood (Figure 36.1). Simultaneously it increases RV afterload which increases right ventricular (RV) cavity pressure promoting right-to-left atrial flow in support of coronary and brain perfusion (8). When these and other compensatory mechanisms fail, asphyxial brain injury may occur. In part, consequent to these fetal changes, hypoxic respiratory failure (HRF) and/or pulmonary hypertension (PH) may accompany HIE. The pathogenesis of this association,

however, is multifactorial and the process itself may be dynamic, evolving with time (disease course) and therapy. It is important to recognize the risk for PH because it is not always clinically apparent (9), although its severity may influence treatment decisions (e.g. continuation of therapeutic hypothermia [TH]) and impact outcomes. The following chapter presents the diverse contributors to HRF in the HIE population, the interaction between HIE and PH and highlights therapeutic considerations unique to these patients.

Pathophysiological contributors to HRF among patients with HIE

Changes which are adaptive to lack of oxygen and perfusion for the fetus are pathological after delivery. Other modifiers which compromise the neonatal transition (e.g. lung disease), factors that reduce the neonate's adaptive capacity to high pulmonary artery pressure (PAP) (e.g. RV dysfunction, adrenal insufficiency) or postnatal therapies that raise PVR further (e.g. TH, pulmonary vasoconstrictors) may all exacerbate disease severity. In addition, neonates with HIE are prone to seizures, which may be difficult to detect in the absence of electroencephalography (EEG) changes, particularly among patients with significant cardiorespiratory illness. Epileptic events should be considered in the differential of vital sign abnormalities, particularly acute hypoxemia. For each patient, there may be multiple inter-related physiological changes which modulate a common endpoint of severe hypoxemia, the most relevant of which will be explored in more detail.

Concurrent lung disease

The population of patients at risk for HIE includes those born following complicated pregnancies which also put them at higher risk for diseases that present with HRF (Table 36.1). Lung

DOI: 10.1201/9780367494018-36

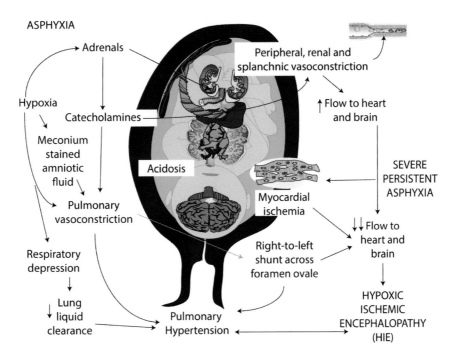

FIGURE 36.1 Hemodynamic consequences of asphyxia. During moderate asphyxia, blood flow to intestines, kidney and lung are decreased. The blood flow to the brain, heart and adrenals is preserved. Release of catecholamines from the adrenals further contributes to pulmonary and peripheral vasoconstriction. Respiratory depression and poor clearance of lung liquid also contribute to increased pulmonary vascular resistance. With persistent asphyxial insult, blood flow to the heart and brain eventually decreases, leading to myocardial necrosis and hypoxic-ischemic encephalopathy (HIE). (Copyright Satyan Lakshminrusimha 2021.)

disease may interfere with gas exchange, alter lung compliance, produce areas of intrapulmonary shunt and therefore independently contributing to raised PVR (10). Even in the absence of specific lung pathology, efficient clearance of fetal lung water requires a forceful inhaled air column to displace the air-fluid interface and create a pressure gradient for fetal lung fluid to be absorbed into the interstitium (11). The asphyxiated neonate who does not initiate respirations is reliant on less effective positive pressure breaths, which may interfere with establishing functional residual capacity.

Impact of asphyxia on the myocardium

Structural and metabolic characteristics of fetal cardiomyocytes confer vulnerability to asphyxia (12). Antioxidant systems are underdeveloped at birth (13). Normally cardiomyocyte metabolism switches almost entirely from glycolytic pathways to oxidation of fatty acids for metabolism (12), to enhance efficiency and adapt to the oxygen-enriched environment. Ischemia upends this change. Myocardial ischemia may be further complicated by

diminished preload, asphyxia induced autonomic dysfunction and/or vasoplegia (14).

Electrocardiography changes following asphyxia have been linked to neurological outcomes in the pre-cooling era (15, 16). Cardiac biomarkers, too have been studied (16–18). CO is lower and cardiac troponin (cTnT) higher following asphyxia compared to healthy controls (17) cTnT is associated with low CO and impaired coronary flow, highlighting the central role of myocardial perfusion (18). On autopsy, 20–30% of neonates with myocardial necrosis have a history of asphyxia (19), making it the most common single cause of myocardial ischemia. As echocardiography becomes increasingly sophisticated, a more robust literature supporting abnormal cardiac function is emerging(20) and being related to biomarkers including cTnT (21). LV myocardial velocities and deformation indices which are lower than expected for age have been reported using Tissue Doppler imaging (TDI) and speckle tracking echocardiography (STE), respectively (20–22). The severity of RV dysfunction, comparatively, may be greater and has been associated with brain injury independent of illness severity (22).

TABLE 36.1 Examples of Pregnancy Complications Commonly Associated with Both Hypoxic Ischemic Encephalopathy and a Second Disorder Contributing to Hypoxemic Respiratory Failure

Pregnancy Complication	Possible Association with HIE	Possible Association with HRF
Impaired glucose metabolism	Cephalo-pelvic disproportion (e.g. LGA)	Respiratory distress syndrome
Chorioamnionitis	Placental dysfunction	Neonatal pneumonia or sepsis
Maternal hypertensive disorders	Placental insufficiency	Intrauterine growth restriction
Prolonged rupture of membranes	Cord prolapse	Neonatal pneumonia or sepsis
Post-dates pregnancy	Placental dysfunction	Delivery without labor (failed transition, retained fetal lung fluid)
Emergency c/s	Fetal distress	Meconium aspiration syndrome

There are several possible explanations for RV predominant disease which relate to the conformation (i.e. large circumferential-area:radius), metabolic demands (i.e. dominant ventricle during transition), nature of coronary circulation and both a vulnerability and exposure to high afterload to which the LV is relatively better suited. Because of an inability of the RV to generate sufficient pressure to achieve normal end-systolic emptying when PVR and PAP are high, RV and right atrial (RA) pressures climb and the RV dilates. This contributes to escalating metabolic requirements, low CO and low aortic root pressure. Coronary circulation to the RV, which depends on an aorta to RA pressure gradient, is thus disadvantaged biologically. Additionally, RV dilation leads to abnormal LV shape and RV dysfunction disadvantages the LV by shared myocardial fibers (i.e. interventricular dependence). Like LV dysfunction, RV disease tends to be worse in the first postnatal days and typically resolves by 96 h (23).

Implications of cardiac dysfunction on adaptation to pulmonary hypertension

Normal RV systolic function is critical for adequate PBF; abnormalities may relate to myocardial ischemia and/or elevated PAP. RV function is dependent on afterload. With increasing PAP, there is a proportional decline in RV systolic function which is governed by the stress-velocity relationship (i.e. RV:PA coupling). Maturational characteristics of the myocardium dictate the decrement in function by unit increase in afterload (24). Echocardiography has been used to approximate this relationship by relating the tricuspid annulus plane systolic excursion (TAPSE) to non-invasive and invasive measures of PVR and PAP. This has relevance because when RV-PA coupling is normal, treatment lowering PVR may also enhance RV performance and normalize RV function.

Although there is limited HIE evidence, 'uncoupling' may occur due to due to coexistence of myocardial ischemic injury (22). RV ischemia may predispose the asphyxiated neonate with elevated PAP to impaired PBF and ultimately low CO. RV dysfunction is, therefore, the catalyst for a cascade of downstream events and self-perpetuating cycle of declining cardiovascular wellbeing which ultimately results in cardiac arrest if untreated (Figure 36.2). Hypoxemia may or may not accompany elevated PAP in the early stages, depending on the degree to which lung disease is interfering with the ability to appropriately match ventilation (V) to perfusion (Q). Ultimately, however, impaired cerebral oxygen delivery occurs even under perfectly V/Q matched conditions because of poor CO. Lung disease may further aggravate the magnitude of hypoxemia via intrapulmonary shunt. Due to impaired cerebral autoregulation, low CO may precipitate ongoing brain injury as may hypoxemia, oxidative stress and fluctuating cerebral perfusion pressure.

Role of adrenal insufficiency

Adrenal insufficiency may also be an important consideration (25). In lamb models, a rapid increase in adrenocorticotropic hormone (ACTH) and cortisol secretion occurs both during acute complete and partial prolonged asphyxia (26, 27). This is in keeping with the fetal adaptative response to centralize blood flow by raising vascular resistance. After 3–5 minutes of umbilical cord occlusion, adaptation fails and cerebral blood flow (CBF) declines, followed by adrenal blood flow (28). While ACTH returns to normal after restoration of blood flow *in utero*, cortisol levels remain high for hours to days (26, 27). Delivery of the fetus followed by neonatal resuscitation is associated with increased adrenal blood flow and elevated cortisol despite low BP (28). Human neonates demonstrate elevated serum cortisol with suppressed dehydro-epiandrosterone sulfate suggesting a redistribution of adrenal production towards the glucocorticoid pathway (29). Together this data suggests an intact stress response and possibly a new cortisol set-point following asphyxia; in a piglet model, however, although cortisol levels were high, a delayed response to adrenocorticotrophin stimulation may occur (30).

The clinical significance of these animal studies is unclear but the role for postnatal glucocorticoid supplementation may, in any case, be independent of adrenal adaptation. Steroids play an important role in upregulating myocardial and vascular adrenoreceptors, increasing circulating catecholamines (inhibited degradation), improving vessel tone and decreasing capillary leak (31). In a placebo-controlled trial of cooled patients with HIE treated with dopamine, those receiving hydrocortisone required a lower dopamine dose and duration, suggesting responsiveness to exogenously administered glucocorticoid (32). In addition, adrenal hemorrhage has been associated with HIE and may be asymptomatic (i.e. if unilateral) or associated with adrenal insufficiency. Adrenal dysfunction should be considered, particularly for neonates with refractory hypotension.

The use of TH as a neuroprotective agent

Clinical trials using TH (33–34°C) have demonstrated meaningful reductions in both mortality (NNT = 11) and risk of neurodevelopmental impairment (NNT = 8) for term infants with HIE (33). The most beneficial effect is among neonates with 'moderate encephalopathy' based on clinical exam with or without amplitude integrated EEG. The biological mechanisms include reduced cellular metabolism, suppression of microglia activation with lower inducible nitric oxide synthase activity, and both lower pro-inflammatory cytokines and phagocyte activity (34, 35). Given TH's widespread use, it is important to understand its effects on hemodynamics, gas exchange and its potential cardioprotective role.

Effects of TH on hemodynamics

Severe (30°C) hypothermia produces a nearly 50% increase in mean PAP (36) in a neonatal lamb and mild (34–35°C) hypothermia has been associated with cardiovascular changes including reduced CO and lower LV function in piglets (37). Cold-induced increase in PVR may be related to peripheral vasoconstriction, release of catecholamines and/or blood viscosity which increases with lower body temperature (38). Clinical studies suggest that some neonates experience an increase in requirement for oxygen (39) and echocardiography evidence of elevated PVR (40) during TH, which reverses on rewarming. Clinical symptoms of increased PVR may or may not be apparent depending on baseline degree of RV dysfunction, which may pre-date TH (40), and degree of V/Q mismatch (hypoxemia) while normothermic. For neonates with substantial pre-existing pulmonary vasoconstriction or RV dysfunction, an increase in PVR by 1% per degree, as suggested by an animal model (41), may have substantial consequences. A marginal increase in afterload may be a tipping point for patients with poor RV function and patients with modest hypoxemia may have increased intrapulmonary shunt, and therefore greater oxygenation impairment. Although a higher incidence of clinical PH was not evident from pooled randomized trial analyzes (42), the value of pulmonary hemodynamics data is questionable; neonates with HRF were largely excluded, corrected mean PaO_2 was maintained

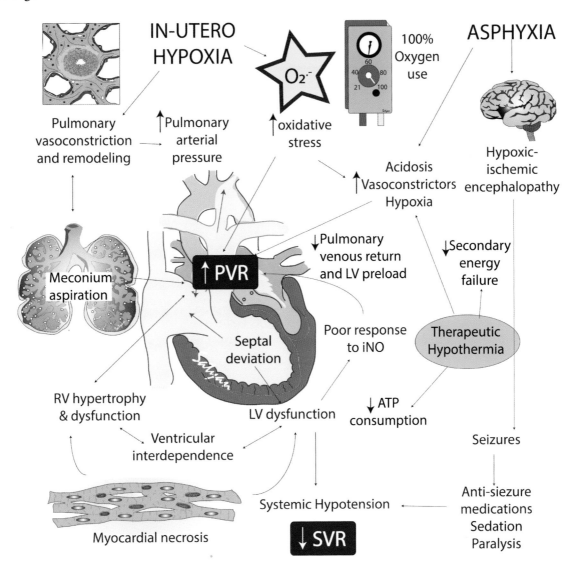

FIGURE 36.2 The vicious cycle of PPHN in asphyxia. *In utero* hypoxia and perinatal asphyxia contribute to pulmonary vascular remodeling and vasoconstriction. Preexisting lung disease such as meconium aspiration syndrome contributes to increased pulmonary vascular resistance (PVR) and right ventricular (RV) hypertrophy and dysfunction. Myocardial ischemia, ventricular interdependence and septal deviation, poor pulmonary venous return (and reduced preload) lead to left ventricular (LV) dysfunction. LV dysfunction, sedation, anti-seizure medications and vasoplegia can contribute to systemic hypotension and reduced systemic vascular resistance (SVR). LV dysfunction and oxidative stress due to hyperoxic ventilation can lead to poor response to inhaled nitric oxide (iNO). Therapeutic hypothermia reduces ATP consumption and prevents secondary energy failure in brain (and possibly myocardium) and improves outcomes but can contribute to pulmonary vasoconstriction and exacerbation of pulmonary hypertension. (Copyright Satyan Lakshminrusimha 2021.)

>70 mmHg during the cooling period (43) and echocardiography was not systematically performed.

Lower CO, related to reduced heart rate with preserved stroke volume, has been identified in multiple neonatal studies (22, 44, 45). Lower superior vena cava (SVC) flow overall (2) with a redistribution of total systemic flow to the central nervous system as reflected by a greater ratio of SVC:LVO (left ventricular output), have been shown to be associated with abnormal MRI (44). This may reflect abnormal cerebral autoregulation but the clinical relevance needs further exploration. One may speculate that bradycardia may either be protective or a response to lower cardiac metabolism. Both LVO and SVC flow increase with rewarming and, given the risk of reperfusion injury, careful monitoring and weaning of cardiovascular drugs should be considered.

Effect of TH on gas exchange

Reduced PBF from TH increases the V/Q ratio. Reduced temperature results in lower partial pressure of gas and increases solubility assuming that the volume the gas is constant (PV = nRT, where P is the pressure of the gas, V is the volume, n is the number of moles of gas, R is a constant and T is the temperature in Kelvin) (46). During whole-body hypothermia, both $PaCO_2$ and PaO_2 decrease; hence, blood gases are corrected for body temperature in most studies evaluating TH. Targeting $PaCO_2$ (temperature-corrected) in the mid-40s is thought to promote CBF resulting in uniform brain cooling. End-tidal CO_2 correlates well with temperature corrected $PaCO_2$ in infants undergoing whole-body TH (47). The oxygen-hemoglobin dissociation curve shifts left as temperature falls. Pulse oximetry does not accurately predict corrected

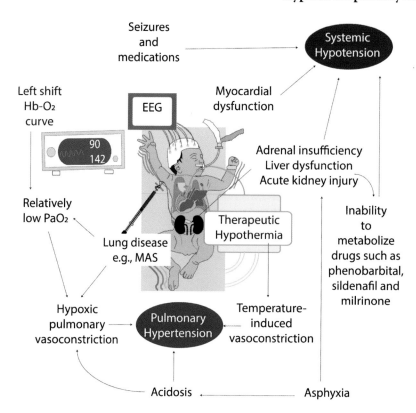

FIGURE 36.3 Hemodynamic effects of therapeutic whole-body hypothermia. Low temperature-induced pulmonary vasoconstriction along with alveolar hypoxia leads to pulmonary hypertension which can be exacerbated by acidosis induced by asphyxia. The leftward shift in oxygen-hemoglobin dissociation curve may mask systemic hypoxia (if blood gases are not temperature-corrected). Adrenal insufficiency can lead to systemic hypotension due to loss of cortisol and catecholamines. Myocardial failure, liver dysfunction and acute kidney injury may limit metabolism of medications such as phenobarbital, sildenafil and milrinone exacerbating systemic hypotension. (Copyright Satyan Lakshminrusimha 2021.)

PaO$_2$, might underestimate hypoxemia and increase the risk of PH. Targeting SpO$_2$ in the 92–98% range results in a PaO$_2$ of 70 mmHg during normothermia but only a PaO$_2$ of 51 mmHg at 33.5°C (47). Frequent arterial blood gas monitoring with a target of corrected PaO$_2$ 50–80 mmHg, and preductal SpO$_2$ ≥ 92% is recommended.

Potential cardioprotective role of TH
Although changes in vascular tone and loading conditions may be deleterious, TH may have relevant cardioprotective effects. In adult cardiac ischemia models of TH, reduced metabolism, energy preservation, and positive inotropy have been shown in some studies (48). Animal models demonstrate lower ATP consumption at 32–34°C and smaller infarcts with lesser post-ischemic dysfunction (49–51). TH may also be used in the post-operative management of congenital heart disease (CHD) (52). Limiting reactive oxygen species, inflammation modulation, and the possible mitigation of mitochondrial damage are other proposed mechanisms (53). Given differences in cardiac metabolism, myocardial composition and mechanism of injury, neonatal data specific to HIE should be considered.

Evaluation of cardiovascular dysfunction in neonates with HIE

Comprehensive consideration of physiology is essential due to multiple possible contributors to hypoxemia, low cardiac output state (LCOS) and hypotension. As previously mentioned,

RV dysfunction may present as low CO alone due to intact V/Q matching with an increased V/Q ratio and catecholamine-induced increased in SVR. A high index of suspicion for abnormal RV function is required as strategies that increase BP by inducing systemic vasoconstriction may be harmful. Characterizing hemodynamic status ("stable/unstable") following asphyxia is challenging, because it may be difficult to separate ongoing from pre-existing organ injury. Plasma lactate and base deficit have been associated more with the severity of the primary injury (54) and, although the rate of decline of lactate has been investigated, it has shown poor relationship with serial noninvasive CO measures (45). Similarly, acute kidney injury (AKI), which impacts up to 70% of neonates with HIE and may be severe (55, 56), may obviate urine output as a marker of cardiovascular health. In adults with normal kidney function, urine output decreased by 5 mL/h/1°C reduction core temperature, making TH another potential confounder (57). Modifications of skin perfusion induced by temperature and centralization of blood flow compound the reliability of capillary refill time and skin color.

The use of BP as a metric, similarly, has challenges. Although it is known that mean BP and CO are not directly related in pre-term infants (58), this relationship has not been studied in term patients with HIE. Given the biological mechanisms involved, however, it is likely that BP is an inconsistent predictor of CO, and therefore CBF, in this population also. In randomized trials of TH, most neonates were treated with non-specific vasoactive agents aiming to increase systemic arterial pressure (SAP).

TABLE 36.2 Elements of a Comprehensive Echocardiogram in Patients with HIE

Pulmonary Pressure	Pulmonary/Systemic Hemodynamics	Cardiac Function	Shunts	Anatomic R/O
• Estimation of RVSp or mPAP based on TR or PI if available • Septal motion (eccentricity index) • Shunt characteristics • Ratio of RVET:PAAT • Presence of PA notching	• Left ventricular output • Right ventricular output • End-organ flow evaluation (MCA, celiac artery Doppler)	• Quantitative RV function (TAPSE, RV-FAC) • Quantitative systolic LV function (EF, Simpson's biplane method) • RV size • LV diastolic function	• Ductal size (characterize restriction) • Ductal direction • Atrial restrictiveness/ direction • Presence/direction VSDs if applicable	• Aortic arch anomalies • Transposition/major duct dependent lesions • Obstructed pulmonary venous drainage

Abbreviations: RVSp, right ventricular systolic pressure; mPAP, mean pulmonary artery pressure; TR, tricuspid regurgitation; PI, pulmonary insufficiency; RVET, right ventricular ejection time; PAAT, pulmonary artery acceleration time; MCA, middle cerebral artery; TAPSE, tricuspid annulus plane systolic excursion; RV-FAC, right ventricular fractional area change; RV, right ventricle; LV, left ventricle; EF, ejection fraction; VSD, ventricular septal defect; R/O, rule out.

It is important to acknowledge, however, that significant practice variability in how clinicians define low SAP in this population (59) exists; also, the contributors to changes in SAP, while often assumed to be vasomotor in origin (60), may actually vary widely. It is also relevant that the optimal SAP, CO, and CBF targets prior to or during TH and upon rewarming are unknown. In the absence of concrete data, the use of a holistic approach that aims to maintain normal or near-normal tissue oxygenation and avoid extreme fluctuations in organ perfusion pressure and blood flow is prudent. Echocardiography and other modalities, such as near infrared spectroscopy (NIRS) may also aid in monitoring of organ-level hemodynamics.

Role of echocardiography

Quantitative echocardiography or Targeted Neonatal Echocardiography (TnECHO) in centers where this is available, may play an important role in delineating physiology and guiding treatment. Direct and indirect measures may be used to quantify the degree of cardiac dysfunction, evaluate the relative contribution of RV and LV disease, objectify pulmonary and systemic blood flow (SBF) and evaluate the patency, and directionality of flow, through shunts. Because of the complexity of the potential contributors to disease, it is essential that comprehensive and standardized evaluation is performed by trained experts. The minimum suggested components of a complete evaluation are indicated in Table 36.2.

Although deranged pulmonary and SBF are expected due to failure of normal transition among patients with HIE, it is important to remember that CHD may concurrently be present. Placental blood flow or sentinel delivery events (e.g. uterine rupture, cord prolapse) are often assumed to be the cause of HIE; however, postnatal cardiovascular collapse due to CHD should remain on the differential and echocardiography of sufficient quality to rule it out be performed. Although many centers have integrated echocardiography into the assessment of neonates with HIE either as a screening or diagnostic tool, the majority report using objective measures of LV but not RV performance and CO remains uncommonly reported except in centers with access to TnECHO (59). Given the prominence of RV disease and the association of abnormal function at 24h post-natal age with adverse outcome (22), quantitative assessment of RV performance (see *Echo of PH* chapter) including TAPSE and fractional area change (FAC) should be measured (22).

Role for cerebral near-infrared spectroscopy

Cerebral Near-Infrared Spectroscopy (NIRS) has been increasingly studied as an adjunctive tool in the last 5 years. NIRS uses

light to quantify cerebral oxygen saturation (CrSO$_2$, combined saturation of the arterial and venous blood components weighted ~25:75%, respectively for volume) and fractional tissue oxygen extraction [(SpO$_2$–CrSO$_2$)/SpO$_2$] and to estimate regional cerebral blood volume (CBV, concentration of oxygenated+deoxygenated hemoglobin) (61). Although >45 studies have been published, small numbers with widely varied methodology and outcome measures make the body of literature challenging to interpret. Several studies suggest that high CrSO$_2$ (62-64) and/or low CrSO$_2$ variation (62) at various time-points in the first 96 postnatal hours portend negative prognosis, which may be biologically interpreted as relating to low cellular metabolism and decreased oxygen utilization. There is inconsistency in studies evaluating CBV; van Bel et al. and others have noted low CBV among neonates with severe HIE in the first 12 h (65, 66) with increasing values and more stability between 12–24 hrs of age (65) in the pre-cooling era. Others equate higher CBV with poor outcome on the first postnatal day, highlighting the importance of continued refinement in this area (67, 68). Also of importance is the consideration of end-organ measurements using NIRS within the context of systemic substrate delivery. For example, although high CrSO$_2$ among patients with more severe brain injury is widely assumed to be related primarily to low oxygen utilization, it is possible that redirection of left ventricular output to the brain (44) may be providing greater delivery, thus reducing the need for extraction and biasing the assessment of CrSO$_2$ (i.e. "luxury perfusion"). One study with both NIRS and simultaneous TnECHO supports the utilization theory (22), however, further study combining modalities is needed; therefore for clinical purposes, both systemic and end-organ monitoring are complimentary and recommended.

Treatment considerations specific to patients with HIE and comorbid cardiovascular instability

Heterogenous disease severity, comorbid PH, lack of consensus regarding normal SAP, effect of TH, and lack of easy access to physiological information in many centers influence decision-making. Most North American units report using **dopamine**, a primary vasoconstrictor as first-line treat patients with PH and HIE (59). Dopamine, however, has been shown to increase PVR>SVR in animal models. In fact, dopamine alone or in combination with epinephrine is associated with an increase in PAP by 94–101% in a piglet asphyxia model (69). The clinical effects of increased PVR may be obvious among patients with concurrent

HRF who have worsening hypoxemia. Among those patients with high PAP, intact V/Q matching and RV dysfunction; however, the effects may be difficult to detect. Progressive tachycardia with declining perfusion may be attributed to disease progression rather than a medication side effect producing RV failure due to increased afterload and low CO-mediated RV ischemia secondary to coronary hypoperfusion. Hypoxemia due to a profoundly LCOS may occur secondarily. Medication administration which is followed by clinical deterioration should be reconsidered; pharmacologic appropriateness and physiology should be reassessed. Given the biological likelihood of RV disease and elevated PAP in this population, it is essential that choices of therapy consider both the underlying physiology, properties of specific drugs/therapies, and characteristics of the patient which may impact drug response and clearance.

Therapeutic considerations in managing hypoxemic respiratory failure

Careful appraisal of lung compliance, carbon dioxide clearance and chest radiography to determine the degree of lung disease prior to initiation of high mean airway pressure (Paw) ventilation is recommended. The open-lung strategy, typically employed in the management of preterm lung disease (70) (adequate recruitment determined by fraction of inspired oxygen ≤30%), only applies if PBF is assumed to be normal. Utilization of high PEEP or high-frequency ventilation with high Paw may be harmful to patients with minimal lung disease. Excessive Paw when lung compliance is good may over-distend alveoli, iatrogenically increase PVR (10) and precipitate acute PH crisis. Surfactant, similarly, should be used judiciously. Although associated with improved PVR and FRC among premature patients with respiratory distress syndrome (71), impaired gas exchange due to transient airway obstruction may impair alveolar ventilation (72) and increase PAP. Stable oxygenation and medical control of PH should be established prior to initiation of TH to avoid precipitating a potentially fatal PH crisis by cold-mediated PVR increase. For patients with refractory hypoxemia while cooled despite aggressive medical therapy, an increase in temperature by 0.5–1°C increments may allow temporary stabilization.

Inhaled nitric oxide (iNO) remains standard of care in HIE-associated PH and should be considered for hypoxic patients if PVR remains high after establishing FRC and alveolar ventilation. Although response to iNO has not been shown different among patients with HIE compared to those with PH for other reasons, resuscitation practices may influence iNO response; asphyxiated lambs resuscitated with 100% oxygen as compared to those resuscitated using 21%, subsequently have an impaired response to iNO (73) This may relate to formation of reactive oxygen species and is one reason why room-air resuscitation is recommended. Sedation and muscle relaxation are not contraindicated for HIE patients, however, morphine and midazolam clearance (74) may be significantly reduced by TH which may lead to systemic hypotension. Additionally, continuous EEG monitoring should be strongly considered for heavily sedated or muscle relaxed patients given the prevalence of seizures and their propensity to present as acute hypoxemia. *Milrinone*, a phosphodiesterase-3-inhibitor, is a commonly used adjunct PH therapy with established pharmacology (75). It acts by increasing intracellular cyclic adenosine monophosphate and has been shown to benefit CO and SBF in animal asphyxia models (14). While this data is promising, milrinone is excreted by the kidneys with little to no metabolism, which raises questions as to clearance among patients with AKI

undergoing TH. Limited pediatric studies suggest prolonged half-life among patients with renal disease (76). Concerningly, preliminary human data suggests that neonates with HIE undergoing TH have a high risk of severe systemic hypotension and need for rapid escalation of vasopressors within 2h of milrinone exposure (77). Caution is advised until this association is more fully explored.

The use of extracorporeal membrane oxygenation (ECMO) has been published for patients with HIE. In a comparison of patients with HIE in the Extracorporeal Life Support Organization (ELSO) registry, the survival and morbidities of neonates who did versus did not receive TH while on respiratory ECMO between 2005 and 2013 were similar (78). This study, however, compared outcomes across epochs; and one would expect that as TH became more common-place and ICU techniques more sophisticated, the rate of morbidity and mortality should improve. A modern single center report indicated a 30% risk of intracranial hemorrhage for HIE patients undergoing TH while on pump (79). Similarly, a secondary analysis of a modern cohort of neonates cooled for non-HIE indications suggested an increased risk of intracranial hemorrhage (40% vs. 15.8%, p=0.012) (80). Optimizing intensive care strategies to avoid the need for ECMO and associated anticoagulation for HIE patients should be strongly considered.

Therapeutic considerations for patients with deranged systemic hemodynamics

Many neonates with HIE have systolic-predominant hypotension related to low CO. TH, hypoxia and acidosis are all associated with increased SVR (38). Unless severe endothelial damage and/or adrenal dysfunction have precipitated a loss of peripheral vascular tone, normal or elevated diastolic due to vasoconstriction and high cardiac afterload is the norm. Because the primary drivers of low SBF include low PBF secondary to high PAP and/or RV dysfunction, drugs whose primary action is non-selective vasoconstriction (e.g. dopamine) are not likely to be beneficial and may induce harm. Importantly, the historical approach to hypotension among patients with acute PH, whereby the goal of care was to achieve "reversal of ductal shunt" by driving the SAP to supra-normal values, is rarely effective and may be particularly damaging in this patient population. Creating supranormal BP in a situation where cerebral autoregulation is compromised may contribute to ischemia-reperfusion brain injury. Additionally, this approach increases RV afterload, which may be poorly tolerated, for the following reasons. *First*, most vasoconstrictors are non-selective with comparable systemic and pulmonary effects. *Second*, in the presence of an open ductus, the ability of the PDA to act as a "pop-off" for the RV is compromised if SAP is also high. Although this approach theoretically may lead to decreased pre/post saturation gradient by reducing right to left flow, the negative effect of increased RV afterload and potential increased V/Q mismatch make this practice physiologically non-desirable. It is important to emphasize that significant RV dysfunction may be present despite apparently normal mean BP, particularly if vasoconstricting medications are given as first line. Echocardiography may be advantageous and should be considered for all HIE patients treated with vasopressors.

Instead, a focus on improving PBF and supporting cardiac function is recommended. As previously mentioned, among patients with HRF, iNO may improve systolic BP on its own by increasing pulmonary venous return. In the absence of HRF, the role of iNO is unstudied. *Dobutamine*, predominantly a β-agonist, which acts to increase CO via increased contractility is a biologically logical first-line therapy. Although chronotropy may precipitate tachycardia at high doses, dobutamine is well suited for mild cardiac dysfunction. *Epinephrine*, a more potent positive inotrope, may be required but is associated with metabolic effects (e.g. increased lactate, hyperglycemia) and should be started at inotropic doses (<0.1 mcg/kg/min) to minimize pulmonary vasoconstriction. For critically unwell neonates with severe RV dysfunction, the pulmonary circulation may be pressure passive and *fluid boluses* may force the circulation forward while other, more long-lasting therapies are instituted. Similarly, for patients with severe metabolic acidosis (pH<7) and significant heart dysfunction, judicious use of sodium bicarbonate may be used to improve pH>7. Neither fluid boluses, nor sodium bicarbonate are recommended with a goal of correcting metabolic or lactic acidosis in isolation; rapid fluctuations in pH or CBF may precipitate further brain injury and these will self-correct over time.

Systemic vasoconstriction may be required if diastolic BP is particularly low (e.g. antiepileptic side effect, concomitant sepsis) to maintain normal coronary perfusion pressure. *Vasopressin* is a logical, but not formally tested, agent which activates V_1 receptors and modulates ATP-sensitive K+ channels. Its vasodilator effects, which predominate in the pulmonary vascular bed among others, are mediated by the activation of endothelial oxytocin receptors which in-turn, trigger activation of nitric oxide synthase (81). Coronary vasodilation may have added benefit, while the merits of relative cerebral vasodilation are uncertain. While improved systemic hemodynamics and cardiac function in piglet models of asphyxia have been demonstrated (82), human HIE data is limited. For patients with severe RV dysfunction, it is common to see mild or moderate LV dysfunction due to interventricular dependence. With severe disease of either ventricle, *prostaglandin E_1* with manipulation of PVR and SVR, as is necessary when managing univentricular physiology, may be required. Avoidance of rapid fluctuations in preductal perfusion pressure and weaning during rewarming as physiological changes reverse are recommended. Although not scientifically proven, until more data is available to adjudicate their contribution to further brain injury, efforts to minimize the risk of postnatal ischemia-reperfusion brain injury may be prudent.

Issues in low-resource settings

In low-resource settings, breathing assistance via stimulation, bag-mask ventilation and advanced resuscitation is required in 15%, 7%, and 1% of deliveries, respectively. Since the introduction of the Helping Babies Breathe campaign in 2010, rates of misclassified stillbirth and neonatal mortality due to asphyxia have been declining (83). Many deliveries, however, occur at home or in poorly equipped facilities with limited access to transport (84) and hospitalization following asphyxia remains common with high mortality (85). TH safety and efficacy are concerns in low-resource settings, particularly absent other intensive care strategies (e.g. ventilation, neuromonitoring). Avoidance of hyperthermia should be practiced and regular core temperature monitoring considered. New devices and practices may allow safe TH in a subset of patients. Ice packs and gloves or bottles with cold water have been used with variable success; however, wide temperature fluctuations occur unless 1:1 nursing is available. Cooling mattresses made of phase-changing material are cost-effective and effectively maintain TH for 24–36 hours (86). It is important to recognize, however, those significant comorbidities,

including thrombocytopenia (55%), coagulopathy (31%), shock (31%), and PH (8%), complicate the course (86).

Conclusions and future research

While the hemodynamic consequences of HIE are widely recognized, circulatory targets to optimize neurological outcomes are unclear. An approach centered on avoiding physiological extremes is recommended. Medications that target the underlying problems and consider the idiosyncrasies of abnormal organ-function, and drug clearance may improve intensive care quality. Comprehensive TnECHO, performed by hemodynamic consultants, may be a useful adjunct to enable enhanced diagnostic precision and longitudinal monitoring. Further research is needed to define "optimal" hemodynamics and CBF, evaluate the impact of physiological deviation from this target and ultimately, develop tools to both minimize abnormal cerebral perfusion and protect the brain during changing conditions, such as on rewarming.

References

1. Report of the American College of Obstetricians and Gynecologists' Task Force on Neonatal Encephalopathy. Obstet Gynecol. 2014; 123(4):896–901.
2. Gebauer CM, et al. Pediatrics. 2006; 117(3):843–850.
3. Kurinczuk JJ, et al. Early Hum Dev. 2010; 86(6):329–338.
4. Gillam-Krakauer M, et al. Birth Asphyxia. In: *StatPearls*. Treasure Island, FL: StatPearls Publishing; 2020.
5. Lawn JE, et al. Health Res Policy Syst. 2007; 5:4.
6. World Health Report. Geneva: WHO; 2007. https://www.who.int/whr/2004/annex/en/
7. Giussani DA. J Physiol. 2016; 594(5):1215–1230.
8. Rudolph AM, et al. Circ Res. 1967; 21(2):163–184.
9. Skinner JR, et al. Arch Dis Child Fetal Neonatal Ed. 1996; 74(1):F26–F32.
10. Creamer KM, et al. Am J Respir Crit Care Med. 1998; 158(4):1114–1119.
11. Hooper SB, et al. FASEB J. 2007; 21(12):3329–3337.
12. Piquereau J, et al. Front Physiol. 2018; 9:959.
13. Gill RS, et al. Can J Physiol Pharmacol. 2012; 90(6):689–695.
14. Joynt C, et al. Front Pediatr. 2018; 6:363.
15. Martin-Ancel A, et al. J Pediatr. 1995; 127(5):786–793.
16. Barberi I, et al. Eur J Pediatr. 1999; 158:742–747.
17. Costa S, et al. Acta Paediatr. 2007; 96(2):181–184.
18. Sehgal A, et al. Eur J Pediatr. 2012; 171(10):1511–1517.
19. Setzer E, et al. J Pediatr. 1980; 96(2):289–294.
20. Nestaas E, et al. Cardiol Young. 2011; 21(1):1–7.
21. Sehgal A, et al. Cardiovasc Ultrasound. 2013; 11:34.
22. Giesinger RE, et al. Am J Respir Crit Care Med. 2019; 200(10):1294–1305.
23. Ahmed MS, et al. J Paediatr Child Health. 2019; 55(7):753–761.
24. Reller MD, et al. Pediatr Res. 1987; 22(6):621–626.
25. Fernandez E, et al. J Perinatol. 2005; 25(2):114–118.
26. Davidson JO, et al. Pediatr Res. 2008; 63(1):51–55.
27. Gardner DS, et al. Endocrinol. 2001; 142(2):589–598.
28. Hernandez-Andrade E, et al. J Matern Fetal Neonatal Med. 2005; 17(2):101–109.
29. Procianoy RS, et al. Acta Paediatr Scand. 1988; 77(5):671–674.
30. Chapados I, et al. Shock. 2010; 33(5):519–525.
31. Giesinger RE, et al. Semin Perinatol. 2016; 40(3):174–188.
32. Kovacs K, et al. J Pediatr. 2019; 211:13.e3–19.e3.
33. Jacobs SE, et al. Cochrane Database Syst Rev. 2007; (4):CD003311.
34. Gibbons H, et al. Brain Res Mol Brain Res. 2003; 110(1):63–75.
35. Kimura T, et al. Cell Mol Neurobiol. 2020. doi: 10.1007/s10571-020-00860-z.
36. Toubas PL, et al. Arch Fr Pediatr. 1978; 35(10 Suppl):84–92.
37. Dudgeon DL, et al. J Pediatr Surg. 1980; 15(6):805–810.
38. Schubert A. J Neurosurg Anesthesiol. 1995; 7(2):139–147.
39. Thoresen M, et al. Pediatrics. 2000; 106(1 Pt 1):92–99.
40. Sehgal A, et al. J Neonatal Perinatal Med. 2019; 12(2):117–125.
41. Rubini A. Eur J Appl Physiol. 2005; 93(4):435–439.
42. Thoresen M. J Pediatr. 2011; 158(2 Suppl):e45–e49.
43. Lakshminrusimha S, et al. J Pediatr. 2018; 196:45–51.e3.
44. Hochwald O, et al. J Pediatr. 2014; 164(5):999.e1–1004.e1.
45. Eriksen VR, et al. PloS One. 2019; 14(3):e0213537.
46. Chandan G, Cascella M. *StatPearls*. Treasure Island, FL: StatPearls Publishing; 2020.
47. Afzal B, et al. Pediatr Crit Care Med. 2019; 20(2):166–171.
48. Weisser J, et al. Basic Res Cardiol. 2001; 96(2):198–205.
49. Jones RN, et al. J Mol Cell Cardiol. 1982; 14 Suppl 3:123–130.
50. Darbera L, et al. Crit Care Med. 2013; 41(12):e457–e465.
51. Dae MW, et al. Am J Physiol Heart Circ Physiol. 2002; 282(5):H1584–H1591.
52. Deakin CD, et al. Anaesthesia. 1998; 53(9):848–853.
53. Kohlhauer M, et al. Arch Cardiovasc Dis. 2016; 109(12):716–722.
54. Shah S, et al. J Perinatol. 2004; 24(1):16–20.

55. Shah P, et al. Arch Dis Child Fetal Neonatal Ed. 2004; 89(2):F152–F155.
56. Bozkurt O, Yucesoy E. Am J Perinatol. 2020. doi: 10.1055/s-0039-1701024.
57. Guluma KZ, et al. Resuscitation. 2010; 81(12):1642–1647.
58. Groves AM, et al. Arch Dis Child Fetal Neonatal Ed. 2008; 93(1):F29–F32.
59. Giesinger RE, et al. Pediatr Res. 2020. doi: 10.1038/s41390-020-01205-8.
60. Pryds O, et al. J Pediatr. 1990; 117(1 Pt 1):119–125.
61. Mitra S, et al. Front Neurol. 2020; 11:393.
62. Arriaga-Redondo M, et al. Ther Hypothermia Temp Manag. 2019; 9(4):243–250.
63. Zaramella P, et al. Early Hum Develop. 2007; 83(8):483–489.
64. Lemmers PM, et al. Pediatr Res. 2013; 74(2):180–185.
65. van Bel F, et al. Pediatrics. 1993; 92(3):365–372.
66. Bale G, et al. Adv Exp Med Biol. 2020; 1232:3–9.
67. Nakamura S, et al. Brain Dev. 2015; 37(10):925–932.
68. Meek JH, et al. Arch Dis Child Fetal Neonatal Ed. 1999; 81(2):F110–F115.
69. Manouchehri N, et al. Pediatr Res. 2013; 73(4 Pt 1):435–442.
70. Tana M, et al. Minerva Anestesiol. 2012; 78(2):151–159.
71. Dinger J, et al. Eur J Pediatr. 2002; 161(9):485–490.
72. Tarawneh A, et al. J Perinatol. 2012; 32(4):270–275.
73. Lakshminrusimha S, et al. Pediatr Res. 2009; 66(5):539–544.
74. Lutz IC, et al. BMJ Paediatr Open. 2020; 4(1):e000685.
75. McNamara PJ, et al. Pediatr Crit Care Med. 2013; 14(1):74–84.
76. Gist KM, et al. J Cardiovasc Pharmacol. 2016; 67(2):175–181.
77. Bischoff AR, et al. Abstract, Pediatric Academic Society Meeting. 2018.
78. Cuevas Guaman M, et al. Am J Perinatol. 2018; 35(3):271–276.
79. Agarwal P, et al. J Perinatol. 2019; 39(5):661–665.
80. Cashen K, et al. Perfusion. 2018; 33(5):354–362.
81. Holmes CL, et al. Chest. 2001; 120(3):989–1002.
82. Cheung DC, et al. Intensive Care Med. 2012; 38(3):491–498.
83. Kamath-Rayne BD, et al. Pediatr Res. 2017; 82(2):194–200.
84. Montaldo P, et al. Semin Fetal Neonatal Med. 2015; 20(2):72–79.
85. Cavallin F, et al. J Matern Fetal Neonatal Med. 2020: 1–6.
86. Prashantha YN, et al. Paediatr Int Child Health. 2019; 39(4):234–239.

SPECIAL CONSIDERATION
HRF in the Preterm

Michelle Baczynski, Amish Jain and Dany E. Weisz

Contents

Introduction

Hypoxemic respiratory failure (HRF) is a common complication among preterm neonates which can occur at various and multiple time points during a neonatal intensive care unit (NICU) stay. The clinical presentation of HRF is an acute and severe impairment of gas exchange resulting from an underlying primary pulmonary or secondary non-pulmonary etiology. While there exist broad consensus regarding the clinical management of term and near-term neonates with HRF, the approach to HRF among preterm neonates is controversial. HRF may occur due to parenchymal lung disease and alterations in pulmonary vascular adaptation during neonatal transition, pathology which occurs with a frequency inversely proportional to gestational age (e.g. respiratory distress syndrome of prematurity caused by surfactant deficiency). Although the initial steps in clinical management of HRF among preterm neonates are similar to that in term neonates, there is considerable uncertainty regarding the optimal management of persistent HRF among preterm neonates, especially in regard to the administration of selective pulmonary vasodilators such as inhaled nitric oxide (iNO). In this chapter, we will focus primarily on HRF in the context of acute pulmonary hypertension (PH) and its determinants in preterm neonates.

Epidemiology of PH in preterm infants

In contrast to term and late-preterm neonates, among whom the incidence of acute PH in the immediate newborn period is 0.2% (1), approximately 8% of extremely preterm infants suffer from acute PH (2). The incidence of acute PH is inversely proportional to GA, affecting 18% of 22–24-week GA neonates and 4% of those born at 27 weeks GA (2). Understanding the true incidence of HRF secondary to acute PH in preterm neonates is challenged by potential information bias related to diagnostic uncertainty. The current standard for diagnosing acute PH is echocardiography, though most centers are limited in the availability of timely echocardiography for preterm infants with HRF. In addition, while normative data exists describing the rate and trajectory of the postnatal decline in PVR among term neonates (3–5), references ranges for preterm infants, and the resultant diagnostic thresholds for acute PH, have not been described. The ubiquitous presence of respiratory distress syndrome owing to surfactant deficiency among many preterm and early term infants with HRF (6) renders the diagnosis of acute PH even more challenging.

Currently, most of our understanding of the epidemiology of acute PH in preterm neonates is derived from large databases and is based on reported utilization of iNO rather than the true incidence of severe oxygenation failure or echocardiography-proven acute PH. There are drawbacks to using iNO as a surrogate to estimate the incidence of acute PH in preterm neonates as the etiology of HRF for which iNO is prescribed by clinicians could either be secondary to acute PH, or to improve ventilation perfusion mismatch in severe oxygen failure not contributory to PH. While the efficacy of iNO in treating preterm neonates has not been established, its off-label use has been well described (7–10). Also, owing to controversy surrounding the use of iNO in preterm neonates, in some centers iNO therapy is withheld irrespective of the etiology of HRF, even in overt acute PH crisis (11). Interestingly, the data in relation to the distribution of iNO use across the range of GA, being highest at the extremes of prematurity and reaching a nadir at 32 weeks before increasing again at term, is similar to the postulated changes in PVR occurring in the fetus throughout gestation (9, 12, 13).

Etiology and pathophysiology of severe hypoxic respiratory failure: Special considerations for preterm infants

Preterm infants experience similar pathophysiology of HRF as term infants and older children (e.g. hypoventilation, V/Q mismatch, intra- and extra-cardiac shunts, and/or impaired alveolar-capillary diffusion). However, prematurity-specific etiologies predominate during perinatal transition. Surfactant deficiency, early onset sepsis, perinatal asphyxia, developmental lung disorders (e.g. pulmonary hypoplasia) and associated sequelae (e.g. pneumothorax) are common causes of HRF in preterm newborns. These etiologies may disrupt the transition from fetal to neonatal pulmonary and systemic circulation, culminating in HRF associated acute PH, which most commonly presents in the perinatal period (14, 15).

Premature birth entails the forced initiation of gas exchange with lungs that may have not reached anatomical and physiological maturity; those born at the border of viability do so during the late canalicular phase or early saccular phase of pulmonary development. At this stage (0.6 term), PVR (and the risk of acute PH associated HRF) is high due to the small number of pulmonary

DOI: 10.1201/9780367494018-37

vessels and lower cross-sectional area of vasculature in the lung. Intra-uterine growth restriction and conditions in which fetal circulating blood volume is increased (e.g. recipient in twin-to-twin transfusion syndrome) may also be associated with acute PH crisis, with the latter occurring due to *in utero* pulmonary vascular remodeling from chronic hypoxia and increased shear stress from increased flow in the pulmonary vascular bed (16–19). Pulmonary hypoplasia secondary to long-standing preterm premature rupture of membranes is the most commonly described pathophysiology associated with an increased risk of acute PH (20–25). Derangements in pulmonary vascular development and arrested alveolar growth and proliferation owing to oligohydramnios and restricted or reduced fetal breathing movements, if complicated by preterm birth, could compromise gas exchange and disrupt circulatory transition. Due to decreased surface area for gas exchange secondary to alveolar underdevelopment, neonates with pulmonary hypoplasia are prone to pneumothoraces, respiratory acidosis, and hypoxemia leading to an increase in PVR. Furthermore, secondary to generalized pulmonary vascular underdevelopment, there may be a fixed component of PH that may be unresponsive to the application of exogenous pulmonary vasodilators.

Endogenous nitric oxide (NO) plays a critical role in the programmed decrease in pulmonary vascular resistance and increase in pulmonary blood flow immediately following birth (17, 26, 27). The substantial increase in pulmonary blood flow is precipitated by lung expansion after birth which gives rise to shearing forces on the pulmonary vascular bed that catalyze the production of endogenous NO and subsequent pulmonary arteriolar vasodilation (28, 29). Aioki et al. identified a subset of preterm neonates requiring mechanical ventilation at birth who subsequently developed HRF and acute PH as having undetectable traces of NO byproducts analyzed from their tracheal aspirates, which remained undetected until exogenous NO administration was initiated (22). In the same cohort, those without HRF but whose mothers had pregnancy-induced hypertension were also missing NO byproducts from their aspirates, suggesting that production and regulation of endogenous NO cannot be the singular determining factor involved in circulatory transition (22). It may instead be a combination of factors, such as a transient deficiency in endogenous NO causing dysregulated pulmonary vascular changes, combined with another underlying pathology, which provoke an acute PH crisis.

While HRF and acute PH occurring beyond the transitional period in preterm infants is phenotypically indistinguishable from acute PH occurring during transition, the etiologies and pathophysiology may be more like those seen among older infants and children. Acute respiratory distress syndrome (ARDS) is characterized by an acute and severe impairment in gas exchange caused by an underlying lung process, pulmonary vascular dysregulation or a combination of both (30). The preterm pulmonary vascular endothelium may be particularly vulnerable to a dysregulated host immune response characterized by circulating and local mediators activated under conditions of pulmonary or systemic inflammation due to pneumonia, sepsis or necrotizing enterocolitis (31). The presence of endothelin-1(ET-1), a potent endogenous vasoconstrictor, in the intestinal mucosa of preterm neonates with necrotizing enterocolitis, and detectable plasma levels measured from newborns with blood culture positive sepsis, would indicate that ET-1 might play a contributory role in the pathophysiology of acute PH (32, 33).

General management principles of HRF in preterm neonates

In addition to the established principles of acute PH management in term infants, management of acute PH in preterm neonates is supportive, aimed at treating the underlying pathology, with a potential role for specific pulmonary vasodilator therapy to treat endogenous NO dysregulation. Table 37.1 details specific management principles and their respective considerations for the preterm neonate.

Echocardiography evaluation in preterm infants with HRF

Echocardiography is a supportive tool in the diagnosis and management of preterm infants with HRF. Occasionally, echocardiography performed due to HRF may unexpectedly identify pericardial tamponade as the cause, often due to extravasation of a central venous catheter, permitting timely and life-saving pericardiocentesis (34). More commonly, echocardiography facilitates the rapid exclusion of acute pulmonary hypertension as a contributory factor to HRF. It permits the reliable, timely, and non-invasive evaluation of pulmonary artery pressure and the characterization of cardiac shunts which may influence pulmonary blood flow and systemic hypoxemia. The identification of exclusively systemic-to-pulmonary ("left-to-right") shunts at the level of the foramen ovale and ductus arteriosus, which are frequently patent among critically ill preterm newborns, indicate sub-systemic pulmonary artery and right ventricular (RV) pressures and implicate non-optimal lung volumes and/or pulmonary parenchymal disease as the primary etiology of HRF. Conversely, similar to term infants with HRF, echocardiography determination of pulmonary hypertension, pulmonary-to-systemic pressure gradients and secondary effects of increased RV afterload on RV performance, provide objective evidence for the employment of intensive care strategies (Table 37.1) and/or intratracheal or intravenous pharmacotherapy to modulate the PVR:SVR ratio, support RV performance and stroke volume, and optimize pulmonary blood flow.

Role of the ductus arteriosus among preterm infants with HRF

During normal transition at birth, the initiation of ventilation in air and umbilical cord clamping result in a decrease in PVR and increase in SVR, respectively. The ductal flow pattern, previously right to left during fetal life, becomes bidirectional and eventually left to right as PVR decreases below systemic arterial pressure. Among preterm neonates with acute PH associated HRF, the ductal shunt is variable in direction, reflecting disordered pulmonary and/or systemic blood flow or perturbations in the programmed postnatal decrease in PVR. The patent ductus arteriosus (PDA) may play a supportive or neutral role in preterm newborns with acute PH, in whom there is a postnatal failure of vasorelaxation of the pulmonary arterioles (due to either abnormal fetal pulmonary development or maladaptive neonatal transition), resulting in persistently elevated PVR. In severe cases, PVR remains suprasystemic and the ductal shunt is from the pulmonary artery to the aorta, supporting the post-ductal systemic blood flow, albeit with deoxygenated blood that results in a difference in oxygen saturation between pre-ductal and post-ductal circulations. Here, though the pulmonary-to-systemic shunt across the PDA potentiates systemic hypoxemia, it also results in reduced RV afterload and may help preserve RV function. In mild cases of PH, the

TABLE 37.1 Principles of Management of Acute Pulmonary Hypertension Associated Hypoxic Respiratory Failure among Preterm Neonates

Management Principle	Biological Rationale	Considerations in Preterm Neonates
Airway management	Establishing a patent airway and a trial of non-invasive ventilation in attempt to improve ventilation and oxygenation may be appropriate, with timely escalation to intubation and invasive mechanical ventilation for impending respiratory failure.	The threshold for intubating a preterm neonate may be less, most often for the purpose of surfactant replacement therapy as treatment for respiratory distress syndrome.
Establish and maintain functional residual capacity (FRC)	Areas of low lung volume or atelectasis can cause compression or twisting of extra-alveolar vessels and conversely, areas with higher volumes or hyperinflation, may cause compression of alveolar vessels. Pulmonary vascular resistance is lowest at FRC.	Maintain alveolar recruitment using the lowest effective mean airway pressure. HRF related to pulmonary hyperinflation and reduced pulmonary blood flow is common, especially in the transitional period when rapid shifts in pulmonary compliance may occur following treatment with exogenous surfactant.
Avoid respiratory acidosis	Acidosis causes pulmonary vasoconstriction and increased PVR. Intracellular acidosis may also impair function of cardiomyocytes.	Avoid large fluctuations in carbon dioxide and maintain targets within a close range between 40–50 mmHg using lung-protective ventilation strategies.
Avoid hypoxia and hyperoxia	Hypoxia causes pulmonary vasoconstriction and may impair cardiomyocyte function. Hyperoxia does not confer any additional benefit and may cause harm.	Maintaining oxygen saturation targets within an accepted standard range for preterm neonates between 91–95% is recommended.
Monitor for signs of systemic hypo-perfusion	Metabolic acidosis causing pulmonary vasoconstriction in combination with decreased venous return and low pulmonary blood flow may worsen gas exchange, leading to further hypoxia. Decreased blood pressure may also compromise cerebral blood flow.	Maintain continuous blood pressure monitoring and a mean arterial blood pressure within the gestational-age specific normative range.
Consider sedation and muscle relaxant	Increased agitation may increase PVR and metabolic demands.	There is a potential of neurological side effects associated with use of these medications and therefore judicious use of sedation and muscle relaxants is indicated.
Administration of exogenous surfactant	HRF associated with respiratory distress syndrome due to surfactant deficiency is common and treatment with exogenous surfactant is recommended prior to treatment with select pulmonary vasodilators such as inhaled nitric oxide (6).	Respiratory distress syndrome occurs in preterm infants with a frequency that is inversely proportional to gestational age.

ductal shunt is bidirectional and may not contribute significantly to either pulmonary overcirculation or RV afterload reduction. Instead the PDA may be an innocuous bystander which provides a valuable non-invasive estimate of the pressure gradient between the pulmonary and systemic circulations.

Among preterm infants with mild or moderate HRF, a large systemic-to-pulmonary shunt from a PDA may be a major contributing factor to oxygenation failure, and echocardiography is a mainstay in the diagnosis and evaluation of the severity of shunt volume. Shunt volume is determined by the pressure gradient between the pulmonary artery and aorta, and by the resistance to transductal flow, which is primarily influenced by ductal diameter and length. Determinants of PVR such as hypocapnemia, hyperoxemia or alkalosis may augment the shunt volume. A large shunt results in volume overload of the pulmonary artery, and subsequent alveolar edema, reduced pulmonary compliance, and increased need for mechanical ventilation. Increased pulmonary blood flow and associated increased shear stress precipitates intimal proliferation and vessel narrowing, leading to increased pulmonary vascular resistance and pulmonary artery pressure, which can exacerbate respiratory insufficiency. Increased blood flow to the left heart results in increased end-diastolic volume of the left atrium and ventricle. Left ventricular dilatation and

impaired diastolic elastance results in pressure loading of the left atrium and contributes to left atrial dilatation. Diastolic flow reversal in the abdominal aorta and systemic arteries (e.g. celiac artery, middle cerebral artery) occurs and may be associated with increased neonatal morbidity (35). The optimal clinical management of preterm infants with HRF and a large PDA shunt is uncertain, however, as few studies have identified echocardiography-based thresholds for medical and/or surgical PDA treatment that improve clinical outcomes (36).

Role of specific pulmonary vasodilators: Inhaled nitric oxide and other therapies for preterm neonates with HRF

There is significant controversy regarding the management of preterm neonates with HRF, especially the administration of iNO. This uncertainty is related to (1) the potential contribution of iNO treatment to the development of early neonatal morbidity among preterm infants with severe HRF, such as intracranial hemorrhage (2, 7) a wide range of evaluation and interpretation of evidence from clinical trials of iNO treatment of preterm infants; (3) heterogeneity in national and international clinical practice guidelines regarding iNO administration (Table 37.2) (37–39), and (4) difficulty in clinically discerning the relative contribution

TABLE 37.2 Summary of Recent Clinical Practice Guidelines Regarding the Use of Inhaled Nitric Oxide in Preterm Neonates with Hypoxic Respiratory Failure and/or Acute Pulmonary Hypertension

Guidelines/Organization	Recommendations
American Academy of Pediatrics (2014) (40)	1. The results of randomized controlled trials, traditional meta-analyses, and an individualized patient data meta-analysis study indicate that neither rescue nor routine use of iNO improves survival in preterm infants with respiratory failure *(Evidence quality, A; Grade of recommendation: strong)*. 2. The preponderance of evidence does not support treating preterm infants who have respiratory failure with iNO for the purpose of preventing/ameliorating BPD, severe intraventricular hemorrhage, or other neonatal morbidities *(Evidence quality, A; Grade of recommendation: strong)*. 3. The incidence of cerebral palsy, neurodevelopmental impairment, or cognitive impairment in preterm infants treated with iNO is similar to that of control infants *(Evidence quality, A)*.
American Heart Association / American Thoracic Society (2015) (38)	1. Lung recruitment strategies can improve the efficacy of iNO therapy and should be performed in patients with PPHN associated with parenchymal lung disease *(Class I; Level of Evidence B)*. 2. iNO can be beneficial for preterm infants with severe hypoxemia that is due primarily to PPHN physiology rather than parenchymal lung disease, particularly if associated with prolonged rupture of membranes and oligohydramnios *(Class IIa; Level of Evidence B)*.
Pediatric Pulmonary Hypertension Network (2016) (39)	1. iNO therapy should not be used in premature infants for the prevention of BPD, as multicenter studies data have failed to consistently demonstrate efficacy for this purpose. 2. iNO therapy can be beneficial for preterm infants with severe hypoxemia that is primarily due to PPHN physiology rather than parenchymal lung disease, particularly if associated with prolonged rupture of membranes and oligohydramnios. 3. iNO is preferred over other pulmonary vasodilators in preterm infants based on a strong safety signal from short- and long-term follow-up of large numbers of patients from multicenter randomized clinical trials for BPD prevention. 4. Placebo controlled trials are not feasible in the target population; therefore, alternate study designs such as the development of multicenter registries, informatics strategies, and other approaches should be used to address issues regarding the efficacy and safety of therapeutic options for preterm infants with life-threatening PPHN physiology.

of surfactant deficiency and other pulmonary parenchymal disease vs. acute PH as the primary etiology of persistent HRF among preterm infants.

Clinical trials of iNO therapy among preterm infants were designed to study the potential role of iNO in the prevention of BPD. No randomized trial has been performed where preterm infants were enrolled based on echocardiography-proven acute pulmonary hypertension. Concern regarding rescue iNO treatment among preterm infants stems predominantly from a statistically non-significant trend toward increased severe IVH identified in a single study (7). On the other hand, there is clinical trial evidence that preterm neonates have a similar therapeutic response to iNO treatment as term/near-term neonates (40), and a growing body of observational literature suggesting effectiveness of iNO among neonates with HRF when acute PH is suspected or confirmed. In preterm neonates, precursors associated with an improvement in oxygenation following iNO initiation include an echocardiography diagnosis of acute PH, severity of oxygenation failure and echocardiography indices of low pulmonary blood flow (41, 42). Further, among those with acute HRF and PH, improved oxygenation after iNO therapy is associated with higher survival rates and better long-term neurodevelopmental outcomes in comparison to those who do not respond (43, 44). In the subpopulation of preterm neonates with pulmonary hypoplasia and acute PH, two studies of note include a large iNO registry which reported increased survival among preterm neonates with iNO responsiveness (45) and a large cohort of preterm neonates with pulmonary hypoplasia and a subgroup with PH treated with iNO that reported a trend towards increased survival (46). In this study, the difference in survival rate among responders and

non responders within this subgroup were not described. Owing to the rarity of this disorder and a loss of equipoise among the neonatal community, which likely stems from anecdotal experience of critically ill infants with HRF who do acutely stabilize following a trial of iNO, a multi-center randomized trial is not anticipated. Differing findings regarding the effects on the most common primary outcome variable, death, or bronchopulmonary dysplasia, has resulted in wide variation in clinical practice and some expert bodies discouraging its use in the preterm population. There does appear to be, however, improvement in survival among preterm neonates who demonstrate an improvement in oxygenation, rendering the withholding of iNO therapy altogether seemingly unjustified. However, it is not known whether the increased mortality in non-responders can be explained by a lack of response and not a worsening secondary to its use.

Despite the controversy in the decision to administer iNO among preterm infants, it remains the dominant selective pulmonary vasodilator used in this population. Adjunct pharmacological agents have the potential for a beneficial effect in improving oxygenation owing to their synergistic mechanism of action. Milrinone and sildenafil are phosphodiesterase inhibitors that facilitate pulmonary arteriolar smooth muscle cell vasodilation by limiting degradation of cyclic adenosine monophosphate and guanine monophosphate, respectively. Bosentan, a competitive antagonist of ET-1 at the ET-A and ET-B receptors, also promotes arteriolar vasodilation primarily by blocking the binding of ET-1 to ET-A which would promote vasoconstriction. Although the pathobiology and pharmacology of these agents may be favorable as adjunctive treatments to iNO, clinical evidence for therapeutic effectiveness in preterm infants is limited to case series (47, 48).

Conclusions/Summary

Acute PH presenting as HRF is a common complication among preterm neonates admitted to NICUs. Preterm neonates, owing to both structural and physiological underdevelopment, are particularly vulnerable to pulmonary vascular dysregulation both following birth and subsequently in the neonatal period. Echocardiography evaluation is a critical tool in characterizing pulmonary and systemic hemodynamics to aid in diagnosis and management. While treatment with inhaled nitric oxide is common, improves short-term oxygenation, and does not cause harm, additional trials enrolling preterm neonates with echocardiography-proven acute PH are required to be confident that treatment improves major clinical outcomes (e.g. survival). Additional evidence is also urgently needed to define diagnostic thresholds and to elucidate the timing, patterns, and underlying mechanisms of acute PH in preterm neonates.

Funding Statement: AJ is supported by a grant from the Heart and Stroke Foundation of Canada for "Improving Management of Pulmonary hypertension and Right heart function In NeonaTes (IMPRINT) research program."

References

1. Walsh-Sukys MC, et al. Pediatrics. 2000; 105(1 Pt 1):14–20.
2. Nakanishi H, et al. Arch Dis Child Fetal Neonatal Ed. 2018; 103(6):F554–F561.
3. Jain A, et al. J Am Soc Echocardiogr 2014; 27(12):1293–1304.
4. Jain A, et al. J Pediatr. 2018; 200:50.e2–57.e2.
5. Popat H, et al. Neonatology. 2012; 101(3):166–171.
6. González A, et al. J Perinatol. 2020. doi: 10.1038/s41372-020-00777-x.
7. Barrington KJ, et al. Cochrane Database Syst Rev. 2017; 1:CD000509.
8. Soraisham AS, et al. Am J Perinatol. 2016; 33(7):715–722.
9. Ellsworth MA, et al. Pediatrics. 2015; 135(4):643–648.
10. Dewhurst C, et al. Acta Paediatr. 2010; 99(6):854–860.
11. Manja V, et al. J Perinatol. 2019; 39(1):86–94.
12. Lakshminrusimha S, et al. J Perinatol. 2016; 36 Suppl 2:S3–S11.
13. Morton SU, et al. Clin Perinatol. 2016; 43(3):395–407.
14. Seth SA, et al. J Matern Fetal Neonatal Med. 2018; 31(23):3147–3152.
15. Rhine WD, et al. Clin Ther. 2019; 41(5):910–919.
16. Goss K. J Physiol. 2019; 597(4):1175–1184.
17. Gao Y, et al. Physiol Rev. 2010; 90(4):1291–1335.
18. Delsing B, et al. Neonatology. 2007; 92(2):134–138.
19. Gijtenbeek M, et al. Neonatology. 2017; 112(4):402–408.
20. Chandrasekharan P, et al. Am J Perinatol. 2017; 34(5):428–440.
21. Shah DM, et al. J Paediatr Child Health. 2011; 47(6):340–345.
22. Aikio O, et al. J Pediatr. 2012; 161(3):397.e1–403.e1.
23. Baczynski M, et al. J Perinatol. 2018; 38(8):1087–1092.
24. Chock VY, et al. Am J Perinatol. 2009; 26(4):317–322.
25. de Waal K, et al. J Pediatr. 2015; 166(5):1113–1120.
26. Fineman JR, et al. J Clin Invest. 1994; 93(6):2675–2683.
27. Abman SH, et al. Am J Physiol. 1990; 259(6 Pt 2):H1921–H1927.
28. Kuchan MJ, et al. Am J Physiol. 1994; 266(3 Pt 1):C628–C636.
29. Sriram K, et al. Biophys J. 2016; 111(1):208–221.
30. Luca DD, et al. Lancet Respir Med. 2017; 5(8):657–666.
31. Pietrasanta C, et al. Front Pediatr. 2019; 7:340.
32. Figueras-Aloy J, et al. J Perinat Med. 2004; 32(6):522–526.
33. Ito Y, et al. Pediatr Res. 2007; 61(2):180–184.
34. Sehgal A, et al. J Perinatol. 2007; 27(5):317–319.
35. Keusters L, et al. J Perinatol. 2020; doi: 10.1038/s41372-020-0663-8.
36. El-Khuffash A, et al. J Pediatr. 2015; 167(6):1354.e2–1361.e2.
37. Abman SH, et al. Circulation. 2015; 132(21):2037–2099.
38. Kinsella JP, et al. J Pediatr. 2016; 170:312–314.
39. Kumar P. Pediatrics. 2014; 133(1):164–170.
40. Van Meurs KP, et al. N Engl J Med. 2005; 353(1):13–22.
41. Dani C, et al Pediatr Pulmonol. 2017; 52(11):1461–1468.
42. Desandes R, et al. Acta Paediatr. 2004; 93(1):66–69.
43. Rallis D, et al. Early Hum Dev. 2018; 127:1–5.
44. Baczynski M, et al. Arch Dis Child Fetal Neonatal Ed. 2017; 102(6):F508–F514.
45. Kettle R, et al. Neonatology. 2019; 116(4):341–346.
46. Ellsworth KR, et al. JAMA Pediatr. 2018; 172(7):e180761.
47. James AT, et al. J Perinatol. 2015; 35(4):268–273.
48. Radicioni M, et al. Eur J Pediatr. 2011; 170(8):1075–1078.

HYPOXEMIC RESPIRATORY FAILURE
Neonatal Cases

Adrianne Rahde Bischoff, Faith Zhu, Amish Jain and Patrick J. McNamara

Contents

Case 1

History

Preterm infant born at 23 weeks with a birth weight of 482 grams presenting with hypoxemic respiratory (HRF) in the third postnatal week. The initial clinical course was significant for respiratory distress syndrome for which he received surfactant and remained intubated on high-frequency jet ventilation (HFJV). He also had a hemodynamically significant patent ductus arteriosus (PDA) for which he received two 3-day courses of acetaminophen, with resolution of the shunt on postnatal day 11. Over the subsequent 2 weeks, he remained intubated on moderate to high ventilator settings on HFJV (Table 38.1). Due to persistent lung disease and inability to wean from the ventilator, he received a dose of late surfactant (calfactant) on day 21. His FiO_2 continued to progressively increase from 0.45–0.50 to 0.75, with worsening pulmonary edema on chest radiograph (Figure 38.1A, B). Given the persistence of HRF, there was a clinical suspicion for acute pulmonary hypertension (PH) for which he was started on inhaled nitric oxide (iNO) at 20 ppm with no clinical response. Mean airway pressure (MAP) was increased to optimize lung recruitment, with no significant improvement in FiO_2. Screening laboratory tests for infection (complete blood count, C-reactive protein) were normal and the infant remained otherwise active and with normal vital signs. Neonatal hemodynamics consultation was requested to assess for PH. At the time of hemodynamics consultation, infant was on high HFJV settings (Table 38.1) and iNO 20 ppm. The remainder of vital signs remained stable (heart rate 160, non-invasive arterial pressure 84/34 mmHg measured on the right arm and 64/33 mmHg measured on the right leg).

Hemodynamics consultation

Targeted neonatal echocardiography (TnECHO) showed a moderate-sized PDA (2 mm) with pulsatile left-to-right shunt. The left atrium (LA) was markedly dilated in relation to the Aorta (Ao) (LA: Ao 2.6) with evidence of left heart volume loading (mitral inflow E/A 0.82, isovolumic relaxation time (IVRT) 23 msec, Left ventricular output (LVO) (400 mL/min/kg). There was diastolic flow reversal in the descending aorta and absent diastolic flow to celiac, superior mesenteric artery and middle cerebral artery. There was no evidence of PH (unable to estimate right ventricular systolic pressure (RVSp) due to incomplete tricuspid regurgitant jet, interventricular septum round throughout the cardiac cycle) and normal biventricular systolic function (Ejection fraction [EF]) 66% by Simpsons biplane, TAPSE 6.4 mm, right ventricular (RV) fractional area change 0.54. RV output (RVO) was estimated to be 100 mL/min/kg and there was a small patent foramen ovale (PFO) with left-to-right shunt. The remainder of the cardiac anatomy was normal. The diagnostic impression was of a moderate sized PDA with high-volume left-to-right shunt; therefore, the clinical team was advised to wean iNO and repeat the echocardiography evaluation.

Management

Upon iNO discontinuation, the FiO_2 progressively decreased to previous baseline of 0.45–0.5 and ventilator settings were weaned due to improvement in blood gases and chest radiograph. Repeat TnECHO evaluation 2 hours after discontinuation of iNO continued to show moderate-sized PDA with high-volume shunt, although markers of shunt significance had somewhat improved (E/A 0.75, IVRT 31 msec, LVO 320 mL/kg/min, RVO

DOI: 10.1201/9780367494018-38

TABLE 38.1 Changes in Mechanical Ventilation Parameters at Baseline, after 18 Hours (Timing of Neonatal Hemodynamics Consultation) and 36 Hours

	Baseline	18 Hours	36 Hours
HFJV			
PIP	38	44	37
PEEP	10	11	11
Rate	480	540	600
iT	0.02	0.02	0.02
IMV			
PIP	21	22	22
Rate	8	10	10
iT	0.5	0.5	0.5
MAP	14	17	16
FiO_2	0.45-0.5	0.8-0.85	0.42
RSS	6.3-7	13.6-14.4	6.7

Abbreviations: HFJV, high-frequency jet ventilation, PIP, peak inspiratory pressure; PEEP, peak end expiratory pressure; iT, inspiratory time; IMV, intermittent mandatory ventilation; MAP, mean airway pressure; FiO_2, fraction of inspired oxygen; RSS, respiratory severity score (MAP × FiO_2).

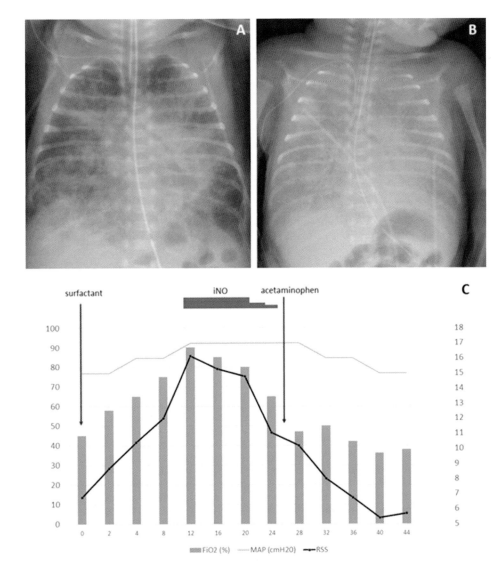

FIGURE 38.1 Case 1. (A) Chest radiograph at baseline; (B) chest radiograph 4 hours after surfactant administration; (C) trends in respiratory status following surfactant, inhaled nitric oxide and acetaminophen. The x-axis depicts hours. (FiO_2, fraction of inspired oxygen; MAP, mean airway pressure; RSS, respiratory severity score – RSS = MAP × FiO_2; iNO, inhaled nitric oxide.)

110 mL/min/kg). A repeat course of acetaminophen was started. Figure 38.1C summarizes the changes in FiO_2, MAP and respiratory severity score (RSS) (calculated as RSS = MAP $\times$ FiO_2) over the clinical course.

Outcome

After 7 days of medical therapy with acetaminophen, there was only marginal improvement in echocardiography markers of shunt significance, so he was referred for definitive percutaneous closure in the catheterization laboratory. He underwent successful PDA closure and had an otherwise unremarkable neonatal course.

Physiological discussion and learning points

- HRF in preterm infants is multifactorial and the underlying physiology may be difficult to discern on the basis of exclusive clinical signs and bedside monitoring (1).
- Late surfactant administration is occasionally used as a rescue for post surfactant slump, particularly in the more immature infants (2–5). Although PDA shunt increases microvascular perfusion and the leakage of plasma proteins into the alveolar space can inhibit surfactant function (6–8), there is no evidence to support surfactant use in the setting of a hemodynamically significant PDA. Rather, administration of late surfactant may lead to hypoxemia due to exacerbated V/Q mismatch or pulmonary circulation secondary to lower pulmonary vascular resistance (PVR).
- Randomized trials of iNO in premature infants have enrolled patients with oxygenation failure but have not consistently reported the presence of PH (9–14). The index case had oxygenation failure due to pulmonary overcirculation secondary to a high-volume PDA shunt, highlighting the importance of echocardiography evaluation prior to administration of a pulmonary vasodilator therapy.
- This case highlights the value of longitudinal echocardiography to enable enhanced differentiation of the causes for hypoxemia (15). Discontinuation of iNO resulted in improvement in respiratory status (Table 38.1, Figure 38.1) as well as markers of shunt significance as described previously.

Case 2

History

Term infant (40 weeks) with a birth weight of 2717 grams presenting with HRF in the setting of hypoxic-ischemic encephalopathy (HIE). The infant was born by assisted delivery with forceps after a history of recurrent variable decelerations during labor. At birth, he required positive pressure ventilation, intubation, chest compressions and one bolus of intravenous epinephrine. Apgar scores were 0, 0, 2, 5, and 7 at 1, 5, 10, 15, and 20 minutes, respectively. The initial arterial gas showed pH 6.9, pCO_2 25 mmHg, base deficit 26 mEq/L, and serum lactic acid of 20 mmol/L. After intubation he continued to require FiO_2 0.8–0.9 and the chest radiograph showed adequate lung recruitment. Inhaled NO (20 ppm) was initiated by the transport team, with minimal change in oxygen requirement (FiO_2 0.75–0.8). On arrival to the tertiary center, the vital signs were unstable with a heart rate of 100 bpm and arterial pressure was 39/19 mmHg (measured invasively on umbilical arterial catheter). He developed rhythmic movements and was treated with phenobarbital for presumed seizure activity. The neurological assessment was consistent with severe HIE for which therapeutic hypothermia (TH) was instituted. Respiratory support was provided with conventional mechanical ventilation on MAP 10, FiO_2 0.8. Laboratory markers showed evidence of myocardial ischemia (troponin 0.67 ng/mL), acute kidney injury (creatinine 0.8 mg/dL), hepatic injury (alanine aminotransferase 952 U/L) and coagulopathy (INR >10, PTT 101). He received 15 mL/kg of fresh frozen plasma.

Evaluation/management

Hemodynamics consultation was requested and TnECHO assessment showed severe RV systolic dysfunction and low cardiac output (Table 38.2, Figure 38.2). The remainder of cardiac anatomy was normal. An intravenous epinephrine infusion was started at 0.05 mcg/kg/min and escalated to 0.08 mcg/kg/min to support heart function. Due to persistent hypotension, in the setting of severe RV dysfunction with profound low cardiac output (LVO 70 mL/min/kg, RVO 27 mL/min/kg), an intravenous vasopressin infusion was also started to support coronary perfusion to the RV. These changes were followed by an improvement in oxygen requirements (FiO_2 0.5) and arterial pressure (60/30 mmHg). Repeat TnECHO was performed while the infant was receiving epinephrine 0.08 mcg/kg/min, iNO 20 ppm and vasopressin 2 milliunits/kg/min. There was interval improvement in RV systolic dysfunction (moderate to severe) and in cardiac output (Table 38.2). The interventricular septum was round throughout the cardiac cycle (eccentricity index at end-systole of 0.99). FiO_2 improved down to 0.3 within the first 4 hours of admission.

Outcome

Over the next 24–48 hours there was significant improvement in cardiovascular status. Arterial pressure remained stable and he was weaned off both epinephrine and vasopressin infusions. The efficacy of oxygenation progressively improved and iNO was discontinued between 2 and 3 days. Repeat echocardiography

TABLE 38.2 Sequential Changes in TnECHO Parameters

	Baseline	3 Hours	24 Hours
TAPSE (mm)	2.5	6.5	12.3
RV-FAC (RV-3Ch)	0.26	0.3	0.35
RV S'	3	4.9	5.3
RVO (mL/min/kg)	27	88	110
EF (Simpsons biplane) (%)	60	65	66
LVO (mL/min/kg)	70	127	132
PDA	0.6 mm, left-to-right	0.6 mm, left-to-right	No transductal shunt

Abbreviations: TAPSE, tricuspid annular plane systolic excursion; RV-FAC, right ventricular fractional area change; 3Ch, right ventricular 3 chamber view; RV S', right ventricular systolic tissue Doppler; RVO, right ventricular output; EF, ejection fraction; LVO, left ventricular output; PDA, patent ductus arteriosus.

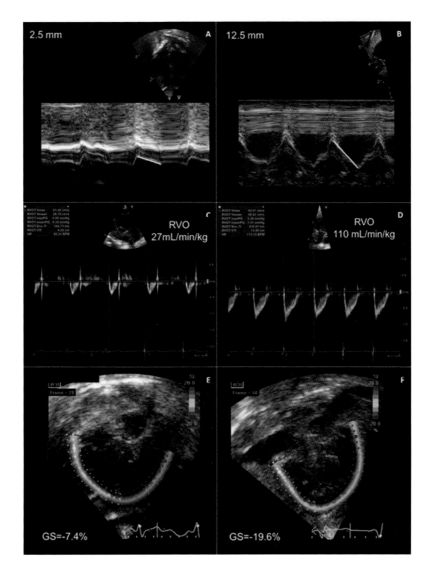

FIGURE 38.2   Case 2. Echocardiography images at baseline (panels A, C and E) and after 24 hours (panels B, D and F). (A) TAPSE at baseline; (B) TAPSE after 24 hours of therapy; (C) RVO at baseline; (D) RVO after 24 hours of therapy; (E) RV-3Ch global strain at baseline; (F) RV-3Ch global strain after 24 hours. TnECHO, targeted neonatal echocardiography; TAPSE, tricuspid annular plane excursion; RVO, right ventricular output; RV-3Ch, right ventricle 3 chamber view; GS, global strain.

evaluation on postnatal day 2 showed normal biventricular systolic function (Table 38.2). His neurological status, however, continued to be severely abnormal and continuous video encephalogram was consistent with severe voltage suppression. After discussion with the family and the likelihood of a devastating neurological prognosis, decision was made to redirect care to end-of-life care.

Physiological discussion and learning points

- Adequate oxygenation is dependent on lung recruitment, pulmonary vascular compliance and resistance, the presence of intra or extra-cardiac shunts and heart function (15). The cardiovascular effects of HIE may include decreased myocardial contractility with or without associated PH secondary to failure of the normal postnatal decline in PVR (16–18). Furthermore, TH induces pulmonary vasoconstriction, which may worsen PH (16, 19). Although frequently associated with pulmonary pathologies such

as meconium aspiration syndrome, sepsis/pneumonia or transient tachypnea of the newborn, HRF may occur in HIE in the absence of lung disease and associated with poor pulmonary blood flow due to PH as well as heart dysfunction (16). More specifically, HIE patients may have both afterload-dependent and -independent mechanisms by which RV function may be diminished. There is data to suggest that RV function becomes uncoupled to afterload, particularly among those with poor neurological outcome (20). TnECHO in this setting aids in the diagnosis of RV dysfunction, in differentiating cases with biventricular/predominant LV systolic dysfunction and in assessing PDA shunt.

- RV systolic dysfunction may be further impacted due to impaired coronary perfusion. Under normal circumstances, the RV is perfused throughout the cardiac cycle due to intrinsically low RV systolic pressure (21). In the setting of HIE with PH, the combination of high central venous pressure and high downstream resistance leads to loss of coronary perfusion during systole. This can be further exacerbated if there is concomitant low aortic root pressure, presenting with low diastolic arterial pressure, and low systemic perfusion (20). Although TH increases systemic vascular resistance, and HIE/TH patients are less likely to present with diastolic hypotension, in the sicker and most severely affected infants it may be important to use a vasopressor to improve coronary perfusion to the RV. It is important to chose a vasopressor that has can increase diastolic arterial pressure with no impact in the pulmonary vasculature such that there is no further worsening of the underlying PH in these patients (22–24).

• The index case demonstrated rapid improvement in RV systolic function, as well as HRF, upon institution of epinephrine and vasopressin which was followed by improvement in pulmonary blood flow leading to enhanced efficacy of oxygenation and cardiac output. Even though the PDA was small, initiation of prostaglandin was not deemed necessary given clinical and echocardiographic improvement. It is important to consider the use of prostaglandins in some circumstances as this may be a beneficial intervention to offload the RV and promote systemic blood flow (25). Prostaglandin may also act as an adjunctive pulmonary vasodilator if there is no improvement with the strategies implemented. Longitudinal and repeat assessments can provide significant insights into mechanism and response to therapies instituted.

Case 3

History

A late preterm, severely growth restricted infant was delivered at 34+6 weeks by emergency C-section. The antenatal history was complicated by maternal type 2 diabetes (treated with insulin), chronic hypertension and large fibroids. The laboring period was complicated by abnormal biophysical profile (2/8) and absent heart rate variability on cardiotocography tracing, prompting delivery. The infant was non-vigorous at birth and required

positive pressure ventilation for the first 3 minutes of life before spontaneous respiratory effort was established. Subsequently, the infant was transitioned to nasal continuous positive airway pressure (CPAP) with peak end expiratory pressure (PEEP) of 7 cmH$_2$O and FiO$_2$ 0.4. The Apgar scores were 1, 5, and 8 at 1, 5, and 10 minutes of life, respectively, and the cord blood gases revealed marked acidosis (arterial cord pH 6.80, base deficit (BD) −13.1 mEq/L). Over the next 2 hours, the infant developed oxygenation failure with a progressive increase in FiO$_2$ requirements reaching 0.7 to 1.0. In addition, a capillary blood gas demonstrated a pH 7.23, pCO$_2$ 59 mmHg, HCO$_3$ 24 mEq/L, BE −4.1 mEq/L, and an elevated lactate of 13 mmol/L, prompting urgent hemodynamic consultation.

Hemodynamics consultation and subsequent management

TnECHO demonstrated evidence of suprasystemic PH, as evidenced by paradoxical interventricular septal movement and bidirectional PDA shunting (4.3 mm; shunting right to left for 63% of the total cardiac cycle duration), and moderate-severe RV dilatation (RV internal diameter in diastole [RVIDd] 11.6 mm, z-score 3.9). The significant RV dilatation was associated with adverse ventricular-ventricular interaction; specifically, leftward deviation of the interventricular septum resulted in a relatively lower LV end-diastolic size ([LVIDd] 15.2 mm, z-score −1.5) (Figure 38.3). Additionally, there was evidence of mild to moderate RV systolic dysfunction (tricuspid annular plane systolic excursion [TAPSE] 5.8 mm; fractional area change [FAC] 0.38) but preserved LV systolic function (fractional shortening [FS] 49%; EF 62% by Simpsons biplane) and normal biventricular cardiac outputs (LVO 219 mL/min/kg, RVO 152 mL/min/kg).

Despite endotracheal intubation, mechanical ventilation with high-frequency oscillation and treatment with iNO, the infant continued to demonstrate severe hypoxemia with an FiO$_2$ of 1.0. Further, the infant's systolic and diastolic blood pressures (BP) dropped below the 3rd centile for gestational age. This was treated with a combination of dobutamine at dose of 5–10 mcg/kg/min (intended to support RV performance) and vasopressin at dose of 0.6–1 milliunits/kg/min (to help increase diastolic BP and

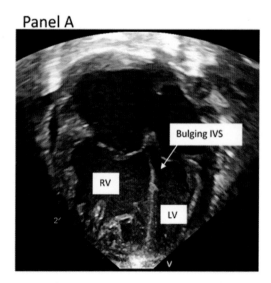
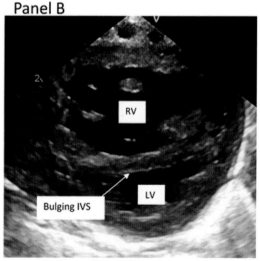

FIGURE 38.3 Case 3 TnECHO. Panels (a) and (b) are echocardiography images obtained from the apical-4-chamber and parasternal short axis views, respectively, showing a dilated right ventricle (RV) with a bulging interventricular septum (IVS) towards the left ventricle (LV).

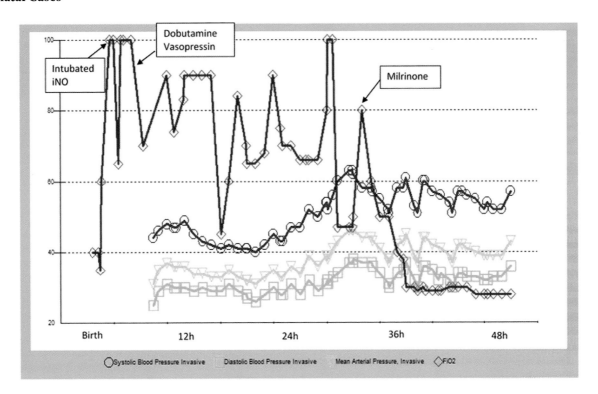

FIGURE 38.4   Case 3 hemodynamics. Blood pressures and FiO$_2$ requirements in the first 48 hours of life. Oxygen requirements (FiO$_2$; Red), invasive systolic (blue), diastolic (green) and mean (blue) arterial blood pressures in the first 48 hours of life in relation to cardiotropic therapies. iNO, inhaled nitric oxide.

support systemic perfusion pressure without adversely affecting PVR). These strategies resulted in normalization of arterial BP.

Over the next 24 hours, although there was overall improvement in the efficacy of oxygenation, FiO$_2$ requirements remained between 0.6 to 0.8. Use of muscle relaxation and increase in MAP to improve alveolar recruitment had little impact. By 36 hours of age the infant was on high-frequency oscillation ventilation (HFOV) with MAP of 18 cmH$_2$O, FiO$_2$ 0.8, and most recent arterial blood gas showing pH 7.14, pCO$_2$ 53 mmHg, HCO$_3$ 18 mEq/L, BE −11.1 mEq/L and serum lactate of 7.0 mmol/L. Follow up TnECHO demonstrated improvement in RV function (TAPSE 8.0 mm, FAC 0.42), mild reduction in RV dilatation (RVIDD 10.8 mm, z-score 3.4) and improvement in LV end-diastolic size (LVIDd 16.1 mm, z-score −0.7). LV function and biventricular outputs continued to be in normal range; however, the PDA continued to shunt bidirectionally, indicating persistence of near-systemic pulmonary pressures. With the intention to induce pulmonary vasodilation, aided by the fact that infant's blood pressures were now normalized, intravenous therapy with infusion with milrinone, a type III phosphodiesterase enzyme inhibitor, was initiated (25 mcg/kg bolus over an hour, followed by a continuous infusion of 0.33 mcg/kg/min). This was associated with a dramatic improvement in oxygenation, with a reduction in FiO$_2$ from 0.8 to 0.3 within 6 hours (Figure 38.4). Subsequently, HRF resolved completely with no further rebound in FiO$_2$ or inotropic requirements. All cardiotropic agents and iNO were subsequently weaned and discontinued by postnatal day 5.

Outcome

The infant was extubated on postnatal day 8 to non-invasive positive pressure ventilation and was transferred to a community level 2 nursery on postnatal day 20.

Physiological discussion and learning points

- Acute PH of the newborn is a complex and variable interplay between high PVR, pulmonary blood flow, right and left ventricular dysfunction and cardiac outputs. While the overall therapeutic goal is to reduce PVR, sequential monitoring and thoughtful titration may be required to ensure restoration of cardiac function and maintenance of systemic organ perfusion pressures.

- Whilst RV dysfunction secondary to PH is well recognized, adverse ventricular-ventricular interactions may be overlooked. The right and left ventricles are interdependent through a number of mechanisms, such as shared myocardial fibers, the interventricular septum and the constraints of space due to unyielding pericardium (26). The latter was observed in this case, where a pressure and volume loaded right ventricle negatively impacted LV geometry, leading to relatively compromised LV end-diastolic volume.

- Right ventricular dilatation, a potentially adaptive mechanism to increased afterload, may be seen in infants with PH. Through the Frank-Starling mechanism, which dictates that higher pre-stretch (preload) of cardiac myocytes results in an increase in force generation and stroke volume (27), RV dilatation may maintain cardiac output in the face of high afterload despite relative pump dysfunction, as seen in this case. Therefore, in the context of RV dilatation, a normal RVO could be falsely reassuring.

- Milrinone, a type III phosphodiesterase inhibitor, has both cardiac and non-selective vasoactive effects; specifically, milrinone inhibits cyclic GMP metabolism in the vascular smooth muscle resulting in vasodilatation of both arteries and veins. On the myocardium, milrinone prevents the breakdown of cyclic AMP which increases phosphorylation of the calcium ion channels and increases calcium availability in the myocytes, thus increasing inotropy, lusitropy (relaxation), and to a lesser extent, chronotropy, resulting in a net improvement in systolic and diastolic function and ultimately cardiac output. Its use in PH, though desirable to reduce PVR, is limited by its undesirable effects of lowering systemic blood pressures (28). Clinicians should ensure a robust blood pressure before initiating therapy with milrinone.

Case 4

History
A preterm infant born at 28+4 weeks, weighing 1240 g, presented with severe refractory HRF shortly after birth. There was previable rupture of membranes at 21 weeks and persistent anhydramnios. The perinatal period was further complicated by maternal vaginal bleeding and significant decelerations on fetal heart rate monitoring, which prompted an emergency caesarean section. The infant was initially apneic at birth with normal heart rate, but spontaneous respiration established shortly thereafter. The Apgar scores were 3 and 8 at 1 and 5 minutes of life, respectively, and the cord pH was 7.24 with a base deficit of −6.3 mEq/L. The infant initially transitioned to nCPAP with a PEEP of 9 cmH$_2$O; however, was electively intubated for persistent oxygenation failure. The FiO$_2$ requirements continued to rise from 0.7 to 1.0 despite invasive ventilation and administration of surfactant. A presumptive clinical diagnosis of PH was made and the infant was commenced on iNO therapy, which did not result in any immediate improvement. Further strategies that were employed unsuccessfully included upsizing the endotracheal tube from size 2.5 mm to 3.0 mm and a step-wise increase in MAP to a maximum of 18 cmH$_2$O. Due to development of low BP at a postnatal age of 4.5 hours, an intravenous infusion dopamine was initiated at 10 mcg/kg/min. A second dose of surfactant was also administered. Improvement in BP was temporarily associated with an improvement in oxygenation (FiO$_2$ reduced from 1.0 to 0.3), which only lasted for ~2 hours. By 8 hours of age, the FiO$_2$ requirements had gradually climbed back to 1.0, despite normal BP. An urgent hemodynamic consultation was requested by the attending physician.

Hemodynamics consultation and subsequent management
At the time of TnECHO evaluation, the infant was receiving HFOV, with a MAP of 16 cmH$_2$O and FiO$_2$ of 1.0 and an acceptable blood gas (pH 7.31, pCO$_2$ 41 mmHg, HCO$_3$ 21 mEq/L, BD −5.4 mEq/L, lactate 3.3 mmol/L). TnECHO findings were consistent with acute PH (bidirectional PDA and PFO shunt, moderate to severe reduction in RV function (TAPSE 2.9 mm, FAC

0.31%), moderate reduction in LV function (EF 45% by Simpsons, FS 33%, IVRT 73 msec), and reduced cardiac outputs (LVO 98 mL/min/kg, RVO 110 mL/min/kg). In addition, qualitatively low end-diastolic volumes were also observed. In order to evaluate the potential impact of relatively high MAP on ventricular filling, the MAP was reduced from 16 cmH$_2$O to 10 cmH$_2$O in one step. This resulted in an immediate improvement in oxygen saturations, allowing for weaning in FiO$_2$ from 1.0 to 0.65. A focused scan repeated 5 minutes later demonstrated qualitative and quantitative improvement in RV chamber size and function (Table 38.3). Additionally, the non-specific vasopressor dopamine was changed to vasopressin, and milrinone infusion was added in order to further support cardiac function, in the context of normal blood pressures at the time. Subsequently, the infant's FiO$_2$ requirements continued to improve, however, blood pressures dropped after 3 hours of milrinone infusion, with no clinical evidence of end-organ dysfunction (Figure 38.5). Repeat TnECHO at 16 hours demonstrated improvement in LV function (FS 35%, EF 60%, IVRT 53 msec) and LVO (128 mL/min/kg) but RV dysfunction (TAPSE 2.4 mm with RVO 77 mL/min/kg). At the time, the infant was receiving ventilation with HFOV in MAP of 10 cmH$_2$O and FiO$_2$ 0.4. The most recent blood gas showed pH 7.32, pCO$_2$ 36 mmHg, BD −6.8 mEq/L, lactate 2.7 mmol/L. Due to low BP, milrinone was stopped and an epinephrine infusion 0.03 mcg/kg/min was started to support RV function. The dose of epinephrine was subsequently increased to a maximum of 0.07 mcg/kg/min, after which BP normalized and FiO$_2$ requirements fell. Repeat TnECHO after 6 hours of epinephrine showed marked improvement in biventricular systolic function (TAPSE 5.2 mm, LV FS 50%) and normal biventricular outputs (LVO 235 mL/min/kg, RVO 218 mL/min/kg).

Outcome
The inotropes and iNO were gradually weaned and stopped on postnatal day 4. Infant was subsequently extubated on postnatal day 5 to noninvasive positive pressure ventilation in an FiO$_2$ of 0.3. The infant's remaining NICU course remained uneventful.

Physiological discussion and learning points
- Changes in intrapleural pressure secondary to mechanical ventilation can adversely affect atrial filling (preload), impedance to ventricular emptying (afterload), heart rate and contractility. Positive pressure ventilation results in an increase in right atrial filling pressures by increasing intrapleural pressure and a reduction in systemic venous return, which depends on the pressure gradient between the extra thoracic veins (driving pressure) and the right atrial pressure (back pressure) (29). Overdistension of the alveoli can lead to an increase in PVR due to compression of the

TABLE 38.3 Echocardiographic Indices of Right Ventricle Function before and after Reducing Mean Airway Pressure from 16 cmH$_2$O to 10 cmH$_2$O

Echocardiography Parameters	MAP 16 cmH$_2$O	5 Minutes after Weaning MAP to 10 cmH$_2$O
RV EDA (cm^2)	0.81	0.91
RV FAC (%)	31	41
RV global longitudinal strain (%)	−8.87	−12.78
RV global systolic strain rate (s^{-1})	−1.88	−3.15
RV early diastolic strain rate (s^{-1})	1.78	3.06
RV late diastolic strain rate (s^{-1})	2.22	3.35

Abbreviations: MAP, mean airway pressure; RV, right ventricle; EDA, end diastolic area; FAC, fractional area change.

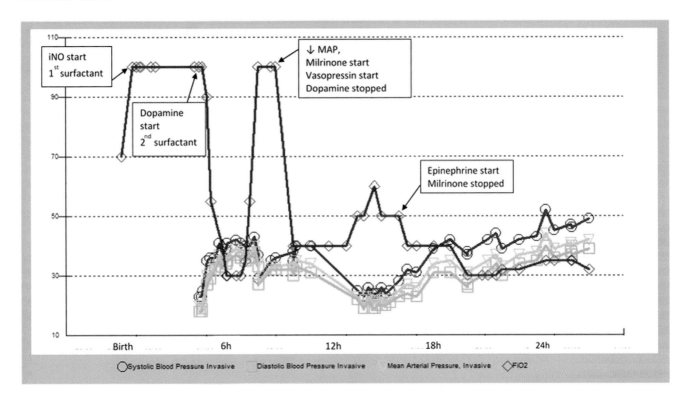

FIGURE 38.5   Case 4. Blood pressures and FiO$_2$ requirements in the first 24 hours of life, in relation to cardiotropic therapies. Oxygen requirements (FiO$_2$; Red), invasive systolic (blue), diastolic (green) and mean (blue) arterial blood pressures in the first 24 hours of life in relation to cardiotropic therapies. iNO: inhaled nitric oxide.

intra-alveolar vessels (30). As a net result, excessive use of mechanical ventilation may worsen RV function, pulmonary blood flow, and oxygenation.

- RV dysfunction and low pulmonary blood flow are important determinants of oxygenation in PH. Severe RV dysfunction may result in a "pressure-passive oxygenation" phenotype (oxygenation changing with systemic blood pressure), where pulmonary blood flow is dependent on systemic venous return and right atrial pressure (31).
- Special attention should be paid to the potential of adverse cardiopulmonary interactions secondary to mechanical ventilation in cases of PH.

References

1. Giesinger RE, et al. Pediatr Res. 2017; 82(6):901–914.
2. Katz LA, et al. J Perinatol. 2006; 26(7):414–422.
3. Sobel DB, et al. J Perinatol. 1994; 14(4):268–274.
4. Ballard PL, et al. Pediatr Res. 2019; 85(3):305–311.
5. Pandit PB, et al. Pediatrics. 1995; 95(6):851–854.
6. Clyman RI. Semin Perinatol. 2013; 37(2):102–107.
7. Merrill JD, et al. Pediatr Res. 2004; 56(6):918–926.
8. Taeusch HW, et al. Pediatr Pathol Mol Med. 2001; 20(6):519–536.
9. Mercier JC, et al. Lancet. 2010; 376(9738):346–354.
10. Srisuparp P, et al. J Med Assoc Thai. 2002; 85 Suppl 2:S469–S478.
11. Su PH, et al. J Perinatol. 2008; 28(2):112–116.
12. Wei QF, et al. Zhongguo Dang Dai Er Ke Za Zhi. 2014; 16(8):805–809.
13. Field D, et al. Pediatrics. 2005; 115(4):926–936.
14. Van Meurs KP, et al. N Engl J Med. 2005; 353(1):13–22.
15. McNamara PJ, et al. In: *Avery's Neonatology: Pathophysiology and Management of the Newborn.* MacDonald, MG Seshia, MMK eds. Philadelphia, PA: Wolters Kluwer; 2016. p. 457–486.
16. Giesinger RE, et al. J Pediatr. 2017; 180:22.e2–30.e2.
17. More KS, et al. Am J Perinatol. 2018; 35(10):979–989.
18. Lakshminrusimha S, et al. J Pediatr. 2018; 196:45.e3–51.e3.
19. Thoresen M, et al. Pediatrics. 2000; 106(1 Pt 1):92–99.
20. Giesinger RE, et al. Am J Respir Crit Care Med. 2019; 200(10):1294–1305.
21. Cassady SJ, et al. Cardiol Clin. 2020; 38(2):243–255.
22. Noori S, et al. Clin Perinatol. 2012; 39(1):221–238.
23. Mohamed AA, et al. J Matern Fetal Neonatal Med. 2020; 1–9.
24. Mohamed A, et al. Pediatr Crit Care Med. 2014; 15(2):148–154.
25. Jain A, et al. Semin Fetal Neonatal Med. 2015; 20(4):262–271.
26. Pinsky MR. Crit Care2016; 20:266..
27. Klabunde R. *Cardiovascular Physiology Concepts.* Philadelphia, PA: Lippincott Williams & Wilkins; 2012. 243 p. ISBN: 9781451113846.
28. Lakshminrusimha S, et al. Semin Perinatol. 2016; 40(3):160–173.
29. Shekerdemian L, et al. Arch Dis Child. 1999; 80(5):475–480.
30. Alviar CL, et al. J Am Coll Cardiol. 2018; 72(13):1532–1553.
31. Zamanian RT, et al. Crit Care Med. 2007; 35(9):2037–2050.

INDEX

Italicized pages refer to figures and **bold** refer to tables.

A

ABO, *see* Air-breathing organs
ACTH, *see* Adrenocorticotropic hormone
Actin cytoskeletal rearrangement, 71–72
Activated protein kinase C (PKC), 111
Acute kidney injury (AKI), 148–149
    aminophylline for, 151
    hyperoxic resuscitation of asphyxiated
        neonates, 150–151
    Neonatal KDIGO definition, 148, **149**
Acute pulmonary hypertension phenotypes,
    208–210, **209**
    of arterial (classic) origin, 208–209
    echocardiography-guided management
        of, 212
    and left ventricular dysfunction, 210
    related to excessive pulmonary blood flow,
        209–210, *210*
Acute respiratory distress syndrome (ARDS),
    51, 54
Adaptations to high altitude
    chronic mountain sickness, 20
    genetic adaptations, *20*, 20–22
    highland populations, phenotypic
        differences in, 19–20, *20*
    overview, 19
Adenosine monophosphate-activated protein
    kinase (AMPK), 85, *85*, 98, 106
Adenosine triphosphate (ATP), 81, 84, 85
    actomyosin crossbridge cycling and, 92
    and energetic intermediates, 98
    from sympathetic nerves, 91
ADMA, *see* Asymmetric dimethylarginine
ADME (absorption, distribution, and
    elimination, through either
    metabolism), 155, 156
ADPribose polymerase (PARP) protein, 26
Adrenocorticotropic hormone (ACTH), 25,
    26, 226
Adventitia, restructured, 72
Air-breathing fish, phylogeny of, 40
Air-breathing organs (ABO), 40
Airway pressure relationships, *200*
Airways development, hypoxia and, 144
Airway smooth muscle (ASM), 142
Alternative oxidase (AOX), 98
Alto Andino, 24, 26, 27
Alveolar development, hypoxia and, 144–145
Alveolar hypoxia, 177–178
Ambystoma mexicanum, 41
American Society of Anesthesiologists (ASA),
    162
Aminophylline, for acute kidney injury, 151
Amphibians
    ontogeny of, 41
    phylogeny of, 40–41
AMPK, *see* Adenosine monophosphate-
    activated protein kinase
Andean highlanders, genetic adaptation in, 21
Anemia, associated with intestinal dysbiosis,
    153
Anemic hypoxia, 179

Anesthesia, for neonate with HRF
    anesthetic agents, 162
    intraoperative management, 162–163
    mechanical ventilation strategies, 161–162
    overview, 160
    pediatric transports, 161
    perioperative assessment, 160–161
    preoperative inotropes and vasopressors, 161
    pulmonary hypertension, management
        of, 163
Angiogenesis in PPHN, role of endothelial cells
    in, 83–85, *84*
    angiogenic signal expression, alterations
        in, 84
    mitochondrial biogenesis and, regulation
        of, 85
    physiologic angiogenesis, regulation of, 84
Animal models of PPHN
    congenital diaphragmatic hernia, 77
    fetal ductal ligation, 76
    hypoxia, 74–75
    lung injury from hyperoxia, 75–76
    pulmonary blood flow, increased, 76
    of pulmonary hypertension, 74–75, 101–105
    reactive oxygen species, 78
    sepsis, 76
    vasoconstrictors, 77–78
Antenatal drug exposure, 172
Antidiuretic hormone (ADH), 149
Apoptosis, 128–129
Arachidonate metabolite thromboxane, 77
ARDS, *see* Acute respiratory distress syndrome
Arginine vasopressin (AVP), 25
Argon, 132
Arterial blood gas (ABG) analysis, 160, 162
Arterial oxygen saturation, in first minutes
    after birth, 62–63
Arterial spin labeled (ASL) perfusion MRI, 137
Asian flu epidemic of 1957, 51
Asphyxia
    birth, 2, 59
    cycle of, *227*
    fetal, 155, 224
    hemodynamic consequences of, *225*
    impact on specific organ functions, **158**
    myocardium, impact on, 225–226
Asphyxiated newborns, physiology of, 59
Asymmetric dimethylarginine (ADMA), 27
Atmospheric partial pressure of O_2 (PO_2), 13
Autophagy, 129
AVP, *see* Arginine vasopressin
Azithromycin, 132

B

Barcroft, Sir Joseph, 1, 24
Barrier function, role of hypoxia in, 153
BAT, *see* Brown adipose tissue
BBB, *see* Blood-brain barrier
Biphasic ventilatory response, to hypoxia, 29
Birds
    ontogeny of, 41
    phylogeny of, 41

Birth asphyxia, 2, 59
Bleomycin treatment, 75–76
Blood-brain barrier (BBB), 135, 137–138
    effects of HI injury on, 137
    impact on pathophysiology of HIE, 138
    neurovascular unit contribute to,
        components of, *138*
    transendothelial electrical resistance, 137
    VEGF and HIF-1α protein, role of, 138
Blood flow
    autoregulation, 180
    ductus arteriosus, 57
    iliac, 20
    microcirculatory, 19
    pulmonary, 2, 17, 57, 76, *see also* Pulmonary
        blood flow
        acute PH phenotype related to,
            209–210, *210*
    pulmonary vascular resistance and, 3
    redirecting, 9
    redistribution, 2, 9, *9*, 25
        in diving mammals during prolonged
            apnea, 34–35
        maternal hypoxia and, 53
Bone marrow-derived macrophages (BMDMs),
    115
Bone morphogenetic protein receptor type 2
    (BMPR2), 120
BPD, *see* Bronchopulmonary dysplasia
Brain
    adjunct therapies for hypoxia ischemia,
        128, 129, 131
    cell death in, 128–129
    development of, effect of hypoxia and
        oxidative stress in, 127–128
        acute or latent or primary phase, *127*,
            127–128
        secondary phase, *127*, 128
        tertiary phase, *127*, 128
    erythropoietin for, 132–133
    latent and secondary phase therapies,
        131–132
    strategies to protect, 129
    tertiary phase therapies, 132–133
    therapeutic hypothermia for, 129, *130*
Brainstem respiratory neurons, sensitivity to
    inflammatory mediators, 15
Breathing, inflammatory-mediated stimulation
    of, 14–15
Bromodomains (BRDs), 116
Bronchial circulation, 72–72
Bronchopulmonary dysplasia (BPD), 63, 64,
    146, 160, 205
    chronic pulmonary hypertension
        phenotypes related to, 211
Brown adipose tissue (BAT), 6
    pH-sensitive, 10
Burrowing mammals, neonates of, 28–33

C

Ca^{++} channels, in HPV, 97
Caffeic acid phenethyl ester (CAPE), 107